Adipokines 2.0

Adipokines 2.0

Special Issue Editor

Christa Buechler

MDPI • Basel • Beijing • Wuhan • Barcelona • Belgrade • Manchester • Tokyo • Cluj • Tianjin

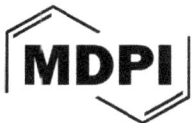

Special Issue Editor
Christa Buechler
Department of Internal Medicine I,
Regensburg University Hospital
Germany

Editorial Office
MDPI
St. Alban-Anlage 66
4052 Basel, Switzerland

This is a reprint of articles from the Special Issue published online in the open access journal *International Journal of Molecular Sciences* (ISSN 1422-0067) (available at: https://www.mdpi.com/journal/ijms/special_issues/adipokines2).

For citation purposes, cite each article independently as indicated on the article page online and as indicated below:

LastName, A.A.; LastName, B.B.; LastName, C.C. Article Title. *Journal Name* **Year**, *Article Number*, Page Range.

ISBN 978-3-03928-586-0 (Pbk)
ISBN 978-3-03928-587-7 (PDF)

Cover image courtesy of Christa Büchler.

© 2020 by the authors. Articles in this book are Open Access and distributed under the Creative Commons Attribution (CC BY) license, which allows users to download, copy and build upon published articles, as long as the author and publisher are properly credited, which ensures maximum dissemination and a wider impact of our publications.
The book as a whole is distributed by MDPI under the terms and conditions of the Creative Commons license CC BY-NC-ND.

Contents

About the Special Issue Editor ix

Christa Buechler
Editorial of Special Issue "Adipokines 2.0"
Reprinted from: *Int. J. Mol. Sci.* **2020**, *21*, 849, doi:10.3390/ijms21030849 1

Thomas Grewal, Carlos Enrich, Carles Rentero and Christa Buechler
Annexins in Adipose Tissue: Novel Players in Obesity
Reprinted from: *Int. J. Mol. Sci.* **2019**, *20*, 3449, doi:10.3390/ijms20143449 5

Birgit Knebel, Pia Fahlbusch, Gereon Poschmann, Matthias Dille, Natalie Wahlers, Kai Stühler, Sonja Hartwig, Stefan Lehr, Martina Schiller, Sylvia Jacob, Ulrike Kettel, Dirk Müller-Wieland and Jörg Kotzka
Adipokinome Signatures in Obese Mouse Models Reflect Adipose Tissue Health and Are Associated with Serum Lipid Composition
Reprinted from: *Int. J. Mol. Sci.* **2019**, *20*, 2559, doi:10.3390/ijms20102559 29

Qi Qiao, Freek G. Bouwman, Marleen A. van Baak, Johan Renes and Edwin C.M. Mariman
Glucose Restriction Plus Refeeding In Vitro Induce Changes of the Human Adipocyte Secretome with an Impact on Complement Factors and Cathepsins
Reprinted from: *Int. J. Mol. Sci.* **2019**, *20*, 4055, doi:10.3390/ijms20164055 45

Christine Graf and Nina Ferrari
Metabolic Health—The Role of Adipo-Myokines
Reprinted from: *Int. J. Mol. Sci.* **2019**, *20*, 6159, doi:10.3390/ijms20246159 63

Żaneta Kimber-Trojnar, Jolanta Patro-Małysza, Marcin Trojnar, Dorota Darmochwał-Kolarz, Jan Oleszczuk and Bożena Leszczyńska-Gorzelak
Umbilical Cord SFRP5 Levels of Term Newborns in Relation to Normal and Excessive Gestational Weight Gain
Reprinted from: *Int. J. Mol. Sci.* **2019**, *20*, 595, doi:10.3390/ijms20030595 85

Jolanta Patro-Małysza, Marcin Trojnar, Katarzyna E. Skórzyńska-Dziduszko, Żaneta Kimber-Trojnar, Dorota Darmochwał-Kolarz, Monika Czuba and Bożena Leszczyńska-Gorzelak
Leptin and Ghrelin in Excessive Gestational Weight Gain—Association between Mothers and Offspring
Reprinted from: *Int. J. Mol. Sci.* **2019**, *20*, 2398, doi:10.3390/ijms20102398 97

Elena Vianello, Elena Dozio, Francesco Bandera, Marco Froldi, Emanuele Micaglio, John Lamont, Lorenza Tacchini, Gerd Schmitz and Massimiliano Marco Corsi Romanelli
Correlative Study on Impaired Prostaglandin E2 Regulation in Epicardial Adipose Tissue and Its Role in Maladaptive Cardiac Remodeling via EPAC2 and ST2 Signaling in Overweight Cardiovascular Disease Subjects
Reprinted from: *Int. J. Mol. Sci.* **2020**, *21*, 520, doi:10.3390/ijms21020520 109

Christa Buechler, Susanne Feder, Elisabeth M. Haberl and Charalampos Aslanidis
Chemerin Isoforms and Activity in Obesity
Reprinted from: *Int. J. Mol. Sci.* **2019**, *20*, 1128, doi:10.3390/ijms20051128 125

Kerry B. Goralski, Ashley E. Jackson, Brendan T. McKeown and Christopher J. Sinal
More Than an Adipokine: The Complex Roles of Chemerin Signaling in Cancer
Reprinted from: *Int. J. Mol. Sci.* **2019**, *20*, 4778, doi:10.3390/ijms20194778 141

Oliver Treeck, Christa Buechler and Olaf Ortmann
Chemerin and Cancer
Reprinted from: *Int. J. Mol. Sci.* **2019**, *20*, 3750, doi:10.3390/ijms20153750 169

Susanne Feder, Arne Kandulski, Doris Schacherer, Thomas S. Weiss and Christa Buechler
Serum Chemerin Does Not Differentiate Colorectal Liver Metastases from Hepatocellular Carcinoma
Reprinted from: *Int. J. Mol. Sci.* **2019**, *20*, 3919, doi:10.3390/ijms20163919 185

Anthony Estienne, Alice Bongrani, Maxime Reverchon, Christelle Ramé, Pierre-Henri Ducluzeau, Pascal Froment and Joëlle Dupont
Involvement of Novel Adipokines, Chemerin, Visfatin, Resistin and Apelin in Reproductive Functions in Normal and Pathological Conditions in Humans and Animal Models
Reprinted from: *Int. J. Mol. Sci.* **2019**, *20*, 4431, doi:10.3390/ijms20184431 199

Nina Smolinska, Marta Kiezun, Kamil Dobrzyn, Edyta Rytelewska, Katarzyna Kisielewska, Marlena Gudelska, Ewa Zaobidna, Krystyna Bogus-Nowakowska, Joanna Wyrebek, Kinga Bors, Grzegorz Kopij, Barbara Kaminska and Tadeusz Kaminski
Expression of Chemerin and Its Receptors in the Porcine Hypothalamus and Plasma Chemerin Levels during the Oestrous Cycle and Early Pregnancy
Reprinted from: *Int. J. Mol. Sci.* **2019**, *20*, 3887, doi:10.3390/ijms20163887 245

Alice Bongrani, Namya Mellouk, Christelle Rame, Marion Cornuau, Fabrice Guérif, Pascal Froment and Joëlle Dupont
Ovarian Expression of Adipokines in Polycystic Ovary Syndrome: A Role for Chemerin, Omentin, and Apelin in Follicular Growth Arrest and Ovulatory Dysfunction?
Reprinted from: *Int. J. Mol. Sci.* **2019**, *20*, 3778, doi:10.3390/ijms20153778 273

Mar Carrión, Klaus W. Frommer, Selene Pérez-García, Ulf Müller-Ladner, Rosa P. Gomariz and Elena Neumann
The Adipokine Network in Rheumatic Joint Diseases
Reprinted from: *Int. J. Mol. Sci.* **2019**, *20*, 4091, doi:10.3390/ijms20174091 295

Elinoar Hoffman, Michal A. Rahat, Joy Feld, Muna Elias, Itzhak Rosner, Lisa Kaly, Idit Lavie, Tal Gazitt and Devy Zisman
Effects of Tocilizumab, an Anti-Interleukin-6 Receptor Antibody, on Serum Lipid and Adipokine Levels in Patients with Rheumatoid Arthritis
Reprinted from: *Int. J. Mol. Sci.* **2019**, *20*, 4633, doi:10.3390/ijms20184633 325

Sven H. Loosen, Alexander Koch, Frank Tacke, Christoph Roderburg and Tom Luedde
The Role of Adipokines as Circulating Biomarkers in Critical Illness and Sepsis
Reprinted from: *Int. J. Mol. Sci.* **2019**, *20*, 4820, doi:10.3390/ijms20194820 335

Hannah Lee, Thai Hien Tu, Byong Seo Park, Sunggu Yang and Jae Geun Kim
Adiponectin Reverses the Hypothalamic Microglial Inflammation during Short-Term Exposure to Fat-Rich Diet
Reprinted from: *Int. J. Mol. Sci.* **2019**, *20*, 5738, doi:10.3390/ijms20225738 347

Thomas Ho-yin Lee, Kenneth King-yip Cheng, Ruby Lai-chong Hoo, Parco Ming-fai Siu and Suk-yu Yau
The Novel Perspectives of Adipokines on Brain Health
Reprinted from: *Int. J. Mol. Sci.* **2019**, *20*, 5638, doi:10.3390/ijms20225638 . . . . **359**

About the Special Issue Editor

Christa Buechler, a scientist at the University Hospital of Regensburg, focuses on research on the role of adipokines in non-alcoholic fatty liver disease and hepatocellular carcinoma since 2003. She obtained a Ph.D. in Biology in 1991 from the University of Regensburg and Stuttgart. In 1994 to 2003, her main research focus was on lipoproteins and reverse cholesterol transport. She was Guest Editor of two Special Issues of the *International Journal of Molecular Science*. Currently, she is member of the Editorial Board of the *International Journal of Molecular Science* and *Biochimica et Biophysica Acta* (BBA) - *Molecular and Cell Biology of Lipids*. She is author of more than 150 scientific publications in international journals, with an H-index of 41. She also contributes to the scientific community as a peer review expert for more than 50 articles per year. She is a member of the German Society for Clinical Chemistry and Laboratory Medicine e.V. (DGKL) and the European *Macrophage and Dendritic Cell Society* (*EMDS*).

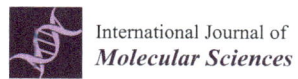

Editorial
Editorial of Special Issue "Adipokines 2.0"

Christa Buechler

Department of Internal Medicine I, Regensburg University Hospital, 93053 Regensburg, Germany; christa.buechler@klinik.uni-regensburg.de; Tel.: +49-0941-944-7009

Received: 21 January 2020; Accepted: 21 January 2020; Published: 28 January 2020

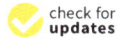

Abstract: This editorial aims to summarize the 19 scientific papers that contributed to the Special Issue "Adipokines 2".

The Special Issue, "Adipokines 2.0" of the International Journal of Molecular Sciences is a follow up of the Special Issue "Adipokines" published two years ago.

Proteins secreted from fat tissues are collectively referred to as adipokines. Circulating levels of these proteins are—with a few exceptions—increased in obesity. Hundreds of adipokines were discovered and annexins, well known as regulators of membrane-related events such as exocytosis, may affect adipokine release from fat tissues [1].

Adipokines promote metabolic and cardiovascular diseases and are biomarkers for obesity-associated comorbidities. Metabolically healthy obesity is associated with an adipokinome similar to that of normal weight mice, providing more evidence for a central role of adipose tissue produced proteins in metabolic diseases [2]. Weight loss improves the parameters of insulin sensitivity and hypertension, but most patients regain weight. Adipocytes cultivated in medium with low, and later on high glucose, showed a different secretome in comparison to the control cells. These differentially released proteins may contribute to worse metabolic parameters in obese patients after weight regain [3].

Physical activity is linked to improved metabolic health in normal weight and obesity. Adipo-myokines are proteins secreted by adipose tissues and skeletal muscle and seem to have a role herein. These molecules may be useful to classify different types of obesity and develop individualized therapeutic strategies [4].

Excessive gestational weight gain increases the risk of neonatal and maternal complications. The adipokine secreted frizzled-related protein 5 (SFRP5) improves metabolic function. Serum as well as umbilical cord blood levels were low in women with an extreme increase in weight during pregnancy [5]. Leptin was higher in the serum and cord blood of male infants born from mothers with excessive gestational weight gain. Such an induction was not observed for female babies [6]. Adipokine levels correlated with neonatal anthropometric measurements and may contribute to greater risk of obesity and metabolic disease in later life [5,6].

Excess body weight is a risk factor for insulin resistance, hypertension, and cardiovascular diseases. Epicardial adipose tissue contributes to cardiac enlargement in the obese and this involves deregulation of prostaglandin E2 [7]. Overweight and obesity are, moreover, linked to a higher risk of different cancers [8,9]. This was studied in detail for the adipokine chemerin. Of note, chemerin was shown to impair and to improve insulin sensitivity, to have pro- and anti-inflammatory activities and to exert pro- and anticancer effects [8–10]. These antagonistic effects may be in part attributed to the different biologic activities of the chemerin isoforms [8]. The role of chemerin in cancer diseases was nicely summarized in two review articles [9,10]. An original investigation tested whether chemerin may serve as a biomarker to discriminate patients with primary and secondary liver tumors. This study identified an association of serum chemerin with hypertension and hypercholesterolemia in the tumor patients [11]. Serum chemerin could, however, not distinguish patients with hepatocellular carcinoma and colorectal liver metastases [11].

Adipokines are involved in the pathogenesis of reproductive disorders. The roles of chemerin, visfatin, resistin, and apelin in fertility and associated diseases were summarized in a review article with various informative and clear illustrations [12].

A potential role of chemerin in reproductive function was supported by the finding that plasma levels as well as the expression of its receptors, chemokine-like receptor 1, G protein-coupled receptor 1, and C-C motif chemokine receptor-like 2 fluctuated throughout the estrous cycle and pregnancy in the porcine hypothalamus [13].

Other approaches have been to determine the release of adipokines by tissues other than fat. One study analyzed the levels of chemerin, apelin, and omentin in follicular fluid and ovarian granulosa cells. Study cohorts were women with polycystic ovary syndrome, women with a polycystic ovary morphology, and the controls. Differential abundance of these adipokines in the patients suggested a possible role in the pathophysiology of polycystic ovary syndrome [14].

Adipokines are expressed by different cells in the joint microenvironment. Locally produced as well as systemic adipokines contribute to osteoarthritis and rheumatoid arthritis. Different studies have analyzed the pathophysiological role of various adipokines (e.g., adiponectin, leptin and so on). These studies were nicely summarized in a review article [15]. Interestingly, the serum levels of most of these adipokines were higher in the patients [15]. A separate study investigated the effect of treatment with the anti-interleukin-6 receptor antibody tocilizumab in patients with rheumatoid arthritis. Four months of therapy was associated with higher resistin levels and lower adiponectin whereas leptin was not altered [16]. After treatment, adiponectin and resistin serum concentrations were similar to the controls, suggesting the normalization of these parameters [16].

Moreover, adipokines were also analyzed as potential biomarkers in sepsis and critical illness. Here, prospective studies are required to finally evaluate the prognostic relevance of the different proteins measured. The heterogeneity of these patient cohorts may limit the diagnostic potential of circulating adipokine levels [17].

The role of adipose tissue in the pathophysiology of most diseases is greatly unknown. There is mounting evidence though that adipokines act in the brain, and the role of leptin in the control of food consumption has been well described. Adiponectin protected mice from high fat diet induced hypothalamic inflammation [18]. Microglia, as the resident macrophages of the central nervous system, expressed both adiponectin receptors and were essential for the protective activity of adiponectin [18].

The neuroprotective effects of the adipokines leptin, adiponectin, chemerin, apelin, and visfatin indicate a potential role for these molecules as therapeutic targets in neurodegenerative diseases [19].

Overall, these 19 contributions published in this Special Issue further strengthen the essential function of adipokines in health and in various diseases. Different adipose tissue depots may have specific functions and detailed analysis of their secretome may provide more insight into the connection between fad pads and physiology.

References

1. Grewal, T.; Enrich, C.; Rentero, C.; Buechler, C. Annexins in Adipose Tissue: Novel Players in Obesity. *Int. J. Mol. Sci.* **2019**, *20*, 3449. [CrossRef] [PubMed]
2. Knebel, B.; Fahlbusch, P.; Poschmann, G.; Dille, M.; Wahlers, N.; Stuhler, K.; Hartwig, S.; Lehr, S.; Schiller, M.; Jacob, S.; et al. Adipokinome Signatures in Obese Mouse Models Reflect Adipose Tissue Health and Are Associated with Serum Lipid Composition. *Int. J. Mol. Sci.* **2019**, *20*, 2559. [CrossRef] [PubMed]
3. Qiao, Q.; Bouwman, F.G.; Baak, M.A.V.; Renes, J.; Mariman, E.C.M. Glucose Restriction Plus Refeeding in Vitro Induce Changes of the Human Adipocyte Secretome with an Impact on Complement Factors and Cathepsins. *Int. J. Mol. Sci.* **2019**, *20*, 4055. [CrossRef] [PubMed]
4. Graf, C.; Ferrari, N. Metabolic Health-The Role of Adipo-Myokines. *Int. J. Mol. Sci.* **2019**, *20*, 6159. [CrossRef] [PubMed]

5. Kimber-Trojnar, Z.; Patro-Malysza, J.; Trojnar, M.; Darmochwal-Kolarz, D.; Oleszczuk, J.; Leszczynska-Gorzelak, B. Umbilical Cord SFRP5 Levels of Term Newborns in Relation to Normal and Excessive Gestational Weight Gain. *Int. J. Mol. Sci.* **2019**, *20*, 595. [CrossRef] [PubMed]
6. Patro-Malysza, J.; Trojnar, M.; Skorzynska-Dziduszko, K.E.; Kimber-Trojnar, Z.; Darmochwal-Kolarz, D.; Czuba, M.; Leszczynska-Gorzelak, B. Leptin and Ghrelin in Excessive Gestational Weight Gain-Association between Mothers and Offspring. *Int. J. Mol. Sci.* **2019**, *20*, 2398. [CrossRef]
7. Vianello, E.; Dozio, E.; Bandera, F.; Froldi, M.; Micaglio, E.; Lamont, J.; Tacchini, L.; Schmitz, G.; Romanelli, A. Correlative Study on Impaired Prostaglandin E2 Regulation in Epicardial Adipose Tissue and its Role in Maladaptive Cardiac Remodeling via EPAC2 and ST2 Signaling in Overweight Cardiovascular Disease Subjects. *Int. J. Mol. Sci.* **2020**, *21*, 520. [CrossRef] [PubMed]
8. Buechler, C.; Feder, S.; Haberl, E.M.; Aslanidis, C. Chemerin Isoforms and Activity in Obesity. *Int. J. Mol. Sci.* **2019**, *20*, 1128. [CrossRef]
9. Goralski, K.B.; Jackson, A.E.; McKeown, B.T.; Sinal, C.J. More Than an Adipokine: The Complex Roles of Chemerin Signaling in Cancer. *Int. J. Mol. Sci.* **2019**, *20*, 4778. [CrossRef] [PubMed]
10. Treeck, O.; Buechler, C.; Ortmann, O. Chemerin and Cancer. *Int. J. Mol. Sci.* **2019**, *20*, 3750. [CrossRef] [PubMed]
11. Feder, S.; Kandulski, A.; Schacherer, D.; Weiss, T.S.; Buechler, C. Serum Chemerin Does Not Differentiate Colorectal Liver Metastases from Hepatocellular Carcinoma. *Int. J. Mol. Sci.* **2019**, *20*, 3919. [CrossRef] [PubMed]
12. Estienne, A.; Bongrani, A.; Reverchon, M.; Rame, C.; Ducluzeau, P.H.; Froment, P.; Dupont, J. Involvement of Novel Adipokines, Chemerin, Visfatin, Resistin and Apelin in Reproductive Functions in Normal and Pathological Conditions in Humans and Animal Models. *Int. J. Mol. Sci.* **2019**, *20*, 4431. [CrossRef] [PubMed]
13. Smolinska, N.; Kiezun, M.; Dobrzyn, K.; Rytelewska, E.; Kisielewska, K.; Gudelska, M.; Zaobidna, E.; Bogus-Nowakowska, K.; Wyrebek, J.; Bors, K.; et al. Expression of Chemerin and Its Receptors in the Porcine Hypothalamus and Plasma Chemerin Levels during the Oestrous Cycle and Early Pregnancy. *Int. J. Mol. Sci.* **2019**, *20*, 3887. [CrossRef] [PubMed]
14. Bongrani, A.; Mellouk, N.; Rame, C.; Cornuau, M.; Guerif, F.; Froment, P.; Dupont, J. Ovarian Expression of Adipokines in Polycystic Ovary Syndrome: A Role for Chemerin, Omentin, and Apelin in Follicular Growth Arrest and Ovulatory Dysfunction? *Int. J. Mol. Sci.* **2019**, *20*, 3778. [CrossRef] [PubMed]
15. Carrion, M.; Frommer, K.W.; Perez-Garcia, S.; Muller-Ladner, U.; Gomariz, R.P.; Neumann, E. The Adipokine Network in Rheumatic Joint Diseases. *Int. J. Mol. Sci.* **2019**, *20*, 4091. [CrossRef] [PubMed]
16. Hoffman, E.; Rahat, M.A.; Feld, J.; Elias, M.; Rosner, I.; Kaly, L.; Lavie, I.; Gazitt, T.; Zisman, D. Effects of Tocilizumab, an Anti-Interleukin-6 Receptor Antibody, on Serum Lipid and Adipokine Levels in Patients with Rheumatoid Arthritis. *Int. J. Mol. Sci.* **2019**, *20*, 4633. [CrossRef] [PubMed]
17. Loosen, S.H.; Koch, A.; Tacke, F.; Roderburg, C.; Luedde, T. The Role of Adipokines as Circulating Biomarkers in Critical Illness and Sepsis. *Int. J. Mol. Sci.* **2019**, *20*, 4820. [CrossRef] [PubMed]
18. Lee, H.; Tu, T.H.; Park, B.S.; Yang, S.; Kim, J.G. Adiponectin Reverses the Hypothalamic Microglial Inflammation during Short-Term Exposure to Fat-Rich Diet. *Int. J. Mol. Sci.* **2019**, *20*, 5738. [CrossRef] [PubMed]
19. Lee, T.H.; Cheng, K.K.; Hoo, R.L.; Siu, P.M.; Yau, S.Y. The Novel Perspectives of Adipokines on Brain Health. *Int. J. Mol. Sci.* **2019**, *20*, 5638. [CrossRef] [PubMed]

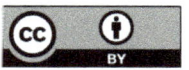

© 2020 by the author. Licensee MDPI, Basel, Switzerland. This article is an open access article distributed under the terms and conditions of the Creative Commons Attribution (CC BY) license (http://creativecommons.org/licenses/by/4.0/).

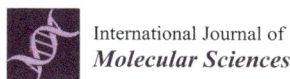

Review

Annexins in Adipose Tissue: Novel Players in Obesity

Thomas Grewal [1], Carlos Enrich [2,3], Carles Rentero [2,3] and Christa Buechler [4,*]

[1] School of Pharmacy, Faculty of Medicine and Health, University of Sydney, Sydney, NSW 2006, Australia
[2] Department of Biomedicine, Unit of Cell Biology, Faculty of Medicine and Health Sciences, University of Barcelona, 08036 Barcelona, Spain
[3] Centre de Recerca Biomèdica CELLEX, Institut d'Investigacions Biomèdiques August Pi i Sunyer (IDIBAPS), 08036 Barcelona, Spain
[4] Department of Internal Medicine I, Regensburg University Hospital, 93053 Regensburg, Germany
* Correspondence: christa.buechler@klinik.uni-regensburg.de; Tel.:+49-941-944-7009

Received: 5 June 2019; Accepted: 11 July 2019; Published: 13 July 2019

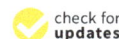

Abstract: Obesity and the associated comorbidities are a growing health threat worldwide. Adipose tissue dysfunction, impaired adipokine activity, and inflammation are central to metabolic diseases related to obesity. In particular, the excess storage of lipids in adipose tissues disturbs cellular homeostasis. Amongst others, organelle function and cell signaling, often related to the altered composition of specialized membrane microdomains (lipid rafts), are affected. Within this context, the conserved family of annexins are well known to associate with membranes in a calcium (Ca^{2+})- and phospholipid-dependent manner in order to regulate membrane-related events, such as trafficking in endo- and exocytosis and membrane microdomain organization. These multiple activities of annexins are facilitated through their diverse interactions with a plethora of lipids and proteins, often in different cellular locations and with consequences for the activity of receptors, transporters, metabolic enzymes, and signaling complexes. While increasing evidence points at the function of annexins in lipid homeostasis and cell metabolism in various cells and organs, their role in adipose tissue, obesity and related metabolic diseases is still not well understood. Annexin A1 (AnxA1) is a potent pro-resolving mediator affecting the regulation of body weight and metabolic health. Relevant for glucose metabolism and fatty acid uptake in adipose tissue, several studies suggest AnxA2 to contribute to coordinate glucose transporter type 4 (GLUT4) translocation and to associate with the fatty acid transporter CD36. On the other hand, AnxA6 has been linked to the control of adipocyte lipolysis and adiponectin release. In addition, several other annexins are expressed in fat tissues, yet their roles in adipocytes are less well examined. The current review article summarizes studies on the expression of annexins in adipocytes and in obesity. Research efforts investigating the potential role of annexins in fat tissue relevant to health and metabolic disease are discussed.

Keywords: annexins; adipose tissue; adiponectin; cholesterol; glucose homeostasis; inflammation; insulin; lipid metabolism; obesity; triglycerides

---

1. Introduction

1.1. Obesity

In most countries, the increasing prevalence of obesity represents a rapidly growing risk factor for chronic liver diseases, type 2 diabetes (T2D), cardiovascular diseases and most types of cancer. The mechanisms contributing to obesity are multifactorial and are far from being completely understood. Moreover, life style changes with less caloric intake and increased energy expenditure appear insufficient to reduce body weight in the long term. Hence, the identification of the multiple processes that contribute to excess adiposity is required to enact innovative strategies to combat this epidemic [1,2].

Some key features and cellular machineries that contribute to increased and dysfunctional fat mass are listed below.

Adipose tissue is central to the development of obesity and is composed of different cell populations including fibroblasts, preadipocytes, mature adipocytes, macrophages, mesenchymal stem cells, endothelial cells, and vascular smooth muscle cells, with cellular function as well as their quantity being affected by obesity [1]. All these different cell types, through various mechanisms, contribute to obesity and associated comorbidities, which has been reviewed in detail elsewhere [1–3]. In brief, storage of nutrients and their mobilization for energy production are critical functions of adipose tissue. Yet, increased lipolysis in obese fat tissue is closely associated with the development of insulin resistance and T2D [1–3]. In addition, the excessive accumulation of fat in adipocytes due to overnutrition can lead to an inflammatory response that creates further metabolic complications [3–5]. In fact, even the physical stress triggered by the swelling that occurs in adipocytes upon increased fat accumulation seems to contribute to inflammation and insulin resistance [6]. In regard to the inflammatory process, macrophages accumulate in adiposity and in response to environmental signals in the fat tissue, undergo polarization to pro-inflammatory M1 macrophages [3]. In addition, in adipose tissue other myeloid cells, as well as T- and B-lymphocytes, have been linked to macrophage homeostasis and the inflammatory process associated with obesity [7]. Moreover, the growing tissue is not appropriately supplied with oxygen causing hypoxia, which contributes to inflammation and fibrosis. This pathological progress, adipose tissue fibrosis, hinders tissue growth and is linked to metabolic impediments [3]. Further complexity is created by truncal or android fat distribution, which was recently identified as an independent risk factor for metabolic diseases in obesity. Also, visceral and subcutaneous adipose tissues differ in blood flow, cellular composition, adipocyte size and endocrine function, thereby contributing differently to whole body physiology [2,3].

Additionally, the identification of brown fat in humans [8–10] has initiated new exciting research in the field over the last decade, as its highly elevated expression of uncoupling proteins leads to the production of heat, which favors weight loss [3,11]. Due to its therapeutic potential, the process of browning has created great interest, where white fat cells become so-called beige or brite adipocytes, acquiring characteristics of brown fat, in particular the upregulation of uncoupling proteins. Hence, molecules targeting brown or brite fat to increase energy expenditure are being investigated for their potential to reduce body weight and improve metabolic health [12]. Actually, besides increased thermodynamic expenditure, the activation of brown adipose tissue additionally accelerated other cardioprotective and clinically relevant events, such as clearance of plasma triglycerides, a process that was dependent on the fatty acid transporter CD36 [13]. Furthermore, brown fat also contributed to lipoprotein processing and the conversion of cholesterol to bile acids in the liver, enabling the removal of excess cholesterol from the body [14]. Moreover, especially under thermogenic stimulation, brown fat releases several bioactive factors with endocrine properties, including insulin-like growth factor I, interleukin-6 (IL-6), or fibroblast growth factor-21, which influence hepatic and cardiac function, contributing to improved glucose tolerance and insulin sensitivity [15–17].

Given that obesity is characterized by an increased accumulation of triglycerides, research in the field over the last two decades has focussed on the dysregulation of the fatty acid metabolism. However, obese adipocytes also accumulate calcium and cholesterol crystals, which was demonstrated to contribute to oxidative stress and cell death [5]. On the other hand, plasma membrane cholesterol was depleted in obese fat cells which probably impaired the function of cholesterol-rich membrane microdomains (lipid rafts), causing an elevated release of C-C motif chemokine ligand 2 (CCL2), a major chemoattractant for monocytes [18]. In other studies, inhibition of the Niemann-Pick type C1 (NPC1) transporter, which facilitates cholesterol export from late endocytic (pre-lysosomal) and lysosomal compartments, impaired insulin signaling and glucose uptake in adipocytes [19]. Cholesterol is also essential for the proper functioning of endo- and exocytic vesicle transport, which control the release of distinct adipokines like adiponectin [20], an anti-inflammatory plasma protein that improves insulin sensitivity, but is reduced in obesity [21].

A more detailed analysis of the various pathways listed above and affected in obese adipose tissues clearly is essential to develop strategies to combat obesity. However, it would go beyond the scope of this review to list all pathways contributing to adipose tissue dysfunction and we refer the reader to other excellent articles [3,4,22]. In the following, we will summarize and focus on the current understanding of how a group of evolutionary conserved proteins, the annexins, may influence fat tissue function in health and disease.

1.2. Annexins

The annexin family in humans and vertebrates consists of twelve structurally related Ca^{2+}- and membrane binding proteins (AnxA1–AnxA11, AnxA13) [23,24]. All annexins contain a variable N-terminus, followed by a conserved C-terminal domain with four (or eight in AnxA6) annexin repeats (Table 1). Each of these repeats encodes for Ca^{2+} binding sites, allowing annexins to rapidly translocate to phospholipid-containing membranes in response to Ca^{2+} elevation [23,25,26]. Hence, annexin functions are intimately dependent on their dynamic and reversible membrane binding behaviour. Nevertheless, their similar structure, phospholipid-binding properties, overlapping localizations, and shared interaction partners have made it difficult to elucidate their precise functions. Yet, despite in vivo studies in knock-out (KO) models strongly suggesting redundancy within the annexin family, specific functions of individual annexins have been identified [23,25–31]. Interestingly, besides often subtle differences in their spatio-temporal and Ca^{2+}-sensitive membrane binding behaviour to negatively charged phospholipids, the diversity of N-terminal interaction partners, affinity to other lipids, including phosphatidylinositol-4,5-bisphosphate, cholesterol and ceramide, posttranslational modifications, and most relevant for this review, their differential expression patterns seem to facilitate opportunities to create functional diversity within the annexin family [23,25–31]. The subsequent chapters will review recent knowledge on the expression of individual annexins in adipose tissue, with quite diverse implications for adipocyte and macrophage function in health and obesity.

Table 1. Domain structure, expression patterns, and potential functions of annexins expressed in adipose tissue. The different length of the N-terminal leader and C-terminal annexin repeats 1–4 (1–8 for AnxA6) for each annexin are indicated. AnxA13a differs from AnxA13b by a 41 amino acid N-terminal deletion [32]. Relevant references for each annexin are listed. AnxA, annexin; GLUT4, glucose transporter type 4; HFD, high-fat diet; HSL, hormone-sensitive lipase; SV, stromal-vascular fraction; TZDs, thiazolidinediones. N/A, not available.

Name	Structure	Adipose Tissue Expression	Function	References
		A. Prominent Annexins in Adipose Tissue.		
AnxA1		adipocytes, SV, visceral fat, subcutaneous fat, obesity ↑, HFD ↑, TZDs ↑	insulin response ↑, obesity ↓, leptin ↓, inflammation ↓	[33–45]
AnxA2		adipocytes, endothelial cells, macrophages, subcutaneous fat, epididymal fat, mesenteric fat, guggulsterone ↑, TZDs ↑	GLUT4 translocation, insulin response, glucose uptake, CD36-mediated fatty acid uptake, inflammation ↑, macrophage infiltration ↑, HSL activation	[46–60]
AnxA6		adipocytes, macrophages, subcutaneous fat, perirenal fat, epididymal fat, visceral fat, brown fat, obesity ↑, HFD ↑, oxidative stress ↑	preadipocyte proliferation ↑, triglyceride storage ↓, adiponectin release ↓, cholesterol-dependent caveolae formation, cholesterol-dependent GLUT4 translocation, cholesterol-dependent adiponectin secretion?	[2,35,47,61–74]

Table 1. Cont.

Name	Structure	Adipose Tissue Expression	Function	References
B. Other Annexins in Adipose Tissue.				
AnxA3		adipocytes, SV, subcutaneous fat, intraabdominal fat	adipocyte differentiation ↓, lipid accumulation?	[75–77], Geo Profiles; DataSet Record GDS2818
AnxA5		SV, subcutaneous fat, intraabdominal fat	fat deposition, storage or mobilization?	[35,78], Geo Profiles; DataSet Record GDS2818
AnxA7		SV, subcutaneous fat, intraabdominal fat	infiltration of immune cells in dysfunctional adipose tissue?	[79–83], Geo Profiles; DataSet Record GDS2818
AnxA8		adipocytes, SV, subcutaneous fat, intraabdominal fat	cholesterol-dependent caveolae formation, cholesterol-dependent GLUT4 translocation, cholesterol-dependent adiponectin secretion?	[84–89], Geo Profiles; DataSet Record GDS2818
C. Insufficiently Studied Annexins in Adipose Tissue.				
AnxA4		N/A	lipolysis?	[90]
AnxA9		N/A	?	
AnxA10		adipocytes, SV, subcutanous fat, intraabdominal fat	?	
AnxA11		adipocytes, SV, subcutanous fat, intraabdominal fat	fatty acid release, adipokine secretion?	[91]
AnxA13a		N/A	?	
AnxA13b		N/A	?	

2. Annexin Expression Patterns in Adipose Tissue and Their Potential Functions in Obesity

2.1. Annexin A1 (AnxA1)

AnxA1 (previously known as lipocortin 1) is expressed in most cell types, and abundant in macrophages, neutrophils, the nervous and endocrine system [23,27,92]. Like other annexins, AnxA1 is found at multiple locations inside cells, including the plasma membrane, endosomal and secretory vesicles, the cytoskeleton and the nucleus, participating in membrane transport, signal transduction, actin dynamics and regulation of metabolic enzymes related to cell growth, differentiation, motility and apoptosis [25,26,92–94]. In addition, AnxA1 has a prominent extracellular function, acting as an anti-inflammatory, pro-resolving protein which exerts its effects via binding to the formyl peptide receptor 2 (FPR2). Both molecules are induced by glucocorticoids and contribute to the beneficial activities of these anti-inflammatory drugs [39,42].

The inflammation-related functions of FPR2 are diverse and complex, with multiple FPR2 ligands exercising various and sometimes opposite activities [36,95]. While the loss of FPR2 reduced inflammation, the overall FPR2 activity in fat tissue in vivo is most likely the net result of the distinct expression patterns and the localized distribution of different FPR2 ligands in this tissue [36]. Importantly, resolvin D1 and lipoxin A$_4$, both bioactive lipid mediators that have been identified in adipose tissue, are agonists of this G-protein coupled receptor [96,97]. These lipids have anti-inflammatory activities and highlight the requirement to fine-tune the balance of ligands with opposing activities, in order to activate the immune response and thereby accelerate the termination of inflammation [96].

Recent studies suggest that the AnxA1/FPR2 axis is highly relevant for obesity and related inflammation, as well as other complications, such as insulin resistance, T2D and atherosclerosis [36,37,41,42,45]. As levels of FPR2 and its ligands critically influence strength of biological response, it is interesting to note that in obese mice, adipose tissue FPR2 mRNA and resolvin D1 levels were decreased [95]. Most relevant for AnxA1 in adipose tissue, the FPR2 peptide agonist WKYMVM, which is derived from the N-terminus of AnxA1, greatly enhanced the insulin response of diet-induced obese mice [45].

Somewhat unexpectedly, FPR2 deficiency improved the metabolic health of mice that were fed a high fat diet [36]. In this study, FPR2 was increased in fat of diet-induced obese mice and diabetic, leptin-receptor mutated, animals. Loss of FPR2 in macrophages blocked polarization into pro-inflammatory M1 macrophages [36]. FPR2 knock-out mice were less obese and higher thermogenesis in skeletal muscle was most likely responsible for enhanced energy expenditure [36]. Although the lack of FPR2 signalling events induced by ligands other than AnxA1 probably also contribute to the phenotype of the FPR2 knock-out mice described above, one can speculate that up- or downregulation of AnxA1 may also have profound effects on FPR2-dependent energy metabolism in adipose tissue.

In this context, it is still unclear which cell types contribute to extracellular AnxA1 levels in adipose tissue. In fat tissues, AnxA1 was more abundant in the stromal-vascular fraction than in adipocytes [43], indicating that infiltrating monocytes and macrophages expressing AnxA1 may represent the main source of extracellular AnxA1 in fat [39]. In support of this hypothesis, when these immune cells became activated, AnxA1 translocated to the cell surface and was secreted [39].

Besides the contribution of non-adipocytes to AnxA1 levels in fat mass, its expression appears tightly regulated during adipocyte differentiation, as murine 3T3-L1 adipogenesis identified AnxA1 mRNA and protein downregulation [44]. In contrast, in mature adipocytes from patients with Simpson Golabi Behmel syndrome, an overgrowth disorder leading to craniofacial, skeletal, cardiac, and renal abnormalities, AnxA1 mRNA and protein amounts were approximately 65-fold higher compared to their corresponding preadipocytes. As FPR2 levels were markedly reduced in this model, it remains to be determined if drastically upregulated AnxA1 expression alters the repertoire and availability of other extracellular FPR2 ligands and impacts on FPR2 activity [38,44]. Simpson Golabi Behmel syndrome is associated with glypican-3 loss-of-function mutations [98], implicating a possible link between adipocyte AnxA1 expression and this poorly characterized cell surface proteoglycan. However, a more likely explanation could be the higher concentration of glucocorticoids used in this study, possibly causing an elevation of AnxA1 levels irrespective of adipogenesis. The analysis of purified preadipocytes and mature cells may be an appropriate approach to better define transcriptional and post-transcriptional regulation of AnxA1 expression during adipogenesis.

The therapeutic potential of AnxA1 is further underscored by its upregulation in the subcutaneous fat of obese men given rosiglitazone for two weeks [33]. Glitazones are insulin sensitizers and agonists of peroxisomal proliferator-activated receptor-γ (PPARγ), a master regulator of adipogenesis [99]. AnxA1 is a target gene of this transcription factor in breast cancer cells [100] and most likely in numerous other cell types [39,101]. Whether this PPARγ-dependent transcriptional control of the AnxA1 promoter also applies for adipocytes needs additional studies.

Further documenting a relationship between AnxA1 and obesity, AnxA1 mRNA was strongly increased in adipose tissue of mice on a high fat diet [34]. This upregulation was observed in both leptin- and IL-6-deficient animals, strongly pointing at transcriptional pathways not directly regulated by these factors being responsible for AnxA1 upregulation in a lipid-rich environment [34]. AnxA1 mRNA expression was also higher in visceral adipose tissues of obese compared to lean children [102]. Proteome assessment of adipocytes isolated from subcutaneous fat of young and old overweight patients revealed higher AnxA1 protein levels in the latter [35]. Hence, as older subjects more often suffer from insulin resistance and cardiovascular disease, these findings further support a function of AnxA1 in metabolic health. Interestingly, under inflammatory conditions, AnxA1 may undergo protease-mediated degradation, leading to pro-inflammatory AnxA1 fragments that lack the FPR2-binding motif in the N-terminal AnxA1 region [103]. Indeed, cleaved AnxA1 was more abundant in adipose tissues of obese individuals independent of their insulin resistance status [40].

Whole body physiology critically influences adipose tissue function and in the following, we will briefly summarize some observations that could impact on AnxA1 levels and functions in fat tissue. In contrast to upregulated adipose AnxA1 levels in obesity-related disease settings listed above [33,34,102], one study identified that circulating levels of AnxA1 were decreased in obesity [38]. Yet, more recent research described that serum AnxA1 amounts increased with body mass index (BMI) and positively correlated with IL-6 [40]. In the same report, an association of serum AnxA1 levels with T2D was not apparent [40]. The opposing outcome of these two studies clearly illustrates that further research is needed to resolve the role of AnxA1 in adiposity and metabolic diseases.

Over the years, many studies have established that dysregulation of the inter-organ cross-talk beween adipose tissue and other metabolic organs contribute to significant changes in energy homeostasis, glucose and lipid metabolism in obesity and associated complications. Adipose tissue releases numerous adipokines that influence liver, muscle and pancreas physiology, which in turn, have potential to modify glucose and lipid handling in fat tissue [3,4]. This may also include alterations in AnxA1 expression, secretion, and protein stability, which may impact on serum AnxA1 levels or influence other AnxA1-related biological activities with indirect effects on adipocytes. For example, non-alcoholic fatty liver disease is commonly diagnosed in the obese and is a spectrum ranging from benign liver steatosis to hepatitis and fibrosis [21]. Hepatic AnxA1 protein expression was reduced in patients with bridging fibrosis when compared to those with mild disease [104]. In mice fed a methionine-choline-deficient diet to induce non-alcoholic steatohepatitis (NASH), hepatic AnxA1 protein levels were nevertheless increased [104]. While these findings may suggest a link between AnxA1 expression levels and hepatic neutral lipid accumulation, oleate-induced lipid storage was normal in AnxA1-overexpressing Huh7 hepatocytes [61]. Accordingly, hepatic triglycerides levels were also comparably induced in murine NASH of wild type and AnxA1-deficient mice [104]. Yet irrespective of neutral lipid storage, liver inflammation and fibrosis were clearly enhanced in AnxA1 KO-animals [104].

AnxA1 was expressed in liver macrophages and contributed to anti-inflammatory M2 macrophage polarization and IL-10 production. Accordingly, macrophages developed into a pro-inflammatory M1 phenotype in the AnxA1 null animals [104]. Galectin-3 is produced by activated macrophages and contributes to liver fibrosis, and recombinant AnxA1 prevented galectin-3 expression [104]. Strikingly, AnxA1 protected the liver from NASH in this experimental model, which is characterized by body weight loss [104]. Furthermore, inhibition of hepatitis C virus replication by AnxA1 showed a protective role in the development of chronic liver disease [105]. Again, steatosis grade was not changed by AnxA1 in the liver cells [105]. Hence, these studies suggest protective roles for AnxA1 in liver function, which could also support a healthy communication with adipose tissue.

Beneficial effects of AnxA1 were also described in muscle and pancreatic beta-cells, both highly relevant for glucose homeostasis [106]. The saturated fatty acid palmitate, which is elevated in the plasma of obese patients, induced insulin resistance and suppressed AnxA1 expression in L6 myotubes [45,107]. On the other hand, AnxA1 released from mesenchymal stromal cells improved the glucose-induced insulin release of human islets in a co-culture model demonstrating protective functions on pancreatic beta-cells [108].

Taken together, most of the data summarized above point towards disease-preventing activities of AnxA1 in obesity (Table 1). In further support of this model, AnxA1 null mice were in fact more obese, had larger adipocytes and increased leptin levels when fed a high fat diet [34]. Common measures that occur with high fat diet feeding, such as upregulation of lipolytic enzymes and downregulation of 11-beta hydroxysteroid dehydrogenase type 1, was only significant in fat tissues of the obese wild type animals [34]. Corticosterone levels were higher in the AnxA1-deficient animals and may have further promoted adiposity in these mice [34]. Moreover, the high fat diet fed AnxA1 KO-mice displayed elevated glucose and insulin levels, and were less insulin-sensitive. Interestingly, despite the prominent anti-inflammatory features of AnxA1 discussed above, adipose tissue inflammation was not induced in these mice [34]. The exacerbation of obesity-associated metabolic diseases in AnxA1 null mice was confirmed in a further study. The treatment of these mice with recombinant human AnxA1 reduced body weight, fat mass, and liver steatosis [41].

Finally, others analyzed AnxA1 null mice fed a control chow diet. Body weight and adipocyte size were normal, whereas epididymal fat mass was reduced in AnxA1-deficient animals [43]. Catecholamine-induced rise in cAMP levels and lipolysis were more pronounced in adipose tissue explants of the control animals [43]. Adipose tissue explants from the AnxA1 KO-mice further displayed a lower production of IL-6, which was not attributed to a decline in the number of macrophages in intra-abdominal fat pads [43].

Overall, the studies summarized above indicate AnxA1 as a metabolism-improving molecule in models of metabolically stressed animals (Figure 1, Table 1). This may provide exciting therapeutic opportunities [37,39,41,42,45,104], but more research—exploring for instance the comparison of energy expenditure measurements in controls and the AnxA1 null mice on chow and high fat diets [34,41]—is still needed to better understand the various molecular pathways regulated by AnxA1 in adipose tissues.

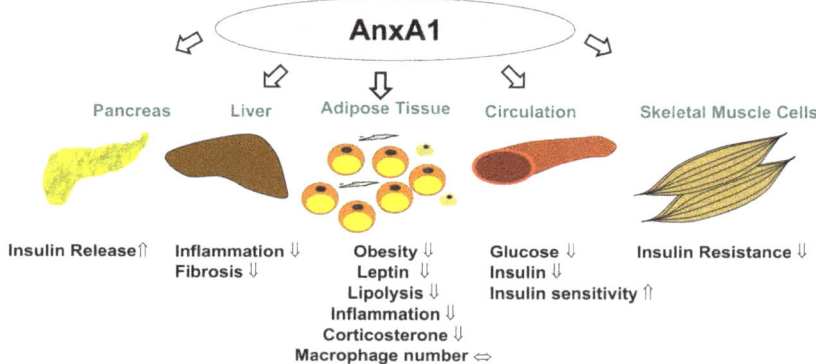

Figure 1. The multiple roles of AnxA1 in metabolism. AnxA1 increased insulin release of pancreatic beta-cells [108] and improved insulin response of skeletal muscle and whole body insulin sensitivity, thus lowering circulating glucose and insulin levels [34,45]. AnxA1 further ameliorated hepatic inflammation and fibrosis in a murine NASH model [104]. AnxA1 null mice were more obese, produced more leptin and had higher adipose tissue lipolysis, inflammation and corticosterone levels. AnxA1 did not alter the recruitment of adipose tissue macrophages [34].

2.2. Annexin A2 (AnxA2)

AnxA2 is ubiquitously expressed and most abundant in endothelial cells, monocytes and macrophages. In addition, AnxA2 is also often upregulated in cancers [23,25,94,109–111]. Most AnxA2 proteins form a heterotetrameric complex with p11, a member of the S100 protein family, at the plasma membrane and intracellular compartments, while only small amounts of AnxA2 monomer are present in the cytosol, endosomes and nucleus. In these multiple locations, AnxA2 contributes to the regulation of endo-/exocytic membrane transport, microdomain organization, membrane repair and nuclear transport, relevant for many different cellular activities [23,25,26,93,94,109]. Also, extracellular AnxA2 activities related to fibrinolysis and not discussed further in this review have been well documented [109–112].

AnxA2 is expressed in the adipose tissues of humans and rodents [53,57] and has been linked with two prominent aspects of adipocyte function (Table 1). Firstly, several studies implicated AnxA2 in glucose homeostasis, in particular the insulin-inducible translocation of GLUT4, the main glucose transporter in adipocytes, from intracellular compartments to the cell surface. In one study, the silencing of AnxA2 in 3T3-L1 adipocytes improved insulin sensitivity and glucose uptake [59]. In striking contrast, others reported that AnxA2 inhibition or depletion, using antibodies or knockdown approaches, strongly reduced insulin-inducible GLUT4 translocation [51]. As insulin exposure promoted GLUT4, but not AnxA2, trafficking to the cell surface [55], it appears unlikely that direct interaction or GLUT4 translocation along AnxA2-positive vesicles occurs. Alternatively, the underlying mechanism could involve a possible role of AnxA2 in insulin signaling through the modulation of insulin receptor internalization [46]. Indeed, the fact that insulin induced AnxA2 phosphorylation [46,56,60], AnxA2 sumoylation [50], and enhanced AnxA2 secretion [60] further indicates that the expression, localization and activity of AnxA2 is closely connected to insulin signaling and glucose handling in adipocytes. Hence, further studies are needed to clarify these current gaps of knowledge and discrepancies.

Secondly, AnxA2 has also been associated with fatty acid accumulation. In fact, in endothelial cells and adipocytes of white adipose tissue, AnxA2 was critical for the cellular uptake of fatty acids. AnxA2 was found to bind prohibitin and the fatty acid transporter CD36 in both cell types, and assembly of this complex at the plasma membrane was enforced by the presence of fatty acids [57]. This protein complex not only improved fatty acid uptake in these two often neighbouring cell types, but also enabled the transport of fatty acids from the endothelium to adipocytes. In further support of these observations, palmitate-inducible expression of inflammatory genes like IL-6, IL-1 beta and tumor necrosis factor alpha was markedly diminished upon AnxA2 suppression, while AnxA2 overexpression amplified the proinflammatory capacity of this saturated fatty acid [59].

Several in vivo studies addressed the aforementioned potential roles of AnxA2 in glucose and fatty acid metabolism (Figure 2). However, AnxA2 null mice had reduced steady-state glucose levels and a normal glucose tolerance [57]. As the glucose uptake of white adipose tissues was comparable in the control and AnxA2-deficient animals, it was concluded that AnxA2 did not have a central function in GLUT4 translocation in vivo. On the other hand, AnxA2-deficient animals had a delayed clearance of infused fatty acids, indicating that the lack of AnxA2 compromised CD36-mediated removal of fatty acids from the bloodstream [57]. Given that thermogenic activation of brown adipose tissue accelerated CD36-dependent clearance of plasma triglycerides [13], and palmitoylation-dependent CD36 localization and trafficking in adipose tissue being sensitive to acute cold exposure [113], testing cold tolerance in AnxA2 KO-mice in future studies could provide further critical insight. Taken together, these findings might point at AnxA2 contributing to a more rapid clearance of lipids and the improvement of postprandial hyperlipidemia.

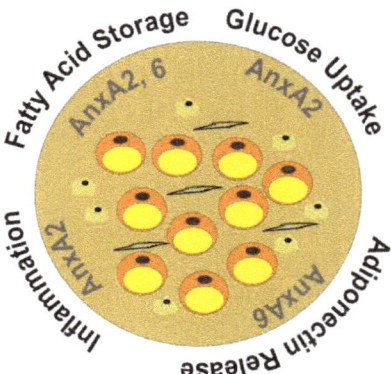

Figure 2. The diverse roles of AnxA2 and AnxA6 in adipose tissue function. AnxA2 improves uptake and storage of fatty acids [57] and may have a role in glucose uptake and adipose tissue inflammation [51,59]. On the other hand, AnxA6 modulates lipolysis and adiponectin secretion [68].

More recently, others investigated adenoviral-mediated AnxA2 up- or downregulation in mice fed a high fat diet. Animals with low AnxA2 levels had reduced body weight at the end of the study, displaying improved fasting blood glucose and insulin levels, as well as glucose and insulin tolerance. Overexpression of AnxA2 did not change any of these parameters. In addition, AnxA2 depletion was associated with less adipose tissue macrophages and inflammation, which was enhanced by AnxA2 overexpression [59]. Hence, several AnxA2 functions observed in cell-based studies might be relevant in stress-induced conditions in vivo, and, as outlined above, cell and animal studies support an involvement of AnxA2 in adipose tissue function. In line with these observations, expression studies in humans and animal models suggest that AnxA2 levels are tightly regulated, often responding to changes in whole body and adipose tissue physiology. For instance, AnxA2 was detected in preadipocytes and was modestly induced during 3T3-L1 adipogenesis [54]. Guggulsterone, a natural drug which inhibits adipocyte differentiation and induces apoptosis, increased AnxA2 expression in these cells [54]. While AnxA2 mRNA remained unchanged, post-translational processing of AnxA2 protein was induced by guggulsterone [54], indicating that truncated AnxA2 isoforms may exert so far unknown inhibitory functions during adipogenesis. However, in another study, troglitazone-induced PPARγ activation, which promotes adipocyte differentiation [99], upregulated AnxA2 mRNA and protein expression in 3T3-L1 adipocytes [51]. Likewise, the PPARγ agonist rosiglitazone also induced AnxA2 levels in subcutaneous fat of obese but otherwise healthy men. Together with the abovementioned studies suggesting AnxA2 to promote glucose and fatty acid uptake, one can speculate that this drug-induced upregulation of AnxA2 may contribute to the beneficial therapeutic effects of the rosiglitazone-induced lowering of fasting insulin, glucose, and free fatty acids in plasma [33].

Interestingly, in murine adipose tissue AnxA2 protein levels were approximately two-fold higher in large compared to small adipocytes. This differential expression pattern was abrogated in fat-specific insulin receptor knock-out mice [47]. As the increased size of adipocytes is associated with an elevated capacity for insulin-inducible neutral lipid storage, this further supports a function of AnxA2 upregulation in insulin-dependent metabolic changes during adipocyte differentiation and growth. Indeed, a comparison of wild type and AnxA2-deficient mice revealed that AnxA2 was essential for adipocyte growth, whereas adipogenesis was unaffected by the loss of AnxA2 [57].

Proteomic approaches to identify changes in weight loss and physical activity identified altered AnxA2 levels in adipose tissue. Although a two-week high-intensity intermittent training of overweight men neither improved BMI nor the parameters of insulin sensitivity, the inflammatory marker IL-6, as well as AnxA2 and fatty acid synthase were significantly reduced in subcutaneous fat [53]. Likewise, dietary changes, such as a low-fat, high-complex carbohydrate diet supplemented with long-chain n-3 polyunsaturated fatty acids not only improved glucose and fatty acid metabolism, but also downregulated AnxA2 expression in subcutaneous fat [52]. In contrast, a five week very low calorie diet improved metabolic health and BMI of obese subjects, yet AnxA2 and GLUT4 levels increased, whereas CD36 expression declined, in subcutaneous adipose tissues [49]. AnxA2 was also higher in subcutaneous fat after weight loss achieved by a very low calorie diet [48]. In summary, the human studies listed here do not consistently imply a common theme that associates similar changes of AnxA2 levels in fat tissues upon weight loss. Likewise, discordant findings were also published on the regulation of AnxA2 expression in murine obesity. Here, AnxA2 was expressed in epididymal and mesenteric fat. Diet-induced obesity led to elevated AnxA2 protein levels in both fat depots, which was also increased in the liver and skeletal muscle [59]. In spite of this, hepatic AnxA2 protein amounts were found to be reduced in mice fed a high fat diet in a separate study [58]. Thus, for a clearer picture of potential AnxA2 functions in fat tissue (Table 1), more studies are needed to improve our understanding of the regulation of AnxA2 protein expression, localization and interaction partners in adipocytes and other cells of fat tissues.

2.3. Annexin A6 (AnxA6)

AnxA6 is found in most cells and tissues, with abundant levels being expressed in endothelial and endocrine cells, hepatocytes and macrophages [23,25–27,114]. The plasma membrane and endocytic compartments represent the most common AnxA6 localizations [26,30,63,66,115–118], but AnxA6 is also found along the secretory pathway [23,25,119], mitochondria [120] and lipid droplets [61,121]. Like other annexins, and depending on the cellular localization and repertoire of interaction partners, AnxA6 participates in many cellular activities, some of which potentially relevant for adipose tissue function, such as endo- and exocytosis, signal transduction, cholesterol homeostasis, stress response [23,25–27,30,64,94,116] and lately, neutral lipid accumulation [61,62].

The multifunctionality of AnxA6 has made it difficult to assign specific AnxA6 functions to particular cell types, but despite a still limited number of studies addressing AnxA6 in adipocyte biology, several cellular processes that are modulated by AnxA6 could possibly be relevant for adipocyte function (Table 1). To begin with, AnxA6 upregulation inhibits cholesterol export from late endosomes, which perturbs cellular cholesterol homeostasis similar to mutations in the late endosomal/lysosomal NPC1 cholesterol transporter. This leads to reduced cholesterol levels in other compartments, such as the plasma membrane, Golgi apparatus and recycling endosomes [63,73]. Consequently, membrane trafficking is compromised, and we initially observed reduced numbers of caveolae due to caveolin-1 accumulation in the Golgi [63]. This could be highly relevant for adipocyte function, as caveolae are most prominent in adipocytes, with roles in endocytosis, cholesterol and fatty acid uptake, lipid droplet formation and signal transduction [122,123]. In follow-up studies, we then identified AnxA6-induced cholesterol imbalance to cause mislocalization and dysfunction of several cholesterol-sensitive SNARE proteins in the secretory pathway [72,73], all of which are fundamental for the metabolic response that facilitates GLUT4 translocation in adipocytes [124]. Also, recent findings from our laboratories indicate that cholesterol accumulation in late endosomes of NPC1 mutants promotes the interaction of AnxA6 with the Rab7-GTPase activating protein TBC1D15 (Rentero, Grewal and Enrich, unpublished results), which has recently been implicated in Rab7-dependent pathways that regulate GLUT4 translocation to the cell surface [125]. Impaired insulin signaling and glucose uptake in 3T3-L1 adipocytes upon NPC1 inhibition [19] extend support for a model of upregulated AnxA6, through cellular cholesterol imbalance, to impact on GLUT4 trafficking.

Secondly, AnxA6 associates with secretory granules in a Ca^{2+}-dependent manner [67], participates in Ca^{2+} homeostasis through store-operated Ca^{2+} entry [70] and alters catecholamine secretion [71], all of which with links to the secretory pathway that enables adiponectin release [126]. Thirdly, the scaffolding function of AnxA6 is critical for the formation and activity of several signalling complexes [26,29,64–66], with roles in GLUT4 translocation and lipolysis [127]. Finally, we recently identified the association of AnxA6 with lipid droplets in hepatocytes to influence their capacity to store neutral lipids [61], which could also be relevant for neutral lipid storage in fat tissue.

Initial insights into AnxA6 functions in fat tissue were lately obtained from the characterization of differentiated 3T3-L1 adipocytes overexpressing or lacking AnxA6. In this model, siRNA-mediated AnxA6 knockdown impaired preadipocyte proliferation. Moreover, maturation of AnxA6-depleted 3T3-L1 adipocytes was associated with increased storage of triglycerides and elevated release of adiponectin [68]. The latter finding was not observed in oleate-loaded cells [68], possibly indicating independent mechanisms that cause changes in triglyceride accumulation and adiponectin release upon AnxA6 depletion. Vice versa, AnxA6 overexpression in 3T3-L1 cells lowered cellular triglycerides and adiponectin release (Figure 2). In addition, the catecholamine-stimulated phosphorylation of hormone-sensitive lipase (HSL) to promote lipolysis was impaired in AnxA6-depleted cells and coincided with AnxA6 localization on lipid droplets in adipocytes, implicating a scaffolding function of AnxA6 at the lipid droplet membrane possibly relevant for HSL phosphorylation and not directly linked to adiponectin release through the secretory pathway [68]. Importantly, this function of HSL is not critical for fatty acid metabolism in non-adipose tissue [128], which might contribute to explain the opposite effects of AnxA6 up- or downregulation on neutral lipid storage in cells from liver and fat tissue [61,68]. Notably, AnxA6 levels did not change lipopolysaccharide response of 3T3-L1 adipocytes, and basal as well as lipopolysaccharide-induced IL-6 levels were comparable in groups with high and low AnxA6 levels [68].

Follow-up studies in AnxA6 KO-mice, which have normal body weight, glucose and insulin levels, support some of the cell-based studies summarized above. In particular, serum adiponectin levels were higher, while reduced amounts of adiponectin were found in the subcutaneous fat of the AnxA6 KO-animals [68]. As cholesterol is critical for the release of adiponectin through the secretory pathway [20], we speculate that the regulatory role of AnxA6 in cholesterol homeostasis [31,63,64,72,73] could be responsible for alterations in adiponectin plasma levels in the AnxA6 KO-animals.

Despite increased lipid storage in AnxA6-depeleted 3T3-L1 adipocytes, circulating triglycerides, free fatty acids and cholesterol were normal in AnxA6 KO-mice [68]. Systemic lipid levels of AnxA6-deficient animals were also comparable to controls after a high fat diet for 17 weeks [61,62]. Most interestingly, AnxA6 KO-mice gained less adipose tissue during high fat feeding [61,62], which might be in line with the impaired proliferation observed in AnxA6-depleted preadipocytes [68]. On the other hand, and in contrast to the cell-based studies described above [68], circulating leptin and adiponectin levels were slightly reduced in high fat diet fed AnxA6 KO-mice [61,62]. Lower fat mass is usually associated with higher adiponectin and improved glucose homeostasis [21]. Such improvements were not observed in the AnxA6 KO-animals [61,62] and AnxA6-related functions in other organs may need to be considered to possibly explain these up till now opposing obervations.

Strikingly, AnxA6 deficiency in mice compromised regulatory steps to downregulate hepatic gluconeogenesis that only became apparent after high fat diet feeding [61,62]. Likewise, dysfunctional hepatic glucose homeostasis in AnxA6-KO mice was also observed after induction of metabolic stress upon partial liver hepatectomy or starvation [129]. Given the prominent role for adipokines in the coordination of hepatic glucose homeostasis, we speculate that so far unidentified changes in the inter-organ metabolic communication beween fat and liver tissues of AnxA6-KO mice may contribute to the fine-tuning of hepatic glucose metabolism, with potential consequences for the systemic control of glucose in health and disease.

The abovementioned and in-part profound effects of AnxA6 up- or downregulation on the central aspects of adipocyte function, including growth, lipid storage, and adiponectin release, suggest that complex mechanisms might be in place to control AnxA6 expression levels in fat tissue. Several studies provide some insight in this matter. AnxA6 protein expression modestly increased during 3T3-L1 cell adipogenesis and was clearly induced in mature human adipocytes when compared to their respective preadipocytes [68]. AnxA6 protein levels were, however, not changed upon lipid loading of adipocytes [68]. Likewise, exposure to high glucose or lipopolysaccharide did not impact on AnxA6 protein levels in 3T3-L1 cells. On the other hand, oxidative stress, which suppresses adiponectin release and contributes to insulin resistance in obese adipose tissues [130], was associated with AnxA6 upregulation in 3T3-L1 adipocytes [68].

AnxA6 was also highly expressed in human monocytes, which can infiltrate fat tissue, and further increased in monocytic cells of overweight patients [74]. How this might impact adipose tissue function is still unclear, but high AnxA6 levels in phagocytes may accompany the process leading to foam cell formation and atherosclerosis [64,74]. Alternatively, AnxA6-induced changes in membrane order at the plasma membrane [131] may influence the distribution and activity of lipoprotein receptors and cholesterol transporters at the cell surface responsible for cholesterol efflux [132]. Of note, adiponectin, which protects from cardiovascular diseases [74,133], reduced AnxA6 protein expression in human monocytic cells [74,133], but not in 3T3-L1 adipocytes [68].

Complex and differential AnxA6 expression patterns have also been observed in animal and human studies. In subcutaneous, perirenal and epididymal adipose tissues from mice fed a high fat diet for 14 weeks, AnxA6 levels were strongly induced [68]. This may in part be related to increased AnxA6 expression in macrophages [74]. Additionally, obese murine adipocytes also displayed higher AnxA6 protein levels [68]. AnxA6 protein amounts remained unchanged in the visceral fat of overweight patients when compared to normal weight patients, illustrating that AnxA6 levels do not increase when body weight and adipocyte size grow in humans [68]. Furthermore, AnxA6 expression was induced in adipocytes during aging [35], which is associated with oxidative stress and a decline in adipocyte function [134]. Hence, increased reactive oxygen species rather than cell hypertrophy seem to mediate the upregulation of AnxA6 in adiposity.

Visceral fat accumulation has deleterious effects [2,68,69] and AnxA6 protein levels were higher in human and murine visceral compared to subcutaneous adipose tissues [2,68,69]. In adipocytes purified from the respective human fat depots, AnxA6 protein amounts were also more abundant in the visceral fat cells [68]. Remarkably, fat depot distribution of AnxA6 changed in obesity. Here,

AnxA6 levels were higher in subcutaneous adipose tissues compared to intraabdominal fat. Such a change in fat depot expression is uncommon and cell-type specific regulation of AnxA6 may need to be evaluated to identify the underlying mechanisms.

In murine epididymal fat, AnxA6 protein levels were approximately 60% higher in large when compared to small adipocytes. This size-dependent change in AnxA6 expression was only detected in insulin receptor knock-out mice but not in the respective control animals [47]. This indicates that adipocyte growth is not associated with higher AnxA6 expression as long as the cells respond to insulin [47]. Whether a differential insulin response of subcutaneous and visceral adipocytes [2] contributes to altered AnxA6 protein needs further studies. Insulin did not change AnxA6 protein levels in 3T3-L1 cells, excluding a direct effect of this hormone [68].

Finally, in brown fat, which is quite distinct from other fat tissues as its main function is to produce heat, AnxA6 protein amounts remained unchanged in obesity [68]. Altogether, AnxA6 is differentially expressed in the various fat depots and in some cases, response to diet was observed (Table 1). Altogether this may indicate differential AnxA6 functions in the various fat tissues, which still need to be resolved in future studies.

2.4. Other Annexins

2.4.1. Annexin A3 (AnxA3)

In comparison to the depth of literature on AnxA1, A2 and A6, up to date only a limited number of studies have examined AnxA3 expression and function (Table 1). AnxA3 is most prominent in neutrophils and macrophages and was detected in heart, lung, placenta, kidney and spleen, with highest levels in murine adipose tissue [77]. Besides its Ca^{2+}-dependent membrane binding behavior, its intra- and extracellular locations and physiological functions are still poorly understood. Most AnxA3-related studies focussed on its potential as a biomarker in several cancers and the association of AnxA3 with chemotherapy resistance [135], with possible roles in the proliferative and invasive properties of cells. Interestingly, a recent study identified the recruitment of AnxA3 to lipid droplets of hepatitis C virus infected Huh7 hepatocytes [76], facilitating the interaction of viral proteins with apolipoprotein E (ApoE) during virus maturation and egress. Given the prominent role of ApoE in mouse and human adipocyte differentiation and lipid accumulation [136], one can speculate that yet to be identified environmental signals may also trigger AnxA3-driven interactions with ApoE or other proteins on the lipid droplet membrane during fat cell differentiation. In fact, one report identified AnxA3 to negatively regulate adipogenesis. In this study, AnxA3 protein was highly expressed in preadipocytes and strongly downregulated during 3T3-L1 cell differentiation [77]. Marked suppression of AnxA3 in early adipogenesis suggested an inhibitory function of AnxA3 in adipocyte differentiation [77]. Indeed, when AnxA3 was depleted by siRNA transfection of preadipocytes, expression of PPARγ2 and lipid droplet accumulation were increased, enhancing terminal adipocyte differentiation [77]. Of note, AnxA3 mRNA levels were comparable in the different white fat depots [77] (Table 2), indicating similar roles in the various fat locations. Interestingly, stromal vascular cell fractions expressed higher AnxA3 mRNA levels compared to adipocytes [75]. Analysis of publicly accessible DNA microarray data confirmed higher AnxA3 mRNA expression in murine stromal vascular cells (Table 2), suggesting that AnxA3 might fulfill multiple cell-specific functions in fat tissue.

2.4.2. Annexin A5 (AnxA5)

AnxA5 is the most abundant annexin and except in neurons, is expressed ubiquitously [25,137]. During proliferation, differentiation and in many cancers, AnxA5 levels are often up- or downregulated [138]. Ca^{2+} elevation triggers AnxA5 binding to various cellular sites [23,139,140] to participate in cell growth and death, Ca^2 signalling and homeostasis, membrane domain organization and transport [23,30,140]. Therapeutically relevant, extracellular AnxA5 binds to outer membrane phosphatidylserine, allowing detection of apoptotic cells [137]. Furthermore, AnxA5 has prominent extracellular roles in blood coagulation, phagocytosis, viral infection, membrane invagination and membrane repair [137,138,141,142].

Although one can envisage several of these intra- and extracellular functions listed above being relevant for the proper functioning of several cell types in adipose tissue, such as macrophages, endothelial and vascular smooth muscle cells as well as adipocytes, current knowldege on AnxA5 function in fat physiology is still insignificant (Table 1). Analysis of publicly available expression data (Geo profiles) revealed that AnxA5 mRNA was mostly expressed in murine adipocytes when compared to the stromal vascular cells in subcutaneous and intraabdominal fat. Whereas adipocytes of both fat depots had similar AnxA5 mRNA levels, stromal vascular cells in subcutaneous fat expressed less AnxA5 mRNA (Table 2). In line with other differentiation models, AnxA5 protein expression was induced in adipocytes during aging [35] and one study demonstrated an association of AnxA5 polymorphisms with obesity in a Korean patient cohort [78], which may suggest a function of AnxA5 directly or indirectly contributing to fat deposition, storage or mobilization.

2.4.3. Annexin A7 (AnxA7)

AnxA7 is the only annexin that contains a long (100 amino acids) and hydrophobic N-terminus. Due to alternative splicing, a 47 kD splice variant is found in most tissues, while a larger 51 kDa isoform is expressed in the brain, heart and skeletal muscle [143]. In these various cells and organs, Ca^{2+}-inducible association of AnxA7 with secretory vesicles, the plasma membrane and the nuclear envelope has been observed [144], with possible roles in Ca^{2+}/GTP-dependent exocytic pathways, prostaglandin synthesis, cardiac remodelling and inflammatory myopathies [81,145,146]. In addition, the GTPase activity of AnxA7 has potential as a tumour suppressor in several cancers [147].

The AnxA7 functions listed above and related to membrane transport, Ca^{2+} signalling and hormone production could be relevant in fat, but very little is still known about potential roles for AnxA7 in adipocytes or other cell types in this tissue (Table 1). Nevertheless, in other cells and tissues, several AnxA7-related tasks may also influence adipose tissue function. For example, one mouse model lacking AnxA7 displayed defects in Ca^{2+} release and Ca^{2+}-dependent signal transduction, affecting insulin secretion [82,83]. On the other hand, another independently generated AnxA7 KO-mouse model was strikingly different and did not reveal a role for AnxA7 in Ca^{2+}-dependent insulin secretion [79]. In addition, in some cell types, AnxA7 negatively regulates cyclooxygenase-dependent prostaglandin E2 formation [80]. Hence, elevated plasma prostaglandin levels in AnxA7 KO-mice may contribute to decreased glucose tolerance and elevated glucose-inducible insulin secretion [81]. Most relevant for fat tissue in obesity, cyclooxygenase-dependent prostaglandin E2 production has been associated with pathologic complications that lead to inflammation and fibrosis, impaired adaptive thermogenesis and lipolysis in obese white adipose tissue [148].

Although the latter might indicate that AnxA7 plays a role in infiltrating immune cells in dysfunctional adipose tissue, at present, very limited information on AnxA7 expression patterns in normal and obese fat tissue is available. AnxA7 mRNA was comparable in adipocytes and stromal vascular cells in subcutaneous and intraabdominal fat (Table 2). Evidently, more studies are needed to possibly identify yet unknown AnxA7 functions in fat tissue.

2.4.4. Annexin A8 (AnxA8)

AnxA8 was first identified in human placenta [149] and, with the exception of acute promyelocyte leukemia [150], is only expressed at low levels in lung, skin, liver, and kidney [151]. Earlier reports described AnxA8 to inhibit blood coagulation [152], but cellular AnxA8 localizations and functions are still not fully understood. AnxA8 may provide opportunities as a biomarker in several cancers [153–155] and more recently, has been linked to the transdifferentiation of retinal pigment epithelial cells [156].

Nonetheless, within the context of adipose tissue function, the unique affinity of AnxA8 towards phosphatidylinositides and F-actin relevant for membrane-cytoskeleton interactions, might be most important. In fact, these distinctive membrane- and actin-binding properties of AnxA8 affect the functioning of late endosomes [84,85] and in endothelial cells, this contributes to control the delivery of CD63 from late endocytic vesicles to the cell surface for leukocyte recruitment and migration [86,89]. In addition, AnxA8 is associated with cholesterol-rich late endosomes, and similarly to AnxA6 overexpression or NPC1 inhibition [19,31,63,64,72,73], AnxA8 depletion results in cholesterol accumulation in this compartment [87]. This may indicate a coordinated mechanism to control AnxA8 and AnxA6 expression levels and their relative amounts in the late endosomal compartment. Along these lines, and as discussed for AnxA6 overexpression and NPC1 deficiency above (see 2.3.), it is tempting to speculate that late endosomal cholesterol accumulation triggered by AnxA8 downregulation might compromise adipocyte function leading to the improper performance of molecular events in caveolae [63,122,123], or related to insulin signaling and GLUT4 translocation [19,72,73,124].

The findings described above suggest that changes in AnxA8 expression levels may cause cellular dysfunction However, little is so far known if AnxA8 expression levels correlate with metabolic complications in obese fat tissue (Table 1). AnxA8 mRNA was expressed in human adipose tissues and was similar in subcutaneous and visceral fat depots of obese men [88]. In mice, AnxA8 mRNA levels were higher in adipocytes than stromal vascular cells. Interestingly, AnxA8 expression in adipocytes was more abundant in subcutanoues fat depots (Table 2). This observation adds AnxA8 to the list of candidate proteins that are differentially expressed in the various fat depots, and possibly relevant to further evaluate the deleterious effects of visceral adiposity [88].

2.4.5. Other Annexins

Up to date, it is unknown if the remaining annexins AnxA4, A9, A10, A11 and A13 contribute to the proper functioning of adipose tissue (Table 1). Out of those annexins, current literature has associated AnxA4 with cAMP production, which could be relevant for lipolysis [90]. Also, roles for AnxA11 in exocytosis and cytokinesis could influence fatty acid release or adipokine secretion [91]. Of note, expression data for AnxA4, AnxA9 and AnxA13 in fat was not publicly available, but AnxA10 and A11 are indeed expressed in fat tissue. AnxA10 expression was similar in adipocytes and stromal vascular cells in subcutaneous and intraabdominal fat (Table 2). AnxA11 was mostly expressed in the stromal vascular cells of subcutaneous adipose tissues when compared to the respective adipocytes and to intraabdominal stromal vascular cells (Table 2). Differential levels of AnxA11 mRNA between the cell populations did not exist in intraabdominal adipose tissue (Table 2). Further studies are evidently required to unravel their possible functions in fat tissue.

Table 2. Expression of annexins AnxA3, A5, A7, A8, A10 and A11 mRNA in murine adipose tissues. Analysis of publicly accessible DNA microarray data (Geo Profiles; DataSet Record GDS2818) was done with unpaired Students t-test. A p-value < 0.05 was regarded as significant. ⇑, ⇓ and ⊟ indicate higher, lower and unchanged mRNA levels, respectively, in adipocytes relative to stromal vascular cells (SVC) or in subcutaneous (sc) fat compared to intraabdominal (intra) fat. The mRNA expression data for AnxA4, AnxA9 and AnxA13 in fat tissue were not available.

	Subcutaneous Fat Adipocyte/SVC	Intrabdominal Fat Adipocyte/SVC	Adipocytes Sc/Intra	SVC Sc/Intra
AnxA3	⇓	⇓	⊟	⊟
AnxA5	⇑	⇑	⊟	⇓
AnxA7	⊟	⊟	⊟	⊟
AnxA8	⇑	⇑	⇑	⇑
AnxA10	⊟	⊟	⊟	⊟
AnxA11	⇓	⊟	⊟	⇑

3. Conclusions

Annexins bind negatively charged phospholipids and cholesterol in a Ca^{2+}-dependent and reversible manner, and together with transient interactions with membrane-associated proteins, this contributes to dynamic changes in the structural and functional organization of membrane domains [23,25–31,64,93,94,109,116,118,137,157]. As outlined in this review, this membrane organizing function of annexins also seems highly relevant for adipose tissue physiology. In particular, AnxA2 has been linked to the insulin-dependent translocation of GLUT4 as well as CD36-mediated fatty acid uptake [51,57,59], the latter providing a protective function in the postprandial state. Likewise, AnxA6 affects signaling events relevant for lipid storage and, importantly, regulates adiponectin release, an essential adipokine in metabolic health [61,62,64,68,70]. Alternatively, the most prominent disease-preventing functions of AnxA1 in adiposity, glucose and lipid homeostasis are facilitated through its extracellular activity as a FPR2 ligand [34,37,39,41,42,45,104]. While functions and mechanistic insights for these three annexins in fat tissue are emerging, up until now all other annexins have been barely studied in the context of obesity, adipocyte physiology, and adipokine production. Future experiments, combining biochemical and imaging techniques in overexpression and knockdown cells and animal models, together with high-throughput and innovative technologies addressing transcriptomics, proteomics, lipidomics, and metabolomics in adipocyte-specific knock-out models may identify the impact of individual annexins in the molecular pathways that contribute to dysregulated adipokine production and fat cell function in obesity.

Author Contributions: Conceptualization, C.B., T.G., writing—review and editing, C.B., T.G., C.E., C.R.

Funding: T.G. is supported by the University of Sydney (U7113, RY253, U3367), Sydney, Australia. C.E. is supported by grants BFU2015-66785-P, Consolider-Ingenio (CSD2009-00016 and BFU2016-81912-REDC) from the Ministerio de Economía y Competitividad (Spain). C.R. is supported by the Serra Húnter Programme (Generalitat de Catalunya). C.B. is supported by the German Research Foundation (BU 1141/13-1).

Acknowledgments: We would like to thank all members of our laboratories, past and present, for their invaluable contributions and apologize to all those researchers whose work could not be discussed owing to space limitations.

Conflicts of Interest: The authors declare no conflict of interest.

References

1. Buechler, C.; Schaffler, A. Does global gene expression analysis in type 2 diabetes provide an opportunity to identify highly promising drug targets? *Endocr. Metab. Immune Disord. Drug Targets* **2007**, *7*, 250–258. [CrossRef] [PubMed]
2. Lee, M.J.; Wu, Y.; Fried, S.K. Adipose tissue heterogeneity: Implication of depot differences in adipose tissue for obesity complications. *Mol. Asp. Med.* **2013**, *34*, 1–11. [CrossRef] [PubMed]
3. Buechler, C.; Krautbauer, S.; Eisinger, K. Adipose tissue fibrosis. *World J. Diabetes* **2015**, *6*, 548–553. [CrossRef] [PubMed]
4. Ghaben, A.L.; Scherer, P.E. Adipogenesis and metabolic health. *Nat. Rev. Mol. Cell Biol.* **2019**, *20*, 242–258. [CrossRef] [PubMed]
5. Giordano, A.; Murano, I.; Mondini, E.; Perugini, J.; Smorlesi, A.; Severi, I.; Barazzoni, R.; Scherer, P.E.; Cinti, S. Obese adipocytes show ultrastructural features of stressed cells and die of pyroptosis. *J. Lipid Res.* **2013**, *54*, 2423–2436. [CrossRef] [PubMed]
6. Ye, L.; Kleiner, S.; Wu, J.; Sah, R.; Gupta, R.K.; Banks, A.S.; Cohen, P.; Khandekar, M.J.; Bostrom, P.; Mepani, R.J.; et al. Trpv4 is a regulator of adipose oxidative metabolism, inflammation, and energy homeostasis. *Cell* **2012**, *151*, 96–110. [CrossRef] [PubMed]
7. Ivanov, S.; Merlin, J.; Lee, M.K.S.; Murphy, A.J.; Guinamard, R.R. Biology and function of adipose tissue macrophages, dendritic cells and b cells. *Atherosclerosis* **2018**, *271*, 102–110. [CrossRef] [PubMed]
8. Saito, M.; Okamatsu-Ogura, Y.; Matsushita, M.; Watanabe, K.; Yoneshiro, T.; Nio-Kobayashi, J.; Iwanaga, T.; Miyagawa, M.; Kameya, T.; Nakada, K.; et al. High incidence of metabolically active brown adipose tissue in healthy adult humans: Effects of cold exposure and adiposity. *Diabetes* **2009**, *58*, 1526–1531. [CrossRef] [PubMed]

9. Van Marken Lichtenbelt, W.D.; Vanhommerig, J.W.; Smulders, N.M.; Drossaerts, J.M.; Kemerink, G.J.; Bouvy, N.D.; Schrauwen, P.; Teule, G.J. Cold-activated brown adipose tissue in healthy men. *N. Engl. J. Med.* **2009**, *360*, 1500–1508. [CrossRef]
10. Virtanen, K.A.; Lidell, M.E.; Orava, J.; Heglind, M.; Westergren, R.; Niemi, T.; Taittonen, M.; Laine, J.; Savisto, N.J.; Enerback, S.; et al. Functional brown adipose tissue in healthy adults. *N. Engl. J. Med.* **2009**, *360*, 1518–1525. [CrossRef]
11. Krautbauer, S.; Eisinger, K.; Hader, Y.; Buechler, C. Free fatty acids and il-6 induce adipocyte galectin-3 which is increased in white and brown adipose tissues of obese mice. *Cytokine* **2014**, *69*, 263–271. [CrossRef] [PubMed]
12. Srivastava, S.; Veech, R.L. Brown and brite: The fat soldiers in the anti-obesity fight. *Front. Physiol.* **2019**, *10*, 38. [CrossRef] [PubMed]
13. Bartelt, A.; Bruns, O.T.; Reimer, R.; Hohenberg, H.; Ittrich, H.; Peldschus, K.; Kaul, M.G.; Tromsdorf, U.I.; Weller, H.; Waurisch, C.; et al. Brown adipose tissue activity controls triglyceride clearance. *Nat. Med.* **2011**, *17*, 200–205. [CrossRef] [PubMed]
14. Worthmann, A.; John, C.; Ruhlemann, M.C.; Baguhl, M.; Heinsen, F.A.; Schaltenberg, N.; Heine, M.; Schlein, C.; Evangelakos, I.; Mineo, C.; et al. Cold-induced conversion of cholesterol to bile acids in mice shapes the gut microbiome and promotes adaptive thermogenesis. *Nat. Med.* **2017**, *23*, 839–849. [CrossRef] [PubMed]
15. Scheja, L.; Heeren, J. Metabolic interplay between white, beige, brown adipocytes and the liver. *J. Hepatol.* **2016**, *64*, 1176–1186. [CrossRef] [PubMed]
16. Villarroya, F.; Cereijo, R.; Villarroya, J.; Giralt, M. Brown adipose tissue as a secretory organ. *Nat. Rev. Endocrinol.* **2017**, *13*, 26–35. [CrossRef] [PubMed]
17. Villarroya, J.; Cereijo, R.; Villarroya, F. An endocrine role for brown adipose tissue? *Am. J. Physiol. Endocrinol. Metab.* **2013**, *305*, E567–E572. [CrossRef]
18. Lu, J.C.; Chiang, Y.T.; Lin, Y.C.; Chang, Y.T.; Lu, C.Y.; Chen, T.Y.; Yeh, C.S. Disruption of lipid raft function increases expression and secretion of monocyte chemoattractant protein-1 in 3t3-l1 adipocytes. *PLoS ONE* **2016**, *11*, e0169005. [CrossRef]
19. Fletcher, R.; Gribben, C.; Ma, X.; Burchfield, J.G.; Thomas, K.C.; Krycer, J.R.; James, D.E.; Fazakerley, D.J. The role of the niemann-pick disease, type c1 protein in adipocyte insulin action. *PLoS ONE* **2014**, *9*, e95598. [CrossRef]
20. Xie, L.; O'Reilly, C.P.; Chapes, S.K.; Mora, S. Adiponectin and leptin are secreted through distinct trafficking pathways in adipocytes. *Biochim. Biophys. Acta* **2008**, *1782*, 99–108. [CrossRef]
21. Buechler, C.; Wanninger, J.; Neumeier, M. Adiponectin, a key adipokine in obesity related liver diseases. *World J. Gastroenterol.* **2011**, *17*, 2801–2811. [PubMed]
22. Cohen, P.; Spiegelman, B.M. Cell biology of fat storage. *Mol. Biol. Cell* **2016**, *27*, 2523–2527. [CrossRef] [PubMed]
23. Gerke, V.; Creutz, C.E.; Moss, S.E. Annexins: Linking Ca^{2+} signalling to membrane dynamics. *Nat. Rev. Mol. Cell Biol.* **2005**, *6*, 449–461. [CrossRef] [PubMed]
24. Moss, S.E.; Morgan, R.O. The annexins. *Genome Biol.* **2004**, *5*, 219. [CrossRef] [PubMed]
25. Gerke, V.; Moss, S.E. Annexins: From structure to function. *Physiol. Rev.* **2002**, *82*, 331–371. [CrossRef] [PubMed]
26. Grewal, T.; Enrich, C. Annexins—Modulators of egf receptor signalling and trafficking. *Cell. Signal.* **2009**, *21*, 847–858. [CrossRef] [PubMed]
27. Grewal, T.; Wason, S.J.; Enrich, C.; Rentero, C. Annexins—Insights from knockout mice. *Biol. Chem.* **2016**, *397*, 1031–1053. [CrossRef]
28. Hayes, M.J.; Rescher, U.; Gerke, V.; Moss, S.E. Annexin-actin interactions. *Traffic* **2004**, *5*, 571–576. [CrossRef] [PubMed]
29. Hoque, M.; Rentero, C.; Cairns, R.; Tebar, F.; Enrich, C.; Grewal, T. Annexins—Scaffolds modulating pkc localization and signaling. *Cell. Signal.* **2014**, *26*, 1213–1225. [CrossRef]
30. Monastyrskaya, K.; Babiychuk, E.B.; Hostettler, A.; Rescher, U.; Draeger, A. Annexins as intracellular calcium sensors. *Cell Calcium* **2007**, *41*, 207–219. [CrossRef]
31. Rentero, C.; Blanco-Munoz, P.; Meneses-Salas, E.; Grewal, T.; Enrich, C. Annexins—Coordinators of cholesterol homeostasis in endocytic pathways. *Int. J. Mol. Sci.* **2018**, *19*, 1444. [CrossRef] [PubMed]

32. Fernandez-Lizarbe, S.; Lecona, E.; Santiago-Gomez, A.; Olmo, N.; Lizarbe, M.A.; Turnay, J. Structural and lipid-binding characterization of human annexin a13a reveals strong differences with its long a13b isoform. *Biol. Chem.* **2017**, *398*, 359–371. [CrossRef] [PubMed]
33. Ahmed, M.; Neville, M.J.; Edelmann, M.J.; Kessler, B.M.; Karpe, F. Proteomic analysis of human adipose tissue after rosiglitazone treatment shows coordinated changes to promote glucose uptake. *Obesity* **2010**, *18*, 27–34. [CrossRef] [PubMed]
34. Akasheh, R.T.; Pini, M.; Pang, J.; Fantuzzi, G. Increased adiposity in annexin a1-deficient mice. *PLoS ONE* **2013**, *8*, e82608. [CrossRef] [PubMed]
35. Alfadda, A.A.; Benabdelkamel, H.; Masood, A.; Moustafa, A.; Sallam, R.; Bassas, A.; Duncan, M. Proteomic analysis of mature adipocytes from obese patients in relation to aging. *Exp. Gerontol.* **2013**, *48*, 1196–1203. [CrossRef] [PubMed]
36. Chen, X.; Zhuo, S.; Zhu, T.; Yao, P.; Yang, M.; Mei, H.; Li, N.; Ma, F.; Wang, J.M.; Chen, S.; et al. Fpr2 deficiency alleviates diet-induced insulin resistance through reducing body weight gain and inhibiting inflammation mediated by macrophage chemotaxis and m1 polarization. *Diabetes* **2019**, *68*, 1130–1142. [CrossRef] [PubMed]
37. Fredman, G.; Kamaly, N.; Spolitu, S.; Milton, J.; Ghorpade, D.; Chiasson, R.; Kuriakose, G.; Perretti, M.; Farokhzad, O.; Tabas, I. Targeted nanoparticles containing the proresolving peptide ac2-26 protect against advanced atherosclerosis in hypercholesterolemic mice. *Sci. Transl. Med.* **2015**, *7*, 275ra220. [CrossRef] [PubMed]
38. Kosicka, A.; Cunliffe, A.D.; Mackenzie, R.; Zariwala, M.G.; Perretti, M.; Flower, R.J.; Renshaw, D. Attenuation of plasma annexin a1 in human obesity. *FASEB J.* **2013**, *27*, 368–378. [CrossRef] [PubMed]
39. Perretti, M.; D'Acquisto, F. Annexin a1 and glucocorticoids as effectors of the resolution of inflammation. *Nat. Rev. Immunol.* **2009**, *9*, 62–70. [CrossRef]
40. Pietrani, N.T.; Ferreira, C.N.; Rodrigues, K.F.; Perucci, L.O.; Carneiro, F.S.; Bosco, A.A.; Oliveira, M.C.; Pereira, S.S.; Teixeira, A.L.; Alvarez-Leite, J.I.; et al. Proresolving protein annexin a1: The role in type 2 diabetes mellitus and obesity. *Biomed. Pharmacother. Biomed. Pharmacother.* **2018**, *103*, 482–489. [CrossRef]
41. Purvis, G.S.D.; Collino, M.; Loiola, R.A.; Baragetti, A.; Chiazza, F.; Brovelli, M.; Sheikh, M.H.; Collotta, D.; Cento, A.; Mastrocola, R.; et al. Identification of annexina1 as an endogenous regulator of rhoa, and its role in the pathophysiology and experimental therapy of type-2 diabetes. *Front. Immunol.* **2019**, *10*, 571. [CrossRef] [PubMed]
42. Soehnlein, O. (Re)solving atherosclerosis. *Sci. Transl. Med.* **2015**, *7*, 275fs7. [CrossRef] [PubMed]
43. Warne, J.P.; John, C.D.; Christian, H.C.; Morris, J.F.; Flower, R.J.; Sugden, D.; Solito, E.; Gillies, G.E.; Buckingham, J.C. Gene deletion reveals roles for annexin a1 in the regulation of lipolysis and il-6 release in epididymal adipose tissue. *Am. J. Physiol. Endocrinol. Metab.* **2006**, *291*, E1264–E1273. [CrossRef] [PubMed]
44. Wong, W.T.; Nick, H.S.; Frost, S.C. Regulation of annexin i in adipogenesis: Camp-independent action of methylisobutylxanthine. *Am. J. Physiol.* **1992**, *262*, C91–C97. [CrossRef] [PubMed]
45. Yoon, J.H.; Kim, D.; Jang, J.H.; Ghim, J.; Park, S.; Song, P.; Kwon, Y.; Kim, J.; Hwang, D.; Bae, Y.S.; et al. Proteomic analysis of the palmitate-induced myotube secretome reveals involvement of the annexin a1-formyl peptide receptor 2 (fpr2) pathway in insulin resistance. *Mol. Cell. Proteom. MCP* **2015**, *14*, 882–892. [CrossRef] [PubMed]
46. Biener, Y.; Feinstein, R.; Mayak, M.; Kaburagi, Y.; Kadowaki, T.; Zick, Y. Annexin ii is a novel player in insulin signal transduction. Possible association between annexin ii phosphorylation and insulin receptor internalization. *J. Biol. Chem.* **1996**, *271*, 29489–29496. [CrossRef] [PubMed]
47. Bluher, M.; Wilson-Fritch, L.; Leszyk, J.; Laustsen, P.G.; Corvera, S.; Kahn, C.R. Role of insulin action and cell size on protein expression patterns in adipocytes. *J. Biol. Chem.* **2004**, *279*, 31902–31909. [CrossRef]
48. Bouwman, F.G.; Claessens, M.; van Baak, M.A.; Noben, J.P.; Wang, P.; Saris, W.H.; Mariman, E.C. The physiologic effects of caloric restriction are reflected in the in vivo adipocyte-enriched proteome of overweight/obese subjects. *J. Proteome Res.* **2009**, *8*, 5532–5540. [CrossRef]
49. Bouwman, F.G.; Wang, P.; van Baak, M.; Saris, W.H.; Mariman, E.C. Increased beta-oxidation with improved glucose uptake capacity in adipose tissue from obese after weight loss and maintenance. *Obesity* **2014**, *22*, 819–827. [CrossRef]
50. Caron, D.; Boutchueng-Djidjou, M.; Tanguay, R.M.; Faure, R.L. Annexin a2 is sumoylated on its n-terminal domain: Regulation by insulin. *FEBS Lett.* **2015**, *589*, 985–991. [CrossRef]

51. Huang, J.; Hsia, S.H.; Imamura, T.; Usui, I.; Olefsky, J.M. Annexin ii is a thiazolidinedione-responsive gene involved in insulin-induced glucose transporter isoform 4 translocation in 3t3-l1 adipocytes. *Endocrinology* **2004**, *145*, 1579–1586. [CrossRef] [PubMed]
52. Jimenez-Gomez, Y.; Cruz-Teno, C.; Rangel-Zuniga, O.A.; Peinado, J.R.; Perez-Martinez, P.; Delgado-Lista, J.; Garcia-Rios, A.; Camargo, A.; Vazquez-Martinez, R.; Ortega-Bellido, M.; et al. Effect of dietary fat modification on subcutaneous white adipose tissue insulin sensitivity in patients with metabolic syndrome. *Mol. Nutr. Food Res.* **2014**, *58*, 2177–2188. [CrossRef] [PubMed]
53. Leggate, M.; Carter, W.G.; Evans, M.J.; Vennard, R.A.; Sribala-Sundaram, S.; Nimmo, M.A. Determination of inflammatory and prominent proteomic changes in plasma and adipose tissue after high-intensity intermittent training in overweight and obese males. *J. Appl. Physiol.* **2012**, *112*, 1353–1360. [CrossRef] [PubMed]
54. Pal, P.; Kanaujiya, J.K.; Lochab, S.; Tripathi, S.B.; Sanyal, S.; Behre, G.; Trivedi, A.K. Proteomic analysis of rosiglitazone and guggulsterone treated 3t3-l1 preadipocytes. *Mol. Cell. Biochem.* **2013**, *376*, 81–93. [CrossRef] [PubMed]
55. Raynal, P.; Pollard, H.B.; Cushman, S.W.; Guerre-Millo, M. Unique subcellular distribution of five annexins in resting and insulin-stimulated rat adipose cells. *Biochem. Biophys. Res. Commun.* **1996**, *225*, 116–121. [CrossRef]
56. Rescher, U.; Ludwig, C.; Konietzko, V.; Kharitonenkov, A.; Gerke, V. Tyrosine phosphorylation of annexin a2 regulates rho-mediated actin rearrangement and cell adhesion. *J. Cell Sci.* **2008**, *121*, 2177–2185. [CrossRef]
57. Salameh, A.; Daquinag, A.C.; Staquicini, D.I.; An, Z.; Hajjar, K.A.; Pasqualini, R.; Arap, W.; Kolonin, M.G. Prohibitin/annexin 2 interaction regulates fatty acid transport in adipose tissue. *JCI Insight* **2016**, *1*. [CrossRef]
58. Song, Y.B.; An, Y.R.; Kim, S.J.; Park, H.W.; Jung, J.W.; Kyung, J.S.; Hwang, S.Y.; Kim, Y.S. Lipid metabolic effect of korean red ginseng extract in mice fed on a high-fat diet. *J. Sci. Food Agric.* **2012**, *92*, 388–396. [CrossRef]
59. Wang, Y.; Cheng, Y.S.; Yin, X.Q.; Yu, G.; Jia, B.L. Anxa2 gene silencing attenuates obesity-induced insulin resistance by suppressing the nf-kappab signaling pathway. *Am. J. Physiol. Cell Physiol.* **2019**, *316*, C223–C234. [CrossRef]
60. Zhao, W.Q.; Chen, G.H.; Chen, H.; Pascale, A.; Ravindranath, L.; Quon, M.J.; Alkon, D.L. Secretion of annexin ii via activation of insulin receptor and insulin-like growth factor receptor. *J. Biol. Chem.* **2003**, *278*, 4205–4215. [CrossRef]
61. Cairns, R.; Alvarez-Guaita, A.; Martinez-Saludes, I.; Wason, S.J.; Hanh, J.; Nagarajan, S.R.; Hosseini-Beheshti, E.; Monastyrskaya, K.; Hoy, A.J.; Buechler, C.; et al. Role of hepatic annexin a6 in fatty acid-induced lipid droplet formation. *Exp. Cell Res.* **2017**, *358*, 397–410. [CrossRef] [PubMed]
62. Cairns, R.; Fischer, A.W.; Blanco-Munoz, P.; Alvarez-Guaita, A.; Meneses-Salas, E.; Egert, A.; Buechler, C.; Hoy, A.J.; Heeren, J.; Enrich, C.; et al. Altered hepatic glucose homeostasis in anxa6-ko mice fed a high-fat diet. *PLoS ONE* **2018**, *13*, e0201310. [CrossRef] [PubMed]
63. Cubells, L.; Vila de Muga, S.; Tebar, F.; Wood, P.; Evans, R.; Ingelmo-Torres, M.; Calvo, M.; Gaus, K.; Pol, A.; Grewal, T.; et al. Annexin a6-induced alterations in cholesterol transport and caveolin export from the golgi complex. *Traffic* **2007**, *8*, 1568–1589. [CrossRef] [PubMed]
64. Enrich, C.; Rentero, C.; de Muga, S.V.; Reverter, M.; Mulay, V.; Wood, P.; Koese, M.; Grewal, T. Annexin a6-linking Ca^{2+} signaling with cholesterol transport. *Biochim. Biophys. Acta* **2011**, *1813*, 935–947. [CrossRef] [PubMed]
65. Enrich, C.; Rentero, C.; Grewal, T. Annexin a6 in the liver: From the endocytic compartment to cellular physiology. *Biochim. Biophys. Acta. Mol. Cell Res.* **2017**, *1864*, 933–946. [CrossRef] [PubMed]
66. Grewal, T.; Evans, R.; Rentero, C.; Tebar, F.; Cubells, L.; de Diego, I.; Kirchhoff, M.F.; Hughes, W.E.; Heeren, J.; Rye, K.A.; et al. Annexin a6 stimulates the membrane recruitment of p120gap to modulate ras and raf-1 activity. *Oncogene* **2005**, *24*, 5809–5820. [CrossRef]
67. Jones, P.G.; Fitzpatrick, S.; Waisman, D.M. Chromaffin granules release calcium on contact with annexin vi: Implications for exocytosis. *Biochemistry* **1994**, *33*, 8180–8187. [CrossRef] [PubMed]
68. Krautbauer, S.; Haberl, E.M.; Eisinger, K.; Pohl, R.; Rein-Fischboeck, L.; Rentero, C.; Alvarez-Guaita, A.; Enrich, C.; Grewal, T.; Buechler, C.; et al. Annexin a6 regulates adipocyte lipid storage and adiponectin release. *Mol. Cell. Endocrinol.* **2017**, *439*, 419–430. [CrossRef]

69. Meier, E.M.; Rein-Fischboeck, L.; Pohl, R.; Wanninger, J.; Hoy, A.J.; Grewal, T.; Eisinger, K.; Krautbauer, S.; Liebisch, G.; Weiss, T.S.; et al. Annexin a6 protein is downregulated in human hepatocellular carcinoma. *Mol. Cell. Biochem.* **2016**, *418*, 81–90. [CrossRef]
70. Monastyrskaya, K.; Babiychuk, E.B.; Hostettler, A.; Wood, P.; Grewal, T.; Draeger, A. Plasma membrane-associated annexin a6 reduces Ca^{2+} entry by stabilizing the cortical actin cytoskeleton. *J. Biol. Chem.* **2009**, *284*, 17227–17242. [CrossRef]
71. Podszywalow-Bartnicka, P.; Kosiorek, M.; Piwocka, K.; Sikora, E.; Zablocki, K.; Pikula, S. Role of annexin a6 isoforms in catecholamine secretion by pc12 cells: Distinct influence on calcium response. *J. Cell. Biochem.* **2010**, *111*, 168–178. [CrossRef] [PubMed]
72. Reverter, M.; Rentero, C.; de Muga, S.V.; Alvarez-Guaita, A.; Mulay, V.; Cairns, R.; Wood, P.; Monastyrskaya, K.; Pol, A.; Tebar, F.; et al. Cholesterol transport from late endosomes to the golgi regulates t-snare trafficking, assembly, and function. *Mol. Biol. Cell* **2011**, *22*, 4108–4123. [CrossRef] [PubMed]
73. Reverter, M.; Rentero, C.; Garcia-Melero, A.; Hoque, M.; Vila de Muga, S.; Alvarez-Guaita, A.; Conway, J.R.; Wood, P.; Cairns, R.; Lykopoulou, L.; et al. Cholesterol regulates syntaxin 6 trafficking at trans-golgi network endosomal boundaries. *Cell Rep.* **2014**, *7*, 883–897. [CrossRef] [PubMed]
74. Stogbauer, F.; Weigert, J.; Neumeier, M.; Wanninger, J.; Sporrer, D.; Weber, M.; Schaffler, A.; Enrich, C.; Wood, P.; Grewal, T.; et al. Annexin a6 is highly abundant in monocytes of obese and type 2 diabetic individuals and is downregulated by adiponectin in vitro. *Exp. Mol. Med.* **2009**, *41*, 501–507. [CrossRef] [PubMed]
75. Gesta, S.; Bluher, M.; Yamamoto, Y.; Norris, A.W.; Berndt, J.; Kralisch, S.; Boucher, J.; Lewis, C.; Kahn, C.R. Evidence for a role of developmental genes in the origin of obesity and body fat distribution. *Proc. Natl. Acad. Sci. USA* **2006**, *103*, 6676–6681. [CrossRef] [PubMed]
76. Rosch, K.; Kwiatkowski, M.; Hofmann, S.; Schobel, A.; Gruttner, C.; Wurlitzer, M.; Schluter, H.; Herker, E. Quantitative lipid droplet proteome analysis identifies annexin a3 as a cofactor for hcv particle production. *Cell Rep.* **2016**, *16*, 3219–3231. [CrossRef] [PubMed]
77. Watanabe, T.; Ito, Y.; Sato, A.; Hosono, T.; Niimi, S.; Ariga, T.; Seki, T. Annexin a3 as a negative regulator of adipocyte differentiation. *J. Biochem.* **2012**, *152*, 355–363. [CrossRef] [PubMed]
78. Seok, H.; Park, H.J.; Lee, B.W.; Kim, J.W.; Jung, M.; Lee, S.R.; Park, K.H.; Park, Y.G.; Baik, H.H.; Chung, J.H. Association of annexin a5 polymorphisms with obesity. *Biomed. Rep.* **2013**, *1*, 654–658. [CrossRef] [PubMed]
79. Herr, C.; Smyth, N.; Ullrich, S.; Yun, F.; Sasse, P.; Hescheler, J.; Fleischmann, B.; Lasek, K.; Brixius, K.; Schwinger, R.H.; et al. Loss of annexin a7 leads to alterations in frequency-induced shortening of isolated murine cardiomyocytes. *Mol. Cell. Biol.* **2001**, *21*, 4119–4128. [CrossRef] [PubMed]
80. Lang, E.; Lang, P.A.; Shumilina, E.; Qadri, S.M.; Kucherenko, Y.; Kempe, D.S.; Foller, M.; Capasso, A.; Wieder, T.; Gulbins, E.; et al. Enhanced eryptosis of erythrocytes from gene-targeted mice lacking annexin a7. *Pflug. Arch. Eur. J. Physiol.* **2010**, *460*, 667–676. [CrossRef]
81. Luo, D.; Fajol, A.; Umbach, A.T.; Noegel, A.A.; Laufer, S.; Lang, F.; Foller, M. Influence of annexin a7 on insulin sensitivity of cellular glucose uptake. *Pflug. Arch. Eur. J. Physiol.* **2015**, *467*, 641–649. [CrossRef] [PubMed]
82. Mears, D.; Zimliki, C.L.; Atwater, I.; Rojas, E.; Glassman, M.; Leighton, X.; Pollard, H.B.; Srivastava, M. The anx7(+/−) knockout mutation alters electrical and secretory responses to Ca^{2+}-mobilizing agents in pancreatic beta-cells. *Cell. Physiol. Biochem. Int. J. Exp. Cell. Physiol. Biochem. Pharmacol.* **2012**, *29*, 697–704. [CrossRef] [PubMed]
83. Srivastava, M.; Atwater, I.; Glasman, M.; Leighton, X.; Goping, G.; Caohuy, H.; Miller, G.; Pichel, J.; Westphal, H.; Mears, D.; et al. Defects in inositol 1,4,5-trisphosphate receptor expression, Ca^{2+} signaling, and insulin secretion in the anx7(+/−) knockout mouse. *Proc. Natl. Acad. Sci. USA* **1999**, *96*, 13783–13788. [CrossRef] [PubMed]
84. Goebeler, V.; Poeter, M.; Zeuschner, D.; Gerke, V.; Rescher, U. Annexin a8 regulates late endosome organization and function. *Mol. Biol. Cell* **2008**, *19*, 5267–5278. [CrossRef] [PubMed]
85. Goebeler, V.; Ruhe, D.; Gerke, V.; Rescher, U. Annexin a8 displays unique phospholipid and f-actin binding properties. *FEBS Lett.* **2006**, *580*, 2430–2434. [CrossRef] [PubMed]
86. Heitzig, N.; Brinkmann, B.F.; Koerdt, S.N.; Rosso, G.; Shahin, V.; Rescher, U. Annexin a8 promotes vegf-a driven endothelial cell sprouting. *Cell Adhes. Migr.* **2017**, *11*, 275–287. [CrossRef]

87. Heitzig, N.; Kuhnl, A.; Grill, D.; Ludewig, K.; Schloer, S.; Galla, H.J.; Grewal, T.; Gerke, V.; Rescher, U. Cooperative binding promotes demand-driven recruitment of anxa8 to cholesterol-containing membranes. *Biochim. Biophys. Acta. Mol. Cell Biol. Lipids* **2018**, *1863*, 349–358. [CrossRef] [PubMed]
88. Linder, K.; Arner, P.; Flores-Morales, A.; Tollet-Egnell, P.; Norstedt, G. Differentially expressed genes in visceral or subcutaneous adipose tissue of obese men and women. *J. Lipid Res.* **2004**, *45*, 148–154. [CrossRef]
89. Poeter, M.; Brandherm, I.; Rossaint, J.; Rosso, G.; Shahin, V.; Skryabin, B.V.; Zarbock, A.; Gerke, V.; Rescher, U. Annexin a8 controls leukocyte recruitment to activated endothelial cells via cell surface delivery of cd63. *Nat. Commun.* **2014**, *5*, 3738. [CrossRef]
90. Heinick, A.; Husser, X.; Himmler, K.; Kirchhefer, U.; Nunes, F.; Schulte, J.S.; Seidl, M.D.; Rolfes, C.; Dedman, J.R.; Kaetzel, M.A.; et al. Annexin a4 is a novel direct regulator of adenylyl cyclase type 5. *FASEB J.* **2015**, *29*, 3773–3787. [CrossRef]
91. Wang, J.; Guo, C.; Liu, S.; Qi, H.; Yin, Y.; Liang, R.; Sun, M.Z.; Greenaway, F.T. Annexin a11 in disease. *Clin. Chim. Acta Int. J. Clin. Chem.* **2014**, *431*, 164–168. [CrossRef] [PubMed]
92. D'Acunto, C.W.; Gbelcova, H.; Festa, M.; Ruml, T. The complex understanding of annexin a1 phosphorylation. *Cell. Signal.* **2014**, *26*, 173–178. [CrossRef] [PubMed]
93. Hayes, M.J.; Moss, S.E. Annexins and disease. *Biochem. Biophys. Res. Commun.* **2004**, *322*, 1166–1170. [CrossRef]
94. Rescher, U.; Gerke, V. Annexins—Unique membrane binding proteins with diverse functions. *J. Cell Sci.* **2004**, *117*, 2631–2639. [CrossRef] [PubMed]
95. Claria, J.; Dalli, J.; Yacoubian, S.; Gao, F.; Serhan, C.N. Resolvin d1 and resolvin d2 govern local inflammatory tone in obese fat. *J. Immunol.* **2012**, *189*, 2597–2605. [CrossRef] [PubMed]
96. Buechler, C.; Pohl, R.; Aslanidis, C. Pro-resolving molecules-new approaches to treat sepsis? *Int. J. Mol. Sci.* **2017**, *18*, 476. [CrossRef] [PubMed]
97. Claria, J.; Nguyen, B.T.; Madenci, A.L.; Ozaki, C.K.; Serhan, C.N. Diversity of lipid mediators in human adipose tissue depots. *Am. J. Physiol. Cell Physiol.* **2013**, *304*, C1141–C1149. [CrossRef] [PubMed]
98. Veugelers, M.; Cat, B.D.; Muyldermans, S.Y.; Reekmans, G.; Delande, N.; Frints, S.; Legius, E.; Fryns, J.P.; Schrander-Stumpel, C.; Weidle, B.; et al. Mutational analysis of the gpc3/gpc4 glypican gene cluster on xq26 in patients with simpson-golabi-behmel syndrome: Identification of loss-of-function mutations in the gpc3 gene. *Hum. Mol. Genet.* **2000**, *9*, 1321–1328. [CrossRef]
99. Debril, M.B.; Renaud, J.P.; Fajas, L.; Auwerx, J. The pleiotropic functions of peroxisome proliferator-activated receptor gamma. *J. Mol. Med.* **2001**, *79*, 30–47. [CrossRef]
100. Chen, L.; Yuan, Y.; Kar, S.; Kanchi, M.M.; Arora, S.; Kim, J.E.; Koh, P.F.; Yousef, E.; Samy, R.P.; Shanmugam, M.K.; et al. Ppargamma ligand-induced annexin a1 expression determines chemotherapy response via deubiquitination of death domain kinase rip in triple-negative breast cancers. *Mol. Cancer Ther.* **2017**, *16*, 2528–2542. [CrossRef]
101. Sawmynaden, P.; Perretti, M. Glucocorticoid upregulation of the annexin-a1 receptor in leukocytes. *Biochem. Biophys. Res. Commun.* **2006**, *349*, 1351–1355. [CrossRef] [PubMed]
102. Aguilera, C.M.; Gomez-Llorente, C.; Tofe, I.; Gil-Campos, M.; Canete, R.; Gil, A. Genome-wide expression in visceral adipose tissue from obese prepubertal children. *Int. J. Mol. Sci.* **2015**, *16*, 7723–7737. [CrossRef] [PubMed]
103. Vong, L.; D'Acquisto, F.; Pederzoli-Ribeil, M.; Lavagno, L.; Flower, R.J.; Witko-Sarsat, V.; Perretti, M. Annexin 1 cleavage in activated neutrophils: A pivotal role for proteinase 3. *J. Biol. Chem.* **2007**, *282*, 29998–30004. [CrossRef] [PubMed]
104. Locatelli, I.; Sutti, S.; Jindal, A.; Vacchiano, M.; Bozzola, C.; Reutelingsperger, C.; Kusters, D.; Bena, S.; Parola, M.; Paternostro, C.; et al. Endogenous annexin a1 is a novel protective determinant in nonalcoholic steatohepatitis in mice. *Hepatology* **2014**, *60*, 531–544. [CrossRef]
105. Hiramoto, H.; Dansako, H.; Takeda, M.; Satoh, S.; Wakita, T.; Ikeda, M.; Kato, N. Annexin a1 negatively regulates viral rna replication of hepatitis c virus. *Acta Med. Okayama* **2015**, *69*, 71–78. [PubMed]
106. Mauvais-Jarvis, F.; Kulkarni, R.N.; Kahn, C.R. Knockout models are useful tools to dissect the pathophysiology and genetics of insulin resistance. *Clin. Endocrinol.* **2002**, *57*, 1–9. [CrossRef]
107. Feng, R.; Luo, C.; Li, C.; Du, S.; Okekunle, A.P.; Li, Y.; Chen, Y.; Zi, T.; Niu, Y. Free fatty acids profile among lean, overweight and obese non-alcoholic fatty liver disease patients: A case-control study. *Lipids Health Disease* **2017**, *16*, 165. [CrossRef]

108. Arzouni, A.A.; Vargas-Seymour, A.; Rackham, C.L.; Dhadda, P.; Huang, G.C.; Choudhary, P.; Nardi, N.; King, A.J.F.; Jones, P.M. Mesenchymal stromal cells improve human islet function through released products and extracellular matrix. *Clin. Sci.* **2017**, *131*, 2835–2845. [CrossRef]
109. Bharadwaj, A.; Bydoun, M.; Holloway, R.; Waisman, D. Annexin a2 heterotetramer: Structure and function. *Int. J. Mol. Sci.* **2013**, *14*, 6259–6305. [CrossRef]
110. Hedhli, N.; Falcone, D.J.; Huang, B.; Cesarman-Maus, G.; Kraemer, R.; Zhai, H.; Tsirka, S.E.; Santambrogio, L.; Hajjar, K.A. The annexin a2/s100a10 system in health and disease: Emerging paradigms. *J. Biomed. Biotechnol.* **2012**, *2012*, 406273. [CrossRef]
111. Bydoun, M.; Waisman, D.M. On the contribution of s100a10 and annexin a2 to plasminogen activation and oncogenesis: An enduring ambiguity. *Future Oncol.* **2014**, *10*, 2469–2479. [CrossRef] [PubMed]
112. Luo, M.; Hajjar, K.A. Annexin a2 system in human biology: Cell surface and beyond. *Semin. Thromb. Hemost.* **2013**, *39*, 338–346. [CrossRef] [PubMed]
113. Wang, J.; Hao, J.W.; Wang, X.; Guo, H.; Sun, H.H.; Lai, X.Y.; Liu, L.Y.; Zhu, M.; Wang, H.Y.; Li, Y.F.; et al. Dhhc4 and dhhc5 facilitate fatty acid uptake by palmitoylating and targeting cd36 to the plasma membrane. *Cell Rep.* **2019**, *26*, 209–221. [CrossRef] [PubMed]
114. Pons, M.; Ihrke, G.; Koch, S.; Biermer, M.; Pol, A.; Grewal, T.; Jackle, S.; Enrich, C. Late endocytic compartments are major sites of annexin vi localization in nrk fibroblasts and polarized wif-b hepatoma cells. *Exp. Cell Res.* **2000**, *257*, 33–47. [CrossRef] [PubMed]
115. de Diego, I.; Schwartz, F.; Siegfried, H.; Dauterstedt, P.; Heeren, J.; Beisiegel, U.; Enrich, C.; Grewal, T. Cholesterol modulates the membrane binding and intracellular distribution of annexin 6. *J. Biol. Chem.* **2002**, *277*, 32187–32194. [CrossRef] [PubMed]
116. Futter, C.E.; White, I.J. Annexins and endocytosis. *Traffic* **2007**, *8*, 951–958. [CrossRef] [PubMed]
117. Grewal, T.; Heeren, J.; Mewawala, D.; Schnitgerhans, T.; Wendt, D.; Salomon, G.; Enrich, C.; Beisiegel, U.; Jackle, S. Annexin vi stimulates endocytosis and is involved in the trafficking of low density lipoprotein to the prelysosomal compartment. *J. Biol. Chem.* **2000**, *275*, 33806–33813. [CrossRef]
118. Skrahina, T.; Piljic, A.; Schultz, C. Heterogeneity and timing of translocation and membrane-mediated assembly of different annexins. *Exp. Cell Res.* **2008**, *314*, 1039–1047. [CrossRef]
119. Freye-Minks, C.; Kretsinger, R.H.; Creutz, C.E. Structural and dynamic changes in human annexin vi induced by a phosphorylation-mimicking mutation, t356d. *Biochemistry* **2003**, *42*, 620–630. [CrossRef]
120. Chlystun, M.; Campanella, M.; Law, A.L.; Duchen, M.R.; Fatimathas, L.; Levine, T.P.; Gerke, V.; Moss, S.E. Regulation of mitochondrial morphogenesis by annexin a6. *PLoS ONE* **2013**, *8*, e53774. [CrossRef]
121. Turro, S.; Ingelmo-Torres, M.; Estanyol, J.M.; Tebar, F.; Fernandez, M.A.; Albor, C.V.; Gaus, K.; Grewal, T.; Enrich, C.; Pol, A. Identification and characterization of associated with lipid droplet protein 1: A novel membrane-associated protein that resides on hepatic lipid droplets. *Traffic* **2006**, *7*, 1254–1269. [CrossRef] [PubMed]
122. Murphy, S.; Martin, S.; Parton, R.G. Lipid droplet-organelle interactions; sharing the fats. *Biochim. Biophys. Acta* **2009**, *1791*, 441–447. [CrossRef] [PubMed]
123. Pani, B.; Singh, B.B. Lipid rafts/caveolae as microdomains of calcium signaling. *Cell Calcium* **2009**, *45*, 625–633. [CrossRef] [PubMed]
124. Kioumourtzoglou, D.; Sadler, J.B.; Black, H.L.; Berends, R.; Wellburn, C.; Bryant, N.J.; Gould, G.W. Studies of the regulated assembly of snare complexes in adipocytes. *Biochem. Soc. Trans.* **2014**, *42*, 1396–1400. [CrossRef] [PubMed]
125. Wu, J.; Cheng, D.; Liu, L.; Lv, Z.; Liu, K. Tbc1d15 affects glucose uptake by regulating glut4 translocation. *Gene* **2019**, *683*, 210–215. [CrossRef] [PubMed]
126. Komai, A.M.; Brannmark, C.; Musovic, S.; Olofsson, C.S. Pka-independent camp stimulation of white adipocyte exocytosis and adipokine secretion: Modulations by Ca^{2+} and atp. *J. Physiol.* **2014**, *592*, 5169–5186. [CrossRef] [PubMed]
127. Kandror, K.V.; Pilch, P.F. The sugar is sirved: Sorting glut4 and its fellow travelers. *Traffic* **2011**, *12*, 665–671. [CrossRef] [PubMed]
128. Fernandez, C.; Lindholm, M.; Krogh, M.; Lucas, S.; Larsson, S.; Osmark, P.; Berger, K.; Boren, J.; Fielding, B.; Frayn, K.; et al. Disturbed cholesterol homeostasis in hormone-sensitive lipase-null mice. *Am. J. Physiol. Endocrinol. Metab.* **2008**, *295*, E820–E831. [CrossRef]

129. Rentero Alfonso, C.; Alvarez-Guaita, A.; Moss, S.E.; Grewal, T.; Enrich, C. Annexin a6 is necessary for liver regeneration and glucose homeostasis in 433 mice. *Hepatology* **2015**, *62*, 239A.
130. Matsuda, M.; Shimomura, I. Roles of adiponectin and oxidative stress in obesity-associated metabolic and cardiovascular diseases. *Rev. Endocr. Metab. Disord.* **2014**, *15*, 1–10. [CrossRef]
131. Alvarez-Guaita, A.; Vila de Muga, S.; Owen, D.M.; Williamson, D.; Magenau, A.; Garcia-Melero, A.; Reverter, M.; Hoque, M.; Cairns, R.; Cornely, R.; et al. Evidence for annexin a6-dependent plasma membrane remodelling of lipid domains. *Br. J. Pharmacol.* **2015**, *172*, 1677–1690. [CrossRef] [PubMed]
132. von Eckardstein, A. Cholesterol efflux from macrophages and other cells. *Curr. Opin. Lipidol.* **1996**, *7*, 308–319. [CrossRef] [PubMed]
133. Sargolzaei, J.; Chamani, E.; Kazemi, T.; Fallah, S.; Soori, H. The role of adiponectin and adipolin as anti-inflammatory adipokines in the formation of macrophage foam cells and their association with cardiovascular diseases. *Clin. Biochem.* **2018**, *54*, 1–10. [CrossRef] [PubMed]
134. Schosserer, M.; Grillari, J.; Wolfrum, C.; Scheideler, M. Age-induced changes in white, brite, and brown adipose depots: A mini-review. *Gerontology* **2018**, *64*, 229–236. [CrossRef] [PubMed]
135. Wu, N.; Liu, S.; Guo, C.; Hou, Z.; Sun, M.Z. The role of annexin a3 playing in cancers. *Clin. Transl. Oncol.* **2013**, *15*, 106–110. [CrossRef]
136. Lasrich, D.; Bartelt, A.; Grewal, T.; Heeren, J. Apolipoprotein e promotes lipid accumulation and differentiation in human adipocytes. *Exp. Cell Res.* **2015**, *337*, 94–102. [CrossRef]
137. Boersma, H.H.; Kietselaer, B.L.; Stolk, L.M.; Bennaghmouch, A.; Hofstra, L.; Narula, J.; Heidendal, G.A.; Reutelingsperger, C.P. Past, present, and future of annexin a5: From protein discovery to clinical applications. *J. Nucl. Med.* **2005**, *46*, 2035–2050.
138. Peng, B.; Guo, C.; Guan, H.; Liu, S.; Sun, M.Z. Annexin a5 as a potential marker in tumors. *Chim. Acta Int. J. Clin. Chem.* **2014**, *427*, 42–48. [CrossRef]
139. Dubois, T.; Mira, J.P.; Feliers, D.; Solito, E.; Russo-Marie, F.; Oudinet, J.P. Annexin v inhibits protein kinase c activity via a mechanism of phospholipid sequestration. *Biochem. J.* **1998**, *330*, 1277–1282. [CrossRef]
140. Ghislat, G.; Aguado, C.; Knecht, E. Annexin a5 stimulates autophagy and inhibits endocytosis. *J. Cell Sci.* **2012**, *125*, 92–107. [CrossRef]
141. Bouter, A.; Gounou, C.; Berat, R.; Tan, S.; Gallois, B.; Granier, T.; d'Estaintot, B.L.; Poschl, E.; Brachvogel, B.; Brisson, A.R. Annexin-a5 assembled into two-dimensional arrays promotes cell membrane repair. *Nat. Commun.* **2011**, *2*, 270. [CrossRef] [PubMed]
142. Rand, J.H.; Wu, X.X.; Quinn, A.S.; Taatjes, D.J. The annexin a5-mediated pathogenic mechanism in the antiphospholipid syndrome: Role in pregnancy losses and thrombosis. *Lupus* **2010**, *19*, 460–469. [CrossRef] [PubMed]
143. Selbert, S.; Fischer, P.; Pongratz, D.; Stewart, M.; Noegel, A.A. Expression and localization of annexin vii (synexin) in muscle cells. *J. Cell Sci.* **1995**, *108*, 85–95. [PubMed]
144. Kuijpers, G.A.; Lee, G.; Pollard, H.B. Immunolocalization of synexin (annexin vii) in adrenal chromaffin granules and chromaffin cells: Evidence for a dynamic role in the secretory process. *Cell Tissue Res.* **1992**, *269*, 323–330. [CrossRef] [PubMed]
145. Gerelsaikhan, T.; Vasa, P.K.; Chander, A. Annexin a7 and snap23 interactions in alveolar type ii cells and in vitro: A role for Ca^{2+} and pkc. *Biochim. Biophys. Acta* **2012**, *1823*, 1796–1806. [CrossRef] [PubMed]
146. Voelkl, J.; Alesutan, I.; Pakladok, T.; Viereck, R.; Feger, M.; Mia, S.; Schonberger, T.; Noegel, A.A.; Gawaz, M.; Lang, F. Annexin a7 deficiency potentiates cardiac nfat activity promoting hypertrophic signaling. *Biochem. Biophys. Res. Commun.* **2014**, *445*, 244–249. [CrossRef]
147. Leighton, X.; Eidelman, O.; Jozwik, C.; Pollard, H.B.; Srivastava, M. Anxa7-gtpase as tumor suppressor: Mechanisms and therapeutic opportunities. *Methods Mol. Biol.* **2017**, *1513*, 23–35. [PubMed]
148. Garcia-Alonso, V.; Titos, E.; Alcaraz-Quiles, J.; Rius, B.; Lopategi, A.; Lopez-Vicario, C.; Jakobsson, P.J.; Delgado, S.; Lozano, J.; Claria, J. Prostaglandin e2 exerts multiple regulatory actions on human obese adipose tissue remodeling, inflammation, adaptive thermogenesis and lipolysis. *PLoS ONE* **2016**, *11*, e0153751. [CrossRef]
149. Pepinsky, R.B.; Hauptmann, R. Detection of vac-beta (annexin-8) in human placenta. *FEBS Lett.* **1992**, *306*, 85–89. [CrossRef]
150. Sarkar, A.; Yang, P.; Fan, Y.H.; Mu, Z.M.; Hauptmann, R.; Adolf, G.R.; Stass, S.A.; Chang, K.S. Regulation of the expression of annexin viii in acute promyelocytic leukemia. *Blood* **1994**, *84*, 279–286.

151. Reutelingsperger, C.P.; van Heerde, W.; Hauptmann, R.; Maassen, C.; van Gool, R.G.; de Leeuw, P.; Tiebosch, A. Differential tissue expression of annexin viii in human. *FEBS Lett.* **1994**, *349*, 120–124. [CrossRef]
152. Hauptmann, R.; Maurer-Fogy, I.; Krystek, E.; Bodo, G.; Andree, H.; Reutelingsperger, C.P. Vascular anticoagulant beta: A novel human Ca^{2+}/phospholipid binding protein that inhibits coagulation and phospholipase a2 activity. Its molecular cloning, expression and comparison with vac-alpha. *Eur. J. Biochem.* **1989**, *185*, 63–71. [CrossRef] [PubMed]
153. Hata, H.; Tatemichi, M.; Nakadate, T. Involvement of annexin a8 in the properties of pancreatic cancer. *Mol. Carcinog.* **2014**, *53*, 181–191. [CrossRef]
154. Iglesias, J.M.; Cairney, C.J.; Ferrier, R.K.; McDonald, L.; Soady, K.; Kendrick, H.; Pringle, M.A.; Morgan, R.O.; Martin, F.; Smalley, M.J.; et al. Annexin a8 identifies a subpopulation of transiently quiescent c-kit positive luminal progenitor cells of the ductal mammary epithelium. *PLoS ONE* **2015**, *10*, e0119718. [CrossRef] [PubMed]
155. Oka, R.; Nakashiro, K.; Goda, H.; Iwamoto, K.; Tokuzen, N.; Hamakawa, H. Annexin a8 is a novel molecular marker for detecting lymph node metastasis in oral squamous cell carcinoma. *Oncotarget* **2016**, *7*, 4882–4889. [CrossRef]
156. Lueck, K.; Carr, A.F.; Stampoulis, D.; Gerke, V.; Rescher, U.; Greenwood, J.; Moss, S.E. Regulation of retinal pigment epithelial cell phenotype by annexin a8. *Sci. Rep.* **2017**, *7*, 4638. [CrossRef] [PubMed]
157. Monastyrskaya, K.; Babiychuk, E.B.; Draeger, A. The annexins: Spatial and temporal coordination of signaling events during cellular stress. *Cell. Mol. Life Sci. CMLS* **2009**, *66*, 2623–2642. [CrossRef]

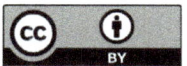

© 2019 by the authors. Licensee MDPI, Basel, Switzerland. This article is an open access article distributed under the terms and conditions of the Creative Commons Attribution (CC BY) license (http://creativecommons.org/licenses/by/4.0/).

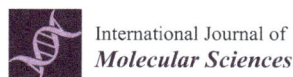

Article

Adipokinome Signatures in Obese Mouse Models Reflect Adipose Tissue Health and Are Associated with Serum Lipid Composition

Birgit Knebel [1,2], Pia Fahlbusch [1,2], Gereon Poschmann [3], Matthias Dille [1,2], Natalie Wahlers [1,2], Kai Stühler [3,4], Sonja Hartwig [1,2], Stefan Lehr [1,2], Martina Schiller [1,2], Sylvia Jacob [1,2], Ulrike Kettel [1,2], Dirk Müller-Wieland [5] and Jörg Kotzka [1,2,*]

[1] Institute of Clinical Biochemistry and Pathobiochemistry, German Diabetes Center at the Heinrich-Heine-University Duesseldorf, Leibniz Center for Diabetes Research; 40225 Duesseldorf, Germany; birgit.knebel@ddz.de (B.K.); pia.fahlbusch@ddz.de (P.F.); matthias.dille@ddz.de (M.D.); nawah101@hhu.de (N.W.); sonja.hartwig@ddz.de (S.H.); stefan.lehr@ddz.de (S.L.); martina.schiller@ddz.de (M.S.); sylvia.jacob@ddz.de (S.J.); ulrike.kettel@ddz.de (U.K.)
[2] German Center for Diabetes Research (DZD), Partner Duesseldorf, 40225 Duesseldorf, Germany
[3] Institute for Molecular Medicine, University Hospital Duesseldorf, Heinrich Heine University Duesseldorf, 40225 Duesseldorf, Germany; gereon.poschmann@hhu.de (G.P.); kai.stuehler@hhu.de (K.S.)
[4] Heinrich-Heine-University Duesseldorf, Molecular Proteomics Laboratory, BMFZ, 40225 Duesseldorf, Germany
[5] Clinical Research Centre, Department of Internal Medicine I, University Hospital Aachen, 52074 Aachen, Germany; dirmueller@ukaachen.de
* Correspondence: joerg.kotzka@ddz.de; Tel.: +49-211-3382-537

Received: 30 April 2019; Accepted: 22 May 2019; Published: 24 May 2019

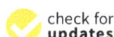

Abstract: Adipocyte and hepatic lipid metabolism govern whole-body metabolic homeostasis, whereas a disbalance of de novo lipogenesis (DNL) in fat and liver might lead to obesity, with severe co-morbidities. Nevertheless, some obese people are metabolically healthy, but the "protective" mechanisms are not yet known in detail. Especially, the adipocyte-derived molecular mediators that indicate adipose functionality are poorly understood. We studied transgenic mice (alb-SREBP-1c) with a "healthy" obese phenotype, and obob mice with hyperphagia-induced "sick" obesity to analyze the impact of the tissue-specific DNL on the secreted proteins, i.e., the adipokinome, of the primary adipose cells by label-free proteomics. Compared to the control mice, adipose DNL is reduced in both obese mouse models. In contrast, the hepatic DNL is reduced in obob but elevated in alb-SREBP-1c mice. To investigate the relationship between lipid metabolism and adipokinomes, we formulated the "liver-to-adipose-tissue DNL" ratio. Knowledge-based analyses of these results revealed adipocyte functionality with proteins, which was involved in tissue remodeling or metabolism in the alb-SREBP-1c mice and in the control mice, but mainly in fibrosis in the obob mice. The adipokinome in "healthy" obesity is similar to that in a normal condition, but it differs from that in "sick" obesity, whereas the serum lipid patterns reflect the "liver-to-adipose-tissue DNL" ratio and are associated with the adipokinome signature.

Keywords: Nonalcoholic fatty liver disease; fatty liver; free fatty acids; label-free proteomic profiling; adipokine; obesity; visceral fat; sick fat

1. Introduction

Obesity is a worldwide health burden. Obesity is prone to severe co-morbidities, including diabetes, cardiovascular disease, and lipotoxicity due to ectopic lipid accumulation. However, some obese individuals do not suffer from obesity-associated syndromes, which is the so-called phenomenon of "fit and fat". This was due to a healthy metabolism and insulin-sensitive adipose tissue, which might increase the likelihood of the incidence of a fatty liver. In contrast, "sick fat" people show an elevated lipid load, inflammation, hyperplasia, insufficient vascularization, and fibrosis of adipose tissue [1–3]. Unfortunately, the "point of no return" from healthy obese people, with functional adipose tissue, to unhealthy obesity, prone to comorbidities, still remains unknown.

There is a close interaction between adipocyte and hepatic lipid metabolism. Adipocytes are essential in whole-body energy homeostasis for the storage of dietary lipids and of lipids generated by de novo lipogenesis (DNL) from alimentary carbohydrates in adipose tissue or the liver. While it is an elementary process for survival, excessive hepatic lipogenesis is a key feature of many models of obesity and diabetes. Therefore, hepatic DNL is thought to be a health burden, as it correlates with ectopic hepatic lipid accumulation and insulin resistance [4–6]. One key regulator of hepatic DNL is the transcription factor sterol regulatory element-binding protein (SREBP)-1. SREBP-1c activity persists even in insulin resistant states, as seen in obesity and T2D. In this context, we have shown that the hepatic overexpression of the transcription active domain of SREBP-1c increases hepatic DNL, without severe insulin resistance, resulting in a fatty liver and a massively increased adipose tissue mass in mouse models [7,8].

In contrast to the liver, adipose tissue stores lipids from blood circulation, without the need for synthesis, and only a marginal amount of lipids is produced by adipose tissue DNL [9]. Therefore, it is unlikely that the role of adipose tissue DNL is primary for lipid storage, but it may act solely for signaling or regulation processes, initiated by the physiological status of the adipose tissue.

It is well accepted that adipose tissue secretes endocrine- and exocrine-acting proteins, i.e., adipokines or adipokinome. These secreted proteins influence food intake, energy metabolism, and insulin sensitivity [10–12]. The alteration of adipokinome in regard to metabolic conditions or diseases has been shown to have an impact on fat mass, either by affecting adipocyte hyperplasia or hypertrophy [13–16]. We recently showed that adipokinomes are correlated with clinical parameters in diabetes [17]. Thus, adipokinome changes in relation to the lipid composition of the adipose tissue and reflects the overall physiological condition of the adipose tissue. Furthermore, there are hints that certain adipokines interfere with the mechanism of hepatic fibrosis [10–12,17].

It is therefore tempting to raise the hypothesis that adipokinome is also involved in the adipose tissue-to-liver interaction for energy homeostasis regulation.

In the present study, we compare the adipokinomes of mice with increased hepatic DNL by the genetic overexpression of the N-terminal domain of SREBP-1c [7], as a model for "healthy" obesity, with hyperphagia-induced morbid obese mice (obob), as model for "sick" adipose tissue or lean mice (C57Bl6) by label-free proteomics.

2. Results

2.1. Physiological Characterization of the Mouse Models

SREBP-1c and obob mice had a marginally higher body weight, fat mass, and liver weight than C57Bl6 animals (Table 1). Blood glucose (BG) and triglycerides (TG) were also increased in the obese mouse models, and additionally, cholesterol was increased in obob mice. Food consumption was comparable in C57Bl6 and alb-SREBP-1c mice and increased in obob animals. Interestingly, the weight gain per unit of food consumed was increased 1.5- to 2-fold in obese mice. Liver enzymes ALT, AST, and GLDH indicated gradual hepatic impairment in the obese mouse models. Overall, alb-SREBP-1c mice were intermediate to obob and C57Bl6 mice. Relevant metabolic hormones showed higher levels of insulin in the obese mice. Leptin was higher in alb-SREBP-1c, compared to C57Bl6, and a leptin deficiency was confirmed in obob. Surrogate parameters for insulin resistance (HOMA-IR) and insulin secretion (HOMA-β%) confirmed a mild insulin resistance (IR) in alb-SREBP-1c and a strong IR in obob mice.

Table 1. Metabolic characterization of the lean mice (C57Bl6), transgenic mice (alb-SREBP-1c) with "healthy" adipose tissue, and of the "sick" adipose tissue obob mice used in the study.

Parameter	C57Bl6	alb-SREBP-1c	obob
body weight [g]	28.62 ± 2.54	35.23 ± 3.44 **	56.82 ± 6.76 **
liver weight [g]	1.56 ± 0.20	2.10 ± 0.30 **	3.72 ± 0.80 **
fat mass [g]	0.40 ± 0.13	1.79 ± 0.57 **	5.31 ± 0.87 **
blood glucose [mg/dL]	148.4 ± 15.24	184.41 ± 10.01 **	769.20 ± 142.31 **
cholesterol [mg/dL]	92.67 ± 12.98	111.18 ± 22.01	140.13 ± 33.70 **
triglycerides [mg/L]	123.60 ± 16.07	244.00 ± 52.86 **	403.60 ± 54.47 **
ALT [U/L]	48.75 ± 22.15	78.45 ± 13.19 **	181.87 ± 46.14 **
AST [U/L]	102.67 ± 24.19	156.36 ± 35.77 **	274.80 ± 102.36 **
GLDH [U/L]	13.46 ± 6.08	29.36 ± 13.68 **	139.75 ± 66.59 **
insulin [ng/mL]	1.06 ± 0.24	3.90 ± 1.39 **	16.51 ± 3.05 **
leptin [ng/mL]	0.90 ± 0.60	12.08 ± 3.48 **	n.d.
HOMA-IR	0.38 ± 0.0.08	2.12 ± 0.36 **	34.43 ± 3.05 **
HOMA-β%	96.26 ± 35.21	324.19 ± 175.06 **	180.71 ± 94.68 **
food uptake/bodyweight (kJ/g)	10.33 ± 2.95	11.84 ± 2.61	16.06 ± 1.79 **
weight gain/food uptake (mg/kJ)	1.55 ± 0.19	2.48 ± 0.25 **	3.14 ± 0.45 **

Data are expressed as mean ± SD ($n = 8$ of each phenotype). * $p < 0.05$, ** $p < 0.01$ ***, and $p < 0.001$, by Student's t-test in comparison to controls.

2.2 Lipid Composition of Serum, Liver, and Adipose Tissue

Serum-free fatty acid (FFA) was increased more than 2-fold in alb-SREBP-1c mice and more than 3-fold in obob mice. However, the total fatty acid (TFA) content of adipose tissue was similar to C57Bl6 mice, independent of the cause of obesity. In contrast, hepatic TFA was increased to a similar degree as free fatty acid in serum (Figure 1A). The change in the lipid composition in serum revealed increased cC16:1 and decreased C18:0 in obese models, compared to controls (Figure 1B). Both obese models differ in C16:0 and C18:0 and show inverse levels for the FFA cC18:1. FFA cC18:2, cC18:3, and cC20:4 were comparably altered. In adipose tissue, lipid composition, compared to controls, indicated, in alb-SREBP-1c mice, an increase in C18:0 and cC18:3 and, in obob mice, a decrease in cC16:1 and an increase in cC18:1. The obesity models differed only in the essential FA cC18:3 (Figure 1B). In the liver, the obese models mainly differed in an increase in cC16:1 and cC18:1 and a reduction of C18:0 and cC20:4, compared to the control mice, whereas the essential FA cC18:2 was more pronounced in the obob mice (Figure 1B).

In further detail, the percentage of serum lipid classes is shown in Figure S1A. The grouping of lipids showed that the amounts of saturated FA (SFA) were decreased, while the unsaturated FA (UFA), mono-UFA (MUFA), poly-UFA (PUFA), or essential FA (EFA) were increased, in the serum of obese mice (Figure S1B). The percentage of adipose tissue lipid classes is shown in Figure S2A. Here, only SFA was changed in both obese mice, compared to the controls, whereas UFA, PUFA, and EFA differed only in the obob mice (Figure S2B). The percentage of liver lipid classes is shown in Figure S3A. In the liver, a decreased SFA and increased UFA and MUFA were present in the obesity models, the latter being the highest in the alb-SREBP-1c mice. Compared to the controls, the content of EFA was higher in the obob and lower in the alb-SREBP-1c mice, and vice versa, for the non-essential FA (NEFA) (Figure S3B).

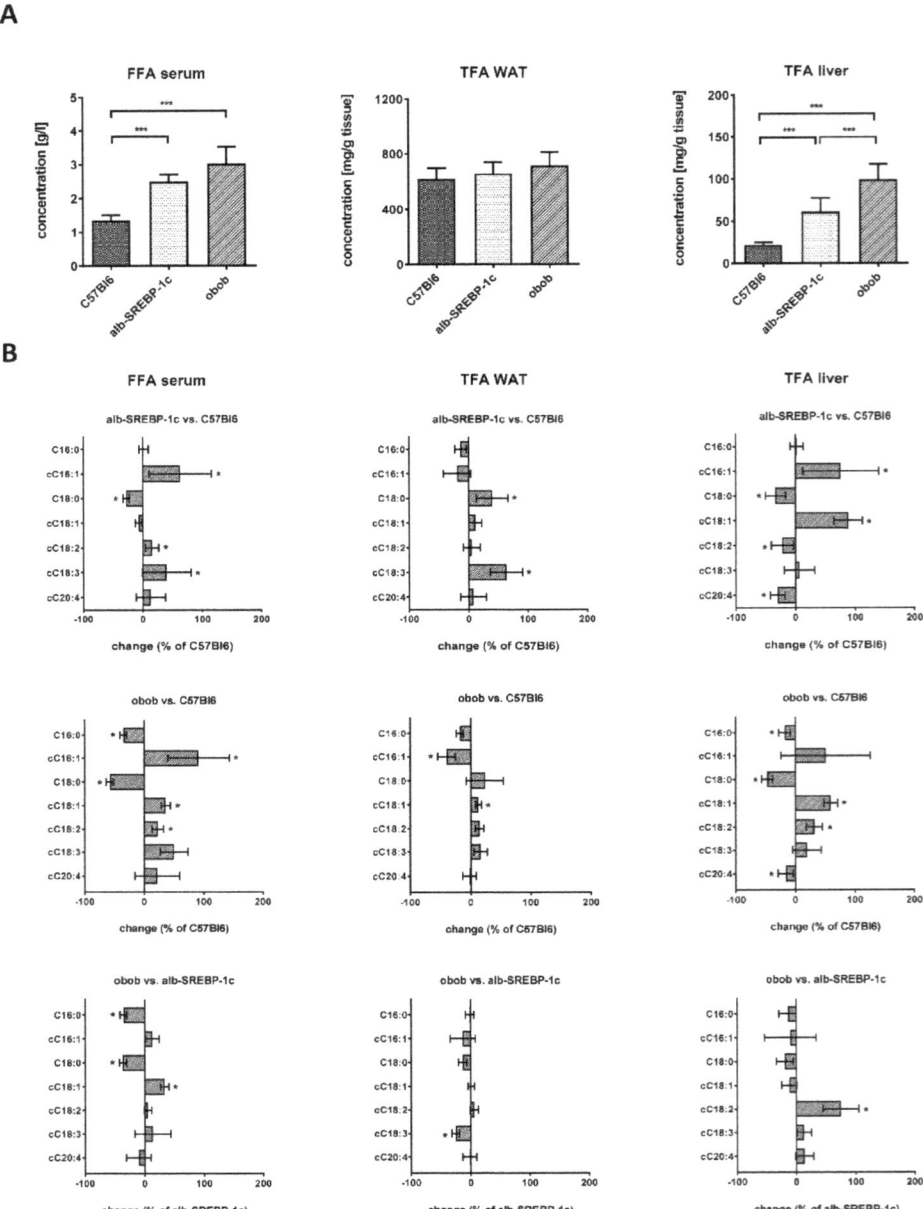

Figure 1. Lipid compositions of the C57Bl6, alb-SREBP-1c, and obob mice. (**A**) Total and specific fractional composition of the serum free fatty acids (FFAs) and the liver or adipose tissue total fatty acids (TFAs); (**B**) the percentage changes in the serum FFA and the liver or adipose tissue TFAs in alb-SREBP-1c vs. C57Bl6, obob vs. C57Bl6, and obob vs. alb-SREBP-1c. Data are expressed as mean ± SD ($n = 8$ of each phenotype). * $p < 0.05$, ** $p < 0.01$, and *** $p < 0.001$, by one-way ANOVA, with a Sidak post-hoc test (A) or students' *t*-test (B).

Lipid indices and surrogate parameters for the enzyme activity in lipid metabolism were calculated based on the lipid compositions determined in the tissues. In WAT (Figure S4A), the Δ6 desaturase activity was reduced in the alb-SREBP-1c mice. However, the elongase activity was elevated in both obese mice. In the liver (Figure S4B), the Δ9 desaturase activity for C16:0 as well as C18:0 was elevated in obese mice. The Δ6 desaturase activity was comparable in the C57Bl6 and obob mice, but lower in the alb-SREBP-1c mice, whereas the Δ5 desaturase activity was comparable in the C57Bl6 and alb-SREBP-1c and higher in the obob mice. Furthermore, a lower elongase activity, compared to controls, was observed in both obese mice.

2.3. Adipose Tissue DNL versus Hepatic DNL

In adipose tissue, DNL declined according to the degree of obesity and insulin resistance status from C57Bl6 (1.21 ± 0.18) to alb-SREBP-1c (0.93 ± 0.07) and obob mice (0.83 ± 0.07) (Figure 2A). Analyses of the hepatic DNL showed that it was higher in alb-SREBP-1c (2.33 ± 0.55) but lower in obob mice (0.96 ± 0.17), compared to the controls (1.62 ± 0.17) (Figure 2B). In regard to the serum lipid levels of cC16:1 and cC18:1, solely a correlation to the adipose tissue DNL in alb-SREBP-1c mice (cC16:1 to DNL: $R = 0.940$, $P = 0.017$; and cC18:1 to DNL: $R = 0.941$, $P = 0.017$), but neither in the lean control nor in the obob mice, was observed. (Table S1). A direct comparison of the adipocyte and hepatic DNL indicated that alb-SREBP-1c mice have the largest difference in "liver-to-adipose-tissue" DNL ratio (2.58 ± 0.67), whereas obob mice have a ratio of 1.14 ± 0.23, which is a comparable DNL-ratio to C57Bl6 mice (1.34 ± 0.3) (Figure 2C).

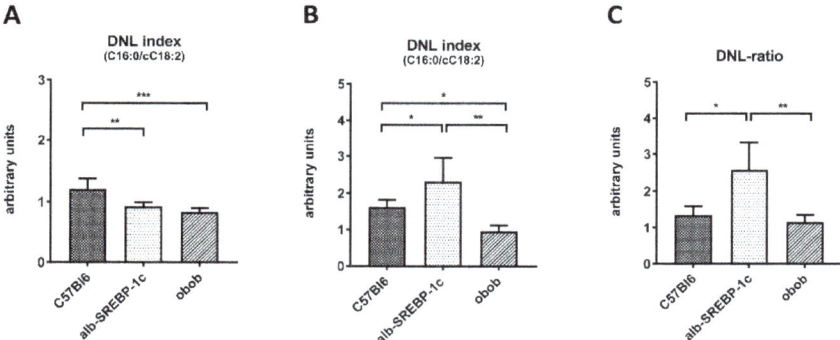

Figure 2. Tissue-specific de novo lipogenesis (DNL). (**A**) The DNL index (C16:0/cC18:2) of adipose tissue; (**B**) DNL index (C16:0/cC18:2) of the liver; and (**C**) "liver-to-adipose-tissue DNL" ratio. Data are expressed as mean ± SD ($n = 8$ of each phenotype). * $p < 0.05$, ** $p < 0.01$, and *** $p < 0.001$, by one-way ANOVA, with a Sidak post-hoc test.

2.4. Adipokinome

The secretome of the isolated adipocytes from visceral fat depots of the mouse models, analyzed by electron spray MS, identified 922 unique proteins. Of all of the proteins, 543 (59%) were predicted as classical or non-classical secreted proteins (SP +/SP−). The remaining 379 proteins identified were not predicted to be secreted (NP) (Table S2).

The intensity patterns of the proteins were predicted to be either classically or non-classically secreted (SP+/SP−) or not predicted to be secreted (NP), and the various mouse models were distinguished in PCA analyses (Figure 3A). Component 1 of the PCA accounted for 30% of the total variance and clearly separated obob from lean mice. The separation of C57Bl6 and alb-SREBP-1c mice was not so clearly achieved in these analyses, as the 95% confidence levels overlapped. Nevertheless, PLS-DA analyses (Figure 3B) and unsupervised cluster analyses segregated mouse models according to phenotype, indicating specific differences in the adipokines patterns.

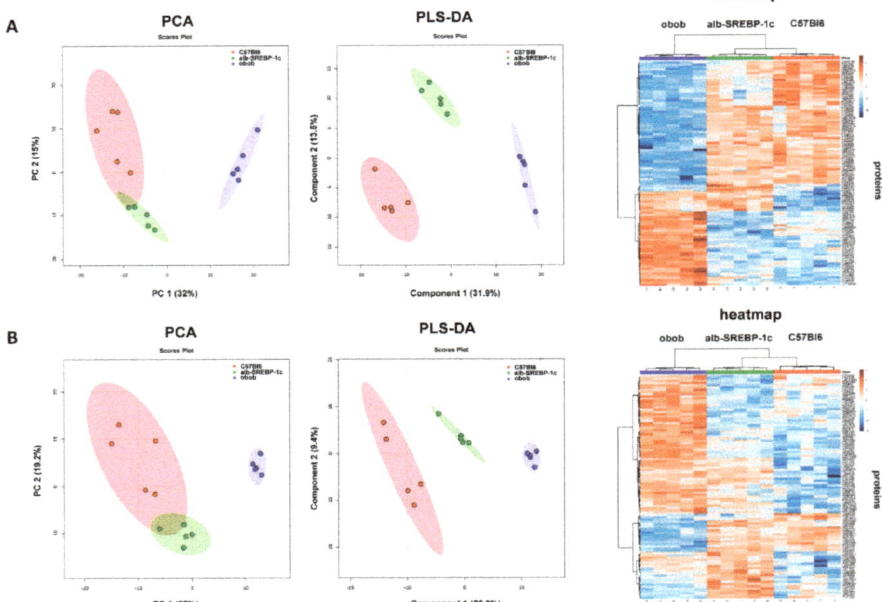

Figure 3. Classification of the mouse models according to the identified differential adipokinomes: (**A**) classically or non-classically secreted (SP+/SP−) proteins and (**B**) NP proteins. Principal component analyses (PCA), partial least square discriminant analyses (PLS-DA), and a heat map of the top 100 proteins with the greatest difference (ANOVA).

2.5. Differential Adipokinomes

Overall, 60% of the SP+/SP− and NP proteins were differentially abundant in the comparisons between C57Bl6 vs. alb-SREBP-1c, C57Bl6 vs. obob, and alb-SREBP-1c vs. obob (Table S3). In the comparison of alb-SREBP-1c and lean C57Bl6 mice secretomes, 121 proteins were identified (70 SP+/SP−; 51 NP) with significantly different secretions. SP+/SP− proteins mainly point to cell cycle modification, including cellular component organization or biogenesis (adjP = 4.67×10^{-5}), actin cytoskeleton organization (adjP = 0.0006), or actin remodeling (adjP = 0.001). Further alterations can solely be annotated to metabolic GO category superfamilies, e.g., cellular process (adjP = 0.0002), but are not specified in more detail. NP adipokines also annotate to cellular modifications, e.g., cellular component organization or biogenesis (adjP = 3.93×10^{-7}), macromolecule localization, (adjP = 8.79×10^{-7}) or inhibitory signaling processes, e.g., inhibitor activity to phospholipase A2 (adjP = 0.0003) or lipase (adjP = 0.0016), with a moderate stringency (Table S4).

The overall comparison C57Bl6 vs. obob identified 376 differentially abundant proteins (235 SP+/SP−; 141 NP). SP+/SP−proteins were involved solely in metabolic pathways, like the preamble cellular process (adjP = 1.22×10^{-13}), and a vast amount of detailed metabolic relevant annotations, including metabolic process (adjP = 7.87×10^{-17}), organic acid metabolic process (adjP = 3.64×10^{-13}), or NAD binding (adjP = 2.63×10^{-8}). Of 141 differentially abundant NP proteins, metabolic processes, e.g., pyridoxal phosphate-binding adjP = 1.33×10^{-5} and the carboxylic acid metabolic process adjP = 6.78×10^{-8}, as well as cell modifying functions, e.g., the protein complex adjP = 8.75×10^{-13}, cellular component biogenesis adjP = 1.00×10^{-6}, or actin-binding adjP = 1.33×10^{-5}, are equally present (Table S4).

A direct comparison of alb-SREBP−1c vs. obob adipocyte secretomes identified 396 different adipokines (156 SP+/SP−; 150 NP). SP+/SP− adipokines were exclusively annotated to metabolic processes (adjP = 4.47×10^{-26}), including, e.g., organic acid metabolic process (adjP = 1.44×10^{-27}) or

NAD binding (adjP = 1.56×10^{-12}). NP adipokines also solely annotate to metabolic processes, e.g., the metabolic carboxylic acid metabolic process (adjP = 1.27×10^{-15}) and oxoacid metabolic process (adjP = 4.68×10^{-15}), or energy-producing organelles (mitochondrion; adjP = 5.10×10^{-16}) (Table S4).

2.6. Knowledge-Based Analyses

Venn analyses revealed comparisons of C57Bl6 and either alb-SREBP-1c or obob, as well as alb-SREBP-1c vs. obob bare overlapping, but also specific different adipokine patterns of SP+/SP− and NP proteins (Figure 4, complete analyses in Table S5).

Knowledge-based analyses of protein interactions indicated the common and individual specificity of all three different adipokinomes. The common pathways affected by secreted SP+/SP− proteins are involved in ECM modeling, inflammation, lipid uptake, and gluconeogenesis or FA degradation. In NP proteins, the transport and glucose metabolism proteins were common, while in SP+/SP− proteins, C57Bl6 and alb-SREBP-1c differed in the proteins involved in class A receptor signaling, and proteins involved in the formation of extracellular matrix proteins dominated in C57Bl6 vs. obob.

No specific pathway can be identified in the NP proteins, compared to the controls. The comparison of both obese models focusses on proteins involved in central metabolic pathways, with a major participation of lipid metabolic processes in SP+/SP− proteins and the proteasome complex formation in NP (Figure 4).

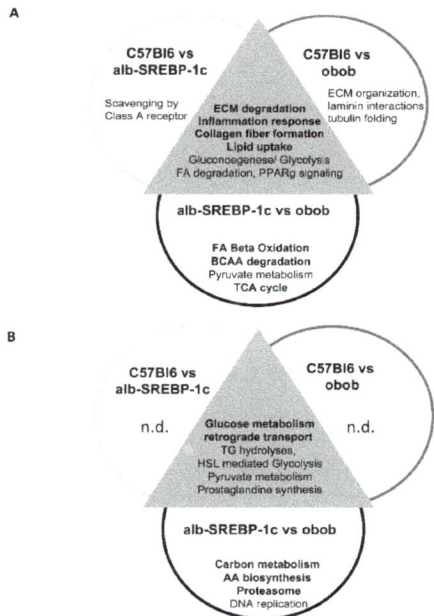

Figure 4. Unique pathways activated by differentially secreted adipokines. The prediction of secretory protein classification as classical SP+/SP− signaling sequences or non-classically secreted proteins was performed with SignalP 4.1 or SecretomeP 2.0, as indicated in the methods section. The functional annotation of differentially abundant proteins was performed separately on (**A**) proteins with classical SP+/SP− signaling sequences and (**B**) non-classically secreted proteins. Abbreviations: AA: amino acids, BCAA: branched chain amino acids; ECM: extracellular matrix; FA: fatty acids; n.d.: not detected, TCA cycle: tricarboxylic acid cycle.

To determine more informative interactions of the different adipokinomes, we used integrative annotation to extend the information to the suggested up- or downstream interactions of the identified proteins. Within these analyses, the most prominent functional overlap was the differential protein patterns per genotype, set to fatty acid metabolism or proteins initially identified to be related to steatosis (Figure 5). There was a differential overlap with fatty acid metabolism in the protein sets of C57Bl6 vs. alb-SREBP-1c ($n = 38$, p-value $= 8.3 \times 10^{-12}$), C57Bl6 vs. obob ($n = 58$, p-value $= 1.9 \times 10^{-17}$), and C57Bl6 vs. alb-SREBP-1c ($n = 72$, p-value $= 8.1 \times 10^{-21}$) (Figure 5). In addition, the number and significance of the proteins related to steatosis processes gradually increased with the severity of obesity in the comparisons of C57Bl6 vs. alb-SREBP-1c ($n = 20$, p-value 3.35×10^{-7}), C57Bl6 vs. obob ($n = 28$, p-value 8.9×10^{-9}), and obob vs. alb-SREBP-1c ($n = 39$, p-value 9.5×10^{-17}) (Figure 5).

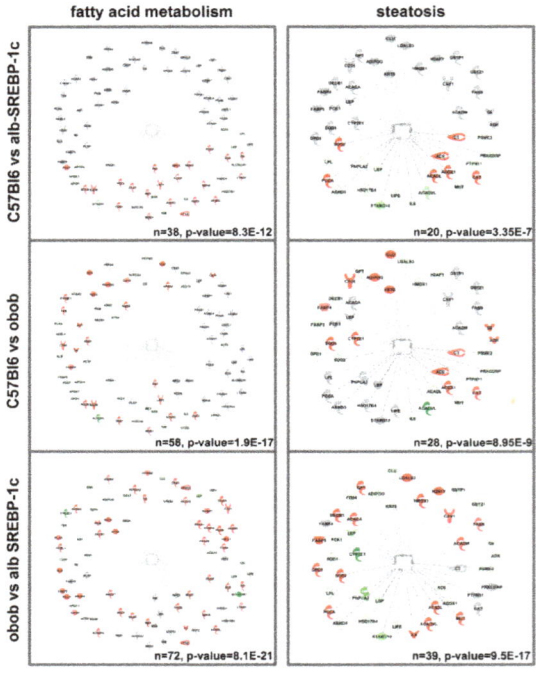

Figure 5. Differential enrichment of FA metabolism and steatosis-related proteins in the adipokinomes. The annotation of specific differentially abundant proteins to lipid metabolism or steatosis is shown. Data were analyzed with IPA® core analyses (default settings). Coloring represents proteins with different abundances in the comparisons C57Bl6 vs. alb-SREBP-1c, C57Bl6 vs. obob, and alb-SREBP-1c vs. obob. (Red: more abundant; green: less abundant; grey: not regulated in the specific comparison).

2.7. Adipokinome—Marker for Tissue-Specific DNL?

To account for the hypothesis that adipokinomes reflected, a marker for adipose tissue functionality and the physiological status of the adipose tissue, we analyzed the different adipokine patterns, identified for correlations, in relation to the specific "liver-to-adipose-tissue DNL" ratio. Of the 922 proteins observed, 55 proteins in C57Bl6 showed a correlation with the "liver-to-adipose-tissue DNL" ratio (Table S1). These included proteins involved in lipid droplet formation, like perilipin, actin-binding or assembly molecules; echinoderm microtubule-associated protein-like 2, plastin-2, -3, or villin molecules; metabolic enzymes, like acyl-CoA dehydrogenase, glycogen phosphorylase, L-lactate dehydrogenase, or NADP(+)-dependent alcohol dehydrogenase; and molecules of the glutathione metabolism involved in ROS clearance.

A total of 50 proteins were correlated with the "liver-to-adipose-tissue DNL" ratio in alb-SREBP-1c and 42 in obob mice. In alb-SREBP-1c mice, more metabolic active molecules were present, e.g., pyruvate kinase; NADPH-cytochrome P450 reductase; fructose-1,6-bisphosphatase; and L-lactate dehydrogenase or the peroxisomal delta(3,5)-delta(2,4)-dienoyl-CoA isomerase (ECH), an auxiliary involved in lipid metabolism. Other proteins were regulatory, like farnesyl pyrophosphate synthase, and protease regulatory subunits were present. In obob mice, the share of relevant correlative metabolic proteins included glycolysis and glyconeogenesis-related proteins, like pyruvate and malat dehydrogenases, and fructose-1,6-bisphosphatase 1, but also proteins involved in redox clearance, like peroxiredoxines, carboxyestherases, lipid droplet formation proteins, and the laminin and catepsin family; or metabolic signaling molecules, like carboxylesterase 1C, 14-3-3 protein, and dipeptidyl peptidase 3.

For the functional annotation, the proteins that correlated with the DNL ratio were used for IPA® core analyses to extend the information to upstream regulating proteins. As our analyses revealed a marked difference in the abundance of proteins known to be regulated by or related to fatty acid metabolism or fibrosis (Figure 6), we generated virtual pathways for all proteins related to these keywords in order to visualize the IPA® analyses. Based on these pathways, lean and healthy obese mice, due to increased hepatic DNL, showed similar patterns, in contrast to the "sick" obese obob mice (Figure 6; differential adipokines and upstream regulator molecules that causes different patterns were summarized in Table S6A,B).

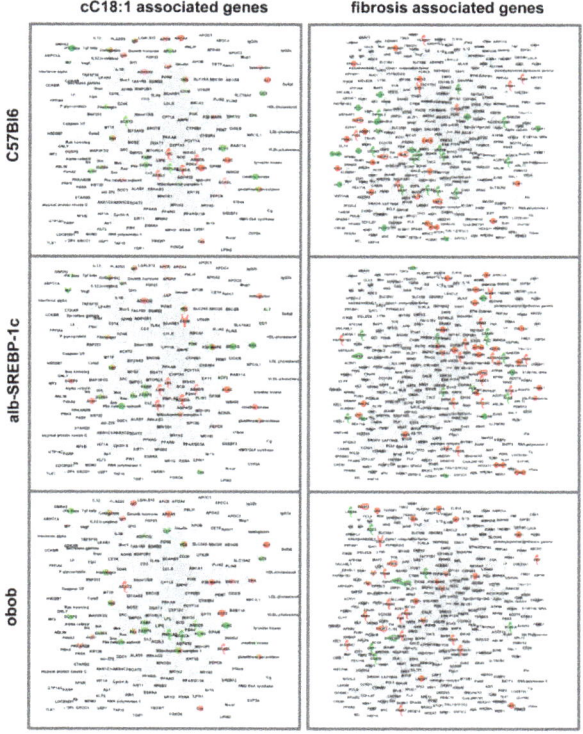

Figure 6. Differential abundance of FA metabolism and steatosis-related proteins in adipokines correlated to the "liver-to-adipose-tissue DNL" ratio. Virtual pathways were generated from proteins related to the keywords to cC18:1 or fibrosis. The proteins that correlated with the "liver-to-adipose-tissue DNL" ratio were used for IPA® core analyses to extend the information to upstream regulating proteins (Supplementary Materials Table S6). Coloring represents the different abundances in the comparisons of C57Bl6 vs. alb-SREBP-1c, C57Bl6 vs. obob, and alb-SREBP-1c vs. obob. (Red: more abundant; green: less abundant; grey: not regulated in the specific comparison).

3. Discussion

In the present study, we provide evidence that (i) the "liver-to-adipose-tissue DNL" ratio shows genotype-specific differences; (ii) this DNL-ratio can be monitored in the serum lipid pattern; and (iii) the pattern of the secreted proteins of adipocyte cells are different, indicated as a shift from secreted proteins, mainly involving tissue remodeling in lean and "healthy" obese mice, to metabolic active adipokines and fibrosis in morbid obese mice, corresponding to the health status of the adipose tissue.

To determine the systemic interaction of liver and adipose tissue in obesity, we choose a mouse model with obesity, according to hyperphagia and leptin deficiency (obob). Obob mice are an accepted morbid obesity model with a fatty liver, which develops cardiovascular complications and increased oxidative stress, including increased macrophage infiltration in adipose tissue and an inflammatory marker concertation [18–20]. On the other hand, we used a transgenic animal with a liver-specific overexpression of human SREBP-1c, which has previously been shown to induce obesity under isocaloric conditions due to increased hepatic DNL [7,8]. In these mice, a fatty liver, as an initial pathophysiological burden, is captured by the massively increasing visceral fat mass. The development of massive obesity in these mice is only accompanied by hepatic insulin resistance (IR), but without signs of inflammation in serum or adipose tissue. Therefore, alb-SREBP-1c mice resemble a "healthy" obesity phenotype, compared to obob mice. In regard to insulin secretion, alb-SREBP-1c mice showed a compensatory beta cells effect, whereas the beta cells failed to offset IR in obob mice. Nevertheless, IR poses a risk, as it increases lipolysis in adipose tissue, resulting in a release of fatty acids to serum, which finally elevates the triglyceride content in the liver [21].

The models showed a characteristic profile, with a decreased saturated C16:0 and C18:0 in the obese model, accompanied by increased levels of desaturated FA in serum. The main sources for the composition of the serum lipid profiles are nutrition, tissue-specific DNL, and the mobilization of FA by lipolysis from adipose tissue [22]. However, the tissue-specific FA patterns we determined in the liver and adipose tissue did not completely account for the different serum lipid patterns. Overall, adipose tissue lipolysis does not seem to be essential for explaining the differences seen in the serum FFA composition. In contrast, alterations observed in the hepatic FA, especially for cC16:1 and cC18:1, were also seen in serum lipids, except in the EFA cC18:2. There is controversy regarding the role of serum cC16:1 in health, as it increases insulin sensitivity in healthy subjects [23,24] but has adverse effects in obesity [25]. On the other hand, insulin resistance or the progression of NAFLD to non-alcoholic liver steatosis is accompanied by an increase of lipids, including cC16:1 and cC18:1 [22]. In NAFLD, cC16:1 and its elongation product, cC18:1, were increased due to the SREBP-1c-regulated increased Δ9 stearoyl-CoA desaturase 1 (SCD-1) activity [22], as seen in the alb-SREBP-1c model. Hepatic DNL was higher in alb-SREBP-1c mice, which is consistent with our previous observation [8]. Especially, the essential cC16:1 is, in general, very present in adipose tissue, making it a direct product and marker for adipose tissue DNL, and its presence in the serum lipid pool favors a role in signaling [23,26,27]. Thus, the data derived support the hypothesis that DNL in adipose or liver tissue might have further physiological functions beyond simple nutrient conversion.

Adipose tissue secretome has been thoroughly studied in metabolic disturbances and has been accepted as a model for various metabolic alterations [10–12,17]. As the FA composition of adipocytes was not grossly altered, thus excluding a predominant lipokine, adipocyte-secreted adipokines might act as a signaling moiety to adjust tissue-specific DNL rates. Overall, analyses of the adipokinome indicated a close relation between the adipokinomes of C57Bl6 and those of alb-SREBP-1c mice. This might indicate the healthy status of the adipose tissue in alb-SREBP-1c mice, in contrast to obob mice.

In proteins with a secretion motive, both obesity models differed in regard to proteins associated with metabolic processes. There was an accumulation of proteins found to be related to or involved in fibrosis-associated processes in obob mice, compared to the controls. This is consistent with the excess accumulation of adipose tissue extra cellular matrix (ECM) components and IR in obesity [28], and to a recent observation of the ECM organization and assembly markers that were increased in obese humans with a high serum FFA mobilization from adipose tissue [29].

Proteins without a secretion signal are probably related to the endomembrane system for vesicular secretion processes [30]. In this context, we have recently shown that adipose tissue-secreted exosomes are enriched in relevant metabolic proteins, without signal peptides [31]. Here, both obesity models differed in proteins related to, e.g., proteosomal degradation processes. In obesity, a proteasome dysfunction further aggravates the cell toxic effects of increased oxidative stress or unfolded protein responses to ER stress in adipocytes. Proteasome function has also been found to maintain insulin sensitivity in adipocytes [32]. In the context of adipose tissue, this might indicate that the fibrosis of the adipose organ is a marker for functionality defects, which is in line with previous observations [10–12].

The most striking difference within the obese mouse models was still that the "healthy" obese alb-SREBP-1c mice showed the largest difference in the "liver-to-adipose-tissue DNL" ratio, and the serum cC16:1 and cC18:1 correlated to adipose tissue DNL solely in the alb-SREBP-1c mice. The correlative adipokines indicated a specific and gradual difference for the obesity models, but the patterns were not conclusive of a certain pathway. Nevertheless, a differential accumulation of cC18:1- and fibrosis-associated proteins in the adipokinome can be determined.

The interaction of adipose tissue and hepatic DNL is in a tight balance in lean healthy conditions, but runs out of control in obesity, IR, or NAFLD [33–35]. In obesity, adipose DNL is reduced [36] and can be restored by caloric restriction [37]. Increased adipocyte DNL seems to be beneficial in regard to IR or glucose homeostasis, independent of obesity in humans [4,13,38]. This idea identified adipocyte-derived lipokines, cC16:1 and cC18:1, as essential systemic mediators that interfere with adipose tissue physiological functionality, with hepatic lipid metabolism and DNL [38,39]. In conclusion, whole body energy homeostasis is mainly dependent on hepatic and adipose tissue communication. The concept of communication by -kines identified cC16:1 and cC18:1 as adipocyte-derived DNL products, as mediators for the adipocyte DNL status to the liver [10–12,27,38].

Our study indicated that the obesity models differ in circulating cC16:1, compared to lean controls, and further by cC18:1, which might act as marker. As the concentration of the lipokine cC18:1 also differs in the serum in the obese models, our observations point to a central role of adipokines as indicators that differentiate healthy and metabolically diseased models. It is noteworthy that a recent study of a mouse model showed that oleate (cC18:1) specifically featured a nuclear accumulation of the master-regulator SREBP-1c of the DNL in hepatocytes, suggesting cC18:1 as central in SREBP-1c-mediated signaling and therefore in DNL [40]. This further supports the hypothesis that an increase in hepatic DNL is essential for maintaining adipose tissue health, and adipokine secretion is part of the systemic regulation.

The composition of the serum lipids reflects the "liver-to-adipose-tissue DNL" ratio. Interestingly, adipokine patterns that correlate with the "liver-to-adipose-tissue DNL" ratio seem to be rather phenotype-specific, as only a marginal overlap can be observed in the models. However, in both obese models, but not in the controls, mitogen-activated protein kinase 14 or isocitrate dehydrogenase show a comparable correlation, whereas acetyl-CoA carboxylase 1, catalyzing the rate-limiting step in the lipid synthesis of malonyl-CoA synthesis from acetyl-CoA, is inversely correlated in healthy and sick obesity. On the other hand, proteins involved in free radical scavenging, like glutathione S-transferase Mu 2, were equally correlated in the healthy obese and the control animals. This, and observation that peroxisomal ECH accounts for alb-SREBP-1c, further supports our previous finding, i.e., that peroxisomal function might play a role in preventing increased hepatic lipid accumulation in metabolic syndrome or diabetes [17,41].

Our data further support the idea that the adipose tissue returns information back to the liver also regarding its status of plasticity and metabolic capacity. Thus, depending on the degree of the "liver-to-adipose-tissue DNL" ratio, adipokinomes show fibrotic pathways as a marker for the beginning of a loss of adipose tissue health.

Conclusion: our analyses features the concept of impaired adipose tissue functionality in obesity. We provide evidence that the "liver-to-adipose-tissue DNL" ratio is a marker for the shift from healthy to diseased adipose tissue. Adipose tissue "health" can be maintained in obesity as long as the hepatic DNL can be increased according to the metabolic requirements. This can be monitored by serum fatty acid cC16:1 and especially cC18:1, as biomarkers, and is accompanied by altered adipose tissue secreted proteins, as the adipokinome of "healthy" or "sick fat" differs in regard to cC16:1 and cC18:1 and fibrosis-dependent proteins.

4. Materials and Methods

4.1. Animals

C57Bl6 (C57Bl6), B6.Cg-Lep^{ob} (obob), and B6-TgN(alb-HA-SREBP-1cNT) (alb-SREBP-1c) [7] mice were bred and maintained under standard conditions (12h light/dark cycle; 22 ± 1 °C, 50% ± 5% humidity). At 6 weeks of age, male littermates of each genotype were kept under standardized conditions, with free access to water and regular laboratory chow (13.7 mJ/kg: 53% carbohydrate, 36% protein, 11% fat (Ssniff, Soest, Germany)). At the age of 18 weeks, the mice were fasted for 6 h and sacrificed by CO_2 asphyxiation (7:00 am). Blood samples were collected by a left ventricular puncture, and organ samples, i.e., the liver and visceral adipose tissue, were removed. The Animal Care Committee of the University Duesseldorf approved the animal care and procedure employed (Approval#84-02.04.2015.A424; 2 April 2015).

4.2. Animal Characterization

Phenotypical characterization; serum diagnostics of clinical measures; as well as the surrogate parameters of insulin resistance, lipid profiling in serum, and liver and adipose tissue by gas chromatography were performed, as previously described [7,42]. Serum-free fatty acids (FFA), hepatic as well as adipose cell total fatty acids (TFA) content, and the specific fractional composition of FAs were determined by gas chromatography. FA data of adipocytes were further used to calculate the Δ5-desaturase index (cC18:2/cC20:4); Δ6-desaturase index (cC18:2/cC18:3); Δ9-desaturase index (cC16:1/C16:0 or cC18:1/C18:0); DNL index (C16:0/cC18:2); elongation index (C18:0/C16:0); as well as the sums of the total FA, non-saturated FA, monounsaturated FA, saturated FA, essential FA (cC18:2+cC18:3), and non-essential FA (C16:0+cC16:1+C18:0+cC18:1) [43]. The nomenclature of FA is given according to IUPAC. The liver-to-adipose-tissue DNL was calculated by the liver DNL/adipose tissue DNL.

4.3. Secretome Profiling by Liquid Chromatography (LC)-Electrospray Ionization (ESI)-MS/MS and Data Analyses

Mature adipocytes were isolated from minced biopsies by collagenase digestion. Adipocytes were cultured (2 days), washed extensively, and supplemented with an FCS-free culture medium to harvest and process the secretome, as previously described [17,44]. Data on all mouse models were acquired in parallel, as described in detail previously [17,45].

4.4. Data Annotation

The functional annotation and prediction of secretory proteins was performed with SignalP 4.1 [46], (http://www.cbs.dtu.dk/services/SignalP/), SecretomeP 2.0. [47], (http://www.cbs.dtu.dk/services/SecretomeP/). We identified 922 individual unique proteins in the secretomes of the mouse models investigated (Supplementary Materials Table S1). Of all proteins, 543 (59%) are characterized as classically or non-classically secreted proteins (SP+/SP−). The remaining 379 identified proteins do not contain classical secretion signals.

4.5. Statistical Analysis

Clinical values are presented as the mean ± SD. Statistical analysis was performed with Student's *t*-test or one-way ANOVA, with a Sidak post hoc test, calculated with Prism 7.04 (GraphPad Software Inc., San Diego, CA, USA), as indicated. Secretome data were further analyzed with the Metabolist 3.0

package [48] or SPSS (IBM Ver. 22). Pearson correlation coefficients, with a two-sided *p*-value, were determined in SPSS (IBM Ver. 22).

4.5. Web-Based Functional Annotation

For the functional annotation, web-based tools from public database sources were used: https://www.ncbi.nlm.nih.gov/, http://www.informatics.jax.org/mgihome/, http://bioinfo.vanderbilt.edu/webgestalt/ [49], https://toppcluster.cchmc.org/ [50], David Bioinformatics Resources 6.8 (https://david.ncifcrf.gov/) [51], and IPA® (Ingenuity™, Qiagen, Hilden, Germany). The fold change of different adipokinome patterns was analyzed, and the *t*-test-derived *p*-values of the comparisons C57Bl6 vs. alb-SREBP-1c, C57Bl6 vs. obob, and alb-SREBP-1c vs. obob were entered for the IPA® analyses. Furthermore, a spearman coefficient and two-sided *p*-value were used. Data were used for core analyses and comparison analyses. The pathways were generated from respective networks, as suggested by IPA®. For expression analyses of different protein sets, an expression fold change (1.5×) and expression differences (*p*-value <0.05) were analyzed, following the core analysis modules. Differentially abundant proteins (1.5× fold difference, *p*-value < 0.05) (one–way ANOVA, posthoc, Welch test) were analyzed separately for C57 vs. obob, C57 vs. alb-SREBP-1c, and alb-SREBP-1c vs. obob mice.

Supplementary Materials: Supplementary Materials can be found at http://www.mdpi.com/1422-0067/20/10/2559/s1.

Author Contributions: B.K. and J.K. were responsible for the experimental design, interpretation, writing, and editing of the manuscript, and they performed the in-silico analyses. G.P., S.H., and U.K. researched the proteomic data. S.L., M.S., K.S. supervised the proteome experiments. S.J., P.F., M.D., and N.W. researched data for the metabolic characterization. D.M.-W. contributed to the experimental design, interpretation of the data, and review and editing of the manuscript. J.K. was the principal investigator of the study.

Funding: This research received no external funding.

Acknowledgments: The work was supported by the German Diabetes Center (DDZ), which is funded by the German Federal Ministry of Health and the Ministry of Innovation, Science, Research, and Technology of the state, North Rhine-Westphalia. This study was supported in part by a grant from the German Federal Ministry of Education and Research (BMBF) to the German Center for Diabetes Research (DZD e. V.).

Conflicts of Interest: The authors declare no conflict of interest.

Abbreviations

ALT	alanine transaminase
AST	aspartate transaminase
BG	blood glucose
BG	blood glucose
DNL	de novo lipogenesis
ECM	extra cellular matrix
EFA	essential FA
ER	endoplasmatic reticulum
FA	fatty acids
FCS	fetal calf serum
FFA	free fatty acids
GLDH	glutamate dehydrogenase
GO	gene ontology
HOMA-%β	Homeostatic model assessment of β -cell function (%)
HOMA-IR	Homeostatic model assessment of insulin resistance
IR	insulin resistance
MS	mass spectrometry
MUFA	monounsaturated fatty acids
NAFLD	nonalcoholic fatty liver disease
NEFA	non-saturated FA

PCA	principal component analysis
PLS-DA	partial least square discriminant analysis
PUFA	poly unsaturated fatty acids
SCD1	Δ9 stearoyl-CoA desaturase 1
SFA	saturated fatty acids
SREBP	sterol regulatory element-binding protein
T2D	type-2 diabetes mellitus
TFA	total fatty acids
TG	triglycerides
UFA	unsaturated fatty acids
WAT	white adipose tissue

References

1. Denis, G.V.; Obin, M.S. Metabolically healthy obesity: Origins and implications. *Mol. Asp. Med.* **2013**, *34*, 59–70. [CrossRef] [PubMed]
2. Jung, C.H.; Lee, W.J.; Song, K.H. Metabolically healthy obesity: A friend or foe? *Korean J. Intern. Med.* **2017**, *32*, 611–621. [CrossRef]
3. Phillips, C.M. Metabolically healthy obesity: Definitions, determinants and clinical implications. *Rev. Endocr. Metab. Disord.* **2013**, *14*, 219–227. [CrossRef]
4. Younossi, Z.; Anstee, Q.M.; Marietti, M.; Hardy, T.; Henry, L.; Eslam, M.; George, J.; Bugianesi, E. Global burden of NAFLD and NASH: Trends, predictions, risk factors and prevention. *Nat. Rev. Gastroenterol. Hepatol.* **2018**, *15*, 11–20. [CrossRef]
5. Samuel, V.T.; Shulman, G.I. Nonalcoholic Fatty Liver Disease as a Nexus of Metabolic and Hepatic Diseases. *Cell Metab.* **2018**, *27*, 22–41. [CrossRef] [PubMed]
6. Eissing, L.; Scherer, T.; Todter, K.; Knippschild, U.; Greve, J.W.; Buurman, W.A.; Pinnschmidt, H.O.; Rensen, S.S.; Wolf, A.M.; Bartelt, A.; et al. De novo lipogenesis in human fat and liver is linked to ChREBP-beta and metabolic health. *Nat. Commun.* **2013**, *4*, 1528. [CrossRef] [PubMed]
7. Knebel, B.; Haas, J.; Hartwig, S.; Jacob, S.; Kollmer, C.; Nitzgen, U.; Muller-Wieland, D.; Kotzka, J. Liver-specific expression of transcriptionally active SREBP-1c is associated with fatty liver and increased visceral fat mass. *PLoS ONE* **2012**, *7*, e31812. [CrossRef] [PubMed]
8. Jelenik, T.; Kaul, K.; Sequaris, G.; Flogel, U.; Phielix, E.; Kotzka, J.; Knebel, B.; Fahlbusch, P.; Horbelt, T.; Lehr, S.; et al. Mechanisms of Insulin Resistance in Primary and Secondary Nonalcoholic Fatty Liver. *Diabetes* **2017**, *66*, 2241–2253. [CrossRef] [PubMed]
9. Song, Z.; Xiaoli, A.M.; Yang, F. Regulation and Metabolic Significance of De Novo Lipogenesis in Adipose Tissues. *Nutrients* **2018**, *10*, 1383. [CrossRef] [PubMed]
10. Adolph, T.E.; Grander, C.; Grabherr, F.; Tilg, H. Adipokines and Non-Alcoholic Fatty Liver Disease: Multiple Interactions. *Int. J. Mol. Sci.* **2017**, *18*, 1649. [CrossRef] [PubMed]
11. Beall, C.; Hanna, L.; Ellacott, K.L.J. CNS Targets of Adipokines. *Compr. Physiol.* **2017**, *7*, 1359–1406.
12. Maira, G.D.I.M.; Pastore, M.; Marra, F. Liver fibrosis in the context of nonalcoholic steatohepatitis: The role of adipokines. *Minerva Gastroenterol. E Dietol.* **2018**, *64*, 39–50.
13. Conde, J.; Scotece, M.; Gomez, R.; Lopez, V.; Gomez-Reino, J.J.; Lago, F.; Gualillo, O. Adipokines: Biofactors from white adipose tissue. A complex hub among inflammation, metabolism, and immunity. *Biofactors* **2011**, *37*, 413–420. [CrossRef]
14. Fasshauer, M.; Bluher, M. Adipokines in health and disease. *Trends Pharmacol. Sci.* **2015**, *36*, 461–470. [CrossRef]
15. Antuna-Puente, B.; Feve, B.; Fellahi, S.; Bastard, J.P. Adipokines: The missing link between insulin resistance and obesity. *Diabetes Metab.* **2008**, *34*, 2–11. [CrossRef]
16. Waki, H.; Tontonoz, P. Endocrine functions of adipose tissue. *Annu. Rev. Pathol.* **2007**, *2*, 31–56. [CrossRef]
17. Knebel, B.; Goeddeke, S.; Poschmann, G.; Markgraf, D.F.; Jacob, S.; Nitzgen, U.; Passlack, W.; Preuss, C.; Dicken, H.D.; Stuhler, K.; et al. Novel Insights into the Adipokinome of Obese and Obese/Diabetic Mouse Models. *Int. J. Mol. Sci.* **2017**, *18*, 1928. [CrossRef]

18. Li, S.Y.; Yang, X.; Ceylan-Isik, A.F.; Du, M.; Sreejayan, N.; Ren, J. Cardiac contractile dysfunction in Lep/Lep obesity is accompanied by NADPH oxidase activation, oxidative modification of sarco(endo)plasmic reticulum Ca2+-ATPase and myosin heavy chain isozyme switch. *Diabetologia* **2006**, *49*, 1434–1446. [CrossRef] [PubMed]
19. Friedman, J.M.; Leibel, R.L.; Siegel, D.S.; Walsh, J.; Bahary, N. Molecular mapping of the mouse ob mutation. *Genomics* **1991**, *11*, 1054–1062. [CrossRef]
20. Zhang, Y.; Proenca, R.; Maffei, M.; Barone, M.; Leopold, L.; Friedman, J.M. Positional cloning of the mouse obese gene and its human homologue. *Nature* **1994**, *372*, 425–432. [CrossRef] [PubMed]
21. Puri, P.; Wiest, M.M.; Cheung, O.; Mirshahi, F.; Sargeant, C.; Min, H.K.; Contos, M.J.; Sterling, R.K.; Fuchs, M.; Zhou, H.; et al. The plasma lipidomic signature of nonalcoholic steatohepatitis. *Hepatology* **2009**, *50*, 1827–1838. [CrossRef]
22. Nielsen, S.; Guo, Z.; Johnson, C.M.; Hensrud, D.D.; Jensen, M.D. Splanchnic lipolysis in human obesity. *J. Clin. Investig.* **2004**, *113*, 1582–1588. [CrossRef] [PubMed]
23. Pinnick, K.E.; Neville, M.J.; Fielding, B.A.; Frayn, K.N.; Karpe, F.; Hodson, L. Gluteofemoral adipose tissue plays a major role in production of the lipokine palmitoleate in humans. *Diabetes* **2012**, *61*, 1399–1403. [CrossRef]
24. Stefan, N.; Kantartzis, K.; Celebi, N.; Staiger, H.; Machann, J.; Schick, F.; Cegan, A.; Elcnerova, M.; Schleicher, E.; Fritsche, A.; et al. Circulating palmitoleate strongly and independently predicts insulin sensitivity in humans. *Diabetes Care* **2010**, *33*, 405–407. [CrossRef] [PubMed]
25. Fabbrini, E.; Magkos, F.; Su, X.; Abumrad, N.A.; Nejedly, N.; Coughlin, C.C.; Okunade, A.L.; Patterson, B.W.; Klein, S.J. Insulin sensitivity is not associated with palmitoleate availability in obese humans. *Lipid Res.* **2011**, *52*, 808–812. [CrossRef] [PubMed]
26. Hodson, L.; Skeaff, C.M.; Fielding, B.A. Fatty acid composition of adipose tissue and blood in humans and its use as a biomarker of dietary intake. *Prog. Lipid Res.* **2008**, *47*, 348–380. [CrossRef]
27. Hodson, L.; Karpe, F. Is there something special about palmitoleate? *Curr. Opin. Clin. Nutr. Metab. Care* **2013**, *16*, 225–231. [CrossRef]
28. Divoux, A.; Tordjman, J.; Lacasa, D.; Veyrie, N.; Hugol, D.; Aissat, A.; Basdevant, A.; Guerre-Millo, M.; Poitou, C.; Zucker, J.D.; et al. Fibrosis in human adipose tissue: Composition, distribution, and link with lipid metabolism and fat mass loss. *Diabetes* **2010**, *59*, 2817–2825. [CrossRef] [PubMed]
29. Van Pelt, D.W.; Guth, L.M.; Wang, A.Y.; Horowitz, J.F. Factors regulating subcutaneous adipose tissue storage, fibrosis, and inflammation may underlie low fatty acid mobilization in insulin-sensitive obese adults. *Am. J. Physiol. Endocrinol. Metab.* **2017**, *313*, E429–E439. [CrossRef]
30. Petersen, T.N.; Brunak, S.; von Heijne, G.; Nielsen, H. SignalP 4.0: Discriminating signal peptides from transmembrane regions. *Nat. Methods* **2011**, *8*, 785–786. [CrossRef]
31. Hartwig, S.; De Filippo, E.; Göddeke, S.; Knebel, B.; Kotzka, J.; Al-Hasani, H.; Roden, M.; Lehr, S.; Sell, H. Exosomal proteins constitute an essential part of the human adipose tissue secretome. *Biochim Biophys Acta Proteins Proteom.* **2018**. [CrossRef]
32. Diaz-Ruiz, A.; Guzman-Ruiz, R.; Moreno, N.R.; Garcia-Rios, A.; Delgado-Casado, N.; Membrives, A.; Tunez, I.; El Bekay, R.; Fernandez-Real, J.M.; Tovar, S.; et al. Proteasome Dysfunction Associated to Oxidative Stress and Proteotoxicity in Adipocytes Compromises Insulin Sensitivity in Human Obesity. *Antioxid. Redox Signal.* **2015**, *23*, 597–612. [CrossRef] [PubMed]
33. Solinas, G.; Boren, J.; Dulloo, A.G. De novo lipogenesis in metabolic homeostasis: More friend than foe? *Mol. Metab.* **2015**, *4*, 367–377. [CrossRef] [PubMed]
34. Shubham, K.; Vinay, L.; Vinod, P.K. Systems-level organization of non-alcoholic fatty liver disease progression network. *Mol. Biosyst.* **2017**, *13*, 1898–1911. [CrossRef] [PubMed]
35. Yamaguchi, K.; Yang, L.; McCall, S.; Huang, J.; Yu, X.X.; Pandey, S.K.; Bhanot, S.; Monia, B.P.; Li, Y.X.; Diehl, A.M. Inhibiting triglyceride synthesis improves hepatic steatosis but exacerbates liver damage and fibrosis in obese mice with nonalcoholic steatohepatitis. *Hepatology* **2007**, *45*, 1366–1374. [CrossRef]
36. Nuotio-Antar, A.M.; Poungvarin, N.; Li, M.; Schupp, M.; Mohammad, M.; Gerard, S.; Zou, F.; Chan, L. FABP4-Cre Mediated Expression of Constitutively Active ChREBP Protects Against Obesity, Fatty Liver, and Insulin Resistance. *Endocrinology* **2015**, *156*, 4020–4032. [CrossRef]

37. Bruss, M.D.; Khambatta, C.F.; Ruby, M.A.; Aggarwal, I.; Hellerstein, M.K. Calorie restriction increases fatty acid synthesis and whole body fat oxidation rates. *Am. J. Physiol. Endocrinol. Metab.* **2010**, *298*, E108–E116. [CrossRef] [PubMed]
38. Cao, H.; Gerhold, K.; Mayers, J.R.; Wiest, M.M.; Watkins, S.M.; Hotamisligil, G.S. Identification of a lipokine, a lipid hormone linking adipose tissue to systemic metabolism. *Cell* **2008**, *134*, 933–944. [CrossRef]
39. Yilmaz, M.; Claiborn, K.C.; Hotamisligil, G.S. De Novo Lipogenesis Products and Endogenous Lipokines. *Diabetes* **2016**, *65*, 1800–1807. [CrossRef]
40. Lounis, M.A.; Bergeron, K.F.; Burhans, M.S.; Ntambi, J.M.; Mounier, C. Oleate activates SREBP-1 signaling activity in SCD1-deficient hepatocytes. *Am. J. Physiol. Endocrinol. Metab.* **2017**, *313*, E710–E720. [CrossRef]
41. Knebel, B.; Goddeke, S.; Hartwig, S.; Horbelt, T.; Fahlbusch, P.; Al-Hasani, H.; Jacob, S.; Koellmer, C.; Nitzgen, U.; Schiller, M.; et al. Alteration of Liver Peroxisomal and Mitochondrial Functionality in the NZO Mouse Model of Metabolic Syndrome. *Proteomics Clin. Appl.* **2018**, *12*. [CrossRef]
42. Kotzka, J.; Knebel, B.; Haas, J.; Kremer, L.; Jacob, S.; Hartwig, S.; Nitzgen, U.; Muller-Wieland, D. Preventing phosphorylation of sterol regulatory element-binding protein 1a by MAP-kinases protects mice from fatty liver and visceral obesity. *PLoS ONE* **2012**, *7*, e32609. [CrossRef]
43. Cinci, G.; Guerranti, R.; Pagani, R.; Carlucci, F.; Terzuoli, L.; Rosi, F.; Marinello, E. Fatty acid composition of phospholipids, triglycerides and cholesterol in serum of castrated and estradiol treated rats. *Life Sci.* **2000**, *66*, 1647–1654. [CrossRef]
44. Goddeke, S.; Kotzka, J.; Lehr, S. Investigating the adipose tissue secretome: A protocol to generate high-quality samples appropriate for comprehensive proteomic profiling. *Methods Mol. Biol* **2015**, *1295*, 43–53.
45. Hartwig, S.; Goeddeke, S.; Poschmann, G.; Dicken, H.D.; Jacob, S.; Nitzgen, U.; Passlack, W.; Stuhler, K.; Ouwens, D.M.; Al-Hasani, H.; et al. Identification of novel adipokines differential regulated in C57BL/Ks and C57BL/6. *Arch. Physiol. Biochem.* **2014**, *120*, 208–215. [CrossRef] [PubMed]
46. Nielsen, H. Predicting Secretory Proteins with SignalP. *Methods Mol. Biol* **2017**, *1611*, 59–73.
47. Bendtsen, J.D.; Nielsen, H.; von Heijne, G.; Brunak, S. Improved prediction of signal peptides: SignalP 3.0. *J. Mol. Biol.* **2004**, *340*, 783–795. [CrossRef] [PubMed]
48. Xia, J.; Sinelnikov, I.V.; Han, B.; Wishart, D.S. MetaboAnalyst 3.0–making metabolomics more meaningful. *Nucleic Acids Res.* **2015**, *43*, W251–W257. [CrossRef]
49. Wang, J.; Vasaikar, S.; Shi, Z.; Greer, M.; Zhang, B. WebGestalt 2017: A more comprehensive, powerful, flexible and interactive gene set enrichment analysis toolkit. *Nucleic Acids Res.* **2017**, *45*, W130–W137. [CrossRef] [PubMed]
50. Kaimal, V.; Bardes, E.E.; Tabar, S.C.; Jegga, A.G.; Aronow, B.J. ToppCluster: A multiple gene list feature analyzer for comparative enrichment clustering and network-based dissection of biological systems. *Nucleic Acids Res.* **2010**, *38*, W96–W102. [CrossRef]
51. Huang, D.W.; Sherman, B.T.; Tan, Q.; Kir, J.; Liu, D.; Bryant, D.; Guo, Y.; Stephens, R.; Baseler, M.W.; Lane, H.C.; et al. DAVID Bioinformatics Resources: Expanded annotation database and novel algorithms to better extract biology from large gene lists. *Nucleic Acids Res.* **2007**, *35*, W169–W175. [CrossRef] [PubMed]

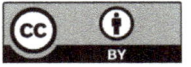

© 2019 by the authors. Licensee MDPI, Basel, Switzerland. This article is an open access article distributed under the terms and conditions of the Creative Commons Attribution (CC BY) license (http://creativecommons.org/licenses/by/4.0/).

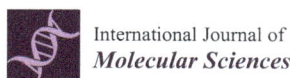

Article

Glucose Restriction Plus Refeeding In Vitro Induce Changes of the Human Adipocyte Secretome with an Impact on Complement Factors and Cathepsins

Qi Qiao, Freek G. Bouwman, Marleen A. van Baak, Johan Renes and Edwin C.M. Mariman *

Department of Human Biology, NUTRIM School of Nutrition and Translational Research in Metabolism, Maastricht University Medical Centre, 6200 MD Maastricht, The Netherlands
* Correspondence: e.mariman@maastrichtuniversity.nl

Received: 27 June 2019; Accepted: 16 August 2019; Published: 20 August 2019

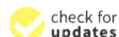

Abstract: Adipose tissue is a major endocrine organ capable of secreting adipokines with a role in whole-body metabolism. Changes in the secretome profile during the development of obesity is suspected to contribute to the risk of health complications such as those associated with weight regain after weight loss. However, the number of studies on weight regain is limited and secretome changes during weight regain have hardly been investigated. In an attempt to generate leads for in vivo studies, we have subjected human Simpson Golabi Behmel Syndrome adipocytes to glucose restriction (GR) followed by refeeding (RF) as an in vitro surrogate for weight regain after weight loss. Using LC-MS/MS, we compared the secreted protein profile after GR plus RF with that of normal feeding (NF) to assess the consequences of GR plus RF. We identified 338 secreted proteins of which 49 were described for the first time as being secreted by adipocytes. In addition, comparison between NF and GR plus RF showed 39 differentially secreted proteins. Functional classification revealed GR plus RF-induced changes of enzymes for extracellular matrix modification, complement system factors, cathepsins, and several proteins related to Alzheimer's disease. These observations can be used as clues to investigate metabolic consequences of weight regain, weight cycling or intermittent fasting.

Keywords: adipokines; SGBS adipocytes; glucose restriction; in vitro fat regain; weight regain; complement factors; cathepsins; extracellular remodeling

1. Introduction

Obesity has become a worldwide critical health issue because it is frequently accompanied by the development of health complications such as type II diabetes, cardiovascular diseases, respiratory problems and certain types of cancer [1]. Obesity is characterized by excess body fat mass, which is mostly stored in the adipose tissue. Additionally, adipose tissue is known as a major endocrine organ capable of secreting various signaling and mediator proteins, termed adipose-derived secreted proteins or adipokines [2]. Studies have shown that the secreted proteins are hormones, cytokines, extracellular matrix related proteins as well as proteins involved in cardiovascular, lipid and glucose metabolism [3]. These adipokines have a variety of effects on homeostasis and metabolism by autocrine, paracrine and endocrine activity, which could contribute to the development of obesity and obesity-associated complications [4,5].

For overweight and obese people, weight loss is an indicated remedy that can reduce the risk for comorbid conditions [6]. A calorie restrictive diet is part of a common practice to try and lose weight. Losing 5% of body weight already results in significant improvement of health parameters such as lower blood pressure, plasma glucose and insulin levels [7]. In parallel, in vitro studies have illustrated that calorie restriction (CR) results in an altered secretion profile of adipocytes, comprised of a less inflammatory phenotype and a reversed expression of detrimental adipokines [8]. However, weight loss is often followed by weight regain. Generally, up to 80% of people who lost weight on CR, regain weight and often return to their original weight or even beyond, within one or two years [9]. Moreover, it has been suggested that weight regain after weight loss could worsen metabolic health [10], possibly mediated by changes in the adipose tissue secretome. Consequently, prevention of weight regain after successful weight loss is a critical challenge for obesity management and it is essential to obtain more knowledge on the causes and consequences of weight regain [11]. So far, the number of biological studies on weight regain has been limited and secretome changes during weight regain are largely unknown.

A growing body of data suggests that Simpson Golabi Behmel Syndrome (SGBS) cells are an excellent tool to study adipokine secretion [3,12–15]. SGBS cells display a much more active differentiation capacity compared with primary pre-adipocytes in culture, and retain this capacity over at least 30 generations while being similar to primary cells in morphology, physiology and biochemistry [12,13]. Moreover, it has been reported that in vitro differentiated SGBS adipocytes behave similar to human primary adipocytes in functions such as glucose transport, lipogenesis and lipolysis [12,15]. Based on their origin and gene expression comparison, differentiated SGBS cells are regarded as subcutaneous white adipocytes [13]. Therefore, SGBS cells have been widely accepted and used for in vitro adipocyte experiments. Using these cells, we have earlier reported on secretome changes induced by glucose restriction (GR) and found several novel adipokines [8,16]. However, the effect of GR plus refeeding (RF) on adipokine secretion has not been investigated. Recently, we established a protocol for GR followed by RF for SGBS cells and examined the influence on the cellular proteome [17]. Here we report on changes in the in vitro secretome when normal feeding (NF) is compared with GR plus RF in an attempt to obtain leads on possible threats to metabolic health as a consequence of weight regain after weight loss.

2. Results

2.1. Proteins Secreted from Human SGBS Adipocytes

In total, 1326 proteins were identified from the collection medium. By filtering these proteins, SignalP 4.1 detected the presence of a signal peptide in 328 proteins. Deeploc recognized 230 secreted proteins by predicting the extracellular location. In total these two groups represented 337 different proteins (Figure 1A; Table S1). 221 out of 337 proteins both contained a signal peptide and were located in the extracellular space, nine proteins (membrane primary amine oxidase (AOC3), cysteine and glycine-rich protein 1 (CSRP1), galectin-1 (LGALS1), D-dopachrome decarboxylase (DDT), trypsin-3 (PRSS3), metallothionein-1G (MT1G), proteasome inhibitor subunit 1 (PSMF1), ectonucleotide pyrophosphatase/phosphodiesterase family member 2 (ENPP2), small proline-rich protein 2G (SPRR2G)) were only predicted by the extracellular space and 107 proteins only had a signal peptide for secretion (Figure 1A). In addition, we manually checked the list of proteins which were not recognized as secreted by SignalP or Deeploc, for proteins known by their function to be secreted. So far, only complement factor 1Q (C1q) was found to be missed by the programs. Thus, C1q was added to our analysis list with a total of 338 secreted proteins (Table S1).

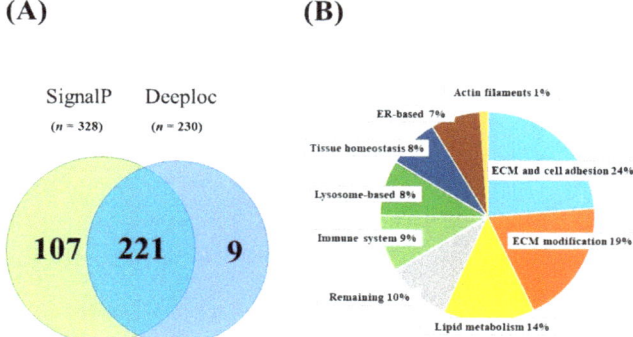

Figure 1. Secreted proteins identified in human Simpson Golabi Behmel Syndrome (SGBS) adipocytes. (**A**) The number of identified secreted proteins by SignalP or Deeploc. (**B**) Pie graph on functional categories of overall identified secreted proteins.

2.2. Newly Identified Secreted Proteins of Human SGBS Adipocytes

Literature on secreted proteins from adipocytes or adipose tissue was searched online and in total 24 research papers and five reviews were found (Table 1) [2,3,8,16,18–42]. Comparing our secretome data set with the data reported in these papers, 49 secreted proteins were identified as novel secreted proteins that had not been described before for adipocytes or adipose tissue (Table 2). Of these proteins, 46 proteins were annotated as classical secreted proteins (S or S + D in Table 2) and three as non-classical secreted proteins (D in Table 2; MT1G, PSMF1, SPRR2G).

Table 1. Literature Reports on Adipocyte Adipokine Profiling.

Order	Reference	Refs	Source	Secreted	Novel
1	Wang et al. (2004)	[18]	Mice (3T3L1 cells)	26	15
2	Chen et al. (2005)	[19]	Rat fat pad	84	53
3	Molina et al. (2009)	[20]	Mice (3T3L1 cells)	147	NA
4	Celis et al. (2005)	[21]	Human adipocytes	359	NA
5	Mutch et al. (2009)	[22]	Human primary preadipocytes	213	NA
6	Alvarez-Llamas et al. (2007)	[23]	Human visceral fat tissue	108	68
7	Zvonic et al. (2007)	[24]	Human adipose-derived stem cells	101	NA
8	Lim J.M. et al. (2008)	[31]	3T3L1 cell line; primary rat adipocytes	97; 203	54; 132
9	Roelofsen H et al. (2009)	[32]	Human omental tissue (control; test)	155; 141	NA
10	Kim et al. (2010)	[25]	Human subcutaneous adipose tissue	307	NA
11	Rosenow et al. (2010)	[3]	Human SGBS cells	80	6
12	Zhong et al. (2010)	[26]	Human adipocytes	420	107
13	Lee M.J. et al. (2010)	[27]	Human adipose tissue derived stem cells	142	NA
14	Rosenow A. et al. (2012)	[16]	Human SGBS cells	40	2
15	Lehr S. et al. (2012)	[28]	Human primary adipocytes	263	44
16	Roca-Rivada A. et al. (2011)	[40]	Rats (visceral; subcutaneous; gonadal fat)	188; 85; 91	NA
17	Sano S. et al. (2014)	[41]	Mice (3T3L1 cells)	231	NA
18	Roca-Rivada A. et al. (2015)	[38]	Human adipose tissue (visceral; subcutaneous)	136; 64	NA
19	Hartwig S. et al. (2018)	[36]	Human adipocytes	884	67
20	Laria A.E. et al. (2018)	[37]	Mice (3T3L1 cells)	839	80
21	Renes J. et al. (2014)	[8]	Human SGBS cells	57	6
22	Li Z.Y. et al. (2014)	[29]	Human SAT/VAT	NA	1
23	Ojima K et al. (2016)	[34]	Mice (3T3L1 cells)	74	NA
24	Ali Khan et al. (2018)	[30]	Mice primary adipocytes	499	NA
25	Mariman et al. (2010)	[33]	(Review)_Human and rodent adipocytes	NA	NA
26	Lehr S; et al. (2012)	[2]	(Review)_Human adipocytes	928	NA
27	Renes J. et al. (2013)	[35]	(Review)_Human and rodent adipocytes	NA	NA
28	Pardo M. et al. (2012)	[39]	(Review)_Human and rat adipocytes	NA	NA
29	Lee M.W. et al. (2019)	[42]	(Review)_Human and rat adipocytes	NA	NA

The number in the "secreted" column refers to the number of identified adipocyte secreted proteins, the "novel" column shows the number of newly reported adipokines in that report. NA: there is no exact number for secreted proteins mentioned in the article or supplemental materials.

Table 2. List of 49 novel adipocyte secreted proteins.

Order	S or D	UniProt	Gene Symbol	Protein Name
1	S	O00763	ACACB	Acetyl-CoA carboxylase 2
2	S + D	P04745	AMY1A	Amylase, Alpha 1A (Salivary)
3	S	O43570	CA12	Carbonic anhydrase 12
4	S	P55287	CDH11	Cadherin-11
5	S	P19022	CDH2	Cadherin-2
6	S + D	Q9BWS9	CHID1	Chitinase domain-containing protein 1
7	S	P26992	CNTFR	Ciliary neurotrophic factor receptor subunit alpha
8	S + D	Q9UI42	CPA4	Carboxypeptidase A4
9	S + D	O75629	CREG1	Protein CREG1
10	S + D	O00602	FCN1	Ficolin-1
11	S	Q10471	GALNT2	Polypeptide N-acetylgalactosaminyltransferase 2
12	S	P23434	GCSH	Glycine cleavage system H protein, mitochondrial
13	S + D	P06280	GLA	Alpha-galactosidase A
14	S + D	Q9UJJ9	GNPTG	N-acetylglucosamine-1-phosphotransferase subunit gamma
15	S	O75487	GPC4	Glypican-4
16	S + D	P35475	IDUA	Alpha-L-iduronidase
17	S + D	P08476	INHBA	Inhibin beta A chain
18	S + D	Q96I82	KAZALD1	Kazal-type serine protease inhibitor domain-containing protein 1
19	S	Q6GTX8	LAIR1	Leukocyte-associated immunoglobulin-like receptor 1
20	S	P38571	LIPA	Lysosomal acid lipase/cholesteryl ester hydrolase
21	S	O75197	LRP5	Low-density lipoprotein receptor-related protein 5
22	S	Q8ND94	LRRN4CL	LRRN4 C-terminal-like protein
23	S	Q5JRA6	MIA3	Transport and Golgi organization protein 1 homolog
24	S + D	P22894	MMP8	Neutrophil collagenase
25	D	P13640	MT1G	Metallothionein-1G
26	S + D	P41271	NBL1	Neuroblastoma suppressor of tumorigenicity 1
27	S	Q04721	NOTCH2	Neurogenic locus notch homolog protein 2
28	S + D	P48745	NOV	Protein NOV homolog
29	S + D	O95897	OLFM2	Noelin-2
30	S + D	Q8NBP7	PCSK9	Proprotein convertase subtilisin/kexin type 9
31	S	P50897	PPT1	Palmitoyl-protein thioesterase 1
32	S + D	P42785	PRCP	Lysosomal Pro-X carboxypeptidase
33	S + D	P07477	PRSS1	Trypsin-1
34	D	Q92530	PSMF1	Proteasome inhibitor subunit 1
35	S	P10586	PTPRF	Receptor-type tyrosine-protein phosphatase F
36	S	Q15274	QPRT	Nicotinate-nucleotide pyrophosphorylase [carboxylating]
37	S	Q6NUM9	RETSAT	All-trans-retinol 13,14-reductase
38	S + D	O00584	RNASET2	Ribonuclease T2
39	S	Q9H173	SIL1	Nucleotide exchange factor SIL1
40	S	Q99523	SORT1	Sortilin
41	D	Q9BYE4	SPRR2G	Small proline-rich protein 2G
42	S + D	P10124	SRGN	Serglycin
43	S + D	A1L4H1	SSC5D	Soluble scavenger receptor cysteine-rich domain-containing protein SSC5D
44	S	Q8NBK3	SUMF1	Sulfatase-modifying factor 1
45	S	Q8NBJ7	SUMF2	Sulfatase-modifying factor 2
46	S	Q5HYA8	TMEM67	Meckelin
47	S + D	Q8WUA8	TSKU	Tsukushin
48	S	Q06418	TYRO3	Tyrosine-protein kinase receptor TYRO3
49	S	P98155	VLDLR	Very low-density lipoprotein receptor

S: secreted proteins identified by SignalP, D: identified by Deeploc, S + D: identified by both software packages.

2.3. Functional Categories of Identified Proteins

To get information of the 338 proteins (Table S1) secreted by SGBS adipocytes, functional classification was done according to information on genes/proteins in databases: GeneCards [43], UniProt [44] and PubMed [45]. Generally, these proteins could be classified into nine categories according to biological function with "extracellular matrix (ECM) and cell adhesion" (80 proteins, 24%) and 'ECM modification' (65 proteins, 19%) representing the largest groups (Figure 1B). Notably, 12 of the 30 proteins in the immune system category appeared to be complement factors and seven of the 29 proteins in the lysosome-based group were cathepsins.

2.4. Adipocyte Secretome Changes after GR Plus RF as Compared with NF

Recently we have reported that the growth rate of fat droplets during NF and during RF after GR shows similar kinetics, which allowed us to investigate the combined influence of GR plus RF on the cellular proteome [17]. In the present study we focused on the secretome of those samples and searched for secreted proteins, of which the abundance was influenced by GR plus RF. For that, protein abundances were quantified by liquid chromatography tandem mass spectrometry (LC-MS/MS) after NF (T18) and after GR plus RF (T22RF). 39 proteins were significantly changed by GR plus RF compared to NF (Table 3) with 18 proteins being up-regulated and 20 proteins being down-regulated. These 39 proteins can be divided into nine functional categories, which seem to parallel the functional categories of the total identified secretome. 13 out of 39 proteins were related to the ECM with seven proteins belonging to the ECM and cell adhesion group and six proteins belonging to ECM modification group. It indicates that GR plus RF induces specific changes to the ECM. Four of the 39 proteins were up-regulated with a FC > 4: complement factor B (CFB), ADAMTS-like protein 1 (ADAMTSL1), target of Nesh-SH3 (ABI3BP), liver carboxylesterase 1 (CES1), and two were down-regulated with a FC > 4: sortilin (SORT1) and dermokine (DMKN). Changes of protein expression during GR plus RF could be due to different mechanisms with major changes either during GR and/or during RF. Therefore, we examined the changes of abundance of the 39 proteins during the separate phases of GR and RF (Table S2). The results confirmed the existence of different regulatory mechanisms. For instance, ADAMTSL1 was up-regulated 10.47× during GR but remained at this level of expression during RF. A similar pattern of expression was observed for prostaglandin-H2 D-isomerase (PTGDS) that was up-regulated 8.44× during GR but only up-regulated 1.51× during RF. ABI3BP did not change during GR, but was 5.04× up-regulated during RF. SORT1 was only slightly down-regulated (1.56×) during GR but 4.07× down-regulated during RF.

Table 3. Proteins significantly different between GR plus RF and NF.

Order	Category	Gene Symbol	Accession	Description	T18-T22RF FC_(GR+RF)/NF	p Value
1	Actin filaments	GSN	P06396	Gelsolin	−1.73	0.007
2	Complement factors	C1Q	Q07021	Complement 1q subcomponent	−2.94	0.030
3		C4B	P0C0L5	Complement C4-B	2.85	0.002
4		CFB	P00751	Complement factor B	4.06	0.018
5		CFD	P00746	Complement factor D	−1.93	0.002
6	ECM and cell adhesion	CDH13	P55290	Cadherin-13	−2.06	0.044
7		COL15A1	P39059	Collagen alpha-1(XV) chain	1.83	0.012
8		COL5A3	P25940	Collagen alpha-3(V) chain	−1.69	0.047
9		LUM	P51884	Lumican	−1.48	0.025
10		MCAM	P43121	Cell surface glycoprotein MUC18	−1.91	0.028
11		NRCAM	Q92823	Neuronal cell adhesion molecule	−2.39	0.046
12		SERPINE2	P07093	Glia-derived nexin	1.58	0.020
13	ECM modification	ADAMTSL1	Q8N6G6	ADAMTS-like protein 1	9.57	0.006
14		MMP2	P08253	72 kDa type IV collagenase	1.48	0.010
15		MMP8	P22894	Neutrophil collagenase	3.72	0.001
16		P4HA1	P13674	Prolyl 4-hydroxylase subunit alpha-1	−1.80	0.004
17		PPIC	P45877	Peptidyl-prolyl cis-trans isomerase C	−1.47	0.012
18		SERPINH1	P50454	Serpin H1	−2.19	0.001
19	ER-based	CALU	O43852	Calumenin	−2.36	0.002
20		HYOU1	Q9Y4L1	Hypoxia up-regulated protein 1	1.78	0.009
21		RCN1	Q15293	Reticulocalbin-1	−2.23	0.002
22		TXNDC5	Q8NBS9	Thioredoxin domain-containing protein 5	−1.39	0.024
23	Lipid metabolism	ACACB	O00763	Acetyl-CoA carboxylase 2	−1.90	0.044
24		AZGP1	P25311	Zinc-alpha-2-glycoprotein	1.59	0.041
25		PCSK9	Q8NBP7	Proprotein convertase subtilisin/kexin type 9	−1.90	0.003
26		PTGDS	P41222	Prostaglandin-H2 D-isomerase	3.67	0.000
27	Lysosome-based	CTSA	P10619	Lysosomal protective protein	2.75	0.009
28		CTSL	P07711	Cathepsin L1	1.24	0.029
29		DNASE2	O00115	Deoxyribonuclease-2-alpha	2.97	0.033
30		SORT1	Q99523	Sortilin	−5.13	0.005
31	Tissue homeostasis	ABI3BP	Q7Z7G0	Target of Nesh-SH3	5.71	0.008
32		GRN	P28799	Granulins	1.73	0.008
33		MYDGF	Q969H8	Myeloid-derived growth factor	−1.93	0.046
34		NRP1	O14786	Neuropilin-1	1.74	0.029
35		RBP4	P02753	Retinol-binding protein 4	−1.91	0.011
36	Remaining	APP	P05067	Amyloid-beta A4 protein	−1.44	0.033
37		CES1	P23141	Liver carboxylesterase 1	4.05	0.008
38		CHI3L2	Q15782	Chitinase-3-like protein 2	3.43	0.005
39		DMKN	Q6E0U4	Dermokine	−5.40	0.000

NF: normal feeding, GR: glucose restriction, RF: refeeding. FC_(GR+RF)/NF: fold change between GR plus RF (T22RF) and NF (T18). When FC >1, the value was described as FC; otherwise, the value was described as −1/FC.

3. Discussion

In the present study, we performed GR followed by RF of SGBS cells as a simple in vitro surrogate for in vivo weight regain after weight loss and investigated the changes of human adipocyte-derived secreted proteins. Comparison between NF and GR plus RF was made to gain information on changes induced to the secretome that could serve as leads to get further insight into the consequences of weight regain for metabolic health. Our results show that GR plus RF induced adipocyte secretome changes involving biological pathways of ECM remodeling, lipid metabolism, complement system, and tissue homeostasis. Furthermore, 49 secreted proteins were described here for the first time as being secreted by adipocytes.

Harvesting secreted proteins from the culture medium inevitable leads to contamination with leaked cellular proteins. We have applied bioinformatics analysis to identify the secreted proteins either as classical secreted proteins, which are typically targeted to the endoplasmic reticulum by a signal peptide, and non-classical secreted proteins without a signal peptide. Till now, SignalP [46] has been a well-accepted method for sorting classical secreted proteins and SecretomeP [47] has been widely used for non-classical secretion. When we first used SignalP in combination with SecretomeP, this yielded 739 potentially secreted proteins in the current study. However, recently Henrik et al. [48] reported that SecretomeP induces more than 20% false positives. Instead, Deeploc obtained the highest accuracy (78% for subcellular localization; 92% for membrane-bound or soluble) on predicting non-classical secreted proteins when compared with other methods [49]. Therefore, in the current study we used the combination of SignalP and Deeploc, which led to 337 secreted protein candidates, of which 66% (221) were ranked as secreted by both programs. Yet, it should be noted that even with our stringent method of selection, a certain level of misclassification cannot be avoided. Additionally, some proteins may be aberrantly classified as non-secreted as observed for complement factor C1q.

The largest change in abundance induced by the combined effects of GR plus RF was the 9.57 × up-regulation of ADAMTSL1. This is a metalloproteinase located in the ECM and known to degrade aggrecan [50]. Two other metalloproteinases (MMP2 and MMP8) are up-regulated as well, suggesting that after GR plus RF, the ECM is in a catabolic state. Moreover, three proteins involved in the maturation of collagens, P4HA1, PPIC and SERPINH1, are down-regulated. Recently we have shown that inside the cells GR leads to an upregulation of certain focal adhesion proteins [17]. It suggests that upon GR plus RF adipocytes intensify the cell-cell interaction while going through a phase of increased ECM flexibility. At the moment, it is not clear whether this also occurs in vivo and whether it would influence weight regain or the metabolic condition after weight regain. Still, in a previous weight loss/follow-up intervention study, expression of the *ADAMTSL1* and *MMP2* genes were significantly up-regulated (FC = 1.09, q = 0.05; FC = 1.24, q < 0.0001, respectively) four weeks after return to a balanced diet [51]. This indicates that ECM adaptations occur also in vivo during weight loss and weight regain.

It is well established that adipose tissue secretes various components of the complement system. During development of overweight and obesity, the secreted levels of complement factors change, which is thought to contribute to the chronic low level inflammation of the adipose tissue and the development of health complications such as insulin resistance, type II diabetes and cardiovascular disorders [1]. In this respect, it has been suggested that modulation of the complement system could be a target for the prevention and therapy of obesity-associated metabolic diseases [11,52–55]. Twelve proteins with an influence on complement activation were identified in our in vitro system and eight of them were complement factors (Table 4). Of those proteins, complement factor B (CFB) and complement factor 4B (C4-B) were significantly increased by GR plus RF, whereas the abundances of C1q and complement factor D (CFD) were significantly reduced. Such changes in vivo after weight loss and weight regain might lead to systemic changes in complement activity, especially in people with a high fat mass [52]. More generally, it could have local effects in the adipose tissue itself. Reduction of C1q and of C1s ($p = 0.13$) indicates a lower classical complement pathway. Yet, the increase of C4-B and mannan-binding lectin serine protease 1 (MASP1) suggest an increase of the C3 convertase C4bC2b.

Together with the strong increase of CFB, a local increase of C3a and C3b could be expected. C3a can be converted to C3desArg (acylation-stimulating protein, ASP) by carboxypeptidases B and N [56]. Here we found that adipocytes secrete carboxypeptide E, which is similarly able to remove arginine from the carboxyterminal tail of proteins. An increase of C3desArg would stimulate triglyceride uptake and glucose transport into adipocytes [57]. In the mouse it has been shown that CFB promotes adipocyte maturation and growth of fat droplets [58]. It is tempting to speculate that GR plus RF could have the same consequence. In addition, C3a has immune-modulatory properties and is often regarded as a pro-inflammatory factor [59]. Factor C3b in interaction with CBb converts C5 into C5a and C5b. C5a has chemotaxis activity and attracts neutrophils, basophils and macrophages. C5b forms with C6–C9 the membrane attack complex, which could be counteracted by the increase of clusterin (FC = 1.40, p = 0.09) [60]. Altogether, our in vitro observations suggest that changes in the complement system through GR plus RF may trigger uptake of triglycerides and glucose by adipocytes and may promote the attraction of immune cells (Figure 2). In fact, in the present study triglyceride content was measured by ORO staining and by measuring the diameter of the five biggest fat droplets [17]. The OD value was higher by about 10%, being 1.55 after NF and 1.69 after GR plus RF (p = 0.13). In line, the diameter was higher by about 14%, being 1.13 µm after NF and 1.29 µm after GR plus RF (p = 0.02). Although this is keeping with the proposed hypothesis, we have no absolute proof to attribute the increased fat content to the influence of complement factors. Regarding the involvement of the innate immune cells, gene expression studies in vivo have indicated that poor ability to reduce myeloid activity from the adipose tissue after weight loss is associated with increased risk of weight regain [11,61].

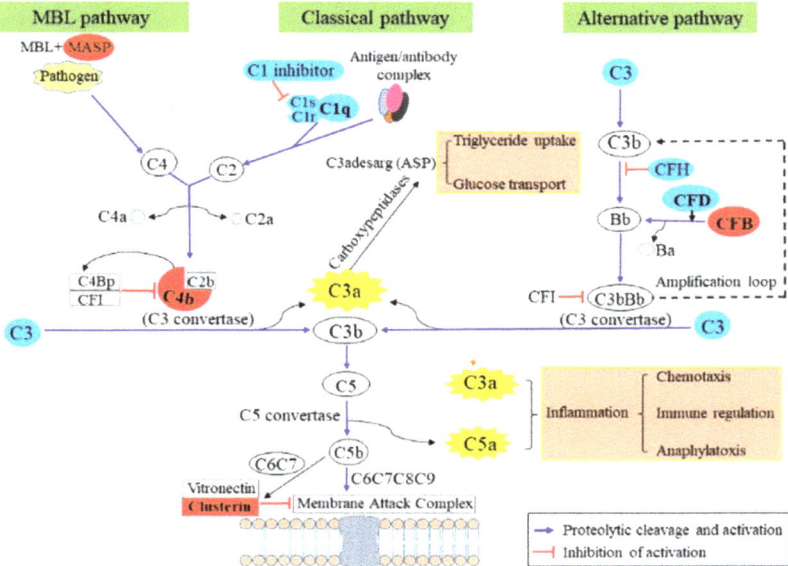

Figure 2. Complement activation pathway comparing GR plus RF with NF. Secreteome changes during GR plus RF vs NF indicate the up regulation of MBL and alternative pathways of the complement system, which may trigger the uptake of triglycerides and glucose by adipocytes on one hand and promote inflammation on the other, which both may have an effect on health after weight regain. Proteins in blue means that the expression was down-regulated (p < 0.1), red means up-regulated (p < 0.1), white are proteins that were not detected in our results. RF: refeeding, NF: normal feeding, GR: glucose restriction. MBL: mannose-binding lectin. MASP: mannose-binding lectin serine protease.

Various lysosome-based proteins were identified by our secretome profiling (Table 4). Lysosomes function as a key degradative compartment of cells, of which lysosomal cathepsins display an essential role in maintaining cell homeostasis by autophagy and extracellular matrix degradation [62–64]. Their extracellular function is mostly associated with pathology and disease including metabolic syndrome in people with obesity [65,66]. In the current study, we observed seven different cathepsins (A, B, D, F, K, L and Z) secreted by adipocytes. Five of the identified cathepsins were up-regulated by trend (Table 4) and two cathepsins were significantly up-regulated (Tables 3 and 4) after GR plus RF versus NF. In detail, cathepsin A (CTSA) and cathepsin L (CTSL) were significantly increased while other cathepsins showed a trend (Table 4). CTSA is able to stabilize the extracellular beta-galactosidase/neuraminidase-1 complex, which is involved in the formation of elastic fibers [67]. In addition, it processes important vascular proteins including endothelin-1, bradykinin and angiotensin I, which are important for the regulation of blood pressure [68]. Pharmacological inhibition indicates a role of CTSL in adipogenesis/fat storage and glucose tolerance. Inhibition of CTSL reduced fibronectin degradation and increased the levels of the beta-subunits of the insulin receptor and insulin-like growth factor-1-receptor [69]. Studies have also shown that CTSL, like cathepsin S (CTSS), has proatherogenic properties [70]. However, those studies did not specifically look at the extracellular function of CTSL. Yet, a literature survey has shown that CTSL is one of the cathepsins involved in extracellular matrix degradation and tissue remodeling [63]. Serum levels of CTSL did not alter following 6-month CR in obese women [71], but were reduced after an 8 week lifestyle intervention [72]. Here we show that GR plus RF significantly increased the extracellular CTSA and CTSL level. It seems therefore warranted to study the in vivo consequences of weight regain on plasma levels of cathepsins and assess the influence on fat storage, blood pressure and glucose tolerance.

Table 4. Complement factors and cathepsins.

Order	UniProt	Gene Symbol	Description	Category	FC	p Value
1	P00736	C1R	Complement C1r subcomponent	Complement factor	−1.00	0.716
2	Q07021	C1Q	Complement C1q subcomponent	Complement factor	−2.96	0.011
3	P09871	C1S	Complement C1s subcomponent	Complement factor	−1.53	0.131
4	P01024	C3	Complement C3	Complement factor	−1.03	0.840
5	P0C0L5	C4B	Complement C4-B	Complement factor	2.85	0.002
6	P00751	CFB	Complement factor B	Complement factor	4.06	0.018
7	P00746	CFD	Complement factor D	Complement factor	−1.93	0.002
8	P08603	CFH	Complement factor H	Complement factor	−1.15	0.277
9	P13987	CD59	CD59 glycoprotein	Complement factor	1.10	0.634
10	O00602	FCN1	Ficolin-1	Complement factor	−4.42	0.578
11	P05155	SERPING1	Plasma protease C1 inhibitor	Complement factor	−1.83	0.190
12	P48740	MASP1	Mannan-binding lectin serine protease 1	Complement factor	2.33	0.196
1	P10619	CTSA	Cathepsin A	Lysosome-based	2.75	0.009
2	P07858	CTSB	Cathepsin B	Lysosome-based	1.19	0.097
3	P07339	CTSD	Cathepsin D	Lysosome-based	1.16	0.309
4	Q9UBX1	CTSF	Cathepsin F	Lysosome-based	1.33	0.239
5	P43235	CTSK	Cathepsin K	Lysosome-based	1.45	NA
6	P07711	CTSL	Cathepsin L1	Lysosome-based	1.24	0.029
7	Q9UBR2	CTSZ	Cathepsin Z	Lysosome-based	1.08	0.466

Fold change (FC) was calculated with the abundance of T22RF/T18. When FC >1, the FC value was described as FC, otherwise the value was described as −1/FC. NA: abundance data available for only one sample. RF: refeeding, NF: normal feeding.

A number of proteins that change abundance significantly between GR plus RF and NF, has been described in relation to Alzheimer's disease. Amyloid-beta A4 protein (APP), which is a major component of the amyloid plaques in the brain of Alzheimer's patients [73], is 1.43× down-regulated. Extracellular SORT1, which has been reported to be involved in plaque formation [74], is 5.13× down-regulated in our study. PTGDS was 3.67× up-regulated due to GR plus RF. Interestingly, an up-regulation of the gene for *PTGDS* after ingestion of soybeans could lead to reduced amyloid-β accumulation and improved cognition [75]. A fourth protein, chitinase-3-like protein 2 (CHI3L2) is 3.43× up-regulated as the consequence of GR plus RF. CHI3L2 is known to bind to glycans, but lacks the required domain for chitinase activity [44]. Recently, it has been reported that the regional expression of

CHI3L2 in the brain of late-onset Alzheimer's patients is altered in comparison to healthy persons [76], but its function is presently unknown. Together, it would be worth to investigate whether weight cycling in humans could influence the expression of those proteins as well.

It should be noted that there are limitations to the present study. Firstly, SGBS cells have widely been used in vitro as a substitute for human white subcutaneous adipocytes since 2001 [13], but a study by Yeo et al. [77] indicated that SGBS cells may also have browning potential. Secondly, arguments including the fact that MS data are based on multiple peptide quantifications per protein, make it convincing that MS quantification is highly accurate [78,79]. Validation by another method has the risk of devaluating the quantitative data. Therefore, such validation was not performed. Thirdly, an in vitro model for weight loss and regain preferably is based on 'obese', hypertrophic fat cells. However, a hypertrophic phenotype of adipocytes differentiated in culture is difficult to define. For the present model it can be said that after 12 days of differentiation, SGBS cells contain 4× as much triglycerides than differentiated primary adipocytes [77]. Here we used 14 days differentiated SGBS cells with a 24% higher diameter of the five biggest fat droplets as compared to day 12 indicating an even higher fat content on day 14. Therefore, we feel confident to regard our findings as valuable clues for the consequences of weight loss and regain in overweight people. This can now be examined in human intervention studies.

4. Materials and Methods

4.1. Cell Culture

Human SGBS cells were obtained from Prof. Dr. M. Wabitsch (University of Ulm, Germany) [12]. SGBS pre-adipocytes were cultured in 6-well plates (Corning, Sigma-Aldrich, Zwijndrecht, The Netherlands) with Gibco™ Dulbecco's Modified Eagle Medium: Nutrient Mixture F-12 (DMEM/F-12, 1:1) media supplemented with 66 mmol/L biotin, 34 mmol/L D-pantothenate, 10% fetal calf serum (Bodinco BV, Alkmaar, The Netherlands) and 1% penicillin and streptomycin (Life Technologies, Thermo Fisher Scientific, Bleiswijk, The Netherlands) as described before [17]. Differentiation started once pre-adipocytes reached 90% confluence. During two weeks of differentiation (T0–T14), SGBS cells first went through four days with quick differentiation medium (serum-free DMEM/F12 medium containing 2 mg/mL human transferrin, 200 µmol/L human insulin, 5 mmol/L Cortisol, 20 µmol/L triiodothyronine, 1 mmol/L 3-isobutyl-1-methylxanthine and 5 mmol/L rosigilitazone). The other 10 days cells remained in 3FC medium (serum-free DMEM/F12 medium containing 2 mg/mL human transferrin, 200 µmol/L human insulin, 5 mmol/L Cortisol, 20 µmol/L triiodothyronine) as described before [17]. All chemicals were purchased from Sigma (Sigma-Aldrich, Zwijndrecht, The Netherlands) unless otherwise stated.

For GR, mature adipocytes on day 14 (T14) were cultured in basic DMEM/F12 medium (without glucose and phenol red (Cell Culture Technologies, Gravesano, Switzerland)), supplemented with 20 nmol/L human insulin and 0.1 mmol/L D-glucose for 96 h (T18GR). As the feeding control, mature adipocytes at T14 originating from the same pre-adipocytes were cultured for 96 h in NF medium (T18): DMEM/F12 medium without glucose and phenol red, but supplemented with 20 nmol/L human insulin and 17.5 mmol/L D-glucose.

For RF, after 96 h of GR, the cells were transferred to DMEM/F12 medium without glucose and phenol red (Cell Culture Technologies) but supplemented with 20 nmol/L human insulin and 17.5 mmol/L D-glucose for another 96 h (T22RF). From T14 onwards, the medium was gently refreshed every second day. Figure 3 provides an overview of the experimental approach.

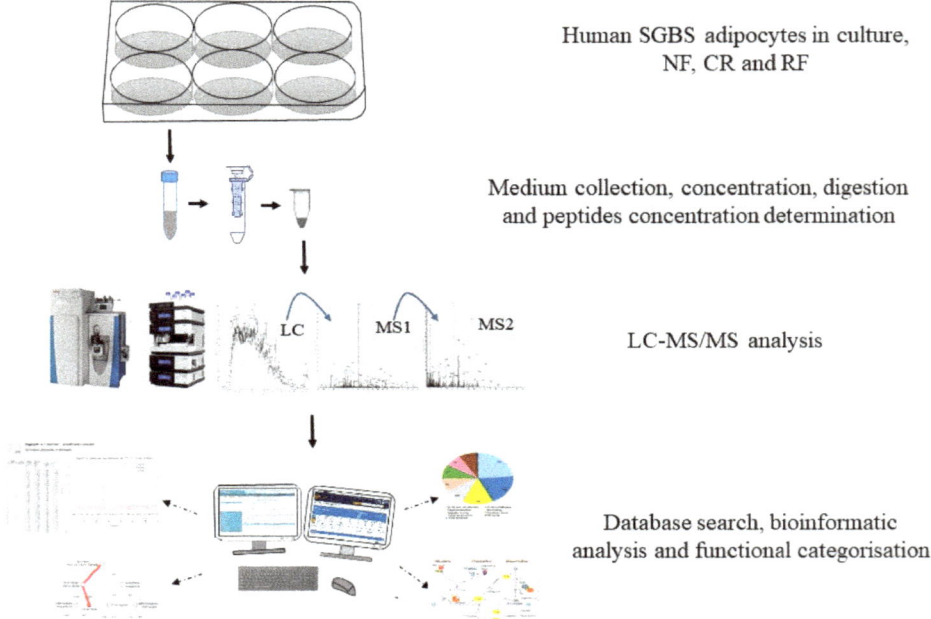

Figure 3. Workflow of the secretome profiling. Firstly, human SGBS adipocytes were cultured and after NF, GR and RF, medium was collected for all the time points. After sample preparation, proteins were identified and quantified by LC-MS/MS. Finally, bioinformatic and statistic analysis were performed for functional interpretation. NF: normal feeding, GR: glucose restriction, RF: refeeding.

4.2. Collection of Secretion Medium

In order to avoid interference of phenol red with MS, for collecting the secretome at T14, adipocyte medium was changed to collection medium: basal medium (DMEM/F12 (1:1) without glucose and phenol red (Cell Culture Technologies, Gravesano, Switzerland)), supplemented with 20 nmol/L human insulin and 17.5 mmol/L glucose for 48 h (T12–T14). The collection medium at T14 was collected in a separate vial for each well. For NF, GR and RF, the medium was already without phenol red from T14 onwards. To collect the secretome after NF, GR and RF, the medium was collected at day 18 (T18 and T18GR) and day 22 (T22RF) from each well separately. The collected medium (4 mL per well) was centrifuged at 5000 rpm for 10 min (Universal 30 RF, Hettich Benelux B.V., The Netherlands). Thereafter, the supernatant was gently moved to a new tube. The whole experiment was performed three times with triplicate samples. The first time the experiment was performed, the triplicate medium samples per time point were pooled to serve proper protocol assessment. For the second and third time that the experiment was performed, the triplicate samples were kept separately. This provided seven replicate samples per time point with in total 28 samples. These were snap-frozen in liquid nitrogen and stored at −80 °C for further analysis.

4.3. Sample Preparation

All samples were treated similarly according to the FASP protocol as described by Wisniewski et al. [80]. In short, after thawing and brief vortexing, the medium of each vial was added to a pre-rinsed filter device (Amicon® Ultra−4 Centrifugal Filter Units, Sigma-Aldrich, Germany), centrifuged at 4000× g at 20 °C for 30 min. The fluid was discarded and the concentrated protein sample on the filter was washed with 3.5 mL 50 mmol/L ammonium bicarbonate and centrifuged at 4000× g at 20 °C for 30 min. For reduction, 15 µL of 200 mmol/L dithiothreitol was added and the filter was incubated at room temperature for 45 min. Next, to accomplish alkylation 18 µL of 400 mmol/L iodoacetamide solution was added and the filter was incubated at room temperature in the darkness for another 45 min. To stop the alkylation, 30 µL of 200 mmol/L dithiothreitol was added and the filter was incubated at room temperature for 45 min.

The alkylated protein sample on the filter was washed with 50 mmol/L ammonium bicarbonate at 4000× g at 20 °C for 40 min. To each concentrated protein sample 3 µg trypsin/Lys-C Mix was added, and after gentle mixing the filter device was incubated at 37 °C overnight. Peptide concentration was measured by the Pierce Quantitative Colorimetric Peptide Assay according to the manufacture's protocol (Thermo Fisher Scientific (#: 23275), Bleiswijk, The Netherlands). Then, digested peptides were diluted to the same final concentration of 0.25 µg/µL by 50 mmol/L ammonium bicarbonate.

4.4. Label-Free Protein Identification and Quantification

The mass analysis was performed using a nanoflow HPLC instrument (Dionex ultimate 3000, Thermo Fisher Scientific, Bleiswijk, The Netherlands), which was coupled on-line to a Q Exactive mass-spectrometer (Thermo Fisher Scientific, Bleiswijk, The Netherlands) with a nano-electrospray Flex ion source (Proxeon, Thermo Fisher Scientific, Bleiswijk, The Netherlands). An equal amount of Pierce Digestion Indicator peptides was added to all peptide samples as internal standard. 5 µL of this mixture was loaded onto a C18-reversed phase column (Acclaim PepMap C18 column, 75 µm inner diameter × 15 cm, 2 µm particle size, Thermo Fisher Scientific, Bleiswijk, The Netherlands). The peptides were separated with a linear gradient of 4–68% buffer B (80% acetonitrile and 0.08% formic acid) at a flow rate of 300 nL/min for 120 min.

MS data were acquired using a data-dependent top-10 method, dynamically choosing the most abundant precursor ions from the survey scan (280–1400 m/z) in positive mode. Survey scans were acquired at a resolution of 70,000 and a maximum injection time of 120 ms. The dynamic exclusion duration was 30 s. Isolation of precursors was performed with a 1.8 m/z window and a maximum injection time of 200 ms. The resolution for HCD spectra was set to 17,500 and the normalized collision energy was 30 eV. The under-fill ratio was defined as 1.0%. The instrument was run with peptide recognition mode enabled, but exclusion of singly charged and charge states of more than five. The entire experiment was repeated three times.

4.5. Database Search and Quantification

The MS data were searched using Proteome Discoverer 2.2 Sequest HT search engine (Thermo Fisher Scientific, Bleiswijk, The Netherlands) based on the UniProt human database [81]. The false discovery rate was set to 0.01 for proteins and peptides, which had to have a minimum length of six amino acids. The precursor mass tolerance was set at 10 ppm and the fragment tolerance at 0.02 Da. One miss-cleavage was tolerated, oxidation of methionine was set as a dynamic modification as well as carbamidomethylation of cysteines. Label free quantitation was conducted using the Minora Feature Detector node in the processing step and the Feature Mapper node combined with the Precursor Ions Quantifier node in the consensus step with default settings within Proteome Discoverer 2.2.

4.6. Data Normalization

The LC-MS-analysis was done in seven runs, each run containing a sample from each time point (T14, T18, T18GR and T22RF). Data normalization was done in two steps.

First, to correct data for possible differences between runs, we chose the 426 proteins, which were present in all of the test samples. We calculated the mean abundance of those 426 proteins in all seven runs (M) and mean abundance of those 426 proteins per run (m_x for run x). Normalization factor 1 for run x ($f1_x$) = M ÷ m_x. Data were firstly corrected (D1) as follows: D1 = $f1_x$ × original tested protein abundance in run x.

Additionally, the Pierce Indicator added to each sample was normalized by f1. The second normalization was then performed to stratify the protein abundances according to the Pierce Indicator. Normalization factor 2 for sample y ($f2_y$) = Pierce's mean abundance from all 28 samples ÷ Pierce abundance in sample y. In general, the second normalization step was: D2 = f2 × D1. More specifically, the abundance of a protein in sample y of run x was normalized as $f1_x$ × $f2_y$ × original tested protein abundance.

4.7. Validation of Secreted Proteins and Imputation of Missing Values

To verify the secreted nature of the identified proteins, their amino acid sequences were obtained from UniProt and analyzed with SignalP and Deeploc. SignalP 4.1 Server [46,82] was used to recognize classical secreted proteins by the fact that they contain a signal peptide for secretion, Deeploc–1.0 [49] was used for prediction of the subcellular localization by creating a recurrent neural network relying on protein sequence information per se. Proteins containing a signal peptide or located in the extracellular space were chosen as secreted proteins for further analysis.

Performing LC-MS analysis of proteins, values could be missing for various reasons [83]. When per time point three or less of the seven samples had missing values, the Multiple Imputation routine of SPSS was used to impute those values. Finally, only proteins recognized as secreted and with no more than three missing values were used for further analysis.

4.8. Statistical Analysis

Data were described as mean ± SEM, variable abundances were log_2-transformed. To determine possible effects over time between NF and RF after GR, two-tailed dependent T-test was carried out with a cut-off for significance of $p < 0.05$. Statistical analyses were conducted using SPSS (version 22.0 Chicago, Illinois, USA). Fold changes (FC) from T18 to T22RF were calculated as follows: FC = 2 (log_2 T22RF − log_2 T18).

5. Conclusions

In summary, in this study we reported for the first time 94 proteins being secreted by adipocytes. In addition, our in vitro study demonstrated that GR followed by return to NF leads to changes in the secretome of adipocytes in comparison with NF alone. Major changes are related to extracellular matrix modification, factors of the complement system, extracellular cathepsins, and several proteins relevant for Alzheimer's disease. These observations can now be used as clues to investigate the metabolic consequences of weight regain, weight cycling or intermittent fasting.

Supplementary Materials: Supplementary materials can be found at http://www.mdpi.com/1422-0067/20/16/4055/s1, (The file contains Tables S1 and S2).

Author Contributions: Conceptualization, E.C.M.M. and Q.Q.; methodology, Q.Q., F.G.B., and J.R.; software, F.G.B. and Q.Q.; formal analysis, E.C.M.M., F.G.B. and Q.Q.; investigation, Q.Q. and F.G.B.; resources, E.C.M.M.; data curation, Q.Q. and E.C.M.M.; writing—original draft preparation, Q.Q.; writing—review and editing, F.G.B., J.R., M.A.v.B. and E.C.M.M.; visualization, Q.Q.; supervision, E.C.M.M.; project administration, E.C.M.M.; funding acquisition, Q.Q.

Funding: Qi Qiao is supported by the China Scholarship Council (File No. 201707720057).

Acknowledgments: We would like to thank med. Martin Wabitsch (University of Ulm in Germany) for kindly donating the human SGBS cell line.

Conflicts of Interest: The authors declare no conflict of interest.

Abbreviations

CR	calorie restriction
SGBS	Simpson Golabi Behmel Syndrome
GR	glucose restriction
RF	refeeding

NF	normal feeding
DMEM/F12	Dulbecco's Modified Eagle Medium: Nutrient Mixture F-12
FC	fold change
C1q	complement factor 1Q
AOC3	membrane primary amine oxidase
CSRP1	cysteine and glycine-rich protein 1
LGALS1	galectin-1
DDT	D-dopachrome decarboxylase
PRSS3	trypsin-3
MT1G	metallothionein-1G
PSMF1	proteasome inhibitor subunit 1
SPRR2G	small proline-rich protein 2G
ENPP2	ectonucleotide pyrophosphatase/phosphodiesterase family member 2
ECM	extracellular matrix
LC-MS/MS	liquid chromatography tandem mass spectrometry
CFB	complement factor B
ADAMTSL1	ADAMTS-like protein 1
AEI3BP	target of Nesh-SH3
CES1	liver carboxylesterase 1
SORT1	sortilin
DMKN	dermokine
PTGDS	prostaglandin-H2 D-isomerase
C4-B	complement factor 4B
CFD	complement factor D
ASP	acylation-stimulating protein
CTSA	cathepsin A
CTSB	cathepsin B
CTSL	cathepsin L
CTSS	cathepsin S
APP	amyloid-beta A4 protein
CHI3L2	chitinase-3-like protein 2
MASP	mannan-binding lectin serine protease

References

1. Fruh, S.M. Obesity: Risk factors, complications, and strategies for sustainable long-term weight management. *J. Am. Assoc. Nurse Pract.* **2017**, *29*, S3–S14. [CrossRef] [PubMed]
2. Lehr, S.; Hartwig, S.; Sell, H. Adipokines: A treasure trove for the discovery of biomarkers for metabolic disorders. *Proteom. Clin. Appl.* **2012**, *6*, 91–101. [CrossRef] [PubMed]
3. Rosenow, A.; Arrey, T.N.; Bouwman, F.G.; Noben, J.P.; Wabitsch, M.; Mariman, E.C.; Karas, M.; Renes, J. Identification of novel human adipocyte secreted proteins by using SGBS cells. *J. Proteome Res.* **2010**, *9*, 5389–5401. [CrossRef] [PubMed]
4. Mohamed-Ali, V.; Pinkney, J.H.; Coppack, S.W. Adipose tissue as an endocrine and paracrine organ. *Int. J. Obes.* **1998**, *22*, 1145–1158. [CrossRef]
5. Ouchi, N.; Parker, J.L.; Lugus, J.J.; Walsh, K. Adipokines in inflammation and metabolic disease. *Nat. Rev. Immunol.* **2011**, *11*, 85–97. [CrossRef] [PubMed]
6. de las Fuentes, L.; Waggoner, A.D.; Mohammed, B.S.; Stein, R.I.; Miller, B.V., 3rd; Foster, G.D.; Wyatt, H.R.; Klein, S.; Davila-Roman, V.G. Effect of moderate diet-induced weight loss and weight regain on cardiovascular structure and function. *J. Am. Coll. Cardiol.* **2009**, *54*, 2376–2381. [CrossRef] [PubMed]
7. Horton, E.S. Effects of Lifestyle Changes to Reduce Risks of Diabetes and Associated Cardiovascular Risks: Results from Large Scale Efficacy Trials. *Obesity* **2009**, *17*, S43–S48. [CrossRef] [PubMed]
8. Renes, J.; Rosenow, A.; Roumans, N.; Noben, J.P.; Mariman, E.C. Calorie restriction-induced changes in the secretome of human adipocytes, comparison with resveratrol-induced secretome effects. *Biochim. Biophys. Acta* **2014**, *1844*, 1511–1522. [CrossRef] [PubMed]

9. Barte, J.C.M.; ter Bogt, N.C.W.; Bogers, R.P.; Teixeira, P.J.; Blissmer, B.; Mori, T.A.; Bemelmans, W.J.E. Maintenance of weight loss after lifestyle interventions for overweight and obesity, a systematic review. *Obes. Rev.* **2010**, *11*, 899–906. [CrossRef]
10. Delahanty, L.M.; Pan, Q.; Jablonski, K.A.; Aroda, V.R.; Watson, K.E.; Bray, G.A.; Kahn, S.E.; Florez, J.C.; Perreault, L.; Franks, P.W.; et al. Effects of weight loss, weight cycling, and weight loss maintenance on diabetes incidence and change in cardiometabolic traits in the Diabetes Prevention Program. *Diabetes Care* **2014**, *37*, 2738–2745. [CrossRef]
11. Van Baak, M.A.; Mariman, E.C.M. Mechanisms of weight regain after weight loss - the role of adipose tissue. *Nat. Rev. Endocrinol.* **2019**, *15*, 274–287. [CrossRef] [PubMed]
12. Wabitsch, M.; Brenner, R.E.; Melzner, I.; Braun, M.; Moller, P.; Heinze, E.; Debatin, K.M.; Hauner, H. Characterization of a human preadipocyte cell strain with high capacity for adipose differentiation. *Int. J. Obes.* **2001**, *25*, 8–15. [CrossRef]
13. Fischer-Posovszky, P.; Newell, F.S.; Wabitsch, M.; Tornqvist, H.E. Human SGBS Cells-a Unique Tool for Studies of Human Fat Cell Biology. *Obes. Facts* **2008**, *1*, 184–189. [CrossRef] [PubMed]
14. Buttner, P.; Bluher, M.; Wabitsch, M.; Kiess, W.; Korner, A. Expression profiles of human adipocyte differentiation using the SGBS cell model. *Horm. Res.* **2008**, *70*, 68.
15. Allott, E.H.; Oliver, E.; Lysaght, J.; Gray, S.G.; Reynolds, J.V.; Roche, H.M.; Pidgeon, G.P. The SGBS cell strain as a model for the in vitro study of obesity and cancer. *Clin. Transl. Oncol.* **2012**, *14*, 774–782. [CrossRef] [PubMed]
16. Rosenow, A.; Noben, J.P.; Jocken, J.; Kallendrusch, S.; Fischer-Posovszky, P.; Mariman, E.C.; Renes, J. Resveratrol-induced changes of the human adipocyte secretion profile. *J. Proteome Res.* **2012**, *11*, 4733–4743. [CrossRef] [PubMed]
17. Qiao, Q.; Bouwman, F.G.; van Baak, M.A.; Roumans, N.J.T.; Vink, R.G.; Coort, S.L.M.; Renes, J.W.; Mariman, E.C.M. Adipocyte abundances of CES1, CRYAB, ENO1 and GANAB are modified in-vitro by glucose restriction and are associated with cellular remodelling during weight regain. *Adipocyte* **2019**, *8*, 190–200. [CrossRef]
18. Wang, P.; Mariman, E.; Keijer, J.; Bouwman, F.; Noben, J.P.; Robben, J.; Renes, J. Profiling of the secreted proteins during 3T3-L1 adipocyte differentiation leads to the identification of novel adipokines. *Cell Mol. Life Sci.* **2004**, *61*, 2405–2417. [CrossRef]
19. Chen, X.L.; Cushman, S.W.; Pannell, L.K.; Hess, S. Quantitative proteomic analysis of the secretory proteins from rat adipose cells using a 2D liquid chromatography-MS/MS approach. *J. Proteome Res.* **2005**, *4*, 570–577. [CrossRef]
20. Molina, H.; Yang, Y.; Ruch, T.; Kim, J.W.; Mortensen, P.; Otto, T.; Nalli, A.; Tang, Q.Q.; Lane, M.D.; Chaerkady, R.; et al. Temporal Profiling of the Adipocyte Proteome during Differentiation Using a Five-Plex SILAC Based Strategy. *J. Proteome Res.* **2009**, *8*, 48–58. [CrossRef]
21. Celis, J.E.; Moreira, J.M.A.; Cabezon, T.; Gromov, P.; Friis, E.; Rank, F.; Gromova, I. Identification of extracellular and intracellular signaling components of the mammary adipose tissue and its interstitial fluid in high risk breast cancer patients—Toward dissecting the molecular circuitry of epithelial-adipocyte stromal cell interactions. *Mol. Cell Proteom.* **2005**, *4*, 492–522. [CrossRef]
22. Mutch, D.M.; Rouault, C.; Keophiphath, M.; Lacasa, D.; Clement, K. Using gene expression to predict the secretome of differentiating human preadipocytes. *Int. J. Obes.* **2009**, *33*, 354–363. [CrossRef] [PubMed]
23. Alvarez-Llamas, G.; Szalowska, E.; de Vries, M.P.; Weening, D.; Landman, K.; Hoek, A.; Wolffenbuttel, B.H.R.; Roelofsen, H.; Vonk, R.J. Characterization of the human visceral adipose tissue secretome. *Mol. Cell Proteom.* **2007**, *6*, 589–600. [CrossRef] [PubMed]
24. Zvonic, S.; Lefevre, M.; Kilroy, G.; Floyd, Z.E.; DeLany, J.P.; Kheterpal, I.; Gravois, A.; Dow, R.; White, A.; Wu, X.Y.; et al. Secretome of primary cultures of human adipose-derived stem cells—Modulation of serpins by adipogenesis. *Mol. Cell Proteom.* **2007**, *6*, 18–28. [CrossRef] [PubMed]
25. Kim, J.; Choi, Y.S.; Lim, S.; Yea, K.; Yoon, J.H.; Jun, D.J.; Ha, S.H.; Kim, J.W.; Kim, J.H.; Suh, P.G.; et al. Comparative analysis of the secretory proteome of human adipose stromal vascular fraction cells during adipogenesis. *Proteomics* **2010**, *10*, 394–405. [CrossRef] [PubMed]
26. Zhong, J.; Krawczyk, S.A.; Chaerkady, R.; Huang, H.L.; Goel, R.; Bader, J.S.; Wong, G.W.; Corkey, B.E.; Pandey, A. Temporal Profiling of the Secretome during Adipogenesis in Humans. *J. Proteome Res.* **2010**, *9*, 5228–5238. [CrossRef] [PubMed]

27. Lee, M.J.; Kim, J.; Kim, M.Y.; Bae, Y.S.; Ryu, S.H.; Lee, T.G.; Kim, J.H. Proteomic Analysis of Tumor Necrosis Factor-alpha-Induced Secretome of Human Adipose Tissue-Derived Mesenchymal Stem Cells. *J. Proteome Res.* **2010**, *9*, 1754–1762. [CrossRef] [PubMed]
28. Lehr, S.; Hartwig, S.; Lamers, D.; Famulla, S.; Muller, S.; Hanisch, F.G.; Cuvelier, C.; Ruige, J.; Eckardt, K.; Ouwens, D.M.; et al. Identification and Validation of Novel Adipokines Released from Primary Human Adipocytes. *Mol. Cell Proteom.* **2012**, *11*. [CrossRef] [PubMed]
29. Li, Z.Y.; Zheng, S.L.; Wang, P.; Xu, T.Y.; Guan, Y.F.; Zhang, Y.J.; Miao, C.Y. Subfatin is a Novel Adipokine and Unlike Meteorin in Adipose and Brain Expression. *CNS Neurosci.* **2014**, *20*, 344–354. [CrossRef] [PubMed]
30. Ali Khan, A.; Hansson, J.; Weber, P.; Foehr, S.; Krijgsveld, J.; Herzig, S.; Scheideler, M. Comparative Secretome Analyses of Primary Murine White and Brown Adipocytes Reveal Novel Adipokines. *Mol. Cell Proteom.* **2018**, *17*, 2358–2370. [CrossRef]
31. Lim, J.M.; Sherling, D.; Teo, C.F.; Hausman, D.B.; Lin, D.W.; Wells, L. Defining the regulated secreted proteome of rodent adipocytes upon the induction of insulin resistance. *J. Proteome Res.* **2008**, *7*, 1251–1263. [CrossRef]
32. Roelofsen, H.; Dijkstra, M.; Weening, D.; de Vries, M.P.; Hoek, A.; Vonk, R.J. Comparison of Isotope-labeled Amino Acid Incorporation Rates (CILAIR) Provides a Quantitative Method to Study Tissue Secretomes. *Mol. Cell Proteom.* **2009**, *8*, 316–324. [CrossRef] [PubMed]
33. Mariman, E.C.; Wang, P. Adipocyte extracellular matrix composition, dynamics and role in obesity. *Cell Mol. Life Sci.* **2010**, *67*, 1277–1292. [CrossRef] [PubMed]
34. Ojima, K.; Oe, M.; Nakajima, I.; Muroya, S.; Nishimura, T. Dynamics of protein secretion during adipocyte differentiation. *FEBS Open Bio* **2016**, *6*, 816–826. [CrossRef] [PubMed]
35. Renes, J.; Mariman, E. Application of proteomics technology in adipocyte biology. *Mol. Biosyst.* **2013**, *9*, 1076–1091. [CrossRef] [PubMed]
36. Hartwig, S.; De Filippo, E.; Goddeke, S.; Knebel, B.; Kotzka, J.; Al-Hasani, H.; Roden, M.; Lehr, S.; Sell, H. Exosomal proteins constitute an essential part of the human adipose tissue secretome. *Biochim. Biophys. Acta Proteins Proteom.* **2018**. [CrossRef]
37. Laria, A.E.; Messineo, S.; Arcidiacono, B.; Varano, M.; Chiefari, E.; Semple, R.K.; Rocha, N.; Russo, D.; Cuda, G.; Gaspari, M.; et al. Secretome Analysis of Hypoxia- Induced 3T3-L1 Adipocytes Uncovers Novel Proteins Potentially Involved in Obesity. *Proteomics* **2018**, *18*. [CrossRef]
38. Roca-Rivada, A.; Bravo, S.B.; Perez-Sotelo, D.; Alonso, J.; Castro, A.I.; Baamonde, I.; Baltar, J.; Casanueva, F.F.; Pardo, M. CILAIR-Based Secretome Analysis of Obese Visceral and Subcutaneous Adipose Tissues Reveals Distinctive ECM Remodeling and Inflammation Mediators. *Sci. Rep.* **2015**, *5*, 12214. [CrossRef]
39. Pardo, M.; Roca-Rivada, A.; Seoane, L.M.; Casanueva, F.F. Obesidomics: Contribution of adipose tissue secretome analysis to obesity research. *Endocrine* **2012**, *41*, 374–383. [CrossRef]
40. Roca-Rivada, A.; Alonso, J.; Al-Massadi, O.; Castelao, C.; Peinado, J.R.; Seoane, L.M.; Casanueva, F.F.; Pardo, M. Secretome analysis of rat adipose tissues shows location-specific roles for each depot type. *J. Proteom.* **2011**, *74*, 1068–1079. [CrossRef]
41. Sano, S.; Izumi, Y.; Yamaguchi, T.; Yamazaki, T.; Tanaka, M.; Shiota, M.; Osada-Oka, M.; Nakamura, Y.; Wei, M.; Wanibuchi, H.; et al. Lipid synthesis is promoted by hypoxic adipocyte-derived exosomes in 3T3-L1 cells. *Biochem. Biophys. Res. Commun.* **2014**, *445*, 327–333. [CrossRef] [PubMed]
42. Lee, M.W.; Lee, M.; Oh, K.J. Adipose Tissue-Derived Signatures for Obesity and Type 2 Diabetes: Adipokines, Batokines and MicroRNAs. *J. Clin. Med.* **2019**, *8*, 854. [CrossRef] [PubMed]
43. GeneCards. Available online: https://www.genecards.org/ (accessed on 19 August 2019).
44. UniProt. Available online: https://www.uniprot.org/ (accessed on 19 August 2019).
45. PubMed. Available online: https://www.ncbi.nlm.nih.gov/pubmed/ (accessed on 19 August 2019).
46. Nielsen, H. Predicting Secretory Proteins with SignalP. *Methods Mol. Biol.* **2017**, *1611*, 59–73. [CrossRef]
47. Bendtsen, J.D.; Jensen, L.J.; Blom, N.; Von Heijne, G.; Brunak, S. Feature-based prediction of non-classical and leaderless protein secretion. *Protein Eng. Des. Sel.* **2004**, *17*, 349–356. [CrossRef] [PubMed]
48. Nielsen, H.; Petsalaki, E.I.; Zhao, L.; Stuhler, K. Predicting eukaryotic protein secretion without signals. *Biochim. Biophys. Acta Proteins Proteom.* **2018**. [CrossRef] [PubMed]
49. Armenteros, J.J.A.; Sonderby, C.K.; Sonderby, S.K.; Nielsen, H.; Winther, O. DeepLoc: Prediction of protein subcellular localization using deep learning. *Bioinformatics* **2017**, *33*, 3387–3395. [CrossRef] [PubMed]

50. Rodriguez-Manzaneque, J.C.; Westling, J.; Thai, S.N.M.; Luque, A.; Knauper, V.; Murphy, G.; Sandy, J.D.; Iruela-Arispe, M. ADAMTS1 cleaves aggrecan at multiple sites and is differentially inhibited by metalloproteinase inhibitors. *Biochem. Biophys. Res. Commun.* **2002**, *293*, 501–508. [CrossRef]
51. Roumans, N.J.T.; Wang, P.; Vink, R.G.; van Baak, M.A.; Mariman, E.C.M. Combined Analysis of Stress- and ECM-Related Genes in Their Effect on Weight Regain. *Obesity* **2018**, *26*, 492–498. [CrossRef] [PubMed]
52. Moreno-Navarrete, J.M.; Fernandez-Real, J.M. The complement system is dysfunctional in metabolic disease: Evidences in plasma and adipose tissue from obese and insulin resistant subjects. *Semin. Cell Dev. Biol.* **2019**, *85*, 164–172. [CrossRef]
53. Kaye, S.; Lokki, A.I.; Hanttu, A.; Nissila, E.; Heinonen, S.; Hakkarainen, A.; Lundbom, J.; Lundbom, N.; Saarinen, L.; Tynninen, O.; et al. Upregulation of Early and Downregulation of Terminal Pathway Complement Genes in Subcutaneous Adipose Tissue and Adipocytes in Acquired Obesity. *Front. Immunol.* **2017**, *8*, 545. [CrossRef]
54. Van Greevenbroek, M.M.J.; Ghosh, S.; van der Kallen, C.J.H.; Brouwers, M.C.G.J.; Schalkwijk, C.G.; Stehouwer, C.D.A. Up-Regulation of the Complement System in Subcutaneous Adipocytes from Nonobese, Hypertriglyceridemic Subjects Is Associated with Adipocyte Insulin Resistance. *J. Clin. Endocr. Metab.* **2012**, *97*, 4742–4752. [CrossRef] [PubMed]
55. Nilsson, B.; Hamad, O.A.; Ahlstrom, H.; Kullberg, J.; Johansson, L.; Lindhagen, L.; Haenni, A.; Ekdahl, K.N.; Lind, L. C3 and C4 are strongly related to adipose tissue variables and cardiovascular risk factors. *Eur. J. Clin. Investig.* **2014**, *44*, 587–596. [CrossRef] [PubMed]
56. Cianflone, K.; Xia, Z.N.; Chen, L.Y. Critical review of acylation-stimulating protein physiology in humans and rodents. *BBA-Biomembr.* **2003**, *1609*, 127–143. [CrossRef]
57. Cui, W.; Paglialunga, S.; Kalant, D.; Lu, H.; Roy, C.; Laplante, M.; Deshaies, Y.; Cianflone, K. Acylation-stimulating protein/C5L2-neutralizing antibodies alter triglyceride metabolism in vitro and in vivo. *Am. J. Physiol.-Endoc. Metab.* **2007**, *293*, E1482–E1491. [CrossRef] [PubMed]
58. Matsunaga, H.; Iwashita, M.; Shinjo, T.; Yamashita, A.; Tsuruta, M.; Nagasaka, S.; Taniguchi, A.; Fukushima, M.; Watanabe, N.; Nishimura, F. Adipose tissue complement factor B promotes adipocyte maturation. *Biochem. Biophys. Res. Commun.* **2018**, *495*, 740–748. [CrossRef] [PubMed]
59. Coulthard, L.G.; Woodruff, T.M. Is the Complement Activation Product C3a a Proinflammatory Molecule? Re-evaluating the Evidence and the Myth. *J. Immunol.* **2015**, *194*, 3542–3548. [CrossRef] [PubMed]
60. Tschopp, J.; Chonn, A.; Hertig, S.; French, L.E. Clusterin, the Human Apolipoprotein and Complement Inhibitor, Binds to Complement-C7, C8-Beta, and the B-Domain of C9. *J. Immunol.* **1993**, *151*, 2159–2165. [PubMed]
61. Roumans, N.J.; Vink, R.G.; Fazelzadeh, P.; van Baak, M.A.; Mariman, E.C. A role for leukocyte integrins and extracellular matrix remodeling of adipose tissue in the risk of weight regain after weight loss. *Am. J. Clin. Nutr.* **2017**, *105*, 1054–1062. [CrossRef] [PubMed]
62. Fonovic, M.; Turk, B. Cysteine cathepsins and extracellular matrix degradation. *BBA-Gen. Subj.* **2014**, *1840*, 2560–2570. [CrossRef] [PubMed]
63. Vidak, E.; Javorsek, U.; Vizovisek, M.; Turk, B. Cysteine Cathepsins and Their Extracellular Roles: Shaping the Microenvironment. *Cells* **2019**, *8*, 264. [CrossRef]
64. Vizovisek, M.; Fonovic, M.; Turk, B. Cysteine cathepsins in extracellular matrix remodeling: Extracellular matrix degradation and beyond. *Matrix Biol.* **2019**, *75–76*, 141–159. [CrossRef] [PubMed]
65. Kramer, L.; Turk, D.; Turk, B. The Future of Cysteine Cathepsins in Disease Management. *Trends Pharm. Sci.* **2017**, *38*, 873–898. [CrossRef] [PubMed]
66. Chen, L.L.; Bin, L.; Yang, Y.H.; Zhang, W.W.; Wang, X.C.; Zhou, H.G.; Wen, J.; Yang, Z.; Hu, R.M. Elevated circulating cathepsin S levels are associated with metabolic syndrome in overweight and obese individuals. *Diabetes-Metab. Res.* **2019**, *35*. [CrossRef] [PubMed]
67. Hinek, A.; Pshezhetsky, A.V.; von Itzstein, M.; Starcher, B. Lysosomal sialidase (neuraminidase-1) is targeted to the cell surface in a multiprotein complex that facilitates elastic fiber assembly. *J. Biol. Chem.* **2006**, *281*, 3698–3710. [CrossRef] [PubMed]
68. Pshezhetsky, A.V.; Hinek, A. Serine Carboxypeptidases in Regulation of Vasoconstriction and Elastogenesis. *Trends Cardiovas. Med.* **2009**, *19*, 11–17. [CrossRef]

69. Yang, M.; Zhang, Y.; Pan, J.; Sun, J.; Liu, J.; Libby, P.; Sukhova, G.K.; Doria, A.; Katunuma, N.; Peroni, O.D.; et al. Cathepsin L activity controls adipogenesis and glucose tolerance. *Nat. Cell Biol.* **2007**, *9*, 970–977. [CrossRef]
70. Lafarge, J.C.; Naour, N.; Clement, K.; Guerre-Millo, M. Cathepsins and cystatin C in atherosclerosis and obesity. *Biochimie* **2010**, *92*, 1580–1586. [CrossRef]
71. Naour, N.; Rouault, C.; Fellahi, S.; Lavoie, M.E.; Poitou, C.; Keophiphath, M.; Eberle, D.; Shoelson, S.; Rizkalla, S.; Bastard, J.P.; et al. Cathepsins in Human Obesity: Changes in Energy Balance Predominantly Affect Cathepsin S in Adipose Tissue and in Circulation. *J. Clin. Endocr. Metab.* **2010**, *95*, 1861–1868. [CrossRef]
72. Larsson, A.; Svensson, M.B.; Ronquist, G.; Akerfeldt, T. Life Style Intervention in Moderately Overweight Individuals Is Associated with Decreased Levels of Cathepsins L and S in Plasma. *Ann. Clin. Lab. Sci.* **2014**, *44*, 283–285.
73. O'Brien, R.J.; Wong, P.C. Amyloid Precursor Protein Processing and Alzheimer's Disease. *Annu. Rev. Neurosci.* **2011**, *34*, 185–204. [CrossRef]
74. Xu, S.Y.; Jiang, J.; Pan, A.; Yan, C.; Yan, X.X. Sortilin: A new player in dementia and Alzheimer-type neuropathology. *Biochem. Cell Biol.* **2018**, *96*, 491–497. [CrossRef] [PubMed]
75. Unno, K.; Konishi, T. Preventive Effect of Soybean on Brain Aging and Amyloid-beta Accumulation: Comprehensive Analysis of Brain Gene Expression. *Recent Pat. Food Nutr. Agric.* **2015**, *7*, 83–91. [CrossRef] [PubMed]
76. Sanfilippo, C.; Malaguarnera, L.; Di Rosa, M. Chitinase expression in Alzheimer's disease and non-demented brains regions. *J. Neurol. Sci.* **2016**, *369*, 242–249. [CrossRef] [PubMed]
77. Yeo, C.R.; Agrawal, M.; Hoon, S.; Shabbir, A.; Shrivastava, M.K.; Huang, S.; Khoo, C.M.; Chhay, V.; Yassin, M.S.; Tai, E.S.; et al. SGBS cells as a model of human adipocyte browning: A comprehensive comparative study with primary human white subcutaneous adipocytes. *Sci. Rep.* **2017**, *7*, 4031. [CrossRef] [PubMed]
78. Aebersold, R.; Burlingame, A.L.; Bradshaw, R.A. Western blots versus selected reaction monitoring assays: Time to turn the tables? *Mol. Cell Proteom.* **2013**, *12*, 2381–2382. [CrossRef] [PubMed]
79. Bults, P.; van de Merbel, N.C.; Bischoff, R. Quantification of biopharmaceuticals and biomarkers in complex biological matrices: A comparison of liquid chromatography coupled to tandem mass spectrometry and ligand binding assays. *Expert Rev. Proteom.* **2015**, *12*, 355–374. [CrossRef] [PubMed]
80. Wisniewski, J.R.; Zougman, A.; Nagaraj, N.; Mann, M. Universal sample preparation method for proteome analysis. *Nat. Methods* **2009**, *6*, 359–362. [CrossRef] [PubMed]
81. UniProt Human Database. Available online: https://www.uniprotKB.org/uniprot/Swiss-Prot/Homosapiens(Human)/ (accessed on 19 August 2019).
82. Petersen, T.N.; Brunak, S.; von Heijne, G.; Nielsen, H. SignalP 4.0: Discriminating signal peptides from transmembrane regions. *Nat. Methods* **2011**, *8*, 785–786. [CrossRef] [PubMed]
83. Karpievitch, Y.V.; Dabney, A.R.; Smith, R.D. Normalization and missing value imputation for label-free LC-MS analysis. *BMC Bioinform.* **2012**, *13*, S5. [CrossRef] [PubMed]

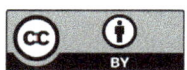

© 2019 by the authors. Licensee MDPI, Basel, Switzerland. This article is an open access article distributed under the terms and conditions of the Creative Commons Attribution (CC BY) license (http://creativecommons.org/licenses/by/4.0/).

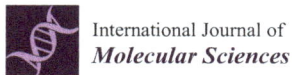

Review

Metabolic Health—The Role of Adipo-Myokines

Christine Graf [1,2,*,†] and Nina Ferrari [2,†]

[1] Department for physical activity in public health, Institute of Movement and Neurosciences, Am Sportpark Müngersdorf 6, German Sport University Cologne, 50933 Cologne, Germany
[2] Cologne Center for Prevention in Childhood and Youth/Heart Center Cologne, University Hospital of Cologne, Kerpener Str. 62, 50937 Cologne, Germany; nina.ferrari@uk-koeln.de
* Correspondence: c.graf@dshs-koeln.de; Tel.: +49-221-49825290
† Authors contributed equally to this work.

Received: 12 November 2019; Accepted: 4 December 2019; Published: 6 December 2019

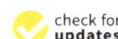

Abstract: Obesity is now a worldwide epidemic. In recent years, different phenotypes of obesity, ranging from metabolically healthy normal weight to metabolically unhealthy obese, were described. Although there is no standardized definition for these phenotypes or for metabolic health, the influence of lifestyle and early-life factors is undisputed. In this context, the ratio of muscle-to-fat tissue seems to play a crucial role. Both adipose tissue and skeletal muscle are highly heterogeneous endocrine organs secreting several hormones, with myokines and adipokines being involved in local autocrine/paracrine interactions and crosstalk with other tissues. Some of these endocrine factors are secreted by both tissues and are, therefore, termed adipo-myokines. High (cardiorespiratory) fitness as a surrogate parameter for an active lifestyle is epidemiologically linked to "better" metabolic health, even in the obese; this may be partly due to the role of adipo-myokines and the crosstalk between adipose and muscle tissue. Therefore, it is essential to consider (cardiovascular) fitness in the definition of metabolically healthy obese/metabolic health and to perform longitudinal studies in this regard. A better understanding of both the (early-life) lifestyle factors and the underlying mechanisms that mediate different phenotypes is necessary for the tailored prevention and personalized treatment of obesity.

Keywords: adipokine; myokine; fitness; metabolically healthy obese; early-life programming

---

1. Introduction

The overall prevalence of obesity increased dramatically over the last few decades [1–3]. The World Health Organization (WHO) reported that more than 1.9 billion adults around the world are overweight, and nearly one-third of the population is obese [4].

From an epidemiological perspective, obesity is linked to so-called non-communicable diseases (NCDs), a set of diseases of long duration and slow progression, including cardiovascular diseases, diabetes mellitus type 2, respiratory diseases, and certain types of cancer [5]. These NCDs kill 41 million people each year, equivalent to 71% of all deaths globally [6]; 1.6 million deaths annually can be attributed to insufficient physical activity [7].

In general, obesity is still defined on the basis of body mass index (BMI), and BMI in itself is generally accepted as a strong predictor of overall early mortality [3]. The increased health risk is particularly linked to high amounts of white and/or visceral fat because of its endocrine activities. Visceral adipose tissue produces more than 600 so-called adipokines that regulate not only metabolic processes such as insulin secretion, hunger and satiety, and energy balance, but inflammatory processes as well [8]. An increasing accumulation of visceral fat in terms of chronic overfeeding results in dysfunctional adipose tissue with excessive adipokine secretion and an altered secretion profile characterized by increased leptin, interleukin (IL)-6, and tumor necrosis factor (TNF)-α levels, as well as increased oxidative stress and a reduction in adiponectin [9], leading to chronic low-grade inflammation.

Whereas physical activity/exercise can be protective against these pathological conditions [10], physical inactivity enhances the inflammatory mechanisms described above [11]. This might be explained by the specific function of skeletal muscle mass. Skeletal muscle is the largest organ in the body; its energy production and consumption are fundamental to metabolic control. Currently, skeletal muscle is also identified as an endocrine organ secreting hundreds of so-called myokines such as myostatin, IL-4, IL-6, IL-7, IL-15, myonectin, follistatin-like 1 (FSTL1), leukemia inhibitory factor, and/or irisin [12,13]. Not only do these myokines act locally in the muscle in an autocrine/paracrine manner, but they are also released into the bloodstream as endocrine factors to regulate physiological processes in other tissues. The release of myokines from contracting muscle is assumed to be at least partly responsible for the health-promoting effects of physical activity that protects against major chronic, low-grade inflammatory diseases like type 2 diabetes, insulin resistance, metabolic syndrome, and many others.

In 2013, Raschke and Eckel [14] described the interplay between muscle and adipose tissue as a two-edged sword. They pointed out that certain cytokines are released by both skeletal muscle and adipose tissue, exhibiting a bioactive effect. The authors suggested calling them adipo-myokines because they are both mediators of exercise and mediators of inflammation. For this reason, as well as for the development of tailored prevention and treatment, it is important to better understand the molecular mechanisms and potential influencing factors that predispose obese (or inactive) individuals to the development of metabolic diseases. Increasing evidence also suggests that early-life exposure to a range of environmental factors, including parental BMI and lifestyle (e.g., maternal nutrition), plays a critical role in defining an offspring's metabolic health. According to the Developmental Origins of Health and Disease hypothesis, environmental exposures during critical periods—such as the preconception, fetal, and early infant phases of life—can influence development and have a persistent impact on metabolic health and gene expression, thereby influencing offspring phenotype and disease risk in later life (Figure 1) [15,16].

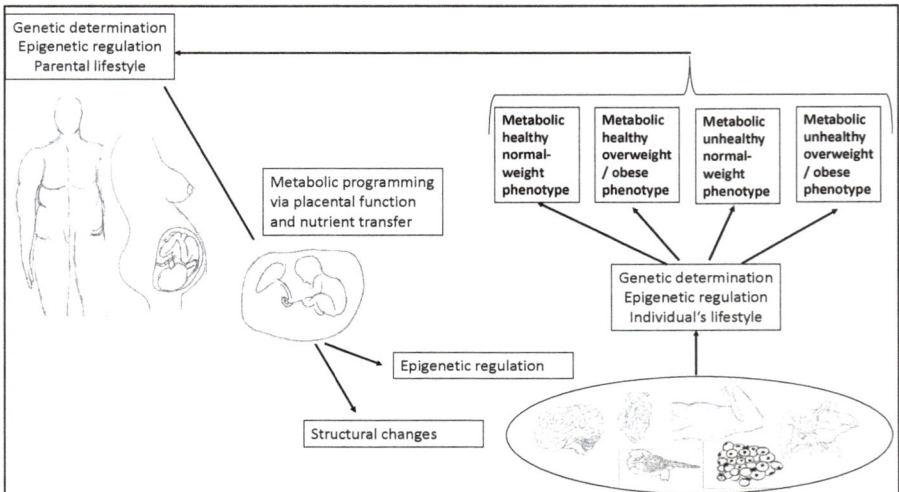

Figure 1. Illustration of the interaction of parental factors on offspring in pregnancy, affecting epigenetic regulation and different organ systems in the development of different obesity phenotypes in terms of metabolic health.

The particular aim of this article is to explore the extent to which biomolecular findings can substantiate the concept of metabolic health and to investigate the role of physical activity/exercise, using cardiorespiratory fitness as a surrogate marker considering early-life factors.

2. Definition and Epidemiological Findings

A striking limitation of BMI is shown by the different phenotypes of obesity. In the early 1980s, Ruderman et al. [17] described the manifestation of cardiometabolic risk factors in non-obese subjects, termed "Metabolically Obese, Normal Weight" (MONW); while they are characterized as having hyperinsulinemia, hyperglycemia, insulin resistance, impaired glucose tolerance, hypercholesterolemia, and hypertriglyceridemia, they have normal adipocyte volume and BMI. On the other hand, obese individuals who showed no health risk factors were also described [18]. This phenomenon—called benign obesity or MHO (metabolically healthy obese)—is characterized by a high BMI or high amount of fat mass in the absence of insulin resistance, increased blood lipids, high blood pressure, or inflammatory dysregulation in contrast to metabolically unhealthy obese (MUO). Discussions about whether the manifestation of MHO is clinically relevant, or whether it might be a form of "honeymoon obesity" (alluding to a temporary absence of metabolic illness), are still ongoing. Nonetheless, it is becoming increasingly clear that a distinction between the various forms of obesity is important given the difference in therapeutic approaches [19]. It is likely that fat distribution and/or body composition play a central role due to different health risks.

To date, there is no uniform classification for this phenotype, while up to 30 different definitions were proposed in several studies (summarized in Reference [20]). Depending on which definition is used, information about the prevalence of MHO varies in the literature [21]. The prevalence of MHO is 3% to 32% in men and 11% to 43% in women using BMI, 6% to 37% in men and 12% to 58% in women using abdominal obesity, and 6% to 43% in men and 12% to 56% in women using body fat as the defining parameter. A similar inconsistency in the literature is found regarding the actual manifestation of the condition. As such, some authors do not recognize the phenomenon as a condition itself but suggest that it is a temporary state which will sooner or later result in a pathological condition [22]. In a meta-analysis, Kramer et al. [23] showed that MHO individuals had an increased risk for cardiovascular events compared with metabolically healthy normal-weight (MHNW) individuals when only studies with 10 or more years of follow-up were considered (+24%). In contrast, all metabolically unhealthy groups had a similar risk: normal weight (risk ratio (RR), 3.14), overweight (RR, 2.70), and obese (RR, 2.65).

Approximately 30% to 50% of MHO individuals seem to convert to the MUO phenotype after four to 20 years of follow-up (summarized in Reference [20]). A major factor in this transition seems to be the development of insulin resistance, which is enhanced by a high BMI, weight gain, older age, and a poor lifestyle index (including physical inactivity).

These controversies underline the need for specific, individualized treatments based on individual diagnostic findings and risk. They further highlight the importance of promoting a healthy, active lifestyle. Moreover, additional factors should be included in health risk assessments. Smith et al. [20] suggest basing the risk on the absence of cardiometabolic diseases and on the cardiometabolic profile, including normal blood lipid, blood pressure, and blood glucose levels, as well as intrahepatic fat content, as advanced criteria. From our point of view, however, body composition and cardiorespiratory fitness would be missing as protective factors in this list of criteria, at least of the advanced type. Similarly, Ruderman et al. [17] noted that physical activity should be added as a therapeutic agent, with maximal oxygen uptake added as a criterion, in reference to MONW. However, Velho et al. [21] demonstrated in the CoLaus Study, a cross-sectional investigation aimed at assessing the prevalence and deciphering the molecular determinants of cardiovascular risk factors in the Caucasian population of Lausanne, that MHO individuals were more physically active. For this reason, Stefan et al. [24] suggested defining MHO using the following six parameters: waist circumference, insulin resistance, blood sugar levels, blood pressure, cholesterol levels, and physical fitness.

3. Physical Activity, Cardiorespiratory Fitness, and/or Sedentary Behavior and Its Relation to MHO

In general, physical activity is defined as any bodily movement that results in energy expenditure [25]. Exercise is a subset of physical activity that is planned, structured, and repetitive, and that has, as a final or an intermediate objective, the improvement or maintenance of physical fitness. The "dose" is expressed as energy expenditure, and the intensity is expressed as the rate of energy consumption in selected activities, usually expressed as a percentage of VO_2 max engaged during exercise (or relative to individual body weight) or metabolic units (METs). Activities with <1.5 METs are classified as sedentary or inactivity [26]. The current physical activity recommendations for adults can be found in Table 1.

Table 1. German physical activity recommendations for adults according to Reference [27].

German Physical Activity Recommendations for Adults
• Adults should be physically active on a regular basis, which can help to achieve significant health effects and to reduce the risk of developing chronic diseases.
• The greatest health benefits take place when individuals who were entirely physically inactive become somewhat more active; this means that all additional physical activity is linked to health benefits and that every single step away from physical inactivity is important, no matter how small, and promotes health.
• To maintain and promote health comprehensively, the following minimum recommendations apply: – adults should have moderate-intensity aerobic physical activity for at least 150 minutes/week, where possible (e.g., 5 × 30 minutes/week); or   – at least 75 minutes/week of vigorous-intensity aerobic physical activity; or   – aerobic physical activity in a corresponding combination of both intensities; and   – should group the overall activity in at least 10-min individual units distributed over days and weeks (e.g., at least 3 × 10 minutes/day on five days per week).
• Adults should also have muscle-strengthening physical activity at least two days per week.
• Adults should avoid long and uninterrupted sitting times and should regularly interrupt sitting with physical activity, where possible.
• Adults can achieve further health effects if they increase the volume and/or intensity of physical activity above the minimum recommendations.

Even though there is a large consensus about the recommended levels of physical activity, the broad range of methods used to measure such activity makes the final decision-making process complex. Studies may use subjective or objective measurements, test endurance, strength, or co-ordination, and different intensities, volumes, and training methods like interval or continuous training in their intervention. Hence, testing cardiorespiratory fitness levels as a surrogate marker may still be the most sensible option. Many studies showed that well-trained individuals have a better prognosis with regard to NCDs than those with lower fitness levels [28,29]. In the concept of fitness instead of fatness, this would also concern overweight and obese individuals [30]. There are, however, only a few studies investigating these connections with MHOs, and most of them are cross-sectional analyses [31]. Between 2010 and 2013, the Maastricht study investigated the relationship between MHO, MUO, metabolically healthy non-obese (MHNO), and metabolically unhealthy non-obese (MUNO) groups, as well as physical activity and sedentary behavior in 2449 men and women aged 40–70 years [31]. Based on accelerometry data, the MHO group was more active (ca. 15 min) and less sedentary (ca. 30 min) than the MUO group. Furthermore, Camhi et al. [32] analyzed National Health and Nutrition

Examination Survey (NHANES) data from obese adolescents and adults from the 2003–2005 cohort. The adult MHO group was 85% more likely to engage in active transportation and nearly three times more likely to be involved in light-intensity, usual daily activity versus sitting (self-reported). A higher level of moderate physical activity was also associated with the MHO group.

In a systematic review and meta-analysis, Ortega et al. [33] explored the differences between physical activity, sedentary behavior, and cardiorespiratory fitness between MHO and MUO individuals, as well as the prognosis of all-cause mortality and cardiovascular disease (CVD) mortality/morbidity in MHO individuals only. The analysis of 67 cross-sectional studies showed that MHO individuals were more active and less sedentary, and they had a higher level of cardiorespiratory fitness. However, cardiorespiratory fitness was only measured in 19 studies, and the difference in VO_2 peak or VO_2 max was usually not more than 1–2 mL/kg body weight. Only one study—the Aerobics Center Longitudinal Study—examined the role of cardiorespiratory fitness in the prognosis of all-cause mortality and cardiovascular disease mortality/morbidity, collecting the data of 43,269 participants. This study explained the differences in the risk of mortality and morbidity between MHO and MHNW subjects through the differences found in cardiorespiratory fitness between both groups. The MHO group had a 30% to 50% lower risk of all-cause mortality, cardiovascular disease, and cancer mortality than the MUO group; no significant differences were observed between the MHO and MHNW groups [34]. The median follow-up period for mortality was 14.3 years, and it was 7.9 years for non-fatal CVD incidence. In another longitudinal study, Pigłowska et al. [35] demonstrated in 101 men that both fat and muscle mass components are important predictors of an individual's metabolic profile. Maintaining regular, high physical activity levels, and a metabolically healthy status throughout young and middle adulthood may have a beneficial influence on body composition parameters and may prevent the age-related decrease of fat-free mass and endothelial dysfunction, defined according to the National Cholesterol Education Program Adult Treatment Panel III (NCEP ATP III) guidelines. Moreover, in a six-year-long cohort study of over 200,000 Taiwanese participants, Martinez-Gomez et al. [36] showed that physical activity can cause a shift in status from MUO to MHO.

4. Myokines, Adipokines, and Adipo-Myokines

The regulation of metabolic health in obese individuals may be mediated by the effects that an active or inactive/sedentary lifestyle have on individual endocrine and inflammatory responses. Myokines, adipokines, and particularly the so-called adipo-myokines are at the crosstalk between muscle and fat tissue. Raschke and Eckel [14], as well as Görgens et al. [37], defined IL-6, TNF-α, visfatin, myostatin, FSTL1, angiopoietin-like protein 4 (ANGPTL4), and monocyte chemoattractant protein-1 (MCP-1) as adipo-myokines. Today, meteorin-like hormone (Metrnl) [38], glypican-4 (GPC-4) [39], and irisin [40] need to be added to the list. Although the number is increasing, only a limited number of cytokines and chemokines were investigated in terms of lifestyle. Main findings are briefly summarized in Tables 2 and 3. In terms of myokines, many other cytokines seem to be involved in the crosstalk between skeletal muscle and adipose tissue. In addition to IL-6 and myostatin, IL-15, irisin, and adiponectin seem to have the decisive role in this "conversation" between adipose tissue and skeletal muscle influencing metabolic health (modified By Reference [41]). A general overview of the already more or less known adipo-myokines, myokines, and adipokines is summarized in Tables 2 and 3.

Table 2. Adipo-myokines, myokines, and adipokines in different tissues, according to References [13,14,37–48].

Name	Effects—Skeletal Muscle	Effects—Adipose Tissue
Adipo-Myokines		
Interleukin-6 (IL-6)	Induces muscle hypertrophy, glucose uptake, glycogen breakdown, and lipolysis; anti-inflammatory effect	Increases lipolysis and free fatty acid (FFA) oxidation in adipocyte, induces adipocyte browning; pro-inflammatory effect
Irisin/fibronectin type III domain-containing protein 5 (FNDC5)	Stimulates glucose uptake and lipid metabolism; involved in muscle growth	Induces adipocyte browning and lipolysis, stimulates glycogenesis, and reduces gluconeogenesis/lipogenesis in liver
IL-15	Stimulates muscle growth and glucose uptake, enhances mitochondrial activity, and exerts anti-oxidative effect	Inhibits lipid accumulation in adipose tissue through adiponectin stimulation
β-aminoiso-butyric acid (BAIBA)	Increases mitochondrial FFA oxidation and ameliorates insulin signaling; anti-inflammatory effect	Increases mitochondria FFA oxidation and browning in adipocytes; reduces hepatic de novo lipogenesis and hepatic endoplasmic reticulum stress
Meteorin-like hormone (Metrnl)	Causes an increase in whole-body energy expenditure; improves glucose tolerance in obese/diabetic mice	Induces adipocyte browning indirectly through regulation of eosinophils
Leukemia inhibitory factor (LIF)	Induces muscle hypertrophy, satellite cell proliferation, regeneration after muscle damage, and glucose uptake	Inhibits adipocyte differentiation
Myostatin	Inhibits muscle hypertrophy	Inhibits myostatin results in adipocyte lipolysis and mitochondrial lipid oxidation; accelerates osteoclast formation
IL-7	Regulates muscle cell development, increases migration of satellite cells	Unknown
Myokines (main effects)		
Fibroblast growth factor 21 (FGF21)	Insulin-responsive myokine involved in the control of glucose homoeostasis, insulin sensitivity, and ketogenesis	Thermogenesis and fat browning in brown (BAT) and white adipose tissue (WAT); increases expression of mitochondrial uncoupling protein 1 (UCP1) and other thermogenic genes in response to cold exposure and β-adrenergic stimulation in both fat depots
Myogenin	Transcription factor; involved in muscle development, myogenesis, and repair	Unknown
Myonectin	Regulates whole-body fatty-acid metabolism	Links skeletal muscle to lipid metabolism adipose tissue and liver
Brain-derived neurotrophic factor (BDNF)	Increases fat oxidation in a 5′ AMP-activated protein kinase (AMPK) -dependent fashion	Size of adipose tissue
Monocyte chemoattractant protein-1 (MCP-1)	Recruitment of monocytes and T lymphocytes; impairs insulin signaling	Involved in low-grade inflammation
Follistatin-like 1 (FSTL1)	Affects glucose metabolism	Correlates with body mass; cardioprotective; improves endothelial function
Angiopoietin-like protein 4 (ANGPTL4)	Increase in FFA	Unknown
Adipokines (main effects)		
Visfatin	Involved in glucose metabolism?	Reduced by exercise?
Resistin	Unknown	Correlates with body fat mass and waist circumference; may cause endothelial dysfunction
Leptin	Increases muscle mass by increasing myocyte cell proliferation and reducing the expression of negative regulators of muscle growth including myostatin, dystrophin, or atrophy markers muscle atrophy F-box (MAFbx) or muscle RING finger 1 (MuRF1); upregulates FNDC5 expression and enhances irisin-induced myocyte proliferation, as well as the muscle growth enhancers myogenin and myonectin; post-exercise decrease	Regulation of energy homeostasis; increases energy expenditure through the stimulation of sympathetic nerve activity in BAT
Adiponectin	Increase fatty-acid oxidation and glucose uptake	Inhibits gluconeogenesis in liver; cardioprotective; increases insulin sensitivity
Tumor necrosis factor alpha (TNF-α)	Reduced after training; increased after very intensive exercise in response to muscle damage; reduced by chronic exercise	Correlates with body fat mass

Table 3. Effect of physical activity in human studies (subject age range 18–65 years).

Name	Effects of Physical Activity
Adipo-Myokines	
IL-6	Plasma concentration of IL-6 increases during muscular exercise. The combination of mode, intensity, and duration of the exercise determines the magnitude of the exercise-induced increase of plasma IL-6 [42]. IL-6 levels were 13.2-fold increased directly after a 35-km long-distance trail run [49].
Irisin/FNDC5	Controversially discussed: Two-fold increase of circulating irisin after 10 weeks of endurance training [40] vs. no increase in irisin after 8 weeks of intermittent sprint running or after 21 weeks of combined endurance and strength training [50,51]. Reduction of circulating irisin in response to 12 weeks of combined endurance and strength training [52] vs. an increase acutely (~1.2-fold) just after acute exercise [52].
IL-15	Controversially discussed: Strength/resistance training leads to an increase in IL-15 messenger RNA (mRNA) level in skeletal muscles dominated by type 2 fibers [53,54]. Short bout of endurance exercise also increases levels of IL-15 in lean subjects, as well as in overweight/obese, subjects [55]. A 2.22-fold increase in serum IL-15 levels following an acute long-distance trail run was also found by Yarcic et al. [49] In contrast, neither sprint interval training (SIT) or combined aerobic and resistance training (A + R) altered IL-15 measured 48 h after exercise in overweight type 2 diabetes (T2D) [56].
BAIBA	Acute aerobic exercise induces a 13% and 20% increase in R-BAIBA and S-BAIBA, respectively [57]. A chronic elevation of 17% was also observed following 20 weeks (3 days/week) of aerobic exercise in previously sedentary and healthy subjects [58].
Metrnl	Lack of data in human studies: Aerobic exercise/swimming (40 min on three non-consecutive days) in temperate (24–25 °C), warm (36.5–37.5 °C), and cold (16.5–17.5 °C) water leads to an increase after exercise in temperate and warm water and a significant decrease in cold water in overweight women [59].
LIF	Aerobic exercise and concentric muscle contractions regulate muscular LIF mRNA expression in humans and lead to an induced expression of LIF in human skeletal muscle [60]. This was also confirmed for resistance exercise [48,61].
Myostatin	Myostatin mRNA expression was reduced in skeletal muscle after acute and long-term exercise and was even further downregulated by acute exercise on top of 12-week training in previously sedentary men [62]. 15 units of a high-intensity circuit training (HICT) program (3×/week for 5 weeks) with own body weight induced the drop of myostatin concentration but significantly only among middle-aged women [63].
IL-7	Lack of data in human studies: Cyclists show higher serum levels of IL-7 compared to less active counterparts [64].
Myokines (main effects)	
FGF21	Increase in serum FGF21 levels in runners after 2 weeks of training [65] and after an acute session of running exercise [66].
Myogenin	Myogenin increases after eccentric resistance training [67,68].
Myonectin	Controversially discussed: Aerobic moderate-intensity exercise leads to a significant reduction in the amount of myonectin in older and younger patients [69]. In contrast, Seldin et al. [44] and Poranjibar et al. [70] found an increase in myonectin expression in muscle and circulation.
BDNF	Increase in BDNF concentrations after aerobic exercise is associated with the amount of aerobic energy required by exercise in a dose-dependent manner [71]. High-intensity and high-volume resistance training lead to elevations in BDNF concentrations [72].
MCP-1	Lack of data in human studies: Low-intensity exercise (walking 10,000 steps/day, 3×/week for 8 weeks) downregulates MCP-1 [73].
FSTL1	Acute sprint interval exercise, as well as acute aerobic exercise, increases FSTL1 [74,75].
ANGPTL4	Controversially discussed: Increase in the gene expression of ANGPTL4 after 4 and 8 h following muscle contraction stimulated in myocytes during exercise using electrical pulse stimulus [76] vs. downregulation of ANGPTL4 in the exercised leg after acute endurance exercise [77].
Adipokines (main effects)	
Visfatin	Lack of data in human studies: Circuit resistance training (3×/week with intensity at 55% of one-repetition maximum) for 8 weeks reduces levels of visfatin [78].
Resistin	Anaerobic exercise might decrease levels of resistin [79]. Resistance training leads to a decrease in resistin after 24 and 48 h compared with baseline and a decline in baseline and immediately after levels compared with pre-training [80].
Leptin	Aerobic exercise leads to lower leptin levels in different population groups (prediabetic/diabetic adults; overweight/obese adults; different age and sex) [81–83].
Adiponectin	Aerobic exercise leads to an increase of adiponectin levels in different population groups (prediabetic/diabetic adults; overweight/obese individuals) [81,82].
TNF-α	Only highly strenuous, prolonged exercise such as marathon running results in a small increase in the plasma concentration of TNF-α [42]. The serum level of TNF-α was significantly downregulated after eccentric resistance exercise in non-athletes [54].

Surprisingly, no investigation in the current literature explicitly investigated the link between the MHO or MUO phenotypes and myokines. Only one study by Carvalho et al. [84] examining 61 adults aged 20–45 years was able to show a correlation between myostatin levels and TNF-α, and between leptin/adiponectin ratio and VO_2 peak [84]. In a different investigation, 10 metabolically healthy obese women had higher cardiorespiratory fitness and lower TNF-α levels than 10 age- and weight-matched women with metabolic syndrome [85]. However, these investigations were cross-sectional analyses, as were most other studies that explored adipokines and myokines in this context. In the Copenhagen Aging and Midlife Biobank, Wedell-Neergaard et al. [86] examined cardiorespiratory fitness levels, plasma levels of cytokines, and high-sensitivity C-reactive protein in 1293 participants aged 49–52 years. Fitness was inversely associated with high-sensitivity C-reactive protein, IL-6, and IL-18, and directly associated with the anti-inflammatory cytokine IL-10, but not associated with TNF-α, interferon gamma, or IL-1β. In a parallel study, lower fitness levels were associated with both abdominal adiposity and low-grade inflammation independent of BMI [87].

Lee et al. [88] analyzed the association between the adipokines IL-6, MCP-1, TNF-α, and adipocyte fatty acid-binding protein (A-FABP) and metabolic health in 456 subjects (303 men and 153 women; mean age 40.5 years). In a model by Wildman et al. [89], participants were separated into four groups: metabolically healthy or unhealthy and obese or non-obese. Differences in TNF-α levels and A-FABP were found between metabolically healthy subjects and MUNW, but no differences were shown in IL-6 and MCP-1 levels. In light of their results, they called for more research to explore these correlations; unfortunately, neither physical activity/exercise nor cardiorespiratory fitness were taken into account.

Arsenault et al. [90] investigated the effect of exercise training on inflammatory markers in hypertensive, postmenopausal, metabolically healthy overweight or obese women. The participants (32.0 ± 5.7 kg/m^2; mean age = 57.3 ± 6.6 years) underwent a six-month exercise intervention program four times per week at 50% VO_2 max. The training significantly increased cardiorespiratory fitness, but no changes were observed for plasma levels of C-reactive protein, IL-6, TNF-α, and adiponectin. A possible explanation for this could be that participants were considered metabolically healthy per se, and that body composition was not considered because BMI and waist circumference were used as parameters. Training intensity may also have been too low. While we can only speculate about the reasons behind the findings, it does underline how much the chosen methodology and study population may influence study results.

In an investigation by Gómez-Ambrosi et al. [91], the inflammatory potential of 222 MHO and 222 MUO individuals was compared with that of 255 matched normal-weight individuals. Both groups showed an increased cardiometabolic risk and no differences in adipokine levels compared with normal-weight subjects. Consequently, the authors asked for a more precise definition of metabolic health. This issue is certainly relevant for most studies presented in this article. For instance, an analysis of sedentary behavior in the English Longitudinal Study of Aging which counted 4931 participants (mean age 65 years) could not show any differences between the MHO, MUO, and MUNW groups [92].

5. Body Composition and Its Influence on Metabolic Health

The previous paragraphs illustrated that exercise and sport are not just means to increase energy consumption, but that the associated development of a high amount of muscle mass elicits the release of myokines, generating an intensive crosstalk between organs. Brown adipose tissue (BAT) and its influence on health may present an important crossover point between fat and muscle mass. In contrast to white adipose tissue (WAT), BAT dissipates lipids in the form of "heat" via β-adrenergic stimulations (e.g., during exercise) or cold exposure. Adipocytes in BAT appear as multilocular cells with small lipid droplets and have a large number of mitochondria and upregulated mitochondrial uncoupling protein 1 (UCP1), which is embedded in the inner membrane of the mitochondrion and uncouples oxidative respiration from ATP synthesis. Whereas classical BAT is observed in specific regions of the body such as the interscapular region and kidney and constitutively sustains its thermogenic activity without any external stimuli, the inducible BAT, known as brite (brown in white), beige, or brown-like adipose tissue, is present within the WAT, and its amount and activity are induced by external stimuli [93].

The adipo-myokine irisin is thought to play a central role in the browning processes. First described by Boström et al. [40], irisin is secreted mainly in skeletal muscle, especially in the perimysium, endomysium, and nuclear parts, although adipose tissue, pancreas, sebaceous glands, and cardiac muscle were identified as secretory tissues [94]. Irisin is secreted into the circulation after transcription from its *FNDC5* gene and proteolytic cleavage at the extracellular surface of cells [40]. This is thought to be triggered by the peroxisome proliferator-activated receptor (PPAR) gamma coactivator 1α (PGC-1α) [95]. Exercise stimulates cell signaling pathways that converge on and increase PGC-1α, a well-known activator of the transcription of mitochondrial transcription factor A (TFAM) and mitochondrial biogenesis [96]. The relationship between physical activity or exercise and PGC-1α and its effects on mitochondrial biogenesis and function are not clear [97–99]. There are some studies [51,52] which investigated the link between PGC-1α with irisin/fibronectin type III domain-containing protein 5 (FNDC5) in muscle in response to acute exercise and showed an increase in muscle FNDC5 messenger RNA (mRNA), while one study [100] detected a positive association of PGC-1α with FNDC5 in muscle. According to chronic exercise, only two studies [52,101] showed increased PGC-1α and FNDC5 mRNA in muscle, while a predominant number of studies [51,102–104] showed no effect of chronic exercise [97,98]. No intervention explored a possible link with MHO. However, Bonfante et al. [105] showed that a higher level of FNDC5/irisin in 20 obese men was associated with better triglyceride levels ($p = 0.01$), lower insulin resistance, risk of type 2 diabetes development, and the tendency to lower serum resistin. Exploring mitochondrial health in this context would exceed the scope of this analysis, and research about metabolic health and sport is sparse. However, a study with 60 participants [106] indicated that MHNW subjects have the most favorable metabolic profiles, while MHO subjects show small alterations, and abnormal diabetic obese individuals have the most unfavorable metabolic profiles [106].

6. Early-Life Programming and the Influence of Different Adipokines, Myokines, and Adipo-Myokines

Today, it is undisputed that early childhood influences metabolic health (see Figure 1). For instance, in the Generation R Study, a population-based prospective cohort investigation among 4871 mothers, fathers, and their children, Gaillard et al. [107] examined the associations of both maternal and paternal pre-pregnancy BMI with childhood body fat distribution and cardiometabolic outcomes six years after birth. Children from obese mothers had a nearly four-fold increased risk of childhood overweight and clustering of cardiometabolic risk factors (odds ratio, 3.00) compared with children from normal-weight women. Furthermore, higher parental pre-pregnancy BMI was associated with higher childhood BMI, total body and abdominal fat mass, systolic blood pressure, and insulin levels, and lower HDL levels.

Cytokines seem to have a central part in this association. In 2016, we published the so-called adipokine–myokine–hepatokine compartment model [108]. Based on the knowledge at the time, the interrelations between skeletal muscle mass, adipose tissue, and maternal liver, and the questionable role of the placenta were investigated in terms of their influence on metabolic regulation in children and how they may be affected by exercise [108]. Knowledge about cytokine and hormone production and secretion of a specific organ is broad, yet little is known about the complex interplay of cytokines, especially with regard to their activities at rest and during different types of physical stress, and how this might affect metabolic health. Below, we explore different biomarkers that are known to be affected by exercise and physical activity during pregnancy, including leptin, brain-derived neurotrophic factor (BDNF), IL-6, irisin, and myostatin. While most studies examined the effect of exercise on those markers, only a few focused on associations taking cardiorespiratory fitness levels or body composition into account.

In a comparative study, we analyzed the long-term effects of an exercise program during pregnancy on metabolism, weight gain, body composition, and changes in leptin and BDNF [109]. Human and animal models were synchronized according to study design, age, and serum parameters. Regular physical activity led to a 6% lower fat mass, 40% lower leptin levels, and an increase of 50% BDNF levels in humans compared with controls, which was not observed in mice. However, with regard to long-term effects, the offspring of exercising mouse dams had significantly lower fat mass and leptin levels than controls. Furthermore, serum BDNF levels were elevated three-fold in the exercise offspring group compared with control [109]. In summary, this shows that lifestyle factors, especially regular physical activity, can shape the metabolic profile of children in the long term.

Because leptin seems to have far-reaching influences in early childhood, this biomarker is discussed in a little bit more detail. According to Vicker et al. [110], leptin is posited to exert programming effects on central and peripheral energy-regulating pathways during a critical period of fetal and infant development. Accordingly, several researchers [111,112] investigated leptin as a candidate prognostic biomarker for obesity risk in later life. It was documented that umbilical cord blood leptin levels are positively correlated with neonatal body weight and fat mass [113]. Moreover, there is evidence that maternal serum concentration of leptin correlates with pre-pregnancy BMI, weight gain during pregnancy, and cord leptin levels [114].

In a follow-up of a cross-sectional study with 76 mother–child pairs, our research group [111] examined the effects of maternal anthropometric, sociodemographic, and lifestyle factors on maternal and cord-blood leptin levels at birth, and on the development of BMI standard deviation scores (SDS) in offspring up to one year of age. We demonstrated that higher maternal and lower cord-blood leptin levels are associated with a higher BMI SDS increase during the first year of life. Maternal leptin is influenced by maternal BMI and weight gain during pregnancy, and cord-blood leptin is influenced by maternal physical activity [111]. These results are in line with findings by Simpson et al. [115], who found that higher cord-blood leptin was associated with higher z-scores of fat mass, waist circumference, and BMI at nine years of age, although they did not take lifestyle factors such as physical activity into account.

The abovementioned myokine BDNF is necessary for placental development, fetal growth, glucose metabolism, and energy homeostasis. It has functions in cognition and neuroplasticity in the hypothalamus and has an influence on appetite regulation and insulin sensitivity in peripheral tissues. Although it is still unknown where exactly BDNF is produced peripherally, BDNF levels in the brain seem to correlate with serum BDNF concentrations [116]. BDNF crosses the blood–brain barrier in a bidirectional manner [117]. Lommatzsch et al. [118] suggested that blood levels of BDNF may reflect brain levels and vice versa. Moreover, we demonstrated in a previous human study that umbilical-cord BDNF is correlated with maternal BDNF levels [119]. In human studies, there is no evidence to date as to how changes in the mother's BDNF values have a long-term effect on the metabolic pattern in the offspring. Camargos et al. [120] evaluated adipokines, cortisol, BDNF, and redox status in 25 overweight/obese infants versus 25 normal-weight peers between six and 24 months of age. Overweight or obese infants presented higher levels of leptin, adiponectin, BDNF, and cortisol and lower levels of thiobarbituric acid-reactive substances (TBARS), as well as catalase and superoxide dismutase activity, than their normal-weight peers. The authors stated that these results indicate neuroendocrine inflammatory response changes in overweight/obese infants. Regarding the effects of physical activity on BDNF levels in children, Walsh et al. [121] examined the associations between changes in diabetes risk factors and changes in BDNF levels after six months of exercise training (aerobic and/or resistance training) in 202 14–18-year-old adolescents with obesity. In this study, exercise-induced reductions in some diabetes risk factors (most notably fasting glucose and beta cell insulin secretory capacity) were associated with increases in BDNF in adolescents with obesity. The authors suggested that exercise training may be an effective strategy to promote metabolic health and increase BDNF. These findings are in line with the results of Mora-Gonzalez et al. [122]; evaluating the effect of physical activity on BDNF levels in 97 overweight or obese children aged eight to 11 years, they found that physical activity was positively correlated with BDNF levels. Although there is currently no evidence about the long-term effects of physical activity during pregnancy on BDNF levels in children, based on the presented results and animal experimental data [123,124], it can be postulated that the metabolic and neurodevelopment profile of children can be shaped in some way.

IL-6 appears to be another important biomarker in early childhood. Our cooperating working group [125] aimed to identify molecular mechanisms of cytokines in the offspring who are affected by maternal exercise during pregnancy. The authors found an almost four-fold increase in serum IL-6 with a clear activation of Janus kinase/signal transducer and activator of transcription signaling in the WAT and hypothalamus of obese offspring, which was completely blunted by maternal exercise during pregnancy. The altered hypothalamic global gene expression in obese offspring showed partial normalization in the obese running offspring group, especially with respect to IL-6 action [125].

In a human-based study of 124 children aged 10.0 ± 0.9 years, Hosick et al. [126] compared markers of inflammation (IL-6, TNF-α) between normal-weight youth of high or low aerobic fitness to obese youth of high or low fitness. They found that higher levels of VO_2 max are associated with lower levels of IL-6, independent of obesity.

Furthermore, irisin may play a crucial role in the interplay between adipokines and myokines during early childhood. It is known that the level of irisin in pregnant women is higher than that of non-pregnant women. Irisin may also contribute to the physiological insulin resistance found in pregnancy [127] and it has an important role in controlling maternal and fetal glucose homeostasis. Low irisin cord-blood levels are associated with newborn growth delay [128] and low proportions of brown fat tissue. Ökdemir et al. [129] aimed to investigate the relationships between irisin, insulin, and leptin levels and maternal weight gain, as well as anthropometric measurements in the newborn. Eighty-four mothers with a mean age of 29.8 ± 5.2 years and their newborns were enrolled in the study. The authors found a negative correlation between the anthropometric measurements of the "appropriate for gestational age" newborns and irisin levels. This correlation was not observed in "small for gestational age" and "large for gestational age" babies. To our knowledge, there are no studies that examined the associations between irisin levels in pregnancy and the development of children in later life. In addition, the association between physical activity during pregnancy and irisin concentrations in the offspring remains to be investigated. Irisin recently became a focus of research in the field of pediatric obesity, because it might play an important pathophysiological role in metabolic dysfunctions and its complications. The positive correlations between leptin levels and anthropometric and metabolic parameters in children with obesity and metabolic syndrome are well known [130,131]. In a cross-sample of 126 Mexican children aged 6–12 years, Gonzales-Gil et al. [132] characterized the association between irisin and adipokines, as well as the cardiometabolic risk factors and anthropometric parameters in children with obesity or metabolic syndrome and in normal-weight children.

They demonstrated that irisin plasma levels were negatively correlated with leptin levels. Furthermore, irisin levels were significantly lower in the obese and metabolic syndrome groups than in the normal-weight group. Stepwise multiple linear regression analysis was conducted to determine whether body composition (lean-fat ratio), metabolic parameters (triglyceride, HDL, and glucose levels), and physical activity in hours per week influenced irisin levels. The lean–fat ratio was found to be the only significant determinant of irisin levels with the model explaining 22.7% of the variance in irisin levels.

Myostatin is secreted during embryonic development, and its function is to limit muscle growth physiologically during development [41]. In the human placenta, the expression of myostatin is negatively correlated with gestational age, and, in placental explants, myostatin acts to facilitate glucose uptake [133]. Myostatin expression is known to be higher in the placenta of pregnancies complicated by preeclampsia [133]. Moreover, Peiris et al. [134] found complications in myostatin protein expression in human placenta from women with gestational diabetes mellitus compared with normal glucose tolerant pregnancies. Compared with lean women, the placentas of obese normal glucose-tolerant women were lower in myostatin dimer expression [134]. The authors concluded that myostatin expression in placental tissue is altered under stress conditions (e.g., obesity and abnormal glucose metabolism) found in pregnancies complicated by gestational diabetes mellitus. In a longitudinal study with 125 infants, De Zegher et al. [135] tested whether large-born infants from non-diabetic mothers develop an early surplus of lean mass while having a lower myostatinemia. They confirmed that breast-fed large-for-gestational-age infants from non-diabetic mothers developed a marked surplus of lean mass at four months of age while maintaining low levels of circulating myostatin. The authors concluded that the fetal–neonatal control of myostatinemia deserves further attention, because it might become a target of interventions aiming to reduce the risk for diabetes in later life by augmenting myogenesis in early life [135]. No studies were conducted to date to investigate the effect of regular physical activity during pregnancy on myostatin in both mother and child. Based on the results of Peiris et al. [134], it might be postulated that placental myostatin could affect glucose homoeostasis and/or cytokine production, which in turn might be influenced by exercise.

7. Discussion

In addition to obesity, physical inactivity/sedentary behavior is a global health problem, and recent data indicate that approximately one-third of the world's adult population is physically inactive. This means that these individuals do not perform the minimum of 150 min per week of moderate-to-vigorous aerobic physical activity recommended by the WHO [27,136]. Importantly, physical inactivity is directly related to higher risk rates for the majority of NCDs. The purpose of this review was to illustrate the association between exercise/physical activity or cardiorespiratory fitness and metabolic health with regard to myokines, adipokines, and adipo-myokines, as well as the influence of early-life factors. Although further research is needed to specifically recommend the type of exercise to be used, as well as corresponding duration, volume, and intensity that would be required to elicit the desired effects, the benefit of exercise in the context of obesity and NCDs remains undisputed. It seems critical that an (exercise) stimulus needs to pass a certain threshold level to be effective [99], but this assumption may be based on a methodological problem. For instance, blood parameters might need to reach a certain level to detect significant differences, although this does not necessarily imply a treatment effect. From a public health perspective, it seems most important to simply "get started", especially because people with a low fitness level will see the greatest health benefits from taking up exercise, particularly in the beginning [10,137]. Regularly performing moderate-to-vigorous intensity, endurance-based activities, for example, walking, jogging, or cycling, leads to an increase of ~10% in "fitness" in different populations (e.g., those who are healthy or obese, or who have coronary artery disease or diabetes) or different obesity phenotypes (e.g., MUO, MHO), which highlights how the majority of adults can acquire clinically important gains in cardiorespiratory fitness. It may not be possible to find an answer as to what is the "right" type of exercise because of the great complexity of the topic. Myokines, for example, were studied for 20 years; many new mechanisms were discovered, some of which we tried to cover in this paper, yet the analysis shows just how many questions are still left unanswered.

There are several limitations to our article. This is a narrative review in which we attempted to explore the interrelations between exercise and, in particular, cardiorespiratory fitness, metabolic health, and obesity, taking into consideration underlying mechanisms and developments in early childhood. We did not perform a systematic literature review about the influence of different types of exercise or training methods. It should be taken into account that the presented results, for example, irisin/FNDC5, may be affected by different subjects' age, conditioning status, and exercise intensity [97,98]. Moreover, different analytical measurements might lead to different results, which were not taken into account. Studies that were included were mostly performed with adult participants. We focused on human interventions and only integrated animal studies to elucidate a specific aspect in more detail. The analysis of adipokines, myokines, and adipo-myokines mentioned herein does not claim to be exhaustive. For instance, epigenetic aspects and/or the role of hepatokines were not taken into consideration. The demand for one uniform definition of metabolically healthy or unhealthy obese individuals (MHO/MUO), or even of metabolic health itself, reflects the difficulties and basic issues involved in this topic and highlights the need for a general consensus. This consensus should consider cardiorespiratory or muscular fitness and should subsequently be tested in future investigations. Equally, interventions should be designed in a manner that allows for an appropriate comparison to make final assumptions. It can only be speculated as to what extent novel techniques such as the secretomic technique can help unravel the underlying mechanisms and their complex interrelations. Mitochondrial biogenesis seems to be one of the central aspects in this issue. Already in 1967, it was shown that physical activity leads to an increased number and improved function of mitochondria [138]; over 50 years later, this issue seems to be more relevant than ever before in light of the rising prevalence of obesity and the adverse changes in body composition toward an unfavorable ratio of fat to muscle mass. As such, there is now an increased focus on sarcopenia, which is usually mentioned in the context of aging and chronic disease [139]. In light of the imminent cost explosion that is to be expected due to the far-reaching consequences of these health issues, it is crucial to understand which patient groups require more or less intensive treatment concepts and prevention. From a practical point of view, it seems sensible to choose an approach that first and foremost focuses on individual tendencies and individual health status to get and keep people physically active. Finally, a political dimension is added to this discussion. Especially in terms of epigenetic aspects, it is crucial to create active living spaces to provide the groundwork for healthy aging. Findings from basic scientific research can help explain and clarify theses connections and their meanings, and facilitate resolving them on a political level.

8. Conclusions

At present, a great body of research on metabolic health and different phenotypes of obesity (MHO/MONW/MUO) exists. However, several questions remain unanswered. Despite the knowledge that different "obesities" exist, no refined metabolic health definition was developed. A better understanding of both the (early-life) lifestyle factors and the underlying mechanisms that mediate different phenotypes is necessary in terms of the tailored prevention and personalized treatment of obesity.

Author Contributions: C.G. and N.F. wrote this article.

Funding: This research received no external funding.

Acknowledgments: We would like to thank Katharina Gross for critically reviewing the manuscript and Selina Müller for the artistic creation of the figure.

Conflicts of Interest: The authors declare no conflicts of interest.

Abbreviations

WHO	World Health Organization
NCDs	Non-Communicable Diseases
BMI	Body Mass Index
MONW	Metabolically Obese, Normal Weight
MUO	Metabolically Unhealth Obese
MHO	Metabolically Healthy Obese
IL	Interleukin
RR	Risk Ratio
METs	Metabolic Units
NHANES	National Health and Nutrition Examination Survey
CVD	Cardiovascular Disease
NCEP APT III	National Cholesterol Education Program Adult Treatment Panel III
FSTL 1	Follistatin-like 1
ANGPTL4	Angiopoietin-like protein 4
MCP-1	Monocyte Chemoattractant Protein-1
Metrnl	Meteorin-like hormone
GPC-4	Glypican-4
TNF-α	Tumor Necrosis Factor alpha
A-FABP	Adipocyte Fatty Acid-Binding Protein
BAT	Brown Adipose Tissue
WAT	White Adipose Tissue

UCP1	Uncoupling protein 1
FNDC5	Fibronectin type III domain-containing protein 5
PPAR gamma	Peroxisome proliferator-activated receptor gamma
PGC-1 alpha	Peroxisome proliferator-activated receptor-gamma coactivator-1 alpha
TFAM	Mitochondrial Transcription Factor A
BDNF	Brain-Derived Neurotrophic Factor
SDS	Standard Deviation Scores
TBARS	Thiobarbituric Acid-Reactive Substances
Jak	Janus kinase
STAT	Signal Transducer and Activator of Transcription
FFA	Free Fatty Acid
MuRF1	muscle RING finger 1
MAFbx	muscle atrophy F-box
AMPK	5′ AMP-activated protein kinase

References

1. The Lancet Public, H. Tackling obesity seriously: The time has come. *Lancet Public Health* **2018**, *3*, e153. [CrossRef]
2. Collaboration, N.C.D.R.F. Worldwide trends in body-mass index, underweight, overweight, and obesity from 1975 to 2016: A pooled analysis of 2416 population-based measurement studies in 128.9 million children, adolescents, and adults. *Lancet* **2017**, *390*, 2627–2642. [CrossRef]
3. Global, B.M.I.M.C.; Di Angelantonio, E.; Bhupathiraju Sh, N.; Wormser, D.; Gao, P.; Kaptoge, S.; Berrington de Gonzalez, A.; Cairns, B.J.; Huxley, R.; Jackson, C.H.L.; et al. Body-mass index and all-cause mortality: Individual-participant-data meta-analysis of 239 prospective studies in four continents. *Lancet* **2016**, *388*, 776–786. [CrossRef]
4. World Health Organization. Obesity and Overweight. Available online: https://www.who.int/news-room/fact-sheets/detail/obesity-and-overweight (accessed on 6 December 2019).
5. Goossens, G.H. The Metabolic Phenotype in Obesity: Fat Mass, Body Fat Distribution, and Adipose Tissue Function. *Obes. Facts* **2017**, *10*, 207–215. [CrossRef]
6. Organisation, W.H. Noncommunicable Diseases. Available online: https://www.who.int/news-room/fact-sheets/detail/noncommunicable-diseases (accessed on 6 November 2019).
7. Collaborators, G.B.D.R.F. Global, regional, and national comparative risk assessment of 79 behavioural, environmental and occupational, and metabolic risks or clusters of risks, 1990-2015: A systematic analysis for the Global Burden of Disease Study 2015. *Lancet* **2016**, *388*, 1659–1724. [CrossRef]
8. Kralisch, S.; Bluher, M.; Paschke, R.; Stumvoll, M.; Fasshauer, M. Adipokines and adipocyte targets in the future management of obesity and the metabolic syndrome. *Mini Rev. Med. Chem.* **2007**, *7*, 39–45. [CrossRef] [PubMed]
9. Mottola, M.F.; Artal, R. Fetal and maternal metabolic responses to exercise during pregnancy. *Early Hum. Dev.* **2016**, *94*, 33–41. [CrossRef] [PubMed]
10. Steell, L.; Ho, F.K.; Sillars, A.; Petermann-Rocha, F.; Li, H.; Lyall, D.M.; Iliodromiti, S.; Welsh, P.; Anderson, J.; MacKay, D.F.; et al. Dose-response associations of cardiorespiratory fitness with all-cause mortality and incidence and mortality of cancer and cardiovascular and respiratory diseases: The UK Biobank cohort study. *Br. J. Sports Med.* **2019**, *53*, 1371–1378. [CrossRef] [PubMed]
11. Handschin, C.; Spiegelman, B.M. The role of exercise and PGC1alpha in inflammation and chronic disease. *Nature* **2008**, *454*, 463–469. [CrossRef]
12. Pedersen, B.K.; Akerstrom, T.C.; Nielsen, A.R.; Fischer, C.P. Role of myokines in exercise and metabolism. *J. Appl. Physiol.* **2007**, *103*, 1093–1098. [CrossRef]
13. Rodriguez, A.; Becerril, S.; Ezquerro, S.; Mendez-Gimenez, L.; Fruhbeck, G. Crosstalk between adipokines and myokines in fat browning. *Acta Physiol. (Oxf.)* **2017**, *219*, 362–381. [CrossRef]
14. Raschke, S.; Eckel, J. Adipo-myokines: Two sides of the same coin–mediators of inflammation and mediators of exercise. *Mediat. Inflamm.* **2013**, *2013*, 320724. [CrossRef]
15. Barker, D.J. Fetal origins of coronary heart disease. *BMJ* **1995**, *311*, 171–174. [CrossRef]
16. Godfrey, K.M.; Barker, D.J. Fetal programming and adult health. *Public Health Nutr.* **2001**, *4*, 611–624. [CrossRef]
17. Ruderman, N.B.; Schneider, S.H.; Berchtold, P. The "metabolically-obese," normal-weight individual. *Am. J. Clin. Nutr.* **1981**, *34*, 1617–1621. [CrossRef]

18. Sims, E.A. Are there persons who are obese, but metabolically healthy? *Metab. Clin. Exp.* **2001**, *50*, 1499–1504. [CrossRef]
19. Bosello, O.; Donataccio, M.P.; Cuzzolaro, M. Obesity or obesities? Controversies on the association between body mass index and premature mortality. *Eat Weight Disord.* **2016**, *21*, 165–174. [CrossRef]
20. Smith, G.I.; Mittendorfer, B.; Klein, S. Metabolically healthy obesity: Facts and fantasies. *J. Clin. Investig.* **2019**, *129*, 3978–3989. [CrossRef]
21. Velho, S.; Paccaud, F.; Waeber, G.; Vollenweider, P.; Marques-Vidal, P. Metabolically healthy obesity: Different prevalences using different criteria. *Eur. J. Clin. Nutr.* **2010**, *64*, 1043–1051. [CrossRef]
22. Iacobini, C.; Pugliese, G.; Blasetti Fantauzzi, C.; Federici, M.; Menini, S. Metabolically healthy versus metabolically unhealthy obesity. *Metab. Clin. Exp.* **2019**, *92*, 51–60. [CrossRef]
23. Kramer, C.K.; Zinman, B.; Retnakaran, R. Are metabolically healthy overweight and obesity benign conditions?: A systematic review and meta-analysis. *Ann. Intern. Med.* **2013**, *159*, 758–769. [CrossRef] [PubMed]
24. Stefan, N.; Haring, H.U.; Hu, F.B.; Schulze, M.B. Metabolically healthy obesity: Epidemiology, mechanisms, and clinical implications. *Lancet Diabetes Endocrinol.* **2013**, *1*, 152–162. [CrossRef]
25. Caspersen, C.J.; Powell, K.E.; Christenson, G.M. Physical activity, exercise, and physical fitness: Definitions and distinctions for health-related research. *Public Health Rep.* **1985**, *100*, 126–131. [PubMed]
26. Gibbs, B.B.; Hergenroeder, A.L.; Katzmarzyk, P.T.; Lee, I.M.; Jakicic, J.M. Definition, measurement, and health risks associated with sedentary behavior. *Med. Sci. Sports Exerc.* **2015**, *47*, 1295–1300. [CrossRef]
27. Pfeifer, K.; Rutten, A. [National Recommendations for Physical Activity and Physical Activity Promotion]. *Gesundheitswesen* **2017**, *79*, S2–S3. [CrossRef]
28. Myers, J.; Prakash, M.; Froelicher, V.; Do, D.; Partington, S.; Atwood, J.E. Exercise capacity and mortality among men referred for exercise testing. *N. Engl. J. Med.* **2002**, *346*, 793–801. [CrossRef]
29. Myers, J.; McAuley, P.; Lavie, C.J.; Despres, J.P.; Arena, R.; Kokkinos, P. Physical activity and cardiorespiratory fitness as major markers of cardiovascular risk: Their independent and interwoven importance to health status. *Prog. Cardiovasc. Dis.* **2015**, *57*, 306–314. [CrossRef]
30. Kennedy, A.B.; Lavie, C.J.; Blair, S.N. Fitness or Fatness: Which Is More Important? *JAMA* **2018**, *319*, 231–232. [CrossRef]
31. De Rooij, B.H.; van der Berg, J.D.; van der Kallen, C.J.; Schram, M.T.; Savelberg, H.H.; Schaper, N.C.; Dagnelie, P.C.; Henry, R.M.; Kroon, A.A.; Stehouwer, C.D.; et al. Physical Activity and Sedentary Behavior in Metabolically Healthy versus Unhealthy Obese and Non-Obese Individuals—The Maastricht Study. *PLoS ONE* **2016**, *11*, e0154358. [CrossRef]
32. Camhi, S.M.; Waring, M.E.; Sisson, S.B.; Hayman, L.L.; Must, A. Physical activity and screen time in metabolically healthy obese phenotypes in adolescents and adults. *J. Obes.* **2013**, *2013*, 984613. [CrossRef]
33. Ortega, F.B.; Cadenas-Sanchez, C.; Migueles, J.H.; Labayen, I.; Ruiz, J.R.; Sui, X.; Blair, S.N.; Martinez-Vizcaino, V.; Lavie, C.J. Role of Physical Activity and Fitness in the Characterization and Prognosis of the Metabolically Healthy Obesity Phenotype: A Systematic Review and Meta-analysis. *Prog. Cardiovasc. Dis.* **2018**, *61*, 190–205. [CrossRef]
34. Ortega, F.B.; Lee, D.C.; Katzmarzyk, P.T.; Ruiz, J.R.; Sui, X.; Church, T.S.; Blair, S.N. The intriguing metabolically healthy but obese phenotype: Cardiovascular prognosis and role of fitness. *Eur. Heart J.* **2013**, *34*, 389–397. [CrossRef]
35. Piglowska, M.; Kostka, T.; Drygas, W.; Jegier, A.; Leszczynska, J.; Bill-Bielecka, M.; Kwasniewska, M. Body composition, nutritional status, and endothelial function in physically active men without metabolic syndrome—A 25 year cohort study. *Lipids Health Dis.* **2016**, *15*, 84. [CrossRef]
36. Martinez-Gomez, D.; Ortega, F.B.; Hamer, M.; Lopez-Garcia, E.; Struijk, E.; Sadarangani, K.P.; Lavie, C.J.; Rodriguez-Artalejo, F. Physical Activity and Risk of Metabolic Phenotypes of Obesity: A Prospective Taiwanese Cohort Study in More Than 200,000 Adults. *Mayo Clin. Proc.* **2019**. [CrossRef]
37. Gorgens, S.W.; Eckardt, K.; Jensen, J.; Drevon, C.A.; Eckel, J. Exercise and Regulation of Adipokine and Myokine Production. *Prog. Mol. Biol. Transl. Sci.* **2015**, *135*, 313–336. [CrossRef]
38. AlKhairi, I.; Cherian, P.; Abu-Farha, M.; Madhoun, A.A.; Nizam, R.; Melhem, M.; Jamal, M.; Al-Sabah, S.; Ali, H.; Tuomilehto, J.; et al. Increased Expression of Meteorin-Like Hormone in Type 2 Diabetes and Obesity and Its Association with Irisin. *Cells* **2019**, *8*, 1283. [CrossRef]
39. Abdolmaleki, F.; Heidarianpour, A. The response of serum Glypican-4 levels and its potential regulatory mechanism to endurance training and chamomile flowers' hydroethanolic extract in streptozotocin-nicotinamide-induced diabetic rats. *Acta Diabetol.* **2018**, *55*, 935–942. [CrossRef]

40. Bostrom, P.; Wu, J.; Jedrychowski, M.P.; Korde, A.; Ye, L.; Lo, J.C.; Rasbach, K.A.; Bostrom, E.A.; Choi, J.H.; Long, J.Z.; et al. A PGC1-alpha-dependent myokine that drives brown-fat-like development of white fat and thermogenesis. *Nature* **2012**, *481*, 463–468. [CrossRef]
41. Leal, L.G.; Lopes, M.A.; Batista, M.L., Jr. Physical Exercise-Induced Myokines and Muscle-Adipose Tissue Crosstalk: A Review of Current Knowledge and the Implications for Health and Metabolic Diseases. *Front. Physiol.* **2018**, *9*, 1307. [CrossRef]
42. Pedersen, B.K.; Febbraio, M.A. Muscles, exercise and obesity: Skeletal muscle as a secretory organ. *Nat. Rev. Endocrinol.* **2012**, *8*, 457–465. [CrossRef]
43. Mattiotti, A.; Prakash, S.; Barnett, P.; van den Hoff, M.J.B. Follistatin-like 1 in development and human diseases. *Cell Mol. Life Sci.* **2018**, *75*, 2339–2354. [CrossRef]
44. Seldin, M.M.; Peterson, J.M.; Byerly, M.S.; Wei, Z.; Wong, G.W. Myonectin (CTRP15), a novel myokine that links skeletal muscle to systemic lipid homeostasis. *J. Biol. Chem.* **2012**, *287*, 11968–11980. [CrossRef] [PubMed]
45. Li, F.; Li, Y.; Duan, Y.; Hu, C.A.; Tang, Y.; Yin, Y. Myokines and adipokines: Involvement in the crosstalk between skeletal muscle and adipose tissue. *Cytokine Growth Factor Rev.* **2017**, *33*, 73–82. [CrossRef] [PubMed]
46. Chung, H.S.; Choi, K.M. Adipokines and Myokines: A Pivotal Role in Metabolic and Cardiovascular Disorders. *Curr. Med. Chem.* **2018**, *25*, 2401–2415. [CrossRef] [PubMed]
47. Trayhurn, P.; Drevon, C.A.; Eckel, J. Secreted proteins from adipose tissue and skeletal muscle—Adipokines, myokines and adipose/muscle cross-talk. *Arch. Physiol. Biochem.* **2011**, *117*, 47–56. [CrossRef] [PubMed]
48. Broholm, C.; Laye, M.J.; Brandt, C.; Vadalasetty, R.; Pilegaard, H.; Pedersen, B.K.; Scheele, C. LIF is a contraction-induced myokine stimulating human myocyte proliferation. *J. Appl. Physiol.* **2011**, *111*, 251–259. [CrossRef]
49. Yargic, M.P.; Torgutalp, S.; Akin, S.; Babayeva, N.; Torgutalp, M.; Demirel, H.A. Acute long-distance trail running increases serum IL-6, IL-15, and Hsp72 levels. *Appl. Physiol. Nutr. Metab. Physiol. Appl. Nutr. Metab.* **2019**, *44*, 627–631. [CrossRef]
50. Huh, J.Y.; Panagiotou, G.; Mougios, V.; Brinkoetter, M.; Vamvini, M.T.; Schneider, B.E.; Mantzoros, C.S. FNDC5 and irisin in humans: I. Predictors of circulating concentrations in serum and plasma and II. mRNA expression and circulating concentrations in response to weight loss and exercise. *Metab. Clin. Exp.* **2012**, *61*, 1725–1738. [CrossRef]
51. Pekkala, S.; Wiklund, P.K.; Hulmi, J.J.; Ahtiainen, J.P.; Horttanainen, M.; Pollanen, E.; Makela, K.A.; Kainulainen, H.; Hakkinen, K.; Nyman, K.; et al. Are skeletal muscle FNDC5 gene expression and irisin release regulated by exercise and related to health? *J. Physiol.* **2013**, *591*, 5393–5400. [CrossRef]
52. Norheim, F.; Langleite, T.M.; Hjorth, M.; Holen, T.; Kielland, A.; Stadheim, H.K.; Gulseth, H.L.; Birkeland, K.I.; Jensen, J.; Drevon, C.A. The effects of acute and chronic exercise on PGC-1alpha, irisin and browning of subcutaneous adipose tissue in humans. *FEBS J.* **2014**, *281*, 739–749. [CrossRef]
53. Nielsen, A.R.; Mounier, R.; Plomgaard, P.; Mortensen, O.H.; Penkowa, M.; Speerschneider, T.; Pilegaard, H.; Pedersen, B.K. Expression of interleukin-15 in human skeletal muscle effect of exercise and muscle fibre type composition. *J. Physiol.* **2007**, *584*, 305–312. [CrossRef] [PubMed]
54. Bazgir, B.; Salesi, M.; Koushki, M.; Amirghofran, Z. Effects of Eccentric and Concentric Emphasized Resistance Exercise on IL-15 Serum Levels and Its Relation to Inflammatory Markers in Athletes and Non-Athletes. *Asian J. Sports Med.* **2015**, *6*, e27980. [CrossRef] [PubMed]
55. Hingorjo, M.R.; Zehra, S.; Saleem, S.; Qureshi, M.A. Serum Interleukin-15 and its relationship with adiposity Indices before and after short-term endurance exercise. *Pak. J. Med. Sci.* **2018**, *34*, 1125–1131. [CrossRef] [PubMed]
56. Banitalebi, E.; Kazemi, A.; Faramarzi, M.; Nasiri, S.; Haghighi, M.M. Effects of sprint interval or combined aerobic and resistance training on myokines in overweight women with type 2 diabetes: A randomized controlled trial. *Life Sci.* **2019**, *217*, 101–109. [CrossRef] [PubMed]
57. Stautemas, J.; Van Kuilenburg, A.B.P.; Stroomer, L.; Vaz, F.; Blancquaert, L.; Lefevere, F.B.D.; Everaert, I.; Derave, W. Acute Aerobic Exercise Leads to Increased Plasma Levels of R- and S-beta-Aminoisobutyric Acid in Humans. *Front. Physiol.* **2019**, *10*, 1240. [CrossRef]
58. Roberts, L.D.; Bostrom, P.; O'Sullivan, J.F.; Schinzel, R.T.; Lewis, G.D.; Dejam, A.; Lee, Y.K.; Palma, M.J.; Calhoun, S.; Georgiadi, A.; et al. beta-Aminoisobutyric acid induces browning of white fat and hepatic beta-oxidation and is inversely correlated with cardiometabolic risk factors. *Cell Metab.* **2014**, *19*, 96–108. [CrossRef]

59. Saghebjoo, M.; Einaloo, A.; Mogharnasi, M.; Ahmadabadi, F. The response of meteorin-like hormone and interleukin-4 in overweight women during exercise in temperate, warm and cold water. *Horm. Mol. Biol. Clin. Investig.* **2018**, *36*. [CrossRef]
60. Broholm, C.; Mortensen, O.H.; Nielsen, S.; Akerstrom, T.; Zankari, A.; Dahl, B.; Pedersen, B.K. Exercise induces expression of leukaemia inhibitory factor in human skeletal muscle. *J. Physiol.* **2008**, *586*, 2195–2201. [CrossRef]
61. Broholm, C.; Pedersen, B.K. Leukaemia inhibitory factor–an exercise-induced myokine. *Exerc. Immunol. Rev.* **2010**, *16*, 77–85.
62. Hjorth, M.; Pourteymour, S.; Gorgens, S.W.; Langleite, T.M.; Lee, S.; Holen, T.; Gulseth, H.L.; Birkeland, K.I.; Jensen, J.; Drevon, C.A.; et al. Myostatin in relation to physical activity and dysglycaemia and its effect on energy metabolism in human skeletal muscle cells. *Acta Physiol. (Oxf.)* **2016**, *217*, 45–60. [CrossRef]
63. Micielska, K.; Gmiat, A.; Zychowska, M.; Kozlowska, M.; Walentukiewicz, A.; Lysak-Radomska, A.; Jaworska, J.; Rodziewicz, E.; Duda-Biernacka, B.; Ziemann, E. The beneficial effects of 15 units of high-intensity circuit training in women is modified by age, baseline insulin resistance and physical capacity. *Diabetes Res. Clin. Pract.* **2019**, *152*, 156–165. [CrossRef] [PubMed]
64. Duggal, N.A.; Pollock, R.D.; Lazarus, N.R.; Harridge, S.; Lord, J.M. Major features of immunesenescence, including reduced thymic output, are ameliorated by high levels of physical activity in adulthood. *Aging Cell* **2018**, *17*. [CrossRef] [PubMed]
65. Cuevas-Ramos, D.; Almeda-Valdes, P.; Meza-Arana, C.E.; Brito-Cordova, G.; Gomez-Perez, F.J.; Mehta, R.; Oseguera-Moguel, J.; Aguilar-Salinas, C.A. Exercise increases serum fibroblast growth factor 21 (FGF21) levels. *PLoS ONE* **2012**, *7*, e38022. [CrossRef] [PubMed]
66. Kim, K.H.; Kim, S.H.; Min, Y.K.; Yang, H.M.; Lee, J.B.; Lee, M.S. Acute exercise induces FGF21 expression in mice and in healthy humans. *PLoS ONE* **2013**, *8*, e63517. [CrossRef] [PubMed]
67. Nederveen, J.P.; Fortino, S.A.; Baker, J.M.; Snijders, T.; Joanisse, S.; McGlory, C.; McKay, B.R.; Kumbhare, D.; Parise, G. Consistent expression pattern of myogenic regulatory factors in whole muscle and isolated human muscle satellite cells after eccentric contractions in humans. *J. Appl. Physiol.* **2019**. [CrossRef] [PubMed]
68. Luk, H.Y.; Levitt, D.E.; Boyett, J.C.; Rojas, S.; Flader, S.M.; McFarlin, B.K.; Vingren, J.L. Resistance exercise-induced hormonal response promotes satellite cell proliferation in untrained men but not in women. *Am. J. Physiol. Endocrinol. Metab.* **2019**, *317*, E421–E432. [CrossRef]
69. Lim, S.; Choi, S.H.; Koo, B.K.; Kang, S.M.; Yoon, J.W.; Jang, H.C.; Choi, S.M.; Lee, M.G.; Lee, W.; Shin, H.; et al. Effects of aerobic exercise training on C1q tumor necrosis factor alpha-related protein isoform 5 (myonectin): Association with insulin resistance and mitochondrial DNA density in women. *J. Clin. Endocrinol. Metab.* **2012**, *97*, E88–E93. [CrossRef]
70. Pourranjbar, M.; Arabnejad, N.; Naderipour, K.; Rafie, F. Effects of Aerobic Exercises on Serum Levels of Myonectin and Insulin Resistance in Obese and Overweight Women. *J. Med. Life* **2018**, *11*, 381–386. [CrossRef]
71. De Assis, G.G.; Gasanov, E.V.; de Sousa, M.B.C.; Kozacz, A.; Murawska-Cialowicz, E. Brain derived neutrophic factor, a link of aerobic metabolism to neuroplasticity. *J. Physiol. Pharmacol. Off. J. Pol. Physiol. Soc.* **2018**, *69*. [CrossRef]
72. Church, D.D.; Hoffman, J.R.; Mangine, G.T.; Jajtner, A.R.; Townsend, J.R.; Beyer, K.S.; Wang, R.; La Monica, M.B.; Fukuda, D.H.; Stout, J.R. Comparison of high-intensity vs. high-volume resistance training on the BDNF response to exercise. *J. Appl. Physiol.* **2016**, *121*, 123–128. [CrossRef]
73. Yakeu, G.; Butcher, L.; Isa, S.; Webb, R.; Roberts, A.W.; Thomas, A.W.; Backx, K.; James, P.E.; Morris, K. Low-intensity exercise enhances expression of markers of alternative activation in circulating leukocytes: Roles of PPARgamma and Th2 cytokines. *Atherosclerosis* **2010**, *212*, 668–673. [CrossRef] [PubMed]
74. Kon, M.; Ebi, Y.; Nakagaki, K. Effects of acute sprint interval exercise on follistatin-like 1 and apelin secretions. *Arch. Physiol. Biochem.* **2019**. [CrossRef] [PubMed]
75. Gorgens, S.W.; Raschke, S.; Holven, K.B.; Jensen, J.; Eckardt, K.; Eckel, J. Regulation of follistatin-like protein 1 expression and secretion in primary human skeletal muscle cells. *Arch. Physiol. Biochem.* **2013**, *119*, 75–80. [CrossRef] [PubMed]
76. Scheler, M.; Irmler, M.; Lehr, S.; Hartwig, S.; Staiger, H.; Al-Hasani, H.; Beckers, J.; de Angelis, M.H.; Haring, H.U.; Weigert, C. Cytokine response of primary human myotubes in an in vitro exercise model. *Am. J. Physiol. Cell Physiol.* **2013**, *305*, C877–C886. [CrossRef] [PubMed]
77. Catoire, M.; Mensink, M.; Kalkhoven, E.; Schrauwen, P.; Kersten, S. Identification of human exercise-induced myokines using secretome analysis. *Physiol. Genom.* **2014**, *46*, 256–267. [CrossRef]

78. Saeidi, A.; Jabbour, G.; Ahmadian, M.; Abbassi-Daloii, A.; Malekian, F.; Hackney, A.C.; Saedmocheshi, S.; Basati, G.; Ben Abderrahman, A.; Zouhal, H. Independent and Combined Effects of Antioxidant Supplementation and Circuit Resistance Training on Selected Adipokines in Postmenopausal Women. *Front. Physiol.* **2019**, *10*, 484. [CrossRef]
79. He, Z.; Tian, Y.; Valenzuela, P.L.; Huang, C.; Zhao, J.; Hong, P.; He, Z.; Yin, S.; Lucia, A. Myokine/Adipokine Response to "Aerobic" Exercise: Is It Just a Matter of Exercise Load? *Front. Physiol.* **2019**, *10*, 691. [CrossRef]
80. Prestes, J.; Shiguemoto, G.; Botero, J.P.; Frollini, A.; Dias, R.; Leite, R.; Pereira, G.; Magosso, R.; Baldissera, V.; Cavaglieri, C.; et al. Effects of resistance training on resistin, leptin, cytokines, and muscle force in elderly post-menopausal women. *J. Sports Sci.* **2009**, *27*, 1607–1615. [CrossRef]
81. Becic, T.; Studenik, C.; Hoffmann, G. Exercise Increases Adiponectin and Reduces Leptin Levels in Prediabetic and Diabetic Individuals: Systematic Review and Meta-Analysis of Randomized Controlled Trials. *Med. Sci. (Basel)* **2018**, *6*, 97. [CrossRef]
82. Yu, N.; Ruan, Y.; Gao, X.; Sun, J. Systematic Review and Meta-Analysis of Randomized, Controlled Trials on the Effect of Exercise on Serum Leptin and Adiponectin in Overweight and Obese Individuals. *Horm. Metab. Res.* **2017**, *49*, 164–173. [CrossRef]
83. Fedewa, M.V.; Hathaway, E.D.; Ward-Ritacco, C.L.; Williams, T.D.; Dobbs, W.C. The Effect of Chronic Exercise Training on Leptin: A Systematic Review and Meta-Analysis of Randomized Controlled Trials. *Sports Med.* **2018**, *48*, 1437–1450. [CrossRef] [PubMed]
84. Carvalho, L.P.; Basso-Vanelli, R.P.; Di Thommazo-Luporini, L.; Mendes, R.G.; Oliveira-Junior, M.C.; Vieira, R.P.; Bonjorno-Junior, J.C.; Oliveira, C.R.; Luporini, R.; Borghi-Silva, A. Myostatin and adipokines: The role of the metabolically unhealthy obese phenotype in muscle function and aerobic capacity in young adults. *Cytokine* **2018**, *107*, 118–124. [CrossRef] [PubMed]
85. Poelkens, F.; Eijsvogels, T.M.; Brussee, P.; Verheggen, R.J.; Tack, C.J.; Hopman, M.T. Physical fitness can partly explain the metabolically healthy obese phenotype in women. *Exp. Clin. Endocrinol. Diabetes Off. J. Ger. Soc. Endocrinol. Ger. Diabetes Assoc.* **2014**, *122*, 87–91. [CrossRef] [PubMed]
86. Wedell-Neergaard, A.S.; Krogh-Madsen, R.; Petersen, G.L.; Hansen, A.M.; Pedersen, B.K.; Lund, R.; Bruunsgaard, H. Cardiorespiratory fitness and the metabolic syndrome: Roles of inflammation and abdominal obesity. *PLoS ONE* **2018**, *13*, e0194991. [CrossRef]
87. Wedell-Neergaard, A.S.; Eriksen, L.; Gronbaek, M.; Pedersen, B.K.; Krogh-Madsen, R.; Tolstrup, J. Low fitness is associated with abdominal adiposity and low-grade inflammation independent of BMI. *PLoS ONE* **2018**, *13*, e0190645. [CrossRef]
88. Lee, T.H.; Jeon, W.S.; Han, K.J.; Lee, S.Y.; Kim, N.H.; Chae, H.B.; Jang, C.M.; Yoo, K.M.; Park, H.J.; Lee, M.K.; et al. Comparison of Serum Adipocytokine Levels according to Metabolic Health and Obesity Status. *Endocrinol. Metab. (Seoul)* **2015**, *30*, 185–194. [CrossRef]
89. Wildman, R.P.; Muntner, P.; Reynolds, K.; McGinn, A.P.; Rajpathak, S.; Wylie-Rosett, J.; Sowers, M.R. The obese without cardiometabolic risk factor clustering and the normal weight with cardiometabolic risk factor clustering: Prevalence and correlates of 2 phenotypes among the US population (NHANES 1999–2004). *Arch. Intern. Med.* **2008**, *168*, 1617–1624. [CrossRef]
90. Arsenault, B.J.; Cote, M.; Cartier, A.; Lemieux, I.; Despres, J.P.; Ross, R.; Earnest, C.P.; Blair, S.N.; Church, T.S. Effect of exercise training on cardiometabolic risk markers among sedentary, but metabolically healthy overweight or obese post-menopausal women with elevated blood pressure. *Atherosclerosis* **2009**, *207*, 530–533. [CrossRef]
91. Gomez-Ambrosi, J.; Catalan, V.; Rodriguez, A.; Andrada, P.; Ramirez, B.; Ibanez, P.; Vila, N.; Romero, S.; Margall, M.A.; Gil, M.J.; et al. Increased cardiometabolic risk factors and inflammation in adipose tissue in obese subjects classified as metabolically healthy. *Diabetes Care* **2014**, *37*, 2813–2821. [CrossRef]
92. Bell, J.A.; Kivimaki, M.; Batty, G.D.; Hamer, M. Metabolically healthy obesity: What is the role of sedentary behaviour? *Prev. Med.* **2014**, *62*, 35–37. [CrossRef]
93. Lee, M.W.; Lee, M.; Oh, K.J. Adipose Tissue-Derived Signatures for Obesity and Type 2 Diabetes: Adipokines, Batokines and MicroRNAs. *J. Clin. Med.* **2019**, *8*, 854. [CrossRef] [PubMed]
94. Martinez Munoz, I.Y.; Camarillo Romero, E.D.S.; Garduno Garcia, J.J. Irisin a Novel Metabolic Biomarker: Present Knowledge and Future Directions. *Int. J. Endocrinol.* **2018**, *2018*, 7816806. [CrossRef] [PubMed]
95. Pilegaard, H.; Saltin, B.; Neufer, P.D. Exercise induces transient transcriptional activation of the PGC-1alpha gene in human skeletal muscle. *J. Physiol.* **2003**, *546*, 851–858. [CrossRef] [PubMed]

96. Fernandez-Marcos, P.J.; Auwerx, J. Regulation of PGC-1alpha, a nodal regulator of mitochondrial biogenesis. *Am. J. Clin. Nutr.* **2011**, *93*, 884S–890S. [CrossRef]
97. Dinas, P.C.; Lahart, I.M.; Timmons, J.A.; Svensson, P.A.; Koutedakis, Y.; Flouris, A.D.; Metsios, G.S. Effects of physical activity on the link between PGC-1a and FNDC5 in muscle, circulating Iotarisin and UCP1 of white adipocytes in humans: A systematic review. *F1000Res* **2017**, *6*, 286. [CrossRef]
98. Fatouros, I.G. Is irisin the new player in exercise-induced adaptations or not? A 2017 update. *Clin. Chem. Lab. Med.* **2018**, *56*, 525–548. [CrossRef]
99. Granata, C.; Jamnick, N.A.; Bishop, D.J. Training-Induced Changes in Mitochondrial Content and Respiratory Function in Human Skeletal Muscle. *Sports Med.* **2018**, *48*, 1809–1828. [CrossRef]
100. Lecker, S.H.; Zavin, A.; Cao, P.; Arena, R.; Allsup, K.; Daniels, K.M.; Joseph, J.; Schulze, P.C.; Forman, D.E. Expression of the irisin precursor FNDC5 in skeletal muscle correlates with aerobic exercise performance in patients with heart failure. *Circ. Heart Fail* **2012**, *5*, 812–818. [CrossRef]
101. Huh, J.Y.; Mougios, V.; Kabasakalis, A.; Fatouros, I.; Siopi, A.; Douroudos, I.I.; Filippaios, A.; Panagiotou, G.; Park, K.H.; Mantzoros, C.S. Exercise-induced irisin secretion is independent of age or fitness level and increased irisin may directly modulate muscle metabolism through AMPK activation. *J. Clin. Endocrinol. Metab.* **2014**, *99*, E2154–E2161. [CrossRef]
102. Alvehus, M.; Boman, N.; Soderlund, K.; Svensson, M.B.; Buren, J. Metabolic adaptations in skeletal muscle, adipose tissue, and whole-body oxidative capacity in response to resistance training. *Eur. J. Appl. Physiol.* **2014**, *114*, 1463–1471. [CrossRef]
103. Ellefsen, S.; Vikmoen, O.; Slettalokken, G.; Whist, J.E.; Nygaard, H.; Hollan, I.; Rauk, I.; Vegge, G.; Strand, T.A.; Raastad, T.; et al. Irisin and FNDC5: Effects of 12-week strength training, and relations to muscle phenotype and body mass composition in untrained women. *Eur. J. Appl. Physiol.* **2014**, *114*, 1875–1888. [CrossRef]
104. Timmons, J.A.; Baar, K.; Davidsen, P.K.; Atherton, P.J. Is irisin a human exercise gene? *Nature* **2012**, *488*, E9–E10, discussion E10–E11. [CrossRef]
105. Bonfante, I.L.P.; Chacon-Mikahil, M.P.T.; Brunelli, D.T.; Gaspari, A.F.; Duft, R.G.; Oliveira, A.G.; Araujo, T.G.; Saad, M.J.A.; Cavaglieri, C.R. Obese with higher FNDC5/Irisin levels have a better metabolic profile, lower lipopolysaccharide levels and type 2 diabetes risk. *Arch. Endocrinol. Metab.* **2017**, *61*, 524–533. [CrossRef]
106. Bhansali, S.; Bhansali, A.; Dhawan, V. Favourable metabolic profile sustains mitophagy and prevents metabolic abnormalities in metabolically healthy obese individuals. *Diabetol. Metab. Syndr.* **2017**, *9*, 99. [CrossRef]
107. Gaillard, R.; Steegers, E.A.; Duijts, L.; Felix, J.F.; Hofman, A.; Franco, O.H.; Jaddoe, V.W. Childhood cardiometabolic outcomes of maternal obesity during pregnancy: The Generation R Study. *Hypertension* **2014**, *63*, 683–691. [CrossRef]
108. Deibert, C.; Ferrari, N.; Flock, A.; Merz, W.M.; Gembruch, U.; Lehmacher, W.; Ehrhardt, C.; Graf, C. Adipokine-myokine-hepatokine compartment-system in mothers and children: An explorative study. *Contemp. Clin. Trials Commun.* **2016**, *3*, 1–5. [CrossRef]
109. Ferrari, N.; Bae-Gartz, I.; Bauer, C.; Janoschek, R.; Koxholt, I.; Mahabir, E.; Appel, S.; Alejandre Alcazar, M.A.; Grossmann, N.; Vohlen, C.; et al. Exercise during pregnancy and its impact on mothers and offspring in humans and mice. *J. Dev. Orig. Health Dis.* **2018**, *9*, 63–76. [CrossRef]
110. Vickers, M.H.; Sloboda, D.M. Leptin as mediator of the effects of developmental programming. *Best Pract. Res. Clin. Endocrinol. Metab.* **2012**, *26*, 677–687. [CrossRef]
111. Telschow, A.; Ferrari, N.; Deibert, C.; Flock, A.; Merz, W.M.; Gembruch, U.; Ehrhardt, C.; Dotsch, J.; Graf, C. High Maternal and Low Cord Blood Leptin Are Associated with BMI-SDS Gain in the First Year of Life. *Obes. Facts* **2019**, *12*, 575–585. [CrossRef]
112. Boeke, C.E.; Mantzoros, C.S.; Hughes, M.D.; Rifas-Shiman, S.; Villamor, E.; Zera, C.A.; Gillman, M.W. Differential associations of leptin with adiposity across early childhood. *Obesity* **2013**, *21*, 1430–1437. [CrossRef]
113. Hassink, S.G.; Sheslow, D.V.; de Lancey, E.; Opentanova, I.; Considine, R.V.; Caro, J.F. Serum leptin in children with obesity: Relationship to gender and development. *Pediatrics* **1996**, *98*, 201–203.
114. Marino-Ortega, L.A.; Molina-Bello, A.; Polanco-Garcia, J.C.; Munoz-Valle, J.F.; Salgado-Bernabe, A.B.; Guzman-Guzman, I.P.; Parra-Rojas, I. Correlation of leptin and soluble leptin receptor levels with anthropometric parameters in mother-newborn pairs. *Int. J. Clin. Exp. Med.* **2015**, *8*, 11260–11267.
115. Simpson, J.; Smith, A.D.; Fraser, A.; Sattar, N.; Lindsay, R.S.; Ring, S.M.; Tilling, K.; Davey Smith, G.; Lawlor, D.A.; Nelson, S.M. Programming of Adiposity in Childhood and Adolescence: Associations With Birth Weight and Cord Blood Adipokines. *J. Clin. Endocrinol. Metab.* **2017**, *102*, 499–506. [CrossRef] [PubMed]

116. Karege, F.; Schwald, M.; Cisse, M. Postnatal developmental profile of brain-derived neurotrophic factor in rat brain and platelets. *Neurosci. Lett.* **2002**, *328*, 261–264. [CrossRef]
117. Pan, W.; Banks, W.A.; Fasold, M.B.; Bluth, J.; Kastin, A.J. Transport of brain-derived neurotrophic factor across the blood-brain barrier. *Neuropharmacology* **1998**, *37*, 1553–1561. [CrossRef]
118. Lommatzsch, M.; Zingler, D.; Schuhbaeck, K.; Schloetcke, K.; Zingler, C.; Schuff-Werner, P.; Virchow, J.C. The impact of age, weight and gender on BDNF levels in human platelets and plasma. *Neurobiol. Aging* **2005**, *26*, 115–123. [CrossRef] [PubMed]
119. Flock, A.; Weber, S.K.; Ferrari, N.; Fietz, C.; Graf, C.; Fimmers, R.; Gembruch, U.; Merz, W.M. Determinants of brain-derived neurotrophic factor (BDNF) in umbilical cord and maternal serum. *Psychoneuroendocrinology* **2016**, *63*, 191–197. [CrossRef]
120. Camargos, A.C.; Mendonca, V.A.; Andrade, C.A.; Oliveira, K.S.; Tossige-Gomes, R.; Rocha-Vieira, E.; Neves, C.D.; Vieira, E.L.; Leite, H.R.; Oliveira, M.X.; et al. Neuroendocrine Inflammatory Responses in Overweight/Obese Infants. *PLoS ONE* **2016**, *11*, e0167593. [CrossRef]
121. Walsh, J.J.; D'Angiulli, A.; Cameron, J.D.; Sigal, R.J.; Kenny, G.P.; Holcik, M.; Doucette, S.; Alberga, A.S.; Prud'homme, D.; Hadjiyannakis, S.; et al. Changes in the Brain-Derived Neurotrophic Factor Are Associated with Improvements in Diabetes Risk Factors after Exercise Training in Adolescents with Obesity: The HEARTY Randomized Controlled Trial. *Neural Plast.* **2018**, *2018*, 7169583. [CrossRef]
122. Mora-Gonzalez, J.; Migueles, J.H.; Esteban-Cornejo, I.; Cadenas-Sanchez, C.; Pastor-Villaescusa, B.; Molina-Garcia, P.; Rodriguez-Ayllon, M.; Rico, M.C.; Gil, A.; Aguilera, C.M.; et al. Sedentarism, Physical Activity, Steps, and Neurotrophic Factors in Obese Children. *Med. Sci. Sports Exerc.* **2019**, *51*, 2325–2333. [CrossRef]
123. Aksu, I.; Baykara, B.; Ozbal, S.; Cetin, F.; Sisman, A.R.; Dayi, A.; Gencoglu, C.; Tas, A.; Buyuk, E.; Gonenc-Arda, S.; et al. Maternal treadmill exercise during pregnancy decreases anxiety and increases prefrontal cortex VEGF and BDNF levels of rat pups in early and late periods of life. *Neurosci. Lett.* **2012**, *516*, 221–225. [CrossRef]
124. Parnpiansil, P.; Jutapakdeegul, N.; Chentanez, T.; Kotchabhakdi, N. Exercise during pregnancy increases hippocampal brain-derived neurotrophic factor mRNA expression and spatial learning in neonatal rat pup. *Neurosci. Lett.* **2003**, *352*, 45–48. [CrossRef] [PubMed]
125. Bae-Gartz, I.; Janoschek, R.; Kloppe, C.S.; Vohlen, C.; Roels, F.; Oberthur, A.; Alejandre Alcazar, M.A.; Lippach, G.; Muether, P.S.; Dinger, K.; et al. Running Exercise in Obese Pregnancies Prevents IL-6 Trans-signaling in Male Offspring. *Med. Sci. Sports Exerc.* **2016**, *48*, 829–838. [CrossRef] [PubMed]
126. Hosick, P.; McMurray, R.; Hackney, A.C.; Battaglini, C.; Combs, T.; Harrell, J. Resting IL-6 and TNF-alpha level in children of different weight and fitness status. *Pediatr. Exerc. Sci.* **2013**, *25*, 238–247. [CrossRef]
127. Garces, M.F.; Peralta, J.J.; Ruiz-Linares, C.E.; Lozano, A.R.; Poveda, N.E.; Torres-Sierra, A.L.; Eslava-Schmalbach, J.H.; Alzate, J.P.; Sanchez, A.Y.; Sanchez, E.; et al. Irisin levels during pregnancy and changes associated with the development of preeclampsia. *J. Clin. Endocrinol. Metab.* **2014**, *99*, 2113–2119. [CrossRef]
128. Briana, D.; Malamitsi-Puchner, A.; Boutsikou, M.; Baka, S.; Ristani, A.; Hassiakos, D.; Gourgiotis, D.; Boutsikou, T. Myokine Irisin is Down-regulated In Fetal Growth Restriction. *Arch. Dis. Child* **2014**, *99* (Suppl. 2), 126. [CrossRef]
129. Okdemir, D.; Hatipoglu, N.; Kurtoglu, S.; Siraz, U.G.; Akar, H.H.; Muhtaroglu, S.; Kutuk, M.S. The Role of Irisin, Insulin and Leptin in Maternal and Fetal Interaction. *J. Clin. Res. Pediatr. Endocrinol.* **2018**, *10*, 307–315. [CrossRef]
130. Gherlan, I.; Vladoiu, S.; Alexiu, F.; Giurcaneanu, M.; Oros, S.; Brehar, A.; Procopiuc, C.; Dumitrache, C. Adipocytokine profile and insulin resistance in childhood obesity. *Maedica (Buchar)* **2012**, *7*, 205–213.
131. Wang, Q.; Yin, J.; Xu, L.; Cheng, H.; Zhao, X.; Xiang, H.; Lam, H.S.; Mi, J.; Li, M. Prevalence of metabolic syndrome in a cohort of Chinese schoolchildren: Comparison of two definitions and assessment of adipokines as components by factor analysis. *BMC Public Health* **2013**, *13*, 249. [CrossRef]
132. Gonzalez-Gil, A.M.; Peschard-Franco, M.; Castillo, E.C.; Gutierrez-DelBosque, G.; Trevino, V.; Silva-Platas, C.; Perez-Villarreal, L.; Garcia-Rivas, G.; Elizondo-Montemayor, L. Myokine-adipokine cross-talk: Potential mechanisms for the association between plasma irisin and adipokines and cardiometabolic risk factors in Mexican children with obesity and the metabolic syndrome. *Diabetol. Metab. Syndr.* **2019**, *11*, 63. [CrossRef]
133. Peiris, H.N.; Salomon, C.; Payton, D.; Ashman, K.; Vaswani, K.; Chan, A.; Rice, G.E.; Mitchell, M.D. Myostatin is localized in extravillous trophoblast and up-regulates migration. *J. Clin. Res. Pediatr. Endocrinol.* **2014**, *99*, E2288–E2297. [CrossRef] [PubMed]
134. Peiris, H.N.; Lappas, M.; Georgiou, H.M.; Vaswani, K.; Salomon, C.; Rice, G.E.; Mitchell, M.D. Myostatin in the placentae of pregnancies complicated with gestational diabetes mellitus. *Placenta* **2015**, *36*, 1–6. [CrossRef] [PubMed]

135. De Zegher, F.; Perez-Cruz, M.; Diaz, M.; Gomez-Roig, M.D.; Lopez-Bermejo, A.; Ibanez, L. Less myostatin and more lean mass in large-born infants from nondiabetic mothers. *J. Clin. Res. Pediatr. Endocrinol.* **2014**, *99*, E2367–E2371. [CrossRef] [PubMed]
136. Ruiz-Casado, A.; Martin-Ruiz, A.; Perez, L.M.; Provencio, M.; Fiuza-Luces, C.; Lucia, A. Exercise and the Hallmarks of Cancer. *Trends Cancer* **2017**, *3*, 423–441. [CrossRef]
137. Kyu, H.H.; Bachman, V.F.; Alexander, L.T.; Mumford, J.E.; Afshin, A.; Estep, K.; Veerman, J.L.; Delwiche, K.; Iannarone, M.L.; Moyer, M.L.; et al. Physical activity and risk of breast cancer, colon cancer, diabetes, ischemic heart disease, and ischemic stroke events: Systematic review and dose-response meta-analysis for the Global Burden of Disease Study 2013. *BMJ* **2016**, *354*, i3857. [CrossRef]
138. Holloszy, J.O. Biochemical adaptations in muscle. Effects of exercise on mitochondrial oxygen uptake and respiratory enzyme activity in skeletal muscle. *J. Biol. Chem.* **1967**, *242*, 2278–2282.
139. Cruz-Jentoft, A.J.; Bahat, G.; Bauer, J.; Boirie, Y.; Bruyere, O.; Cederholm, T.; Cooper, C.; Landi, F.; Rolland, Y.; Sayer, A.A.; et al. Sarcopenia: Revised European consensus on definition and diagnosis. *Age Ageing* **2019**, *48*, 16–31. [CrossRef]

© 2019 by the authors. Licensee MDPI, Basel, Switzerland. This article is an open access article distributed under the terms and conditions of the Creative Commons Attribution (CC BY) license (http://creativecommons.org/licenses/by/4.0/).

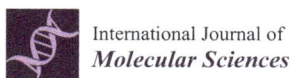

Article

Umbilical Cord SFRP5 Levels of Term Newborns in Relation to Normal and Excessive Gestational Weight Gain

Żaneta Kimber-Trojnar [1,*], Jolanta Patro-Małysza [1], Marcin Trojnar [2], Dorota Darmochwał-Kolarz [3], Jan Oleszczuk [1] and Bożena Leszczyńska-Gorzelak [1]

[1] Chair and Department of Obstetrics and Perinatology, Medical University of Lublin, Lublin 20-090, Poland; jolapatro@wp.pl (J.P.-M.); jan.oleszczuk@umlub.pl (J.O.); b.leszczynska@umlub.pl (B.L.-G.)
[2] Chair and Department of Internal Medicine, Medical University of Lublin, Lublin 20-081, Poland; marcin.trojnar@umlub.pl
[3] Department of Gynecology and Obstetrics, Institute of Clinical and Experimental Medicine, Medical Faculty, University of Rzeszow, Rzeszów 35-959, Poland; ddarmochwal@ur.edu.pl
* Correspondence: zkimber@poczta.onet.pl; Tel.: +48-81-7244-769

Received: 14 January 2019; Accepted: 28 January 2019; Published: 30 January 2019

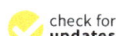

Abstract: Among the new adipokines, secreted frizzled-related protein 5 (SFRP5) is considered to prevent obesity and insulin resistance. The umbilical cord SFRP5 levels have not yet been investigated. The main aim of the study was to investigate whether the umbilical cord SFRP5 concentrations are altered in term neonates born to mothers with excessive gestational weight gain (EGWG). Two groups of subjects were selected depending on their gestational weight gain, i.e., 28 controls and 38 patients with EGWG. Umbilical cord and maternal serum SFRP5 levels were lower in the EGWG group. Umbilical cord SFRP5 concentrations were directly associated with the maternal serum SFRP5, hemoglobin A1c and lean tissue index, umbilical cord leptin levels, as well as newborns' anthropometric measurements in the EGWG subjects. In multiple linear regression models performed in all the study participants, umbilical cord SFRP5 concentrations depended positively on the maternal serum SFRP5, ghrelin, and leptin levels and negatively on the umbilical cord ghrelin levels, low-density lipoprotein cholesterol, pre-pregnancy body mass index, and gestational weight gain. EGWG is associated with disturbances in SFRP5 concentrations. Obstetricians and midwives should pay attention to nutrition and weight management during pregnancy.

Keywords: adipokines; secreted frizzled-related protein 5; leptin; ghrelin; excessive gestational weight gain; neonatal anthropometry; obesity

1. Introduction

As a novel adipokine mainly secreted from the adipose tissue, secreted frizzled-related protein 5 (SFRP5) contains a cysteine rich domain as well as a netrin-like function domain, and it plays a regulatory role in the wingless-type Mouse Mammary Tumor Virus (MMTV) integration site family member (Wnt) signaling pathways [1–3]. Preliminary clinical and basic research reveals that the biologic function of SFRP5 may be similar to adiponectin, which exerts an anti-inflammatory effect in the metabolic homeostasis [1,2]. SFRP5 has been reported to be implicated in obesity, insulin resistance, dyslipidemia, and metabolic syndromes [4–10]. Circulating concentrations of SFRP5 have been measured in healthy and diseased individuals in several studies, but there are still limited data concerning SFRP5 in obstetric aspects [3,11–14].

As far as we know, there is no reported study investigating the SFRP5 concentrations in the human umbilical cord blood. We hypothesized that SFRP5 concentrations would probably be impaired in the umbilical cord of full-term neonates born to excessive gestational weight gain (EGWG) mothers. The aim of this study was also to investigate whether the umbilical cord SFRP5 levels correlate with selected maternal parameters and neonatal anthropometric measurements.

2. Results

Compared with the healthy study participants, the EGWG mothers had comparable age and pre-pregnancy BMIs, but they presented significantly higher BMIs at and after delivery. The EGWG women were also characterized by increased levels of hemoglobin A1c (HgbA1c), triglycerides and indexes of fat (FTI) and lean (LTI) tissues as well as lower concentrations of high-density lipoprotein cholesterol (HDL). The maternal SFRP5 levels were decreased in the serum in the EGWG group. Lower SFRP5 concentrations as well as higher ghrelin and leptin levels were observed in the umbilical cord blood of neonates born to the EGWG mothers. No significant differences were noticed between the groups with regard to other analyzed parameters, including the maternal serum ghrelin and leptin levels as well as neonatal anthropometric measurements (Table 1).

Table 1. Comparison of characteristics of the study subjects.

Variables	Control Group (n = 28)	EGWG Group (n = 38)	p
Maternal characteristics			
age, years	29 (24–38)	29 (28–32)	NS
pre-pregnancy BMI, kg/m^2	20.3 (19.5–24.4)	23.2 (21.6–24.09)	NS
gestational weight gain, kg	15 (11.5–15.6)	23.9 (21–26)	<0.001
gestational BMI gain, kg/m^2	5.4 (3.0–5.6)	8.4 (7.07–9.4)	<0.001
BMI at delivery, kg/m^2	26.3 (24.2–29.1)	31.3 (29.7–32.05)	<0.001
cesarean delivery, %	14	26	NS
BMI after delivery, kg/m^2	22 (21–23.9)	28.6 (26.2–29.7)	<0.001
FTI after delivery, kg/m^2	10.1 (9.1–13.8)	14.7 (13.2–17.2)	<0.001
LTI after delivery, kg/m^2	10.1. (9.4–13.1)	12.9 (11.2–13.9)	<0.01
Maternal Serum			
albumin, g/dL	3.68 (3.43–3.73)	3.55 (3.41–3.81)	NS
total cholesterol, mg/dL	249 (188–287)	225 (197–249)	NS
HDL, mg/dL	78 (75–82)	71 (59–79)	<0.05
LDL, mg/dL	129 (93–152)	106 (87–128)	NS
triglycerides, mg/dL	177 (150–254)	204 (178–258)	<0.05
HgbA1c, %	5.3 (4.6–5.4)	5.5 (5.0–5.5)	<0.05
SFRP5, ng/mL	3.1 (2.62–8.0)	2.47 (1.2–5.0)	<0.05
ghrelin, ng/mL	0.933 (0.646–1.115)	1.187 (0.343–2.433)	NS
leptin, ng/mL	10.43 (6.04–14.9)	14.87 (12.6–47.6)	NS
Umbilical Cord Blood			
SFRP5, ng/mL	5.08 (3.74–5.69)	3.33 (2.3–4.25)	<0.01
ghrelin, ng/mL	0.0195 (0.187–0.282)	0.525 (0.265–1.826)	<0.001
leptin, ng/mL	7.53 (4.9–14.01)	10.99 (8.5–13.4)	<0.001
Neonatal Anthropometric Measurements			
birth weight, g	3630 (3200–3920)	3520 (3400–3650)	NS
birth body length, cm	56 (55–57)	55 (54–56)	NS
head circumference, cm	34 (33–35)	34 (33–35)	NS
chest circumference, cm	34 (34–35)	34 (33–35)	NS

The results are shown as the median (interquartile range: 25–75%). Statistically significant values are given in bold. BMI—body mass index; EGWG—excessive gestational weight gain; FTI—fat tissue index; HDL—high-density lipoprotein cholesterol; HgbA1c—hemoglobin A1c; LDL—low-density lipoprotein cholesterol; LTI—lean tissue index; SFRP5—secreted frizzled-related protein 5.

In the control group, the umbilical cord SFRP5 concentrations correlated positively with the maternal serum HgbA1c, SFRP5, ghrelin and leptin levels, and the neonatal chest circumference. We found negative correlations between the umbilical cord SFRP5 and BMIs (pre-pregnancy, at and after delivery), total cholesterol, and umbilical cord ghrelin levels in the control subjects (Table 2).

Table 2. Correlation coefficient between the umbilical cord SFRP5 levels and clinical parameters in the control and EGWG groups.

Variables	Umbilical Cord SFRP5	
	Control Group	EGWG Group
Maternal Characteristics		
pre-pregnancy BMI	**−0.829 *****	0.152
gestational weight gain	0.371	**−0.435 ***
gestational BMI gain	0.143	**−0.442 ***
BMI at delivery	**−0.6 ****	−0.105
BMI after delivery	**−0.486 ***	0.074
FTI after delivery	0.086	−0.342
LTI after delivery	−0.086	**0.527 ****
Maternal Serum		
albumin	−0.143	**−0.603 ****
total cholesterol	**−0.406 ***	**−0.436 ***
HDL	0.058	**−0.567 ****
LDL	−0.371	−0.087
triglycerides	−0.058	−0.081
HgbA1c	**0.667 *****	**0.636 *****
SFRP5	**0.429 ***	**0.452 ***
ghrelin	**0.771 *****	−0.394
leptin	**0.6 ****	−0.171
Umbilical Cord Blood		
ghrelin	**−0.657 *****	**−0.817 *****
leptin	−0.086	**0.495 ***
Neonatal Anthropometric Measurements		
birth weight	−0.2	**0.781 *****
birth body length	−0.309	**0.739 *****
head circumference	−0.206	**0.532 ****
chest circumference	**0.494 ***	**0.516 ****

Statistically significant values are given in the bold type. * $p < 0.05$; ** $p < 0.01$; *** $p < 0.001$. BMI—body mass index; EGWG—excessive gestational weight gain; FTI—fat tissue index; HDL—high-density lipoprotein cholesterol; HgbA1c—hemoglobin A1c; LDL—low-density lipoprotein cholesterol; LTI—lean tissue index; SFRP5—secreted frizzled-related protein 5.

In the EGWG group, we observed a direct correlation between the umbilical cord SFRP5 and the maternal serum HgbA1c, SFRP5 and LTI after delivery, the umbilical cord leptin levels, and all four newborns' anthropometric measurements (i.e., with neonatal birth weight, birth body length, and head and chest circumference). Negative correlations were revealed between the umbilical cord SFRP5 concentrations and gestational weight and BMI gains, albumin, total cholesterol, HDL, and the umbilical cord ghrelin levels in the EGWG subjects (Table 2).

In multiple linear regression models performed in all the study participants, after adjustment for the maternal serum SFRP5 levels, the serum and umbilical cord ghrelin and leptin levels, maternal low-density lipoprotein cholesterol (LDL), triglycerides, HgbA1c, gestational weight gain, pre-pregnancy BMI, BMI at delivery and gestational BMI gain, we noted that the umbilical cord SFRP5 concentrations were positively dependent on the maternal serum SFRP5, ghrelin and leptin levels as well as negatively dependent on the umbilical cord ghrelin levels, LDL, pre-pregnancy BMI and gestational weight gain (Table 3).

The Benjamini–Hochberg correction for false positive results revealed that all of the originally significant associations were still significant.

Table 3. Multiple linear regression analyses for the umbilical cord SFRP5 levels.

Independent Variable	B	β	95% CI	p
maternal serum SFRP5	0.33	0.50	0.32–0.69	<0.001
maternal serum ghrelin	0.12	0.39	0.19–0.59	<0.001
umbilical cord ghrelin	−0.26	−0.79	−0.99–(−0.59)	<0.001
maternal serum leptin	0.06	0.72	0.52–0.92	<0.001
maternal LDL	−0.01	−0.23	−0.38–(−0.07)	<0.01
pre-pregnancy BMI	−0.12	−0.27	−0.47–(−0.06)	<0.05
gestational weight gain	−0.08	−0.29	−0.48–(−0.11)	<0.01

Adjusted for the serum SFRP5 levels, the serum and umbilical cord ghrelin and leptin levels, maternal LDL, triglycerides, HgbA1c, gestational weight gain, pre-pregnancy BMI, BMI at delivery and gestational BMI gain. Unstandardized β coefficients with 95% confidence interval and B linear regression coefficients are shown. Statistically significant values are given in the bold type. BMI—body mass index; LDL—low-density lipoprotein cholesterol; SFRP5—secreted frizzled-related protein 5.

3. Discussion

We decided to choose EGWG and not pre-pregnant obese women, as EGWG is mainly linked to overnutrition during a relatively short period of time (with regard to life expectancy), i.e. within the last nine months. Gestational weight guidelines of the Institute of Medicine (IOM) [15] provide ranges of recommended weight gain for specific pre-pregnancy body mass index (BMI) categories in relation to the least risk of adverse perinatal outcomes. It is recommended that in order to prevent adverse maternal as well as infant outcomes, women with normal weight at the time of conception should limit their total weight gain in pregnancy to 11.5–16 kg, overweight women to 7–11.5 kg, and obese women to 5–9 kg [15]. Goldstein et al. revealed in a systematic review of 23 cohort studies in 1.3 million women that 47% of women exceeded the upper limit of IOM-recommended weight gain [16]. EGWG, which is usually due to improper nutrition during the pregnancy period, has been regarded as a potentially modifiable, independent risk factor not only for the development of maternal overweight and obesity but childhood adiposity as well [17,18]. EGWG may expose the developing fetus to persistently raised concentrations of glucose, insulin, amino acids, and lipids as well as imbalance between pro- and anti-inflammatory adipokines derived from maternal adipose tissue [19,20].

SFRP5 is an anti-inflammatory adipokine that regulates metabolic homeostasis [5,21]. The classical molecular mechanism of SFRP5 is designated to inhibit the combination of Wnt protein with its cell membrane receptors (frizzled protein) and block the downstream Wnt signaling pathways through binding with the extracellular Wnt-5a or Wnt-3a [2,22,23]. *Sfrp5* knockout mice fed a high fat diet developed adipose macrophage infiltration, severe glucose intolerance, and hepatic steatosis [1,2,24].

SFRP5 is an inhibitor of Wnt signaling, the crucial signaling pathway in the placental vascular development. Placental angiogenesis is a pivotal process that establishes feto-maternal circulation, ensures efficient materno-fetal exchanges and contributes to the overall development of the placenta throughout pregnancy. Any failure in these processes will definitely result in the development of many gestational complications such as preeclampsia, GDM, and intrauterine growth restriction [25–27]. Nevertheless, there are limited data concerning SFRP5 in the obstetric aspects. A previous study demonstrated that first trimester serum SFRP5 levels were significantly lower in the pregnant women who subsequently developed GDM in comparison to the healthy pregnant women [3]. Based on the mechanism that SFRP5 is an inhibitor of the Wnt signaling pathway, which is implicated in the regulation of insulin resistance, inflammation, and placental vasculature, it was suggested that altered levels of SFRP5 may contribute to the development of GDM [3,28,29].

It is worth highlighting that some of the previous studies evaluating the levels of various adipokines in the umbilical cord blood did not take into consideration the maternal BMI and weight gain during pregnancy [30–33]. Our study comprised both participants with normal pre-pregnancy BMI and different gestational weight gain; i.e. an excessive increase in body weight during pregnancy in the EGWG group and an appropriate gestational weight gain in the control group and their offspring. Our results revealed differences at the periparturient period not only in the gestational weight and

BMI gains between these two groups of mothers but in the laboratory results as well. Lower levels of HDL as well as higher HgbA1c and triglycerides concentrations were present in the EGWG group. It seems that in many ways the pregnancies of women with EGWG resemble pregnancies complicated by gestational diabetes mellitus (GDM). What is important in this context is that the women with a history of GDM exhibit altered risk factors of cardiovascular diseases, including lower HDL concentrations, when compared with mothers with healthy pregnancies [34–36].

Nonetheless, the offspring of our control and EGWG groups had comparable anthropometric measurements, including birth weight. However, in light of the previous studies, the fetal metabolic programming may occur within normal birth weight ranges [37,38]. Lawrence et al. [39] reported a potential role of genetics for the existing association between the maternal weight gain during pregnancy and offspring BMI change. The association between the gestational weight gain and offspring BMI change attenuated by 28% when a genetic score was added, but the offspring's genetic variation did not play a role in the association. The authors speculate that epigenetics may underlie this finding [40]. DNA microarray analyses on the placental junctional zones performed by Gao et al. [13] revealed that the *Sfrp5* expression was decreased in the rats fed a low protein diet, which may activate non-canonical Wnt signaling. Christodoulides et al. [41] reported that *Sfrp5* mediated epigenetic silencing of the Wnt signaling pathway in the white adipose tissue could lead to an increased adipogenesis with a significant likelihood of increasing susceptibility to diet-induced obesity in the mice models. In addition, SFRP5 has been demonstrated to inhibit the activation of c-JunN-terminal kinase (JNK) downstream of the Wnt signaling pathway [1,5,42].

To the best of our knowledge, this study is the first report evaluating the umbilical cord SFRP5 in the offspring of healthy mothers as well as of women with excessive gestational weight gain. We also investigated associations between its levels in the umbilical cord and in the maternal serum. Our study revealed that the umbilical cord SFRP5 levels were lower in the offspring of the EGWG mothers. However, what is also extremely important is that the studied mothers with EGWG, when compared with the healthy controls, presented lower SFRP5 concentrations in the serum. The umbilical cord SFRP5 levels were positively associated with the maternal serum SFRP5 levels in both groups. Apart from this, we performed multiple linear analyses that revealed the dependence of the umbilical cord SFRP5 concentrations on its levels in the maternal serum. Each 1 ng/mL decrease in the maternal serum SFRP5 concentration was associated with a decrease in the umbilical cord SFRP5 level by 0.33 ng/mL.

The study of Prats-Puig et al. [43] reported concomitantly decreased concentrations of SFRP5 in obesity markers of prepubertal children. The cited authors found that lower serum SFRP5 potentiated the association between Wnt-5A and insulin resistance. Previous studies showed that circulating SFRP5 was decreased in patients with impaired glucose tolerance or T2DM and was associated with various obesity-related metabolic parameters [8,9,43]. SFRP5 sequesters Wnt-5A, thereby attenuating the activation of c-Jun N-terminal kinase 1 [43–45]. Prats-Puig et al. [43] concluded that SFRP5 may be an anti-inflammatory adipokine that could be negatively regulated during obesity development, leading to a less-favorable metabolic phenotype. Their results also suggested that a failure to upregulate SFRP5 in obesity may lead to unrestrained pro-inflammatory actions of Wnt-5A, resulting in metabolic dysfunction [1,43,46].

The expression of *Sfrp5* is slowly induced in the process of differentiation of white and brown adipocytes and increased in mature adipocytes [47]. Lower SFRP5 levels have been detected in obese subjects in contrast with lean subjects in studies analyzing correlations between SFRP5 and adiposity indicators such as BMI, waist–hip ratio, body fat percentage, and lipid profile [9]. In our study, a positive correlation was found between the umbilical cord serum SFRP5 concentrations and maternal LTI, but only in the EGWG group. LTI, which is defined as the lean tissue mass divided by the square of the body height, expresses the muscle mass [48]. Mori et al. [49] revealed that SFRP5 promotes adipocyte growth by repressing Wnt signaling and decreasing oxidative metabolism as an endogenous suppressor of adipogenesis. Rulifson et al. [50] and Van Camp et al. [51] found that a significant increase in *Sfrp5* expression was observed amongst adipose tissues in obese mice and that genetic variation in *Sfrp5* could determine the distribution and volume of both subcutaneous and abdominal fat in obese males, respectively.

As far as progressive metabolic complications are concerned, it should be pointed out that SFRP5 levels decreased with age in the prepubertal children [43]. On the other hand, increased leptin concentrations during puberty were found to be a reliable indicator of insulin resistance associated with increasing age [52]. Thus, the possibility that reduced SFRP5 levels may contribute to the state of insulin resistance associated with increasing age and pubertal development cannot be excluded [43,53].

In this study, we evaluated the concentrations of leptin and ghrelin, which were higher in the umbilical cord blood of EGWG patients than in the control subjects. However, concentrations of the maternal serum ghrelin and leptin were similar in both studied groups. The previous results suggested that ghrelin may play a role in the fetal adaptation to intrauterine malnutrition [54]. Moreover, it is interesting to point out a negative correlation between SFRP5 and ghrelin concentrations in the umbilical cord of both the control and EGWG newborns. What is more, we were also able to find a positive association between the umbilical cord SFRP5 and leptin levels but only in the EGWG group.

We observed that the SFRP5 umbilical cord levels were associated with the maternal BMI values. We found out that the umbilical cord SFRP5 negatively correlated with the maternal BMIs (pre-pregnancy, at and after delivery) in the control subjects as well as with the gestational weight and BMI gains in the EGWG group. Besides, multiple linear regression models performed in all the study participants revealed that the umbilical cord SFRP5 concentrations were negatively dependent on the pre-pregnancy BMI and gestational weight gain. It is noteworthy that every 1 kg of gestational weight gain was linked to a decrease in the umbilical cord SFRP5 concentration by 0.08 ng/mL. Similarly, we made an observation that the umbilical cord SFRP5 levels correlated with the maternal concentrations of total cholesterol and HgbA1c and were negatively dependent on LDL. These results seem to confirm the impact of maternal weight and metabolic imbalance on SFRP5 in newborns. We cannot relate our results to the previous ones because no such results are available. However, a comparison with the observations made in non-pregnant humans concerning the serum SFRP5 levels negatively associated with BMI values [3,8,9] as well as with insulin resistance and lipid profile [5,9,28] might confirm the existence of a feto-maternal unit and fetal dependence on the maternal nourishment status.

Our study methodology relied on an accurate selection of the study subjects. We decided to choose EGWG and not pre-pregnant obese women. In the case of pre-pregnancy obesity the analysis of the results would have to take into consideration the influence of modulators such as dyslipidemia, hypertension, insulin resistance, pre-pregnancy treatment of obesity, and disorders of the carbohydrate–lipid balance. Because we chose the EGWG group, we were able to reduce the number of interfering and confounding factors in the analysis of the study results. The study groups were formed on the basis of women's similar age, normal pre-pregnancy BMIs, and term pregnancies. Selected women were to be free of any chronic and gestational diseases and receive only vitamins throughout their pregnancy period. On the other hand, this study has an important limitation as a small sample study. Our results require further verification. It also appears of great clinical significance to monitor the circulating SFRP5 levels in all trimesters of pregnancies as well as in future life of children.

4. Materials and Methods

The study comprised infants of mothers who were in a singleton term pregnancy (after 37 weeks of gestation) and delivered at the Chair and Department of Obstetrics and Perinatology, the Medical University of Lublin. The data collection was performed between March 2016 and February 2017. All the study subjects included in this study were Caucasian. The study included women receiving only vitamin-iron supplementation during pregnancy, without any exclusion criteria given below, with normal pre-pregnancy BMI values and three normal results of the two-hour, 75 g oral glucose tolerance test at 24–28 weeks of gestation [55,56]. Depending on the achieved gestational weight gain, two groups were strictly selected:

- healthy controls—28 pregnant women with normal gestational weight gain;
- patients with EGWG—38 pregnant subjects with excessive gestational weight gain.

Exclusion criteria from the study were as follows: multiple pregnancy, chronic infectious diseases, urinary infections, anemia, metabolic disorders (except for improper gestational weight gain for the EGWG group), mental illness, cancer, liver diseases, cardiovascular disorders, fetal malformation, premature membrane rupture, and intrauterine growth retardation. We had to rule out, among others, all females with gestational hypertension, which is a common complication observed in patients with high BMI values in the third trimester of pregnancy.

Anthropometric measurements of the mothers were performed immediately before and after delivery. Calculation of pre-pregnancy BMIs values were based on body weight measured at the first prenatal visit, occurring in the first trimester (before 10 weeks of gestation). We defined total gestational weight gain as the difference between the mother's weight at delivery and her pre-pregnancy weight. We calculated gestational BMI gain as well. Neonatal anthropometric measurements, including birth weight, body length, and head and chest circumferences, were performed immediately after birth. The maternal serum levels of albumin, HgbA1c, and lipid profile were measured at a certified laboratory. The cord blood samples were taken during delivery but without any interference with its course. The maternal serum samples were taken after delivery, taking into account a 6 h fasting period. After centrifugation, all the collected cord blood serum as well as maternal serum samples were stored at $-80\ °C$. Concentrations of SFRP5 and ghrelin in these materials were determined using commercially available kits and in compliance with the manufacturer's instructions (Wuhan EIAab Science Co., Wuhan, China) via traditional enzyme-linked immunosorbent assay (ELISA). Concentrations of leptin in the cord blood serum and maternal serum were determined using commercially available kits and in compliance with the manufacturer's instructions (R&D Systems, Inc., Minneapolis, MN, USA) via ELISA. The survey was performed in duplicates for each patient.

Maternal body composition (LTI and FTI) were evaluated by the bioelectrical impedance analysis (BIA) method with the use of a body composition monitor (BCM) (Fresenius Medical Care) in the early post-partum period (i.e. 48 h after delivery).

All the patients were informed about the study protocol and a detailed written consent was obtained from each patient who agreed to participate in the study. A separate information sheet was prepared for the parents of newborns. Written signed consent from each infant's legal guardians (mothers) was obtained after informed consent.

The study protocol received approval of the Bioethics Committee of the Medical University of Lublin (no. KE-0254/221/2015 (25th June 2015) and no. KE-0254/348/2016 (15th December 2016)).

All values were reported as the median (interquartile range 25–75%) or numbers and percentages. Differences between groups were tested for significance using the Mann–Whitney U test. The Spearman's coefficient test was used for the correlation analyses. Categorical data were compared using the chi-square test. The Benjamini–Hochberg correction for false positive results was performed. Multiple linear regression model was used to examine the association between the umbilical cord SFRP5 levels and the selected biophysical and biochemical parameters of the mothers and their offspring. Regression models were adjusted for the serum SFRP5 levels, the serum and umbilical cord ghrelin and leptin levels, LDL, triglycerides, HgbA1c, gestational weight gain, pre-pregnancy BMI, BMI at delivery, and gestational BMI gain. All analyses were performed using Statistical Package for the Social Sciences software (version 19; SPSS Inc., Chicago, IL, USA). A p-value of <0.05 was considered statistically significant.

5. Conclusions

In light of our study results, it becomes understandable that maternal condition, including gestational weight gain, should be of utmost importance when doing further research into the umbilical cord SFRP5 concentrations and investigating their relationship with the fetal and neonatal anthropometry and metabolic state. Evaluation of the umbilical cord SFRP5 levels in the offspring of EGWG mothers as well as of the relationships between the umbilical cord SFRP5 levels, maternal laboratory results, and neonatal anthropometric measurements is a new idea.

It is also quite obvious that obstetricians and midwives should pay attention to nutrition and weight management of their pregnant patients and should educate them on the dangers of overnutrition and on how it predisposes not only them but also their children to metabolic disorders later in life. On the other hand, it should be emphasized that, in order to avoid potential future metabolic complications, the offspring of mothers with excessive gestational weight gain during pregnancy should be carefully monitored by their pediatricians.

Author Contributions: Conceptualization, Ż.K.-T.; methodology, Ż.K.-T. and J.P.-M.; software, Ż.K.-T. and J.P.-M.; validation, Ż.K.-T., J.P.-M., M.T., and D.D.-K.; formal analysis, M.T.; investigation, Ż.K.-T. and J.P.-M.; data curation, M.T.; writing—original draft preparation, Ż.K.-T. and M.T.; writing—review and editing, Ż.K.-T.; visualization, Ż.K.-T. and J.P.-M.; supervision, J.O. and B.L.-G.; project administration, Ż.K.-T.

Funding: This study was supported by the Medical University of Lublin, grant no. 335.

Conflicts of Interest: The authors declare no conflict of interest.

References

1. Ouchi, N.; Higuchi, A.; Ohashi, K.; Oshima, Y.; Gokce, N.; Shibata, R.; Akasaki, Y.; Shimono, A.; Walsh, K. Sfrp5 is an anti-inflammatory adipokine that modulates metabolic dysfunction in obesity. *Science* **2010**, *329*, 454–457. [CrossRef] [PubMed]
2. Chen, L.; Zhao, X.; Liang, G.; Sun, J.; Lin, Z.; Hu, R.; Chen, P.; Zhang, Z.; Zhou, L.; Li, Y. Recombinant SFRP5 protein significantly alleviated intrahepatic inflammation of nonalcoholic steatohepatitis. *Nutr. Metab.* **2017**, *14*, 56. [CrossRef] [PubMed]
3. Oztas, E.; Ozler, S.; Ersoy, E.; Ersoy, A.O.; Tokmak, A.; Ergin, M.; Uygur, D.; Danisman, N. Prediction of gestational diabetes mellitus by first trimester serum secreted frizzle-related protein-5 levels. *J. Matern. Fetal Neonatal Med.* **2016**, *29*, 1515–1519. [CrossRef] [PubMed]
4. Teliewubai, J.; Bai, B.; Zhou, Y.; Lu, Y.; Yu, S.; Chi, C.; Li, J.; Blacher, J.; Xu, Y.; Zhang, Y. Association of asymptomatic target organ damage with secreted frizzled related protein 5 in the elderly: The Northern Shanghai Study. *Clin. Interv. Aging* **2018**, *13*, 389–395. [CrossRef] [PubMed]
5. Liu, L.B.; Chen, X.D.; Zhou, X.Y.; Zhu, Q. The Wnt antagonist and secreted frizzled-related protein 5: Implications on lipid metabolism, inflammation, and type 2 diabetes mellitus. *Biosci. Rep.* **2018**, *38*, BSR20180011. [CrossRef] [PubMed]
6. Carstensen-Kirberg, M.; Kannenberg, J.M.; Huth, C.; Meisinger, C.; Koenig, W.; Heier, M.; Peters, A.; Rathmann, W.; Roden, M.; Herder, C.; et al. Inverse associations between serum levels of secreted frizzled-related protein-5 (SFRP5) and multiple cardiometabolic risk factors: KORA F4 study. *Cardiovasc. Diabetol.* **2017**, *16*, 109. [CrossRef] [PubMed]
7. Carstensen-Kirberg, M.; Hatziagelaki, E.; Tsiavou, A.; Chounta, A.; Nowotny, P.; Pacini, G.; Dimitriadis, G.; Roden, M.; Herder, C. Sfrp5 associates with beta-cell function in humans. *Eur. J. Clin. Investig.* **2016**, *46*, 535–543. [CrossRef]
8. Hu, Z.; Deng, H.; Qu, H. Plasma SFRP5 levels are decreased in Chinese subjects with obesity and type 2 diabetes and negatively correlated with parameters of insulin resistance. *Diabetes Res. Clin. Pract.* **2013**, *99*, 391–395. [CrossRef]
9. Hu, W.; Li, L.; Yang, M.; Luo, X.; Ran, W.; Liu, D.; Xiong, Z.; Liu, H.; Yang, G. Circulating Sfrp5 is a signature of obesity-related metabolic disorders and is regulated by glucose and liraglutide in humans. *J. Clin. Endocrinol. Metab.* **2013**, *98*, 290–298. [CrossRef]
10. Xu, Q.; Wang, H.; Li, Y.; Wang, J.; Lai, Y.; Gao, L.; Lei, L.; Yang, G.; Liao, X.; Fang, X.; et al. Plasma Sfrp5 levels correlate with determinants of the metabolic syndrome in Chinese adults. *Diabetes Metab. Res. Rev.* **2017**, *33*. [CrossRef]
11. Yokota, T.; Oritani, K.; Sudo, T.; Ishibashi, T.; Doi, Y.; Habuchi, Y.; Ichii, M.; Fukushima, K.; Okuzaki, D.; Tomizuka, K.; et al. Estrogen-inducible sFRP5 inhibits early B-lymphopoiesis in vivo, but not during pregnancy. *Eur. J. Immunol.* **2015**, *45*, 1390–1401. [CrossRef] [PubMed]

12. Dahlhoff, M.; Pfister, S.; Blutke, A.; Rozman, J.; Klingenspor, M.; Deutsch, M.J.; Rathkolb, B.; Fink, B.; Gimpfl, M.; Hrabě de Angelis, M.; et al. Peri-conceptional obesogenic exposure induces sex-specific programming of disease susceptibilities in adult mouse offspring. *Biochim. Biophys. Acta* **2014**, *1842*, 304–317. [CrossRef]
13. Gao, H.; Tanchico, D.; Yallampalli, U.; Yallampalli, C. Sfrp5 expression is reduced in placental junctional zone in pregnant rats fed a low protein diet. *Placenta* **2014**, *35*, 77. [CrossRef]
14. Atli, M.O.; Guzeloglu, A.; Dinc, D.A. Expression of wingless type (WNT) genes and their antagonists at mRNA levels in equine endometrium during the estrous cycle and early pregnancy. *Anim. Reprod. Sci.* **2011**, *125*, 94–102. [CrossRef] [PubMed]
15. Institute of Medicine (US) and National Research Council (US) Committee to Reexamine IOM Pregnancy Weight Guidelines; Rasmussen, K.M.; Yaktine, A.L. *Weight Gain during Pregnancy: Reexamining the Guidelines*; National Academies Press: Washington, DC, USA, 2009.
16. Goldstein, R.F.; Abell, S.K.; Ranasinha, S.; Misso, M.; Boyle, J.A.; Black, M.H.; Li, N.; Hu, G.; Corrado, F.; Rode, L.; et al. Association of Gestational Weight Gain with Maternal and Infant Outcomes: A Systematic Review and Meta-analysis. *JAMA* **2017**, *317*, 2207–2225. [CrossRef]
17. Guo, L.; Liu, J.; Ye, R.; Liu, J.; Zhuang, Z.; Ren, A. Gestational Weight Gain and Overweight in Children Aged 3–6 Years. *J. Epidemiol.* **2015**, *25*, 536–543. [CrossRef]
18. Diesel, J.C.; Eckhardt, C.L.; Day, N.L.; Brooks, M.M.; Arslanian, S.A.; Bodnar, L.M. Gestational Weight Gain and Offspring Longitudinal Growth in Early Life. *Ann. Nutr. Metab.* **2015**, *67*, 49–57. [CrossRef]
19. Estampador, A.C.; Pomeroy, J.; Renström, F.; Nelson, S.M.; Mogren, I.; Persson, M.; Sattar, N.; Domellöf, M.; Franks, P.W. Infant body composition and adipokine concentrations in relation to maternal gestational weight gain. *Diabetes Care* **2014**, *37*, 1432–1438. [CrossRef]
20. Walsh, J.M.; McGowan, C.A.; Mahony, R.M.; Foley, M.E.; McAuliffe, F.M. Obstetric and metabolic implications of excessive gestational weight gain in pregnancy. *Obesity* **2014**, *22*, 1594–1600. [CrossRef]
21. Lu, Y.C.; Wang, C.P.; Hsu, C.C.; Chiu, C.A.; Yu, T.H.; Hung, W.C.; Lu, L.F.; Chung, F.M.; Tsai, I.T.; Lin, H.C.; et al. Circulating secreted frizzled-related protein 5 (Sfrp5) and wingless-type MMTV integration site family member 5a (Wnt5a) levels in patients with type 2 diabetes mellitus. *Diabetes Metab. Res. Rev.* **2013**, *29*, 551–556. [CrossRef]
22. McDowall, M.D.; Scott, M.S.; Barton, G.J. PIPs: Human protein-protein interaction prediction database. *Nucleic Acids Res.* **2009**, *37*, D651–D656. [CrossRef] [PubMed]
23. Li, Y.; Rankin, S.A.; Sinner, D.; Kenny, A.P.; Krieg, P.A.; Zorn, A.M. Sfrp5 coordinates foregut specification and morphogenesis by antagonizing both canonical and noncanonical Wnt11 signaling. *Genes Dev.* **2008**, *22*, 3050–3063. [CrossRef] [PubMed]
24. Rauch, A.; Mandrup, S. Lighting the fat furnace without SFRP5. *J. Clin. Investig.* **2012**, *122*, 2349–2352. [CrossRef] [PubMed]
25. Marciniak, A.; Patro-Małysza, J.; Kimber-Trojnar, Ż.; Marciniak, B.; Oleszczuk, J.; Leszczyńska-Gorzelak, B. Fetal programming of the metabolic syndrome. *Taiwan J. Obstet. Gynecol.* **2017**, *56*, 133–138. [CrossRef] [PubMed]
26. Kwon, E.J.; Kim, Y.J. What is fetal programming?: A lifetime health is under the control of in utero health. *Obstet. Gynecol. Sci.* **2017**, *60*, 506–519. [CrossRef] [PubMed]
27. Zhang, S.; Regnault, T.R.; Barker, P.L.; Botting, K.J.; McMillen, I.C.; McMillan, C.M.; Roberts, C.T.; Morrison, J.L. Placental adaptations in growth restriction. *Nutrients* **2015**, *7*, 360–389. [CrossRef] [PubMed]
28. Almario, R.U.; Karakas, S.E. Roles of circulating WNT-signaling proteins and WNT-inhibitors in human adiposity, insulin resistance, insulin secretion, and inflammation. *Horm. Metab. Res.* **2015**, *47*, 152–157. [CrossRef] [PubMed]
29. Yilmaz, H.; Celik, H.T.; Namuslu, M.; Inan, O.; Onaran, Y.; Karakurt, F.; Ayyildiz, A.; Bilgic, M.A.; Bavbek, N.; Akcay, A. Benefits of the neutrophil-to-lymphocyte ratio for the prediction of gestational diabetes mellitus in pregnant women. *Exp. Clin. Endocrinol. Diabetes* **2014**, *122*, 39–43. [CrossRef] [PubMed]
30. Kharb, S.; Bala, J.; Nanda, S. Markers of obesity and growth in preeclamptic and normotensive pregnant women. *J. Obstet. Gynaecol.* **2017**, *37*, 610–615. [CrossRef] [PubMed]

31. Treviño-Garza, C.; Villarreal-Martínez, L.; Estrada-Zúñiga, C.M.; Leal-Treviño, M.; Rodríguez-Balderrama, I.; Nieto-Sanjuanero, A.; Cárdenas-Del Castillo, B.; Montes-Tapia, F.F.; de la O-Cavazos, M. Leptin, IL-6 and TNF-α levels in umbilical cord blood of healthy term newborns in relation to mode of delivery. *J. Obstet. Gynaecol.* **2016**, *36*, 719–721. [CrossRef] [PubMed]
32. Boutsikou, T.; Briana, D.D.; Boutsikou, M.; Kafalidis, G.; Piatopoulou, D.; Baka, S.; Hassiakos, D.; Gourgiotis, D.; Malamitsi-Puchner, A. Cord blood nesfatin-1 in large for gestational age pregnancies. *Cytokine* **2013**, *61*, 591–594. [CrossRef] [PubMed]
33. Martos-Moreno, G.A.; Barrios, V.; Sáenz de Pipaón, M.; Pozo, J.; Dorronsoro, I.; Martínez-Biarge, M.; Quero, J.; Argente, J. Influence of prematurity and growth restriction on the adipokine profile, IGF1, and ghrelin levels in cord blood: Relationship with glucose metabolism. *Eur. J. Endocrinol.* **2009**, *161*, 381–389. [CrossRef] [PubMed]
34. Kimber-Trojnar, Ż.; Patro-Małysza, J.; Skórzyńska-Dziduszko, K.E.; Oleszczuk, J.; Trojnar, M.; Mierzyński, R.; Leszczyńska-Gorzelak, B. Ghrelin in Serum and Urine of Post-Partum Women with Gestational Diabetes Mellitus. *Int. J. Mol. Sci.* **2018**, *19*, 3001. [CrossRef] [PubMed]
35. Huopio, H.; Hakkarainen, H.; Pääkkönen, M.; Kuulasmaa, T.; Voutilainen, R.; Heinonen, S.; Cederberg, H. Long-Term changes in glucose metabolism after gestational diabetes: A double cohort study. *BMC Pregnancy Childbirth* **2014**, *14*, 296. [CrossRef] [PubMed]
36. Bellamy, L.; Casas, J.; Hingorani, A.; Williams, D. Type 2 diabetes mellitus after gestational diabetes: A systematic review and meta-analysis. *Lancet* **2009**, *373*, 1773–1779. [CrossRef]
37. Luo, Z.C.; Bilodeau, J.F.; Nuyt, A.M.; Fraser, W.D.; Julien, P.; Audibert, F.; Xiao, L.; Garofalo, C.; Levy, E. Perinatal Oxidative Stress May Affect Fetal Ghrelin Levels in Humans. *Sci. Rep.* **2015**, *5*, 17881. [CrossRef] [PubMed]
38. Gluckman, P.D.; Hanson, M.A. Living with the past: Evolution, development, and patterns of disease. *Science* **2004**, *305*, 1733–1736. [CrossRef]
39. Lawrence, G.M.; Shulman, S.; Friedlander, Y.; Sitlani, C.M.; Burger, A.; Savitsky, B.; Granot-Hershkovitz, E.; Lumley, T.; Kwok, P.Y.; Hesselson, S.; et al. Associations of maternal pre-pregnancy and gestational body size with offspring longitudinal change in BMI. *Obesity* **2014**, *22*, 1165–1171. [CrossRef]
40. Van Rossem, L.; Wijga, A.H.; Gehring, U.; Koppelman, G.H.; Smit, H.A. Maternal Gestational and Postdelivery Weight Gain and Child Weight. *Pediatrics* **2015**, *136*, e1294–e1301. [CrossRef]
41. Christodoulides, C.; Lagathu, C.; Sethi, J.K.; Vidal-Puig, A. Adipogenesis and WNT signalling. *Trends Endocrinol. Metab.* **2009**, *20*, 16–24. [CrossRef]
42. Schulte, D.M.; Kragelund, D.; Müller, N.; Hagen, I.; Elke, G.; Titz, A.; Schädler, D.; Schumacher, J.; Weiler, N.; Bewig, B.; et al. The wingless-related integration site-5a/secreted frizzled-related protein-5 system is dysregulated in human sepsis. *Clin. Exp. Immunol.* **2015**, *180*, 90–97. [CrossRef] [PubMed]
43. Prats-Puig, A.; Soriano-Rodríguez, P.; Carreras-Badosa, G.; Riera-Pérez, E.; Ros-Miquel, M.; Gomila-Borja, A.; de Zegher, F.; Ibáñez, L.; Bassols, J.; López-Bermejo, A. Balanced duo of anti-inflammatory SFRP5 and proinflammatory WNT5A in children. *Pediatr. Res.* **2014**, *75*, 793–797. [CrossRef] [PubMed]
44. Bilkovski, R.; Schulte, D.M.; Oberhauser, F.; Gomolka, M.; Udelhoven, M.; Hettich, M.M.; Roth, B.; Heidenreich, A.; Gutschow, C.; Krone, W.; et al. Role of WNT-5a in the determination of human mesenchymal stem cells into preadipocytes. *J. Biol. Chem.* **2010**, *285*, 6170–6178. [CrossRef] [PubMed]
45. Almind, K.; Kahn, C.R. Genetic determinants of energy expenditure and insulin resistance in diet-induced obesity in mice. *Diabetes* **2004**, *53*, 3274–3285. [CrossRef] [PubMed]
46. Schulte, D.M.; Müller, N.; Neumann, K.; Oberhäuser, F.; Faust, M.; Güdelhöfer, H.; Brandt, B.; Krone, W.; Laudes, M. Pro-inflammatory wnt5a and anti-inflammatory sFRP5 are differentially regulated by nutritional factors in obese human subjects. *PLoS ONE* **2012**, *7*, e32437. [CrossRef]
47. Wang, R.; Hong, J.; Liu, R.; Chen, M.; Xu, M.; Gu, W.; Zhang, Y.; Ma, Q.; Wang, F.; Shi, J.; et al. SFRP5 acts as a mature adipocyte marker but not as a regulator in adipogenesis. *J. Mol. Endocrinol.* **2014**, *53*, 405–415. [CrossRef] [PubMed]
48. Wang, Y.W.; Lin, T.Y.; Peng, C.H.; Huang, J.L.; Hung, S.C. Factors Associated with Decreased Lean Tissue Index in Patients with Chronic Kidney Disease. *Nutrients* **2017**, *9*, 434. [CrossRef]
49. Mori, H.; Prestwich, T.C.; Reid, M.A.; Longo, K.A.; Gerin, I.; Cawthorn, W.P.; Susulic, V.S.; Krishnan, V.; Greenfield, A.; Macdougald, O.A. Secreted frizzled-related protein 5 suppresses adipocyte mitochondrial metabolism through WNT inhibition. *J. Clin. Investig.* **2012**, *122*, 2405–2416. [CrossRef]

50. Rulifson, I.C.; Majeti, J.Z.; Xiong, Y.; Hamburger, A.; Lee, K.J.; Miao, L.; Lu, M.; Gardner, J.; Gong, Y.; Wu, H.; et al. Inhibition of secreted frizzled-related protein 5 improves glucose metabolism. *Am. J. Physiol. Endocrinol. Metab.* **2014**, *307*, E1144–E1152. [CrossRef]
51. Van Camp, J.K.; Beckers, S.; Zegers, D.; Verrijken, A.; Van Gaal, L.F.; Van Hul, W. Common genetic variation in sFRP5 is associated with fat distribution in men. *Endocrine* **2014**, *46*, 477–484. [CrossRef]
52. Xu, L.; Li, M.; Yin, J.; Cheng, H.; Yu, M.; Zhao, X.; Xiao, X.; Mi, J. Change of Body Composition and Adipokines and Their Relationship with Insulin Resistance across Pubertal Development in Obese and Nonobese Chinese Children: The BCAMS Study. *Int. J. Endocrinol.* **2012**, *2012*, 389108. [CrossRef] [PubMed]
53. Bush, N.C.; Darnell, B.E.; Oster, R.A.; Goran, M.I.; Gower, B.A. Adiponectin is lower among African Americans and is independently related to insulin sensitivity in children and adolescents. *Diabetes* **2005**, *54*, 2772–2778. [CrossRef] [PubMed]
54. Chiesa, C.; Osborn, J.F.; Haass, C.; Natale, F.; Spinelli, M.; Scapillati, E.; Spinelli, A.; Pacifico, L. Ghrelin, leptin, IGF-1, IGFBP-3, and insulin concentrations at birth: Is there a relationship with fetal growth and neonatal anthropometry? *Clin. Chem.* **2008**, *54*, 550–558. [CrossRef] [PubMed]
55. International Association of Diabetes and Pregnancy Study Groups Consensus Panel. International association of diabetes and pregnancy study groups recommendations on the diagnosis and classification of hyperglycemia in pregnancy. *Diabetes Care* **2010**, *33*, 676–682. [CrossRef] [PubMed]
56. Diabetes Poland (Polish Diabetes Association). 2018 Guidelines on the management of diabetic patients. A position of Diabetes Poland. *Clin. Diabetol.* **2018**, *7*, 1–90. [CrossRef]

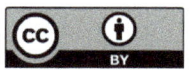

© 2019 by the authors. Licensee MDPI, Basel, Switzerland. This article is an open access article distributed under the terms and conditions of the Creative Commons Attribution (CC BY) license (http://creativecommons.org/licenses/by/4.0/).

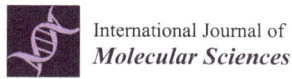

Article

Leptin and Ghrelin in Excessive Gestational Weight Gain—Association between Mothers and Offspring

Jolanta Patro-Małysza [1,*], Marcin Trojnar [2], Katarzyna E. Skórzyńska-Dziduszko [3], Żaneta Kimber-Trojnar [1], Dorota Darmochwał-Kolarz [4], Monika Czuba [1] and Bożena Leszczyńska-Gorzelak [1]

[1] Chair and Department of Obstetrics and Perinatology, Medical University of Lublin, Lublin 20-090, Poland; zkimber@poczta.onet.pl (Ż.K.-T.); monikaczuba77@o2.pl (M.C.); b.leszczynska@umlub.pl (B.L.-G.)
[2] Chair and Department of Internal Medicine, Medical University of Lublin, Lublin 20-081, Poland; marcin.trojnar@umlub.pl
[3] Chair and Department of Human Physiology, Medical University of Lublin, Lublin 20-080, Poland; katarzyna.skorzynska-dziduszko@umlub.pl
[4] Department of Gynecology and Obstetrics, Institute of Clinical and Experimental Medicine, Medical Faculty, University of Rzeszow, Rzeszów 35-959, Poland; ddarmochwal@ur.edu.pl
* Correspondence: jolapatro@wp.pl; Tel.: +48-81-7244-769; Fax: +48-81-7244-841

Received: 13 March 2019; Accepted: 13 May 2019; Published: 15 May 2019

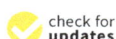

Abstract: Two-thirds of pregnant women exceed gestational weight gain recommendations. Excessive gestational weight gain (EGWG) appears to be associated with offspring's complications induced by mechanisms that are still unclear. The aim of this study was to investigate whether umbilical cord leptin (UCL) and ghrelin (UCG) concentrations are altered in full-term neonates born to EGWG mothers and whether neonatal anthropometric measurements correlate with UCL and UCG levels and maternal serum ghrelin and leptin as well as urine ghrelin concentrations. The study subjects were divided into two groups, 28 healthy controls and 38 patients with EGWG. Lower UCL and UCG levels were observed in neonates born to healthy mothers but only in male newborns. In the control group UCG concentrations correlated positively with neonatal birth weight, body length and head circumference. In the control group maternal serum ghrelin levels correlated negatively with neonatal birth weight, body length and head circumference as well as positively with chest circumference. In the EGWG group UCG concentrations correlated negatively with neonatal birth weight and birth body length. UCL correlated positively with birth body length in EGWG group and negatively with head circumference in the control group. In conclusion, EGWG is associated with disturbances in UCL and UCG concentrations.

Keywords: excessive gestational weight gain; neonatal anthropometry; leptin; ghrelin

1. Introduction

According to the current state of knowledge, excessive gestational weight gain (EGWG) as well as pre-pregnancy obesity appear to be associated with long-term sequelae in the offspring. Prenatal life may be of importance as a 'critical period' since it is the time when the risk of development and persistence of dyslipidemia, overweight, obesity, impairments in cognition, neuropsychiatric disorders, cardiovascular diseases and metabolic syndrome in the future life of the offspring is increased [1–4]. Maternal hyperinsulinemia, hyperleptinemia and inflammation are associated with excessive nutrient transport at the placental level. EGWG, which is usually due to improper nutrition during the pregnancy period, has been regarded as a potentially modifiable, independent risk factor for excessive offspring growth and serious metabolic disorders [3,5].

Gestational weight guidelines of the Institute of Medicine (IOM) [6] provide ranges of recommended weight gain for specific pre-pregnancy body mass index (BMI) categories in relation to the least risk of adverse perinatal outcomes. In order to minimize the risk of maternal and infant complications it has been suggested that weight gain in pregnancy should not exceed 11.5–16, 7–11.5 and 5–9 kg in women with normal pre-pregnancy BMI, overweight and obese subjects, respectively [6]. More than two-thirds of pregnant women exceed gestational weight gain recommendations of the IOM [7].

Leptin, an adipocyte-derived satiety factor, is known to reduce food intake and raise/boost energy expenditure. However, due to the increase of leptin levels in the maternal blood in the second half of pregnancy, leptin resistance develops [8,9], which, especially in late pregnancy, is thought to be mediated by the placental secretion hormones, i.e., prolactin and placental lactogen family of the molecules [10,11].

Ghrelin, an acylated peptide hormone, plays a crucial role in energy homeostasis and it has been demonstrated to stimulate fetal development by binding to the growth hormone receptors [12]. Ghrelin is also an important factor linking the central nervous system with the peripheral tissues that regulate energy homeostasis and lipid metabolism [12]. A physiological increase of maternal and fetal ghrelin levels has been observed during pregnancy in mammals (including humans) [13,14]. In light of this, it seems plausible that ghrelin is likely to be one of many peptides engaged in the process of fertilization as well as in preimplantation embryo development and implantation; intragestational ghrelin participates in reproductive fetal programming [15]. Ghrelin levels can be affected by multiple factors, including diet composition, exercise, environment and lifestyle [12].

Disrupted leptin and ghrelin secretion homeostasis may result in production of improper hypothalamic signals, thereby bringing a feeling of hunger, which will lead to excessive food consumption and lipogenesis. All of this has been displayed in both animal and human models [11].

Even though numerous studies have performed leptin and ghrelin blood concentration measurements in both healthy and unhealthy individuals [11–13], the data on the relative role of maternal and fetal leptin and ghrelin in the fetal growth are still patchy. The aim of this study was to investigate whether the umbilical cord leptin and ghrelin concentrations are altered in full-term neonates born to EGWG mothers and whether neonatal anthropometric measurements correlate with the umbilical cord blood and maternal serum leptin and ghrelin levels as well as with the maternal urine ghrelin levels. This statistical analysis was also performed taking into consideration the infants' genders.

2. Results

Comparative characteristics of the study groups are presented in Tables S1 and S2. Data presented in Table 1 revealed that higher umbilical cord blood leptin and ghrelin concentrations were observed in the neonates born to the EGWG mothers. We compared the levels of leptin and ghrelin in all the tested materials depending on the sex of the newborns. Higher umbilical cord blood concentrations of leptin and ghrelin in the EGWG group were observed in the male neonates, while no such observations were made in the female infants. In the EGWG group, the mothers of the male newborns had significantly higher serum leptin levels (Table 1).

We checked correlations between the neonatal anthropometric measurements and leptin and ghrelin levels. Taking into consideration the relatively small group of female infants in our study, we performed the correlation analysis only on male newborns in the EGWG and control groups. In the EGWG group the umbilical cord ghrelin levels correlated negatively with the neonatal birth weight and birth body length in all infants (Table 2) as well as in the male subjects (Table 3). Negative correlations were also found between the maternal urine ghrelin levels and neonatal birth weight and chest circumference in all studied infants in the EGWG group (Table 2), whereas in the male subjects only the chest circumference was negatively associated with the maternal urine ghrelin level (Table 3).

The birth body length correlated positively with the umbilical cord leptin levels in the EGWG group (Table 2). This relation was not observed in the male subgroup (Table 3).

Table 1. Comparison of the study groups.

Variables	EGWG Group (n = 38)	Control Group (n = 28)	p
Male infant, n (%)	24 (63.2)	20 (71.4)	0.66
Female infant, n (%)	14 (36.8)	8 (28.6)	0.66
Cord blood ghrelin, ng/mL	0.52 (0.26–1.83)	0.19 (0.19–0.28)	**0.00001**
Male	0.49 (0.27–0.8)	0.19 (0.19–0.2)	**0.0001**
Female	0.56 (0.25–20.11)	0.28 (0.23–0.29)	0.44
Cord blood leptin, ng/mL	10.99 (8.5–13.4)	7.53 (4.9–14.01)	**0.00003**
Male	10.8 (8.7–12.6)	7.3 (4.9–7.8)	**0.03**
Female	21 (8.2–22.3)	14 (11.7–14.6)	0.36
Maternal serum ghrelin, ng/mL	1.19 (0.34–2.43)	0.93 (0.65–1.12)	0.63
Male	1.1 (0.44–1.73)	0.97 (0.9–1.1)	0.42
Female	2.7 (0.2–16.7)	0.25 (0.21–0.39)	0.34
Maternal urine ghrelin, ng/mL	0.12 (0.04–0.3)	0.1 (0.1–0.29)	0.75
Male	0.25 (0.05–0.34)	0.1 (0.1–0.29)	0.92
Female	0.08 (0.03–0.12)	0.1 (0.1–0.25)	0.26
Maternal serum leptin, ng/mL	14.87 (12.6–47.6)	10.43 (6.04–14.9)	0.06
Male	15 (14.6–61.7)	14.6 (6.04–14.9)	**0.01**
Female	12.3 (11.8–33.4)	6.5 (6.3–7.3)	0.09

The results are shown as the median (interquartile range 25–75%). Statistically significant values are given in bold. EGWG—Excessive gestational weight gain.

Table 2. Correlations of neonatal anthropometric measurements in the EGWG group (Spearman's rho coefficient).

Variables	Birth Weight	Birth Body Length	Head Circumference	Chest Circumference
Umbilical cord ghrelin level	**−0.560 ***	**−0.727 ***	−0.203	−0.331
Maternal serum ghrelin level	-0.105	-0.309	-0.170	0.001
Maternal urine ghrelin level	**−0.452 ***	-0.320	-0.174	**−0.596 ***
Umbilical cord leptin level	0.326	**0.572 ***	0.063	−0.044
Maternal serum leptin level	−0.151	−0.133	0.066	−0.228

Statistically significant values are given in bold. * $p < 0.05$; *** $p < 0.0001$; EGWG—excessive gestational weight gain.

The controls presented umbilical cord ghrelin levels correlating positively with the neonatal birth weight, birth body length and head circumference (Table 4); whereas only with the head circumference measurements in the male subjects (Table 5). The maternal serum ghrelin levels correlated negatively with all these parameters but positively with the chest circumference in all control newborns (Table 4). In the male subgroup the maternal serum ghrelin level was negatively connected to the neonatal head circumference (Table 5). The urine ghrelin correlated negatively with all the anthropometric parameters of the neonates of the healthy group (Table 4), but in male subjects except for the head circumference measurements (Table 5). Positive correlations were found between the maternal serum leptin levels and all the neonatal anthropometric measurements except the head circumference, which correlated negatively with the umbilical cord leptin levels. These associations were statistically significant in all newborns in the control group (Table 4) as well as in the male subjects of this group (Table 5).

Table 3. Correlations of neonatal anthropometric measurements in the EGWG group in male subjects (Spearman's rho coefficient).

Variables	Birth weight	Birth Body Length	Head Circumference	Chest Circumference
Umbilical cord ghrelin level	−0.733 **	−0.829 ***	−0.271	−0.747 **
Maternal serum ghrelin level	−0.300	−0.393	−0.140	−0.378
Maternal urine ghrelin level	−0.450	−0.419	−0.420	−0.615 *
Umbilical cord leptin level	0.445	0.445	0.437	0.413
Maternal serum leptin level	−0.133	−0.265	0.061	−0.351

Statistically significant values are given in bold. * $p < 0.05$; ** $p < 0.001$; *** $p < 0.0001$; EGWG—excessive gestational weight gain.

Table 4. Correlations of neonatal anthropometric measurements in the control group (Spearman's rho coefficient).

Variables	Birth Weight	Birth Body Length	Head Circumference	Chest Circumference
Umbilical cord ghrelin level	0.486 *	0.525 *	0.794 ***	−0.278
Maternal serum ghrelin level	−0.543 *	−0.617 *	−0.706 **	0.432 *
Maternal urine ghrelin level	−0.771 ***	−0.833 ***	−0.441 *	−0.463 *
Umbilical cord leptin level	−0.286	−0.092	−0.559 *	0.061
Maternal serum leptin level	0.600 *	0.494 *	0.294	0.833 ***

Statistically significant values are given in bold. * $p < 0.05$; ** $p < 0.001$; *** $p < 0.0001$.

Table 5. Correlations of neonatal anthropometric measurements in the control group in male subjects (Spearman's rho coefficient).

Variables	Birth Weight	Birth Body Length	Head Circumference	Chest Circumference
Umbilical cord ghrelin level	0.200	0.289	0.669 *	−0.335
Maternal serum ghrelin level	−0.200	−0.289	−0.667 *	0.335
Maternal urine ghrelin level	−0.700 **	−0.866 ***	−0.205	−0.671 **
Umbilical cord leptin level	−0.500 *	−0.577 *	−0.820 ***	0.112
Maternal serum leptin level	0.900 ***	0.866 ***	0.410	0.783 ***

Statistically significant values are given in bold. * $p < 0.05$; ** $p < 0.001$; *** $p < 0.0001$.

3. Discussion

Maternal pre-pregnancy BMI as well as gestational weight gain, connected to nutrition, have both independent and interacting effects not only on the fetal growth [4]. The majority of studies have investigated the relationship between the umbilical cord leptin and ghrelin and neonatal anthropometric measurements [9,16–21], however, their associations with the maternal serum and urine ghrelin concentrations are less studied. To the best of our knowledge, this study is the first to show the umbilical cord, maternal serum and urine ghrelin levels as well as the umbilical cord and maternal serum leptin levels in women with EGWG and the relationship of these parameters to the neonatal anthropometric measurements.

Our study showed that levels of leptin and ghrelin in the umbilical cord blood were statistically higher in male infants of the EGWG group in comparison to healthy subjects. We hypothesize that these differences can be connected to disparities in body composition and hydration status. Our previous study revealed that mothers with EGWG were characterized by increased fat and lean tissues in the bioelectrical impedance analysis [22]. Unfortunately, the evaluation of these parameters seems to not be feasible in the case of newborns.

Lecoutre et al. [23] observed a link between maternal obesity and adult rat offspring, where the latter were sensitized by the obese mother to increased visceral adiposity in a sex-specific manner. The cited authors demonstrated that maternal obesity programs visceral depots only in the male offspring in the group with a high-fat diet (HF; containing 60% lipids). Perirenal fat pads, yet not gonadal ones, were found to be involved in determining features in HF male offspring. On the basis of previous studies, the heterogeneity of the adipose lineage was proposed. It has been demonstrated that adipogenic stem cells and adipocytes act differently in the course of adipogenesis [24,25].

Previous studies revealed that females tended to have higher serum leptin levels than males [26]. Similar findings were observed in our study. Karakosta et al. [27] observed gender-specific differences in leptin levels in the umbilical cord blood of approximately 400 healthy neonates. The cited authors revealed that female subjects were characterized by higher levels of this adipokine than males [27]. It has also been observed that later in life the leptin levels are consistently higher in females in comparison to males [28,29].

Many authors are of the opinion that leptin concentration is higher in the mother than in the newborn [17,18,23,30]. Similar results were observed in the present study in all studied subjects and in groups of male infants. In both studied groups the leptin concentration was about 1.4 times higher in the blood of the mothers in comparison with the leptin concentration in the newborns. The discrepancy between leptin levels in the maternal serum and cord blood of male and female subjects can be connected to the phenomenon typical of this period of life when infants may be affected by an energy imbalance correlating with leptin levels [31]. Interestingly, a higher level of leptin was observed in the umbilical cord blood than in mothers in the group of female newborns. A similar dependence was described by Okdemir et al. [32] in the large for gestational age babies, however, these authors did not take into account the division of the group by sex of children.

Previous studies reported high ghrelin concentrations in the umbilical cord blood of pre-term and small-for-gestational-age infants. It was also reported that ghrelin levels were increased in the offspring of those women who had cigarette smoking habits and suffered from hypertension during pregnancy [33,34]. A limited and contrary amount of data is available on the umbilical cord ghrelin concentrations in the offspring of mothers with metabolic disturbances. Hehir et al. [35] did not detect a significant difference between healthy and type 1 diabetic pregnant women in this respect. However, Karakulak et al. [36] found that the umbilical cord blood ghrelin levels were decreased in the offspring of the gestational diabetes mellitus (GDM) women even after adjustment for birth weight, whereas Kara et al. [20] were able to notice similar ghrelin and leptin concentrations in the serum of the control and GDM mothers' newborns. It has been suggested that ghrelin may play a role in the fetal adaptation to intrauterine malnutrition [34]. Our previous study detected lower serum and higher urine ghrelin concentrations in the early post-partum period when GDM women were compared with the health control group [37]. It is presumed that ghrelin in the cord blood is mainly secreted by the fetus. It is worth noting, however, that ghrelin is mainly secreted by the pancreas during the perinatal period rather than by the fundus of the stomach, which is typical of adult humans and rodents [38]. On the other hand, our findings of significant correlations between maternal serum and urine ghrelin levels and neonatal anthropomorphic measurements seem to be connected to the fact that a pregnant woman and her child may be perceived as a functional, complex unit. We decided to focus on urine as an easily obtainable biological material. Nonetheless, we are aware of the fact that small groups of participants represent a study limitation and we are not able to discuss these results in detail. Furthermore, it is not possible to relate our observations to the previously published papers of other authors since no such data exists.

There are many studies showing higher umbilical cord leptin levels in neonates born to obese mothers [17,21] but there are still limited data about leptin concentrations in women with EGWG.

Previous studies concentrated on gestational weight gain in the first two trimesters of pregnancy, where EGWG was associated with higher levels of leptin and other parameters in the cord blood [8,39]. Allbrand et al. [21] observed increased level of the umbilical cord leptin and C-peptide in the infants born to obese versus normal-weight women. The present results confirm that the level of leptin in the umbilical cord blood was significantly higher in the EGWG patients than in the controls. These findings are similar to those reported by Biesiada et al. [17] who observed that leptin concentrations in the large for gestational age (LGA) children born to obese mothers were higher than in the LGA children born to mothers with normal BMI.

It is worth highlighting that many of the above-quoted studies did not take into consideration the maternal BMI and weight gain during pregnancy. The results of our study revealed differences not only in the gestational weight gain between two groups of mothers but in the laboratory results as well. Lower levels of high-density lipoprotein cholesterol (HDL) as well as higher HgbA1c and triglycerides concentrations were present in the EGWG group. These results are consistent with the observations reported by other authors. Nonetheless, the offspring of the mothers from both studied groups presented similar anthropometric measurements, and their birth weight was also comparable. However, previous studies seem to confirm that the fetal metabolic programming may occur within normal birth weight ranges [40,41].

Researchers studying the relationship between ghrelin and anthropometric measurements revealed an inverse correlation between ghrelin concentrations and birth weight, height as well as BMI [42–46]. In their study, in which blood samples of diabetic mothers' newborns were taken after birth before feeding, Kara et al. [20] found that only serum ghrelin negatively correlated with the birth weight. The authors concluded that this negative correlation of ghrelin, which seems to be a regulator of appetite, body fat mass, and energy balance, could potentially be advantageous to infants since appetite reduction might prevent postnatal excessive food intake and subsequent weight gain. Ding et al. [16] also suggested that ghrelin may play a role in regulation of body weight and energy homeostasis from the fetal period to adulthood. In our study the umbilical cord ghrelin levels negatively correlated with birth weight and birth body length in the EGWG group, they were also positively associated with the birth weight, birth body length, and head circumference in the control group. In the literature there is no clear evidence of consistent relationship between the ghrelin levels and neonatal anthropometry. There are also studies in which no correlation whatsoever has been reported [19,47–49].

The positive association detected in this study between the leptin concentration in the maternal serum and umbilical cord and neonatal anthropometric measurements confirms what was reported in the previous studies [9,17,30,50]. Schubring et al. [30] detected a significant correlation between leptin levels in the umbilical vein and artery and birth weight of the neonates. Biesiada at al. [17] observed moderate correlations between leptin concentrations and Ponderal Index, birth weight and the placenta weight. Samano et al. [9], similar to our findings in the control group, showed a correlation between the maternal leptin concentration and length of the newborn. This positive correlation between the cord blood leptin levels and birth weight could be indicative of leptin as a regulating factor responsible for fetal weight and its development.

As other studies have reported, in our study the mean leptin concentrations were also higher in female neonates than in male neonates even though the birth weight in both sexes was similar. This may suggest participation of sex hormones in leptin secretion [17,50,51]. This is contrary to the study results published by Palcevska-Kocevsa et al. [50], who found no differences in the leptin concentrations between the male and female infants. In our study we observed significantly higher levels of leptin in the female neonates only in the control group. Similar levels of leptin between the males and females in the EGWG group may result from the fact that the male newborns had statistically higher levels of leptin in the umbilical cord blood in the group of patients with EGWGthan in the control group. Similar relationships, however, were not observed in the female newborns.

Our results seem to highlight the importance of maternal condition, including gestational weight gain, in further research into the umbilical cord ghrelin and leptin concentrations and their relationship with the fetal and/or neonatal anthropometry and metabolic state.

The strength of this study lies in its novelty—the evaluation of the umbilical cord ghrelin levels of the EGWG mothers' offspring as well as their associations with the maternal laboratory results and neonatal anthropometric measurements is an innovative approach. Nevertheless, the presented study has certain limitations. Firstly, it is indeed a relatively small-sample study. Secondly, we measured the levels of ghrelin and leptin in all the material only once. Therefore, it would be interesting to check how they change in time both in the mothers and in their offspring, which is quite motivating for us to continue our research into this issue and verify our results.

4. Materials and Methods

4.1. Study Population

The study consisted of Caucasian, singleton-term-pregnancy mothers (who completed 37 weeks of pregnancy) and infants delivered at the Chair and Department of Obstetrics and Perinatology, the medical University of Lublin, Poland. The study material was obtained between March 2016 and February 2017. The women were recruited at the time of delivery. We took into account only those in full-term pregnancy, i.e., after the completed 37th week of pregnancy calculated on the basis of the date of the last menstrual period or ultrasound examination in case the date of the last menstrual period was unknown. Two groups were selected on the basis of gestational weight gain: one group included women with normal gestational weight gain (11.5–16 kg; $n = 28$), while the other consisted of those with excessive gestational weight gain (≥ 20 kg; $n = 38$). Informed consent was obtained from each study subject and infant mother.

Characteristics of the study subjects also included: normal pre-pregnancy BMI values and three consecutive correct/normal results of 2 h-75 g-oral glucose tolerance test performed at 24–28 weeks of pregnancy [52,53], no concomitant diseases, and only vitamin-iron supplementation.

Exclusion criteria from the study included: multiple pregnancy, chronic infectious diseases, current urinary infections, abnormal laboratory results (e.g., the complete blood count, creatinine, glomerular filtration rate (GFR) findings); metabolic disorders (except improper gestational weight gain for the EGWG group), mental illness, cancer, liver diseases, cardiovascular disorders, fetal malformation, premature membrane rupture and intrauterine growth retardation.

The study protocol received approval of the Bioethics Committee of the Medical University of Lublin (no. KE-0254/221/2015 [25 June 2015] and no. KE-0254/348/2016 [15 December 2016]).

4.2. Measurements and Data Collection

Anthropometric measurements of mothers were performed shortly prior to and after delivery. Pre-pregnancy BMI values were determined during the first visits in the out-patients clinic, which were carried out up to 10 weeks of gestation. The following formula was used to calculate the gestational weight gain: the mother's pre-pregnancy body mass subtracted from the weight at the day of delivery. We calculated gestational BMI gain as well. We defined gestational BMI loss as the difference between the mother's BMI after delivery (during 48 h after delivery) and her BMI shortly prior to delivery. The newborn weights, lengths as well as the head and chest circumferences were measured right after delivery.

The cord blood samples' collection was performed during delivery causing no hinderance to its course. The maternal serum and urine samples were taken after delivery, taking into account a 6 h fasting period. Samples were centrifuged at 1000× g, at 20 °C for 15 min. After centrifugation all the collected cord blood serum as well as the serum and urine samples obtained from the studied mothers were stored at −80 °C. Ghrelin concentrations were determined with the use of kits available on the market and in agreement with the manufacturer's instructions (Wuhan EIAab Science Co., Wuhan,

China) via traditional enzyme-linked immunosorbent assay (ELISA). Detection range for ghrelin was 0.156–10 ng/mL. Concentrations of leptin in cord blood serum and maternal serum and urine were measured by means of commercially available kits and in agreement with the manufacturer's instructions (R&D Systems, Inc., Minneapolis, MN, USA) via ELISA. The threshold of leptin sensitivity was equal to 7.8 pg/mL, while the reference range for women was 3877–77,273 pg/mL. Since the leptin urine levels in the majority of the studied subjects were below the threshold of sensitivity of the ELISA test, the "urine leptin" parameter was not included in our study results. The measurements of maternal serum levels of albumin, fasting blood glucose (FBG), hemoglobin A1c (HgbA1c) as well as the lipid profile were performed by an authorized laboratory.

This is the second analysis based on subjects from the control group that was previously used in our study [37]. In the cited study we compared women diagnosed with gestational diabetes mellitus (GDM) with the aforementioned control group [37]. The cohort analyzed in the present study was used to measure SFRP5 and was described in our previous study [22]. Comparative characteristics of the study groups are presented in Tables S1 and S2.

4.3. Statistical Analysis

All the obtained results are presented as the median (interquartile range 25–75%) or as numbers and percentages. Differential significance test was conducted by means of Mann–Whitney U test. Correlation analyses used Spearman's coefficient test and were performed with the use of Statistical Package for the Social Sciences software (version 19; SPSS Inc., Chicago, IL, USA); $p < 0.005$ was assumed to be statistically significant.

5. Conclusions

Our study revealed that the umbilical cord leptin and ghrelin levels were significantly higher in the offspring of the EGWG mothers, but only in the male newborns. Our study results indicate that the condition of the mother, i.e., her BMI values both in the periconceptional and periparturient periods as well as her metabolic parameters (e.g., her lipid profile), may affect her offspring's ghrelin and leptin concentrations at delivery.

Differences in the correlations between the leptin and ghrelin concentrations (both in the umbilical cord blood and maternal serum as well as in urine) and the anthropometric results of the neonates are dependent on the studied group. This can be exemplified by the umbilical cord ghrelin which correlates negatively with the birth weight and birth body length in the EGWG group, while its correlation with the birth weight, birth body length and head circumference is positive in the control group. These significant correlation differences result from different levels of ghrelin in the umbilical cord blood (significantly higher level in the EGWG group, at $p < 0.0001$) with comparable birth measurements in both studied groups. However, the possibility of fetal metabolic programming occurrence within the normal birth weight ranges, as has previously been reported by other authors [40,41], should be stressed once more.

Supplementary Materials: Supplementary materials can be found at http://www.mdpi.com/1422-0067/20/10/2398/s1.

Author Contributions: Conceptualization: J.P.-M. and Ż.K.-T.; methodology: J.P.-M..; validation: J.P.-M. and K.E.S.-D.; formal analysis: J.P.-M., M.T. and D.D.-K.; investigation: M.C., Ż.K.-T. and J.P.-M.; data curation: J.P.-M. and Ż.K.-T; writing: J.P.-M. and M.T.; visualization: J.P.-M.; supervision: B.L.-G.

Funding: This study was supported by the Medical University of Lublin, grant no. 335.

Conflicts of Interest: The authors declare no conflict of interest.

References

1. Bianchi, C.; de Gennaro, G.; Romano, M.; Aragona, M.; Battini, L.; del Prato, S.; Bertolotto, A. Pre-pregnancy obesity, gestational diabetes or gestational weight gain: Which is the strongest predictor of pregnancy outcomes? *Diabetes Res. Clin. Pract.* **2018**, *144*, 286–293. [CrossRef]
2. Bellamy, L.; Casas, J.; Hingorani, A.; Williams, D. Type 2 diabetes mellitus after gestational diabetes: A systematic review and meta-analysis. *Lancet* **2009**, *373*, 1773–1779. [CrossRef]
3. Jin, W.Y.; Lv, Y.; Bao, Y.; Tang, L.; Zhu, Z.W.; Shao, J.; Zhao, Z.Y. Independent and Combined Effects of Maternal Prepregnancy Body Mass Index and Gestational Weight Gain on Offspring Growth at 0–3 Years of Age. *Biomed. Res. Int.* **2016**, *2016*, 4720785. [CrossRef] [PubMed]
4. Marciniak, A.; Patro-Małysza, J.; Kimber-Trojnar, Ż.; Marciniak, B.; Oleszczuk, J.; Leszczyńska-Gorzelak, B. Fetal programming of the metabolic syndrome. *Taiwan. J. Obstet. Gynecol.* **2017**, *56*, 133–138. [CrossRef] [PubMed]
5. Hrolfsdottir, L.; Schalkwijk, C.G.; Birgisdottir, B.E.; Gunnarsdottir, I.; Maslova, E.; Granström, C.; Strøm, M.; Olsen, S.F.; Halldorsson, T.I. Maternal diet, gestational weight gain, and inflammatory markers during pregnancy. *Obesity* **2016**, *24*, 2133–2139. [CrossRef] [PubMed]
6. Institute of Medicine (US) and National Research Council (US) Committee to Reexamine IOM Pregnancy Weight Guidelines; Rasmussen, K.M.; Yaktine, A.L. *Weight Gain during Pregnancy: Reexamining the Guidelines*; National Academies Press: Washington, DC, USA, 2009.
7. Goldstein, R.F.; Abell, S.K.; Ranasinha, S.; Misso, M.; Boyle, J.A.; Black, M.H.; Li, N.; Hu, G.; Corrado, F.; Rode, L.; et al. Association of Gestational Weight Gain with Maternal and Infant Outcomes: A Systematic Review and Meta-Analysis. *JAMA* **2017**, *317*, 2207–2225. [CrossRef]
8. Lacroix, M.; Battista, M.; Doyon, M.; Moreau, J.; Patenaude, J.; Guillemette, L.; Ménard, J.; Ardilouze, J.; Perron, P.; Hivert, M. Higher maternal leptin levels at second trimester are associated with subsequent greater gestational weight gain in late pregnancy. *BMC Pregnancy Childbirth* **2016**, *16*, 62. [CrossRef] [PubMed]
9. Sámano, R.; Martínez-Rojano, H.; Chico-Barba, G.; Godínez-Martínez, E.; Sánchez-Jiménez, B.; Montiel-Ojeda, D.; Tolentino, M. Serum Concentration of Leptin in Pregnant Adolescents Correlated with Gestational Weight Gain, Postpartum Weight Retention and Newborn Weight/Length. *Nutrients* **2017**, *9*, 1067. [CrossRef]
10. Cassidy, F.C.; Charalambous, M. Genomic imprinting, growth and maternal-fetal interactions. *J. Exp. Biol.* **2018**, *221*, jeb164517. [CrossRef]
11. Kisioglu, B.; Nergiz-Unal, R. Potential effect of maternal dietary sucrose or fructose syrup on CD36, leptin, and ghrelin-mediated fetal programming of obesity. *Nutr. Neurosci.* **2018**, *1*, 1–11. [CrossRef] [PubMed]
12. Lv, Y.; Liang, T.; Wang, G.; Li, Z. Ghrelin, a gastrointestinal hormone, regulates energy balance and lipid metabolism. *Biosci. Rep.* **2018**, BSR20181061. [CrossRef]
13. Palik, E.; Baranyi, E.; Melczer, Z.; Audikovszky, M.; Szöcs, A.; Winkler, G.; Cseh, K. Elevated serum acylated (biologically active) ghrelin and resistin levels associate with pregnancy-induced weight gain and insulin resistance. *Diabetes Res. Clin. Pract.* **2007**, *76*, 351–357. [CrossRef] [PubMed]
14. Harrison, J.L.; Adam, C.L.; Brown, Y.A.; Wallace, J.M.; Aitken, R.P.; Lea, R.G.; Miller, D.W. An immunohistochemical study of the localization and developmental expression of ghrelin and its functional receptor in the ovine placenta. *Reprod. Biol. Endocrinol.* **2007**, *5*, 25. [CrossRef] [PubMed]
15. Torres, P.J.; Luque, E.M.; Ponzio, M.F.; Cantarelli, V.; Diez, M.; Figueroa, S.; Vincenti, L.M.; Carlini, V.P.; Martini, A.C. The role of intragestational ghrelin on postnatal development and reproductive programming in mice. *Reproduction* **2018**, REP-18-0192. [CrossRef] [PubMed]
16. Ding, H.; Pan, Y.; Yu, Y.; Gu, P. Cord ghrelin levels are decreased in large-for-gestational-age neonates. *Clin. Obes.* **2012**, *2*, 50–56. [CrossRef]
17. Biesiada, L.A.; Głowacka, E.; Krekora, M.; Sobantka, S.; Krokocka, A.; Krasomski, G. The impact of excessive maternal weight on the nutritional status of the fetus—The role of leptin. *Arch. Med. Sci.* **2016**, *12*, 394–401. [CrossRef] [PubMed]
18. Ozdemir, U.; Gulturk, S.; Aker, A.; Guvenal, T.; Imir, G.; Erselcan, T. Correlation between birth weight, leptin, zinc and copper levels in maternal and cord blood. *J. Physiol. Biochem.* **2007**, *63*, 121–128. [CrossRef]

19. Imam, S.S.; Kandil, M.E.; Shoman, M.; Baker, S.I.; Bahier, R. Umbilical cord ghrelin in term and preterm newborns and its relation to metabolic hormones and anthropometric measurements. *Pak. J. Biol. Sci.* **2009**, *12*, 1548–1555.
20. Kara, M.; Orbak, Z.; Döneray, H.; Ozkan, B.; Akcay, F. The Relationship Between Skinfold Thickness and Leptin, Ghrelin, Adiponectin, and Resistin Levels in Infants of Diabetic Mothers. *Fetal Pediatr. Pathol.* **2017**, *36*, 1–7. [CrossRef]
21. Allbrand, M.; Åman, J.; Lodefalk, M. Placental ghrelin and leptin expression and cord blood ghrelin, adiponectin, leptin, and C-peptide levels in severe maternal obesity. *J. Matern. Fetal Neonatal Med.* **2018**, *31*, 2839–2846. [CrossRef]
22. Kimber-Trojnar, Ż.; Patro-Małysza, J.; Trojnar, M.; Darmochwał-Kolarz, D.; Oleszczuk, J.; Leszczyńska-Gorzelak, B. Umbilical Cord SFRP5 Levels of Term Newborns in Relation to Normal and Excessive Gestational Weight Gain. *Int. J. Mol. Sci.* **2019**, *20*, 595. [CrossRef]
23. Lecoutre, S.; Deracinois, B.; Laborie, C.; Eberlé, D.; Guinez, C.; Panchenko, P.E.; Lesage, J.; Vieau, D.; Junien, C.; Gabory, A.; et al. Depot- and sex-specific effects of maternal obesity in offspring's adipose tissue. *J. Endocrinol.* **2016**, *230*, 39–53. [CrossRef]
24. Yamamoto, Y.; Gesta, S.; Lee, K.Y.; Tran, T.T.; Saadatirad, P.; Kahn, C.R. Adipose depots possess unique developmental gene signatures. *Obesity* **2010**, *18*, 872–878. [CrossRef]
25. Berry, D.C.; Stenesen, D.; Zeve, D.; Graff, J.M. The developmental origins of adipose tissue. *Development* **2013**, *140*, 3939–3949. [CrossRef]
26. Savino, F.; Rossi, L.; Benetti, S.; Petrucci, E.; Sorrenti, M.; Silvestro, L. Serum reference values for leptin in healthy infants. *PLoS ONE* **2014**, *9*, e113024. [CrossRef]
27. Karakosta, P.; Georgiou, V.; Fthenou, E.; Margioris, A.; Castanas, E.; Kogevinas, M.; Kampa, M.; Chatzi, L. Gender-specific reference intervals for cord blood leptin in Crete, Greece. *Eur. J. Pediatr.* **2012**, *171*, 1563–1566. [CrossRef]
28. Kawamata, R.; Suzuki, Y.; Yada, Y.; Koike, Y.; Kono, Y.; Yada, T.; Takahashi, N. Gut hormone profiles in preterm and term infants during the first 2 months of life. *J. Pediatr. Endocrinol. Metab.* **2014**, *27*, 717–723. [CrossRef]
29. Wilasco, M.I.; Goldani, H.A.; Dornelles, C.T.; Maurer, R.L.; Kieling, C.O.; Porowski, M.; Silveira, T.R. Ghrelin, leptin and insulin in healthy children: Relationship with anthropometry, gender, and age distribution. *Regul. Pept.* **2012**, *173*, 21–26. [CrossRef]
30. Schubring, C.; Kiess, W.; Englaro, P.; Rascher, W.; Dötsch, J.; Hanitsch, S.; Attanasio, A.; Blum, W.F. Levels of leptin in maternal serum, amniotic fluid, and arterial and venous cord blood: relation to neonatal and placental weight. *J. Clin. Endocrinol. Metab.* **1997**, *82*, 1480–1483. [CrossRef]
31. Mansoub, S.; Chan, M.K.; Adeli, K. Gap analysis of pediatric reference intervals for risk biomarkers of cardiovascular disease and the metabolic syndrome. *Clin. Biochem.* **2006**, *39*, 569–587. [CrossRef]
32. Ökdemir, D.; Hatipoğlu, N.; Kurtoğlu, S.; Siraz, Ü.G.; Akar, H.H.; Muhtaroğlu, S.; Kütük, M.S. The Role of Irisin, Insulin and Leptin in Maternal and Fetal Interaction. *J. Clin. Res. Pediatr. Endocrinol.* **2018**, *10*, 307–315. [CrossRef]
33. Farquhar, J.; Heiman, M.; Wong, A.C.; Wach, R.; Chessex, P.; Chanoine, J.P. Elevated umbilical cord ghrelin concentrations in small for gestational age neonates. *J. Clin. Endocrinol. Metab.* **2003**, *88*, 4324–4327. [CrossRef]
34. Chiesa, C.; Osborn, J.F.; Haass, C.; Natale, F.; Spinelli, M.; Scapillati, E.; Spinelli, A.; Pacifico, L. Ghrelin, leptin, IGF-1, IGFBP-3, and insulin concentrations at birth: Is there a relationship with fetal growth and neonatal anthropometry? *Clin. Chem.* **2008**, *54*, 550–558. [CrossRef]
35. Hehir, M.P.; Laursen, H.; Higgins, M.F.; Brennan, D.J.; O'Connor, D.P.; McAuliffe, F.M. Ghrelin concentrations in maternal and cord blood of type 1 diabetic and non-diabetic pregnancies at term. *Endocrine* **2013**, *43*, 233–235. [CrossRef]
36. Karakulak, M.; Saygili, U.; Temur, M.; Yilmaz, Ö.; Özün Özbay, P.; Calan, M.; Coşar, H. Comparison of umbilical cord ghrelin concentrations in full-term pregnant women with or without gestational diabetes. *Endocr. Res.* **2017**, *42*, 79–85. [CrossRef]
37. Kimber-Trojnar, Ż.; Patro-Małysza, J.; Skórzyńska-Dziduszko, K.E.; Oleszczuk, J.; Trojnar, M.; Mierzyński, R.; Leszczyńska-Gorzelak, B. Ghrelin in Serum and Urine of Post-Partum Women with Gestational Diabetes Mellitus. *Int J Mol Sci* **2018**, *19*, 3001. [CrossRef]

38. Chanoine, J.P.; de Waele, K.; Walia, P. Ghrelin and the growth hormone secretagogue receptor in growth and development. *Int. J. Obes.* **2009**, *33*, S48–S52. [CrossRef]
39. Rifas-Shiman, S.L.; Fleisch, A.; Hivert, M.F.; Mantzoros, C.; Gillman, M.W.; Oken, E. First and second trimester gestational weight gains are most strongly associated with cord blood levels of hormones at delivery important for glycemic control and somatic growth. *Metabolism* **2017**, *69*, 112–119. [CrossRef]
40. Gluckman, P.D.; Hanson, M.A. Living with the past: evolution, development, and patterns of disease. *Science* **2004**, *305*, 1733–1736. [CrossRef]
41. Luo, Z.C.; Bilodeau, J.F.; Nuyt, A.M.; Fraser, W.D.; Julien, P.; Audibert, F.; Xiao, L.; Garofalo, C.; Levy, E. Perinatal Oxidative Stress May Affect Fetal Ghrelin Levels in Humans. *Sci. Rep.* **2015**, *5*, 17881. [CrossRef]
42. Onal, E.E.; Cinaz, P.; Atalay, Y.; Türkyilmaz, C.; Bideci, A.; Aktürk, A.; Okumuş, N.; Unal, S.; Koç, E.; Ergenekon, E. Umbilical cord ghrelin concentrations in small- and appropriate-for-gestational age newborn infants: relationship to anthropometric markers. *J. Endocrinol.* **2004**, *180*, 267–271. [CrossRef]
43. Kitamura, S.; Yokota, I.; Hosoda, H.; Kotani, Y.; Matsuda, J.; Naito, E.; Ito, M.; Kangawa, K.; Kuroda, Y. Ghrelin concentration in cord and neonatal blood: Relation to fetal growth and energy balance. *J. Clin. Endocrinol. Metab.* **2003**, *88*, 5473–5477. [CrossRef]
44. Soriano-Guillén, L.; Barrios, V.; Campos-Barros, A.; Argente, J. Ghrelin levels in obesity and anorexia nervosa: Effect of weight reduction or recuperation. *J. Pediatr.* **2004**, *144*, 36–42. [CrossRef]
45. Cortelazzi, D.; Cappiello, V.; Morpurgo, P.S.; Ronzoni, S.; Nobile de Santis, M.S.; Cetin, I.; Beck-Peccoz, P.; Spada, A. Circulating levels of ghrelin in human fetuses. *Eur. J. Endocrinol.* **2003**, *149*, 111–116. [CrossRef]
46. Wu, H.; Sui, C.; Xia, F.; Zhai, H.; Zhang, H.; Xu, H.; Weng, P.; Lu, Y. Effects of exenatide therapy on insulin resistance in the skeletal muscles of high-fat diet and low-dose streptozotocin-induced diabetic rats. *Endocr. Res.* **2016**, *41*, 1–7. [CrossRef]
47. James, R.J.; Drewett, R.F.; Cheetham, T.D. Low cord ghrelin levels in term infants are associated with slow weight gain over the first 3 months of life. *J. Clin. Endocrinol. Metab.* **2004**, *89*, 3847–3850. [CrossRef]
48. Bellone, S.; Rapa, A.; Vivenza, D.; Vercellotti, A.; Petri, A.; Radetti, G.; Bellone, J.; Broglio, F.; Ghigo, E.; Bona, G. Circulating ghrelin levels in the newborn are positively associated with gestational age. *Clin. Endocrinol.* **2004**, *60*, 613–617. [CrossRef]
49. Pirazzoli, P.; Lanari, M.; Zucchini, S.; Gennari, M.; Pagotto, U.; de Iasio, R.; Pasquali, R.; Cassio, A.; Cicognani, A.; Cacciari, E. Active and total ghrelin concentrations in the newborn. *J. Pediatr. Endocrinol. Metab.* **2005**, *18*, 379–384. [CrossRef]
50. Palcevska-Kocevska, S.; Aluloska, N.; Krstevska, M.; Shukarova-Angelovska, E.; Kojik, L.; Zisovska, E.; Kocevski, D.; Kocova, M. Correlation of serum adiponectin and leptin concentrations with anthropometric parameters in newborns. *Srp. Arh. Celok. Lek.* **2012**, *140*, 595–599. [CrossRef]
51. Hauguel-de Mouzon, S.; Lepercq, J.; Catalano, P. The known and unknown of leptin in pregnancy. *Am. J. Obstet. Gynecol.* **2006**, *194*, 1537–15345. [CrossRef]
52. International Association of Diabetes and Pregnancy Study Groups Consensus Panel. International association of diabetes and pregnancy study groups recommendations on the diagnosis and classification of hyperglycemia in pregnancy. *Diabetes Care* **2010**, *33*, 676–682. [CrossRef]
53. Diabetes Poland (Polish Diabetes Association). 2018 Guidelines on the management of diabetic patients. A position of Diabetes Poland. *Clin. Diabetol.* **2018**, *7*, 1–90. [CrossRef]

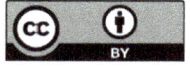

© 2019 by the authors. Licensee MDPI, Basel, Switzerland. This article is an open access article distributed under the terms and conditions of the Creative Commons Attribution (CC BY) license (http://creativecommons.org/licenses/by/4.0/).

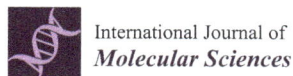

Article

Correlative Study on Impaired Prostaglandin E2 Regulation in Epicardial Adipose Tissue and Its Role in Maladaptive Cardiac Remodeling via EPAC2 and ST2 Signaling in Overweight Cardiovascular Disease Subjects

Elena Vianello [1,*], Elena Dozio [1], Francesco Bandera [1,2], Marco Froldi [3,4], Emanuele Micaglio [5], John Lamont [6], Lorenza Tacchini [1], Gerd Schmitz [7] and Massimiliano Marco Corsi Romanelli [1,5]

1. Department of Biomedical Sciences for Health, University of Milan, 20133 Milan, Italy; elena.dozio@unimi.it (E.D.); francesco.bandera@unimi.it (F.B.); lorenza.tacchini@unimi.it (L.T.); mmcorsi@unimi.it (M.M.C.R.)
2. Cardiology University Department, Heart Failure Unit, IRCCS Policlinico San Donato, 20097 Milan, Italy
3. Department of Clinical Sciences and Community Health, University of Milan, 20122 Milan, Italy; marco.froldi@unimi.it
4. Internal Medicine Unit IRCCS Policlinico San Donato, San Donato Milanese, 20097 Milan, Italy
5. U.O.C. SMEL-1 of Clinical Pathology, IRCCS Policlinico San Donato, San Donato Milanese, 20097 Milan, Italy; emanuele.micaglio@grupposandonato.it
6. Randox Laboratories LTD, R&D, Crumlin-Antrim, Belfast, BT29, Northen Ireland, UK; john.lamont@randox.com
7. Department of Clinical Chemistry and Laboratory Medicine, University Hospital Regensburg, 93053 Regensburg, Germany; Gerd.Schmitz@ukr.de
* Correspondence: elena.vianello@unimi.it; Tel.: +39-02-50315342

Received: 23 December 2019; Accepted: 12 January 2020; Published: 14 January 2020

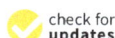

Abstract: There is recent evidence that the dysfunctional responses of a peculiar visceral fat deposit known as epicardial adipose tissue (EAT) can directly promote cardiac enlargement in the case of obesity. Here, we observed a newer molecular pattern associated with LV dysfunction mediated by prostaglandin E2 (PGE_2) deregulation in EAT in a cardiovascular disease (CVD) population. A series of 33 overweight CVD males were enrolled and their EAT thickness, LV mass, and volumes were measured by echocardiography. Blood, plasma, EAT, and SAT biopsies were collected for molecular and proteomic assays. Our data show that PGE_2 biosynthetic enzyme (PTGES-2) correlates with echocardiographic parameters of LV enlargement: LV diameters, LV end diastolic volume, and LV masses. Moreover, PTGES-2 is directly associated with EPAC2 gene (r = 0.70, $p < 0.0001$), known as a molecular inducer of ST2/IL-33 mediators involved in maladaptive heart remodelling. Furthermore, PGE_2 receptor 3 (PTGER3) results are downregulated and its expression is inversely associated with ST2/IL-33 expression. Contrarily, PGE_2 receptor 4 (PTGER4) is upregulated in EAT and directly correlates with ST2 molecular expression. Our data suggest that excessive body fatness can shift the EAT transcriptome to a pro-tissue remodelling profile, may be driven by PGE_2 deregulation, with consequent promotion of EPAC2 and ST2 signalling.

Keywords: epicardial adipose tissue (EAT); prostaglandin E2 (PGE_2); EP3 receptor; EP4 receptor; exchange protein directly activated by cAMP isoform 2 (EPAC2); stimulating growth factor 2 (ST2); interleukin(IL)-33; Cardiovascular Diseases (CVDs); fat mass

1. Introduction

Perturbations of signaling in the heart and vessels of the body are the leading causes of cardiovascular disorders including coronary artery diseases (CAD) and valve heart diseases (VHD) [1]. Among different stimuli which can contribute to alter cardiac and vessel molecular responses, excessive fat body can be considered one of the primary causes associated with maladaptive heart response [2]. Obese patients are at increased risk of cardiovascular disease (CVD) and heart failure (HF) due to the hemodynamic stresses related to abnormal body mass and increase of volume overload [3]. The excessive hemodynamic stresses lead to cardiac microvascular rarefaction and fibrosis, especially with abnormalities of cardiac diastolic filling [4].

The first effect of chronic volume overload on left ventricle (LV), directly related to fatness, is characterized by typically LV and left atria (LA) dilation, with a preserved ejection fraction (EF), suggesting proportional expansion of plasma volume with body mass. For this reason, the capacity of LV to dilate in response to hydrodynamic volume overload is impaired and disproportionate.

Since overweight is the most deputed cause of these cardiac outcomes, it is assumed that visceral adiposity drives both vessels derangements and heart fibrosis [5], but the molecular patterns relating to these abnormalities are not fully understood. There is recent evidence suggesting that during maladaptive adipose tissue remodeling, dysfunctional fat responses of a particular visceral fat closely surrounding the heart and all arteries- known as epicardial adipose tissue (EAT)-can be a metabolic transducer of both local and systemic inflammation, through the direct release into myocardial microcirculation of bioactive fibro-adipokines [6,7] involved in heart metabolism [8–13]. EAT thickness varies 1 mm to a maximum of almost 23 mm [13]. This wide range probably reflects the substantial differences in abdominal visceral fat distribution [13]. Previous studies found median epicardial fat thicknesses of 7 mm in men and 6.5 mm in women in a large population of patients who were examined by transthoracic echocardiography for standard clinical indication [13]. Variations in EAT size can be considered a potential cardiovascular risk factor due to the shift in the production of active cardiometabolic mediators. Among these, one peculiar adipokine known as soluble stimulating growth factor 2 (sST2) [14] has attracted attention on account of both fat mass enlargement and maladaptive heart response due to its role in silencing the main mechanosensitive system [15,16] expressed and activated both in adipose tissue and in the heart [17]; this comprises by two immune mediators, the transmembrane isoform of ST2 (ST2L) and its natural ligand, the interleukin (IL)-33, one of the main alarmin proteins in the body [18]. The IL-33/ST2L system in adipose tissue tries to maintain the size of the fat mass, controlling intracellular nuclear factors that regulate adipocytes number and size of the adipocytes [19,20]. In the heart IL-33/ST2L system has cardioprotective effects since under biomechanical stress it promotes cell survival and prevents apoptosis and fibrosis [21]. However, in pathological conditions such as obesity and cardiovascular disorders, both adipocytes and cardiac cells release larger amount of sST2; this functions as a decoy receptor, sequestering IL-33, losing its cardio-fat protection properties through ST2L binding, and consequently promoting an increase in fat mass, and heart damage [14,16,19,22]. In a previous study [23] we identified as potential molecular inducer of this system in EAT, the exchange proteins directly activated by cAMP (EPACs), which are the main effectors of the second messenger in the body, the cycle adenine monophosphate(cAMP) [23,24]. The EPAC protein family is composed of EPAC1 and EPAC2 which in adipose tissue control adipogenesis and lipolysis and are induced by cAMP [25,26]. We reported that when EAT thickness increases, the local upregulation of EPAC2 promotes an alarm profile associated with maladaptive remodeling in which ST2 gene, encoding for both cardiac stretch proteins, ST2L and sST2, correlated with local expression of EPAC2 [23].

Prostaglandin E2 (PGE$_2$) appears to have a crucial role in intracellular cAMP concentration in visceral fat [27–29]. PGE$_2$ is a potent lipid mediator secreted by various cell types in visceral adipose tissue and it appears to be implicated in the regulation of inflammation and adipocytes functions [30]. Different studies have noted that the excess accumulation of visceral fat depends on depot-specific expression of key enzymes involved in adipose tissue functions, including PGE$_2$ biosynthesis-related enzymes [31].

PGE$_2$ is the principal prostaglandin produced by visceral adipose tissue including EAT deposit [27], which regulates energy metabolism and, particularly in obesity, contributes to fat-inflammation and obesity-related insulin resistance, through the activation of prostaglandin-endoperoxide synthase 2 (PTGES-2) [32], known also as cyclooxygenase 2. PGE$_2$ regulates adipose functions and exerts its biological effects through its four receptors (EP1, EP2, EP3 and EP4) [27]. The EP1 receptor is involved in intracellular Ca^{2+} level. The EP3 receptor is designed to lower intracellular cAMP concentration through the inhibition of adenylyl cyclases (ADCYs), thus promoting adipogenesis [33,34]. EP2 and especially EP4 have opposite effects, stimulating the increase of intracellular cAMP levels with the promotion of lipolysis [35–38]. The different role of PGE$_2$ receptors in the control of intracellular cAMP concentration, led to them being considered the master regulators of adipogenic and lipolytic processes, and their deregulation can be associated with obesity-related disorders. By eliciting signaling through cAMP and its effectors, the EPACs proteins, PGE$_2$ can potentiate the expression of mechanosensitive system IL-33/ST2L in immune cells [39].

Due to the importance of ST2 gene both in heart and fat metabolism, we set out to identify a new molecular gap among PGE$_2$ metabolism in EAT of overweight CVD persons and the expression of ST2 cardiac stretch mediator via EPAC2 gene, as new potential molecular pattern of maladaptive heart response.

2. Results

2.1. CVD Patients' Main Characteristics and Echocardiography

Anthropometric, clinical data and body fatness measurements are set out in Table 1. The CVD subjects had higher indices of body fatness and different in BMI (27.95 ± 5.19 vs normal range 18.50–24.99), waist circumference (106.70 ± 15.08 cm vs normal reference value less than 94 cm) and waist:hip ratio (WHR) (0.98 ± 0.13 normal cut off less than 0.95), indicating that CVD patients were overweight.

Biochemical parameters associated with body fatness were intra-male reference ranges except for N-terminal pro B-type natriuretic peptide (NT-pro-BNP) (453.92 ± 596 pg/mL) and C-reactive protein (CRP) (0.98 ± 0.38 mg/100 mL) which are the clinical parameters currently most used for cardiac stress assessment and body inflammation.

Echocardiography parameters of our CVD subjects are reported in Table 2. EAT thickness was evaluated both in end-diastolic and end-systolic echocardiographic frames and we used the end-systolic frame as EAT measurement because it is considered the best cardiac moment to detect EAT thickness [13,40]. The average EAT was about 7 mm. A normal upper-limit value for EAT thickness has yet not been established.

Echocardiography showed that overweight CVD subjects typically had left ventricle (LV) and atria (LA) dilation, with a preserved ejection fraction (EF), CVD subjects presented an eccentric LV hypertrophy (relative wall thickness: RTW < 0.42% and indexed LV mass: LVM/BSA ≥115 g/m^2), the first effect of chronic volume overload on LV, directly related to fatness [7].

Table 1. Cardiovascular disease (CVD) patients' main details and echocardiographic assessment.

Cardiovascular Patients	Mean	SD	Reference Range
Age (years)	66.86	10.47	/
Systolic blood pressure (mmHg)	130.6	9.66	115–120
Diastolic blood pressure (mmHg)	73.53	4.92	75–80
BMI	27.95	5.19	18.50–24.99
Weight (kg)	83.29	20.48	/
Height (m)	1.71	0.06	/
Waist (cm)	106.70	15.08	<94
Hip (cm)	110.5	25.22	/
HOMA	2.36	2.38	<2.50
WHR	0.98	0.127	<0.95
Family history			
Hypertension	3	/	/
Diabetes	2	/	/
CAD	4	/	/
Biochemical parameters			
Creatinine (mg/dL)	0.99	0.38	0.60–1.30
Fasting glucose (mg/dL)	46.11	45.04	60–99
HbA1c (%)	4.55	1.43	<6.30
NT-PRO BNP (pg/mL)	453.92	567	<300
Total cholesterol (mg/dL)	155.9	28.86	<200
HDL (mg/dL)	42.48	11.4	40–59
Triglycerides (mg/dL)	132	52.47	<150
Acid uric (mg/dL)	6.64	1.44	4.0–8.0
CRP (mg/100 mL)	0.98	0.38	0.50
ALT (U/L)	28.09	24.67	9.0–60.0
AST (U/L)	32.32	37.33	10.0–40.0
Bilirubin (total) (mg/dL)	0.57	0.31	0.3–1.00

Table 2. Echocardiographic assessment of the overweight CVD subjects.

Echocardiographic Data	Mean	SD	Reference Range
EAT thickness in systole (mm)	6.73	2.164	/
LV internal dimension			
LV diastolic diameter (cm)	5.68	0.91	4.2–5.8
LV systolic diameter (cm)	3.99	1.13	2.5–4.0
LV volumes (biplane)			
LV EDV (mL)	147.5	80.64	62.15
LV ESV (mL)	71.06	49.07	21–61
LV volumes normalized by BSA			
LV EDV (mL/m^2)	75.97	37.04	34–74
LV ESV (mL/m^2)	35.71	24.25	11.31
LV EF function			
LV EF (%)	55.65	11.38	52–72
LV mass by 2D method			
septal wall thickness (cm)	1.22	0.2	0.60–1.00
RWT (%)	0.41	0.11	<0.42
LV mass (g)	294.3	119.5	88–224
LV mass/BSA (g/m^2)	146.9	53.15	49–115
LA size			
LA (cm)	4.2	0.67	<4
RV function			
TAPSE (mm)	23.2	5.71	>17
Pulmonary artery pressure			
PAP (mmHg)	32.23	13.53	<35–40

2.2. Anthropometric Measures of Body Fatness Are Associated with Maladaptive Heart Remodeling in Overweight CVD Subjects

The acknowledged parameters of fat body distribution as BMI and waist circumference, directly correlate with echocardiographic indexes of heart maladaptation (Table 3). BMI is not only a predicting factor of insulin resistance due to the positive correlations with Homeostatic Model Assessment for Insulin Resistance (HOMA), fast insulin, waist circumference and an inverse relation with HDL cholesterol. It also directly correlates with both the diameters and volumes of LV, with its mass and LA size. The LA enlargement and dysfunction are the most predictors of (HF) in overweight patients with CVD. The alternative measure that reflects abdominal adiposity waist circumference, which has been suggested as superior to BMI in predicting CVD outcomes, is directly related to EAT thickness and with the indexes predicting insulin resistance. Waist circumference is also related to both LV and LA enlargement.

Table 3. Anthropometric measures of body fatness are associated with maladaptive heart remodeling in overweight CVD subjects.

BMI (x)	Spearman r	p Value
LV diastolic diameter (cm)	0.48	0.02
LV systolic diameter (cm)	0.47	0.03
LV EDV (mL)	0.48	0.03
LV ESV (mL)	0.47	0.04
LVM (g)	0.40	0.05
LA (cm)	0.53	0.03
Insulin resistance predicting factors		
Waist (cm)	0.70	0.0004
Fasting insulin (microU/mL)	0.62	0.005
HOMA	0.53	0.02
HDL (mg/dL)	−0.43	0.05
Waist (x)	**Spearman r**	**p value**
EAT thickness in systole (mm)	0.48	0.02
LV diastolic diameter (cm)	0.45	0.03
LVM (g)	0.45	0.03
LA (cm)	0.60	0.01
Insulin resistance predicting factors		
BMI	0.70	0.0004
Fasting glucose (mg/dL)	0.46	0.03
Fasting insulin (microU/mL)	0.58	0.001
Triglycerides (mg/dL)	0.43	0.04

2.3. Prostaglandin-Endoperoxide Synthase 2 (PTGES-2) Expression in EAT is Directly Related to Maladaptive Heart Remodeling Indexes in Overweight CVD Subjects

In view the importance of body fatness on heart maladaptation, we investigated the PGE_2 molecular alterations in EAT from overweight CVD patients. Considering the role of PTGES-2 as a mediator of adiposity and its involvement in fat-inflammation and obesity-related disorders, including cardiovascular complications, we ran a correlation analysis between PTGES-2 molecular expression and echocardiographic parameters of heart remodeling (Figure 1). There were linear correlations among PTGES-2 molecular expression in EAT and the diameters (diastolic and systolic), volume (EDV) and mass (LVM and LVM/BSA); this suggests that PGE_2 biosynthesis in EAT of overweight CVD people is involved in maladaptive cardiac responses.

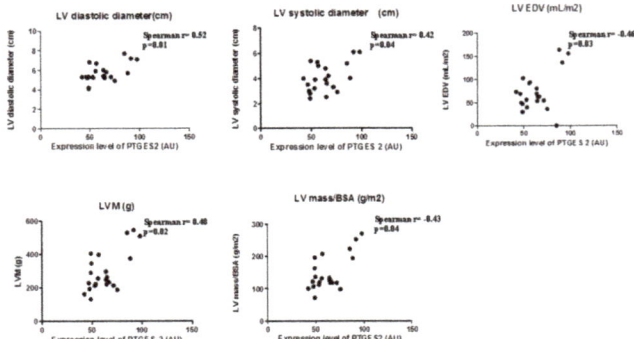

Figure 1. PTGES-2 molecular expression level in epicardial adipose tissue (EAT) of overweight CVD subjects.

2.4. EP3 Receptor Molecular Expression in EAT Correlates with Body Fatness of Overweight CVD People

EP3 expression correlated substantially with body fatness and waist circumference (Spearman r = 0.43, p = 0.05) and WHR (Spearman r = 0.44, p = 0.04); and also with factors predicting insulin resistance, such as triglycerides (Spearman r = 0.46, p = 0.04) and fasting glucose (Spearman r = 0.50, p = 0.03). This suggests that EP3 molecular expression in EAT is related to the increase of body fatness in overweight CVD subjects (Figure 2).

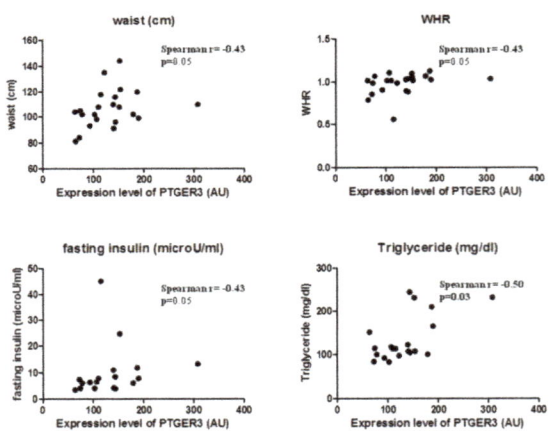

Figure 2. EP3 molecular expression in EAT is associated with body fatness.

2.5. EP3, EP4, and PTGES-2 Are Involved Differently in cAMP Production in EAT

Since PGE_2 drives both adipogenesis and lipolysis in visceral adipose tissue, acting on intracellular cAMP production by silencing adenylyl cyclase (ADCY) enzymes through its receptors, we ran a correlational analysis between the PTGES-2, EP3 and 4 receptors and the molecular expression of ADCYs in EAT to clarify their effects on cAMP intracellular concentrations in case of excessive (Table 4). PTGES-2 and EP4 were mostly associated with the increase of intracellular cAMP due to the positive correlations between them and ADCY isoforms, suggesting their pro-lipolytic effect on EAT when fat mass increases. In contrast, EP3 molecular expression in EAT seems to be related to anti-lipolytic signaling due to the inverse associations with the main ADCY isoforms in cAMP production, suggesting a protective role against lipolysis during fat mass increase (Table 4).

Table 4. EP3, EP4, and PTGES-2 are involved differently in cAMP production in EAT.

PTGES-2	Spearman r	p Value	EP3	Spearman r	p Value	EP4	Spearman r	p Value
ADCY1	0.73	<0.0001	ADCY1	−0.37	0.04	ADCY1	0.47	0.01
ADCY2	0.66	<0.0001	ADCY2	−0.45	0.01	ADCY2	0.51	0.002
ADCY3	0.04	0.84	ADCY3	−0.34	0.05	ADCY3	−0.19	0.27
ADCY4	−0.13	0.47	ADCY4	−0.11	0.56	ADCY4	0.02	0.89
ADCY5	0.58	0.0005	ADCY5	−0.40	0.02	ADCY5	0.43	0.01
ADCY6	−0.41	0.02	ADCY6	0.62	0.0001	ADCY6	−0.42	0.01
ADCY7	−0.39	0.02	ADCY7	−0.64	<0.0001	ADCY7	0.24	0.16
ADCY8	0.74	<0.0001	ADCY8	−0.46	0.01	ADCY8	0.53	0.001
ADCY9	0.55	0.001	ADCY9	−0.54	0.0011	ADCY9	0.11	0.52
ADCY10	0.78	<0.0001	ADCY10	−0.36	0.04	ADCY10	0.45	0.01

2.6. The PTGES-2 Gene Correlates Directly with EPAC2 as the Molecular Inducer of the ST2/IL-33 Mechanosensitive System

Considering the role of PGE_2 in the regulation of cAMP concentrations in visceral adipose tissue, and of EPAC2 cAMP effector in the control of cardiac stretch genes such as ST2 and IL-33, we explored the relations between the expression of PTGES-2 and EPAC2 cAMP effector gene (Figure 3a).

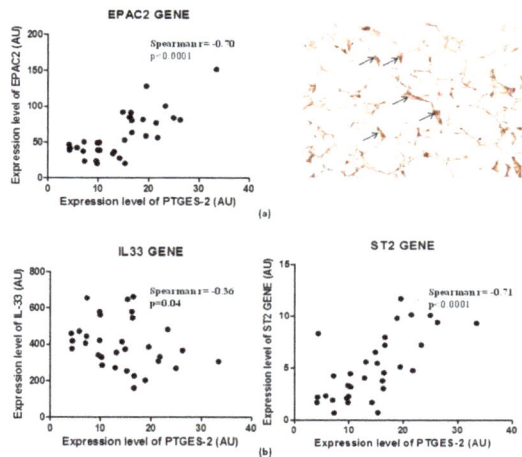

Figure 3. PTGES-2 gene directly correlates with EPAC2 inducer of ST2/IL-33 mechanosensitive system in overweight CVD patients. (a) The expression level of PTGES-2 directly correlates with the local expression gene of EPAC2 cAMP effector, powerful inducer of ST2/IL33 mechanosensitive system in immune cells. The local immunolocalization of EPAC2 cAMP effector in EAT biopsies of overweight CVD subjects is demonstrated by EPAC2$^+$ cells in the stroma region (black arrows; magnification 20×). (b) The PTGES-2 controller of cAMP effectors directly correlates with ST2/IL-33 mechanosensitive genes associated with fat and cardiac maladaptation.

PTGES-2 correlates positively with the local expression of EPAC2 (Spearman r = 0.70, p < 0.0001) which was recently recognized as one of the main inducers of ST2 gene in EAT. The local protein production of EPAC2 in EAT biopsy suggests active control of EPAC2 in adipocytes due to the stroma immune-localization of EPAC positive cells (black arrows).

That PTGES-2 is involved in sST2/ST2/IL-33 cardiac stretch mediators is further confirmed by the molecular relations between PTGES-2 and ST2, IL-33 gene expression in EAT (Figure 3b). PTGES-2 directly correlates with ST2 gene (Spearman r = 0.70, p < 0.0001) which encodes for both ST2 cardiac stretch mediators (ST2L and sST2) and inversely with IL-33 gene (Spearman r = −0.36, p = 0.04), which transducer for the main alarmin in the body able to block the circulating isoform of ST2 gene, promoting cardiac cell survival and preventing fibrosis and heart remodeling.

2.7. Increase of EAT Mass Deregulates EP3 and EP4 Molecular Expression with Direct Induction of ST2 Gene via EPAC2 cAMP Effector

In the light of the opposite effects of EP3 and EP4 in cAMP intracellular concentrations and the PGE_2's role in the induction of sST2/ST2/IL-33 cardiac stretch mediators in immune cells through EPAC2 cAMP effector, we explored the molecular interaction between EP3 and EP4 and EPAC2 and sST2/ST2/IL-33 mediators in EAT of overweight people (Figure 4). Regarding EP4 receptor, which is closely involved in lipolytic processes, gave a positive relation between EPAC2 cAMP effector (Spearman r = 0.46, p = 0.001) and ST2 gene (Spearman r = 0.63, p = 0.002), and an inverse relation with IL-33 molecular expression, although close to the statistical significance (Spearman r = −0.36, p = 0.05) (Figure 4a). Noteworthy, there is a positive association between EP4 molecular expression and EAT thickness (Spearman r = 0.70, p = 0.0003) (Figure 4a). There was an interesting inverse relation between EP3 adipogenic receptor and ST2 gene (Spearman = −0.37, p < 0.03) and the soluble protein of ST2 receptor sST2 (Spearman R = −0.60, p = 0.008) (Figure 4b) which is a powerful mediator of maladaptive heart remodeling released in response to cardiac overload. The EP3 receptor was inversely related to EPAC2 as cAMP effector and inducer of ST2 gene (Spearman r = −0.47, p = 0.006) (Figure 4b).

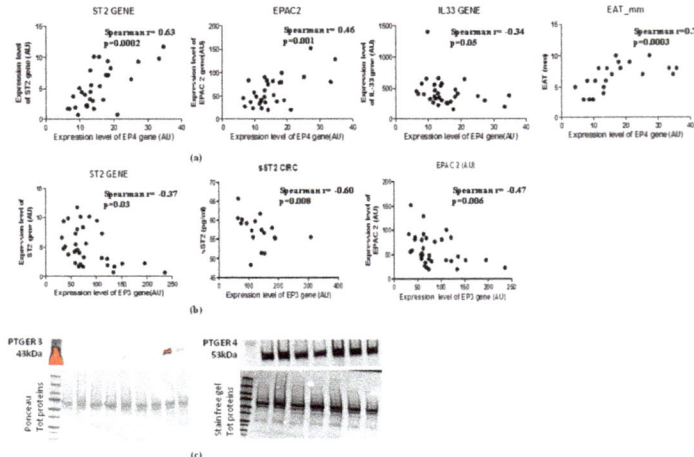

Figure 4. EAT mass increase deregulates EP3 and EP4 molecular expression levels with direct induction of ST2 gene via the EPAC2 cAMP effector. (**a**) EP4 lipolytic PGE_2 receptor directly correlates with genes associated with mechano-tissue responses including EPAC2 cAMP effector (Spearman r = 0.46, p = 0.001) and ST2 gene (Spearman r = 0.63, p = 0.002) and inversely with IL-33 molecular expression, although close to the statistical significance (Spearman r = −0.36, p = 0.05). (**b**) EP3 anti- lipolytic PGE_2 receptor correlates inversely with both ST2 isoforms and with EPAC2 cAMP effector. (**c**) EP4 pro-lipolytic isoform of PGE_2 receptors is more present than the EP3 anti-lipolytic PGE_2 receptor.

To verify whether the increased EAT mass in overweight persons influences the local protein expression of PGE_2 receptors, we used western blot analysis to quantify EP3 and EP4 proteins in EAT (Figure 4c). The EAT of overweight persons produced less EP3 anti-lipolytic receptor than EP4 pro-lipolytic receptor, suggesting that an increase of EAT mass can deregulate PGE_2 control on lipolytic processes via EP3 reduction, contributing to a local increase in cAMP.

3. Discussion

EAT is a transducer in obesity and inflammation due to the release of different adipokines that can influence the metabolism of neighboring tissues, especially of the myocardium, on account its anatomical position [41]. In obesity, EAT changes its biological characteristics, with consequent structural and functional abnormalities, leading to impaired myocardial microcirculation, increased LV volume and size, and LA dilatation [41,42], as in our overweight CVD subjects. The anthropometric parameters of abdominal obesity—BMI and waist circumference—are currently used for predicting CVD events associated with insulin resistance [7]. We observed associations between body fatness and echocardiographic parameters of heart maladaptation. The waist circumference, recognized as the best anthropometric measurement of abdominal fat, directly correlates with EAT thickness and both LV and LA dilatation as predictive factor of maladaptive heart response in overweight CVD patients [43]. The question whether the molecular pattern of EAT can shift to a dysfunctional state when abdominal fat mass increases, with the promotion of maladaptive LV structural changes, could be partly answered by our molecular study, where PGE_2 molecular regulation is pivotal in the activation of ST2 cardiac stretch mediator via EPAC2 cAMP effector.

PGE_2 is a potent lipid mediator secreted by various cell types in visceral adipose tissue and it appears to be implicated in the regulation of inflammation and adipocytes functions. Different studies have noted that the excess accumulation of visceral fat depends on depot-specific expression of key enzymes involved in adipose tissue functions, including PGE_2 biosynthesis-related enzymes [38]. In obesity, PTGES-2 promotes adipose tissue dysfunction, with sustained inflammation and fibrosis, impaired adaptative thermogenesis and increased lipolysis. PTGES-2, also known as cyclooxygenase-2, has in fact been shown to be linked to the early onset of type 2 diabetes and insulin resistance in chronic low-grade inflammation state, especially through the production of PGE_2 [38]. In view of the involvement of body fatness in heart metabolism, we explored PTGES-2 expression in EAT from overweight CVD patients and echocardiographic parameters of LV enlargement. Our overweight CVD subjects showed a linear correlation between PTGES-2 molecular expression in EAT and cardiac abnormalities associated with LV remodeling, denoting a possible involvement of dysfunctional EAT metabolism and maladaptive heart response. Since adipogenic and lipolytic processes are driven by intracellular cAMP concentrations under PGE_2 control, we examined the molecular relation between PGE_2 metabolism in EAT and the expression of genes linked to adenylyl cyclases. There was a positive association between PTGES-2 and the main isoforms of adenylyl cyclases responsible for cAMP synthesis, underling its involvement in intracellular cAMP concentrations during fat mass increase. This is confirmed by the molecular association of PGE_2 receptors with ADCYs genes. There was an interesting inverse relation between EP3 receptor and ADCY isoforms, confirming its involvement in adipogenic processes, and noteworthy direct associations between EP4 and ADCYs involved in intracellular cAMP increases. The increase of lipolysis driven by cAMP intracellular level, may be one of the factors contributing to obesity-related insulin resistance controlled by PGE_2 receptors in visceral adipose tissue. The EP3 receptor leads to lower rates of lipolysis and in adipose tissue its deletion may promote an obese phenotype in adult mice [27]. We found EP3 molecular expression correlated positively with the factor predicting insulin resistance, suggesting its potential protective role against obesity-related disorders in overweight CVD subjects. In view of the role of cAMP intracellular levels in the regulation of adipogenic and lipolytic processes driven by PGE_2 metabolism, and the pivotal role of PTGE-2 in obesity-related disorders, we investigated the involvement of PTGES-2 in the expression of EPAC2, known as a cAMP effector and recently associated with ST2/IL-33 mechanosensitive system involved in the maladaptive heart response. We previously demonstrated when there is an increase in EAT mass, EPAC2 can upregulate ST2 gene, which is a powerful inducer of both cardiac and fat remodeling [23]. Through alternative splicing this gene can transduce for ST2L and sST2 proteins with opposite biological effects: the transmembrane isoform, ST2L can promote cell survival and anti-fibrotic signaling through binding with the IL-33 alarmin protein in cardiac and fat cells [15,18]. In contrast, the truncated soluble isoform, sST2, functioning as a decoy receptor, sequesters IL-33 alarmin protein into extracellular space, preventing ST2L/IL-33 signaling and promoting cardiac and fat tissue maladaptive responses [18]. In view of the role PTGES-2 in obesity and in the control of intracellular cAMP concentrations through PGE_2 receptors [30,32], we investigate the possible association between PTGES-2 and EPAC2 cAMP effector and ST2/IL-33 mechanosensitive genes. We found active expression of EPAC2 in EAT from overweight CVD subjects and an interesting direct association between PTGES-2 and EPAC2 genes EAT mass increases. Moreover, PTGES-2 inversely correlates with IL-33 alarmin expression and positively with the ST2 gene, reinforcing the hypothesis that PGE_2 metabolism, which controls intracellular cAMP levels, can also influence the molecular expression of the ST2/IL-33 mechanosensitive genes, through EPAC2. Since in a murine model of macrophages PGE_2 played a pivotal role in production of IL-33 through EP4-cAMP-EPAC [39] dependent pathway, we looked into the molecular involvement of EP3 and EP4 expression in EAT from overweight CVD subjects and ST2 and IL-33 expression as molecular transducers of maladaptive tissue response. The EP4 receptor correlated directly with EAT thickness, suggesting that EAT mass increase promotes EP4 local expression. Moreover, EP4 directly correlated with EPAC2 and ST2 genes and inversely with IL-33, suggesting its involvement in maladaptive tissue response through EPAC2/ST2 signaling. In contrast, EP3 seems involved in ST2L local expression in case of EAT mass increase and inversely correlates with total sST2 circulating levels, suggesting its possible role in the prevention of maladaptive tissue responses. The local protein production of EP3 and EP4 receptors is expressed differently in EAT from overweight CVD patients. EP4—implicated in lipolytic processes—are more present than EP3 receptor protein, suggesting that when EAT mass increases, deregulated PGE_2 metabolism seems to be addressed to increased intracellular cAMP level, with consequent upregulation of EPAC2 cAMP effector which is closely involved in ST2 gene expression.

4. Materials and Methods

4.1. Study Population

This study is conducted on 33 male CVDs patients enrolled at I.R.C.C.S. Policlinico San Donato (San Donato Milanese, Milan, Italy) who underwent open heart surgery. Patients with recent acute myocardial infarction, malignant disease, prior major abdominal surgery, renal failure, end-stage heart failure (HF) and more than 3% variation in body weight in the previous 3 months were excluded. Demographic, anthropometric and clinical data including age, sex, and family history of hypertension, diabetes and CAD are recorded. In accordance to the preoperative coronary angiographic examination, 23 were ischemic patients with CAD undergoing elective coronary artery bypass grafting surgery and 10 were VHD patients receiving valvular replacement. Before surgery, EAT thickness was evaluated by echocardiography. The study protocol was approved by the local Ethics Committee (ASL Milano Due, protocol number 2516; date: 28 December 2009) and patients gave their written informed consent to the examination protocol, conducted in accordance with the Declaration of Helsinki, as revised in 2013. A flow chart which shows the experimental procedure of the study setting is included as Supplementary Figure S1.

4.2. Blood Collection and Measurements

Blood samples were collected after overnight fasting into pyrogen-free tubes with ethylenediaminetetraacetic acid as anticoagulant. Plasma samples were separated after centrifugation at $1000\times g$ for 15 min and were stored at $-20\ °C$ until analysis. Fasting glucose, glycated hemoglobin (HbA1c), creatinine and N-terminal pro B-type natriuretic peptide (NT-pro BNP) were quantified with commercial kits using Cobas 6000 analyzer (Roche Diagnostics, Milan, Italy). Plasmatic level of sST2 was assayed by enzyme-linked immunosorbent assays (ELISA) (R&D Systems, Minneapolis, MN, USA).

4.3. Quantification of EAT and SAT Collection

Pre-surgical EAT quantification was quantified by echocardiography with a 2.5- to 3.5-MHz transducer probe (Vingmed-System Five; General Electric, Horten, Norway). EAT thickness was measured along the free wall of the right ventricle from both parasternal long-and short-axis views as previously reported [13]. This point is where EAT generally shows the major thickness and is measurable more easily [13]. EAT thickness at level of the right ventricle free wall is normally 7 mm in both male and female healthy lean individuals; no clinical cut of value is currently validated. EAT biopsy samples were harvested adjacent to the proximal right coronary artery prior to initiation of cardiopulmonary bypass pumping. For gene expression analysis, EAT biopsies were stored in Allprotect Tissue Reagent (Qiagen, Hilden, Germany) at −20 °C until RNA and protein extraction. For immunohistochemical staining assays, EAT biopsies were immediately fixed in paraformaldehyde 4%. To validate RT-PCR assay we collected subcutaneous fat depot (SAT) as control tissue and SAT biopsies were treated like EAT (Supplementary Figure S2).

4.4. Echocardiography Data of Left Ventricular Mass (LV)

Pre-surgical resting echocardiography (Vingmed-System Five; General Electric, Horten, Norway) was performed to assess systolic, diastolic and valvular morphology and function. LV hypertrophy was defined according the current guidelines for echocardiographic chambers quantification.

The outcome measures were LV diastolic diameter (reference values (RV): male 4.2–5.8 cm), LV systolic diameter (RV: male 2.5–4.0 cm), LV end diastolic volume (EDV) (RV: male 62–150 mL), LV end systolic volume (ESV) (RV: male 21–61 mL), LV ejection fraction (EF) (RV: male 52–75%), septal wall thickness (RV: male 0.6–1.0 cm), relative wall thickness (RWT) (RV: male < 0.42%), LV mass (RV: male 88–224 g), indexed LV (LVM/BSA) (RV: male 49–115 g/m^2), left atria (LA) (RV: male < 4 cm), tricuspid annular plane systolic excursion (TAPSE) (RV: male > 17 mm) and pulmonary artery pressure (PAP) (RV: male < 35–40 mmHg).

4.5 DNA Microarray Chip Array Expression Assay

Total RNA was extracted from EAT biopsies with the RNeasy Lipid Tissue Kit (Qiagen). RNA concentration was quantified by NanoDrop 2000 (ThermoScientific, Wilmington, Germany) and RNA integrity was assessed using the Agilent RNA 6000 Nano kit and the Agilent 2100 Bioanalyzer (Agilent Technologies, Santa Clara, CA, USA). Gene expression analysis was performed by one color microarray platform (Agilent). 50 ng of total RNA was labelled with Cy3 using the Agilent LowInput Quick-Amp Labeling kit-1 color, according to manufacturer's instructions. RNA was purified with the RNeasy Lipid Tissue Mini Kit (Qiagen) and the amount and labelling efficiency were measured with NanoDrop. Hybridization was performed using Agilent Gene Expression hybridisation Kit and scanning with Agilent G2565CA Microarray Scanner System. Data were processed using Agilent Feature Extraction Software (10.7) with the single-color gene expression protocol and raw data were analyzed with ChipInspector Software (Genomatix, Munich, Germany). In brief, raw data were normalized on single probe level based on the array mean intensities and statistics were calculated based on the SAM algorithm by Tusher. From microarray chip analysis, the gene expression of RAPGEF3 (encoding for EPAC1), RAPGEF4 (encoding for EPAC2), gene associated with PGE2 signaling including PTGES-2 (encoding for PTGES-2 enzyme), PTGER3 and 4 (encoding for EP3 and E4 respectively genes, and remodeling mediators including IL1RL1 (encoding for ST2L and sST2) and IL-33 were evaluated and expressed in arbitrary unit (AU).

4.6. Real Time Reverse-Transcription PCR (RT-PCR) Assay

To validate our microarray results, we performed RT-PCR assay for only our target genes. Briefly, total RNA was extracted as previously described in the above section. First strand cDNA was synthesized using RT^2 first strand kit (Qiagen). Quantitative PCR analysis was then performed with

RT^2 SYBR Green Fast Mastermix (Qiagen) and PCR technology (Rotor Gene Q, Qiagen). Relative quantification of mRNA expression in the gene of interest was calculated using the comparative threshold cycle number and the difference between EAT and SAT was evaluated using $2^{-\Delta CT}$ method. Data were normalized by GAPDH levels and expressed as percentage relative to controls. All PCRs were performed at least in triplicate for each experimental condition. GAPDH (Qiagen, PPH00150F), PTGER3 (Qiagen, PPH01838B), PTGER4 (Qiagen, PPH02677A), PTGES2 (Qiagen, PPH16120A), IL1RL1 encoding for ST2 (Qiagen, PPH01076A), IL-33 (Qiagen, PPH17375E), RAPGEF3 encoding for EPAC1 (Qiagen, PPH02838A) and RAPGEF4 encoding for EPAC2 (Qiagen, PPH10495C) genes were measured.

4.7. Western Blot Analysis

EAT tissue was homogenized using Minute™ Total Protein Extraction kit for Adipose Tissue/Cultured Adipocytes kit (Invent Biotechnologies, Inc), according to the manufacturer's instructions. Aliquots of 30 µg of total proteins were electrophoresed on SDS Mini-PROTEAN® TGX™ Stain-Free Precast Gels (BIO RAD, Hercules, CA, USA) and transferred to nitrocellulose membrane of Trans-Blot® Tranfer System Transfer Pack (BIO RAD) on Trans Blot® Turbo™ device (BIO RAD). Membranes first blocked with 5% nonfat dry milk/TBS with 0.1% (Vol/Vol) Tween 20 for 1 h and then incubated overnight at 4 °C with primary antibodies for: vinculin (Cell Signaling, Denver, MA, USA; 1:1000), PTGER3 (Proteintech, Manchester, United Kingdom; dilution 1:500) and PTGER4 (Proteintech, Manchester, United Kingdom, dilution 1:700). After washing, membranes are incubated with appropriate horseradish peroxidase (HRP)-labeled secondary antibodies for 2 h at room temperature. Immunoreactive protein bands were then detected using ECL chemiluminescence kit (BIO RAD) using ChemiDoc MP Imaging System (BIO RAD). Desitometric analyses were performed using Image Lab 5.2.1 software (BIO RAD). Data were normalized on total protein quantity after stain-free blot or ponceau staining and presented as percentage density volume (%). All Western Blots were performed at least in duplicate. The full blots were provided in Supplementary Figure S3.

4.8. EPAC2 Immunohistochemical Staining in EAT Sections

Deparaffinised EAT sections were rehydrated and antigen retrieval was performed by autoclaving in sodium citrate buffer 0.01 M pH 6 for 5 min at 120 °C. After rinsing in PBS 1X, quenching of endogenous peroxidases activity was performed in 0.3% H_2O_2 in PBS for 20 min. To block unspecific binding, sections were incubated with normal swine serum (Dako Cytomation) and then with the following primary antibody: mouse monoclonal anti-human EPAC2 (diluted 1:400 in PBS, Cell Signaling) overnight and overnight. Sections were then rinsed in PBS and processed for the amplification of immune signal using anti-mouse HRP-polymer complex (MACH 1 Universal HRP-Polymer detection, Biocare Medical, Concord, CA, USA). BIOCARE's Betazoid DAB was used for color development Sections were counterstained with Mayer's hematoxylin and mounted with Mowiol 4–88.

Immunohistochemical reactions were observed with a Nikon Eclipse 80i microscope and images acquired by the digital camera and the image acquisition software.

4.9. Statistical Analysis

Data were expressed as mean ± standard (SD) and analyzed by GraphPad Prism 5.0 biochemical statistical package (GraphPad Software, Inc., San Diego, CA, USA). The normality of data distribution was assessed by the Kolmogrov-Smirnoff test. Comparison between groups was performed using two-tailed unpaired Student *t* test or Mann-Whitney U-test as appropriate. Spearman or Pearson correlation analyses were used to examine the association between different variables. All differences with $p < 0.05$ was considered statistically significant.

5. Conclusions

In summary, our data reinforce the current knowledge on PGE$_2$ control of cAMP levels through EP3 and EP4 receptors, and, in case of EAT mass increase, EP3 deregulation seems to be associated with the increase in lipolytic processes with consequent molecular upregulation of the newer inducer of ST2/IL-33 mechanosensitive system, the EPAC2 cAMP effector, in overweight CVD subjects. Further research is now needed to clarify the role of PGE_2 metabolism in the induction of ST2/IL-33 so as to pave the way to potential therapeutic strategies to prevent cardiac/fat tissue maladaptation driven by obesity.

Supplementary Materials: The following are available online at http://www.mdpi.com/1422-0067/21/2/520/s1.

Author Contributions: Conceptualization, E.V.; methodology, E.V.; software, G.S.; validation, G.S., E.V. and E.D.; formal analysis, E.D., E.M., and G.S.; investigation, E.V.; resources, E.V. and E.D.; data F.B. and M.F.; writing—original draft preparation, E.V.; writing—review and editing, E.D., J.L. and M.M.C.R.; visualization, L.T. and J.L.; supervision, M.M.C.R. and L.T.; project administration, E.V.; funding acquisition, M.M.C.R. All authors have read and agreed to the published version of the manuscript.

Funding: This research was funded by the Italian Ministry of Health "Ricerca Corrente" IRCCS Policlinico San Donato, and by Fondazione E. A. Fiera Internazionale di Milano to Università degli Studi di Milano.

Acknowledgments: Authors thank L. Menicanti for EAT biopsies collection at I.R.C.C.S. Policlinico San Donato; A. Fiorani for excellent coordination between surgical rooms and researchers; T. Konovalova from University of Regensburg, for bioinformatic support.

Conflicts of Interest: The authors declare no conflict of interest.

Abbreviations

CAD	Coronary artery disease
VHD	Valve heart disease
EAT	Epicardial adipose tissue
sST2	soluble stimulating growth factor 2
ST2L	Transmembrane isoform of ST2
IL-33	Interleukin-33
EPACs	Echange proteins directly activated by cAMP
EPAC1	Echange proteins directly activated by cAMP isoform 1
EPAC2	Echange proteins directly activated by cAMP isoform 2
PGE_2	Prostaglandin E2
PTGES-2	prostaglandin-endoperoxide synthase 2
BMI	Body mass index
CVD	Cardiovascular disease
EF	Ejection fraction
LV	Left ventricle
LA	Left atria
EDV	LV end diastolic volume
IL-33	Interleukin-33
LVM	Left ventricular mass
LVM/BSA	Indexed left ventricular mass
BSA	Body surface area
NT-pro BNP	N-terminal pro B-type natriuretic peptide
CRP	C reactive protein
HF	Heart failure
RTW	Relative wall thickness
HOMA	Homeostatic Model Assessment for Insulin Resistance
WHR	Waist hip ratio
ADCYs	Adenylyl cyclases
RV	Reference value
ESV	LV end systolic volume
TAFSE	Trycuspid annular plane systolic excursion
PAPs	Pulmonary artery pressure
RAPGEF3	Gene encoding for EPAC1

RAPGEF4	Gene encoding for EPAC2
PTGER3	Gene encoding for EP3 receptor
PTGER4	Gene encoding for EP4 receptor
ILRL1	Gene encoding for ST2 proteins
AU	Arbitrary unit
PBS	Phosphate buffered saline
SAT	Subcutaneous adipose tissue

References

1. Cavalera, M.; Wang, J.; Frangogiannis, N.G. Obesity, metabolic dysfunction, and cardiac fibrosis: Pathophysiological pathways, molecular mechanisms, and therapeutic opportunities. *Transl. Res.* **2014**, *164*, 323–335. [CrossRef] [PubMed]
2. Fuster, J.J.; Ouchi, N.; Gokce, N.; Walsh, K. Obesity-Induced Changes in Adipose Tissue Microenvironment and Their Impact on Cardiovascular Disease. *Circ. Res.* **2016**, *118*, 1786–1807. [CrossRef] [PubMed]
3. Manna, P.; Jain, S.K. Obesity, Oxidative Stress, Adipose Tissue Dysfunction, and the Associated Health Risks: Causes and Therapeutic Strategies. *Metab. Syndr. Relat. Disord.* **2015**, *13*, 423–444. [CrossRef] [PubMed]
4. Walpot, J.; Inacio, J.R.; Massalha, S.; El Mais, H.; Hossain, A.; Shiau, J.; Small, G.R.; Crean, A.M.; Yam, Y.; Rybicki, F.; et al. Early LV remodelling patterns in overweight and obesity: Feasibility of cardiac CT to detect early geometric left ventricular changes. *Obes. Res. Clin. Pract.* **2019**, *13*, 478–485. [CrossRef] [PubMed]
5. Fernandes-Silva, M.M.; Shah, A.M.; Claggett, B.; Cheng, S.; Tanaka, H.; Silvestre, O.M.; Nadruz, W.; Borlaug, B.A.; Solomon, S.D. Adiposity, body composition and ventricular-arterial stiffness in the elderly: The Atherosclerosis Risk in Communities Study. *Eur. J. Heart Fail.* **2018**, *20*, 1191–1201. [CrossRef] [PubMed]
6. Gruzdeva, O.; Uchasova, E.; Dyleva, Y.; Borodkina, D.; Akbasheva, O.; Belik, E.; Karetnikova, V.; Brel, N.; Kokov, A.; Kashtalap, V.; et al. Relationships between epicardial adipose tissue thickness and adipo-fibrokine indicator profiles post-myocardial infarction. *Cardiovasc. Diabetol.* **2018**, *17*, 40. [CrossRef] [PubMed]
7. Packer, M. Epicardial Adipose Tissue May Mediate Deleterious Effects of Obesity and Inflammation on the Myocardium. *J. Am. Coll. Cardiol.* **2018**, *71*, 2360–2372. [CrossRef]
8. Venteclef, N.; Guglielmi, V.; Balse, E.; Gaborit, B.; Cotillard, A.; Atassi, F.; Amour, J.; Leprince, P.; Dutour, A.; Clement, K.; et al. Human epicardial adipose tissue induces fibrosis of the atrial myocardium through the secretion of adipo-fibrokines. *Eur. Heart J.* **2015**, *36*, 795–805. [CrossRef]
9. McAninch, E.A.; Fonseca, T.L.; Poggioli, R.; Panos, A.L.; Salerno, T.A.; Deng, Y.; Li, Y.; Bianco, A.C.; Iacobellis, G. Epicardial adipose tissue has a unique transcriptome modified in severe coronary artery disease. *Obesity (Silver Spring)* **2015**, *23*, 1267–1278. [CrossRef]
10. Ng, A.C.T.; Strudwick, M.; van der Geest, R.J.; Ng, A.C.C.; Gillinder, L.; Goo, S.Y.; Cowin, G.; Delgado, V.; Wang, W.Y.S.; Bax, J.J. Impact of Epicardial Adipose Tissue, Left Ventricular Myocardial Fat Content, and Interstitial Fibrosis on Myocardial Contractile Function. *Circ. Cardiovasc. Imaging* **2018**, *11*, e007372. [CrossRef]
11. Guglielmi, V.; Sbraccia, P. Epicardial adipose tissue: At the heart of the obesity complications. *Acta Diabetol.* **2017**, *54*, 805–812. [CrossRef] [PubMed]
12. Iacobellis, G.; Ribaudo, M.C.; Zappaterreno, A.; Iannucci, C.V.; Leonetti, F. Relation between epicardial adipose tissue and left ventricular mass. *Am. J. Cardiol.* **2004**, *94*, 1084–1087. [CrossRef] [PubMed]
13. Iacobellis, G.; Willens, H.J. Echocardiographic epicardial fat: A review of research and clinical applications. *J. Am. Soc. Echocardiogr.* **2009**, *22*, 1311–1319. [CrossRef] [PubMed]
14. Martinez-Martinez, E.; Miana, M.; Jurado-Lopez, R.; Rousseau, E.; Rossignol, P.; Zannad, F.; Cachofeiro, V.; Lopez-Andres, N. A role for soluble ST2 in vascular remodeling associated with obesity in rats. *PLoS ONE* **2013**, *8*, e79176. [CrossRef]
15. Sanada, S.; Hakuno, D.; Higgins, L.J.; Schreiter, E.R.; McKenzie, A.N.; Lee, R.T. IL-33 and ST2 comprise a critical biomechanically induced and cardioprotective signaling system. *J. Clin. Investig.* **2007**, *117*, 1538–1549. [CrossRef] [PubMed]
16. Gao, Q.; Li, Y.; Li, M. The potential role of IL-33/ST2 signaling in fibrotic diseases. *J. Leukoc. Biol.* **2015**, *98*, 15–22. [CrossRef]

17. Ragusa, R.; Cabiati, M.; Guzzardi, M.A.; D'Amico, A.; Giannessi, D.; Del Ry, S.; Caselli, C. Effects of obesity on IL-33/ST2 system in heart, adipose tissue and liver: Study in the experimental model of Zucker rats. *Exp. Mol. Pathol.* **2017**, *102*, 354–359. [CrossRef]
18. Hu, Z.Q.; Zhao, W.H. The IL-33/ST2 axis is specifically required for development of adipose tissue-resident regulatory T cells. *Cell. Mol. Immunol.* **2015**, *12*, 521. [CrossRef]
19. Han, J.M.; Wu, D.; Denroche, H.C.; Yao, Y.; Verchere, C.B.; Levings, M.K. IL-33 Reverses an Obesity-Induced Deficit in Visceral Adipose Tissue ST2+ T Regulatory Cells and Ameliorates Adipose Tissue Inflammation and Insulin Resistance. *J. Immunol.* **2015**, *194*, 4777–4783. [CrossRef]
20. Xu, Z.; Wang, G.; Zhu, Y.; Liu, R.; Song, J.; Ni, Y.; Sun, H.; Yang, B.; Hou, M.; Chen, L.; et al. PPAR-gamma agonist ameliorates liver pathology accompanied by increasing regulatory B and T cells in high-fat-diet mice. *Obesity (Silver Spring)* **2017**, *25*, 581–590. [CrossRef]
21. Garbern, J.C.; Williams, J.; Kristl, A.C.; Malick, A.; Rachmin, I.; Gaeta, B.; Ahmed, N.; Vujic, A.; Libby, P.; Lee, R.T. Dysregulation of IL-33/ST2 signaling and myocardial periarteriolar fibrosis. *J. Mol. Cell. Cardiol.* **2019**, *128*, 179–186. [CrossRef] [PubMed]
22. Zeyda, M.; Wernly, B.; Demyanets, S.; Kaun, C.; Hammerle, M.; Hantusch, B.; Schranz, M.; Neuhofer, A.; Itariu, B.K.; Keck, M.; et al. Severe obesity increases adipose tissue expression of interleukin-33 and its receptor ST2, both predominantly detectable in endothelial cells of human adipose tissue. *Int. J. Obes.* **2013**, *37*, 658. [CrossRef] [PubMed]
23. Vianello, E.; Dozio, E.; Bandera, F.; Schmitz, G.; Nebuloni, M.; Longhi, E.; Tacchini, L.; Guazzi, M.; Romanelli, M.M.C. Dysfunctional EAT thickness may promote maladaptive heart remodeling in CVD patients through the ST2-IL33 system, directly related to EPAC protein expression. *Sci. Rep.* **2019**, *9*, 1–11. [CrossRef] [PubMed]
24. Lezoualc'h, F.; Fazal, L.; Laudette, M.; Conte, C. Cyclic AMP Sensor EPAC Proteins and Their Role in Cardiovascular Function and Disease. *Circ. Res.* **2016**, *118*, 881–897. [CrossRef]
25. Bisserier, M.; Blondeau, J.P.; Lezoualc'h, F. Epac proteins: Specific ligands and role in cardiac remodelling. *Biochem. Soc. Trans.* **2014**, *42*, 257–264. [CrossRef]
26. Madsen, L.; Kristiansen, K. The importance of dietary modulation of cAMP and insulin signaling in adipose tissue and the development of obesity. *Ann. N. Y. Acad. Sci.* **2010**, *1190*, 1–14. [CrossRef]
27. Xu, H.; Fu, J.L.; Miao, Y.F.; Wang, C.J.; Han, Q.F.; Li, S.; Huang, S.Z.; Du, S.N.; Qiu, Y.X.; Yang, J.C.; et al. Prostaglandin E2 receptor EP3 regulates both adipogenesis and lipolysis in mouse white adipose tissue. *J. Mol. Cell Biol.* **2016**, *8*, 518–529. [CrossRef]
28. Pierre, C.; Guillebaud, F.; Airault, C.; Baril, N.; Barbouche, R.; Save, E.; Gaige, S.; Bariohay, B.; Dallaporta, M.; Troadec, J.D. Invalidation of Microsomal Prostaglandin E Synthase-1 (mPGES-1) Reduces Diet-Induced Low-Grade Inflammation and Adiposity. *Front. Physiol* **2018**, *9*, 1358. [CrossRef]
29. Zhang, A.J.X.; Zhu, H.; Chen, Y.; Li, C.; Li, C.; Chu, H.; Gozali, L.; Lee, A.C.Y.; To, K.K.W.; Hung, I.F.N.; et al. Prostaglandin E2-Mediated Impairment of Innate Immune Response to A(H1N1)pdm09 Infection in Diet-Induced Obese Mice Could Be Restored by Paracetamol. *J. Infect. Dis.* **2019**, *219*, 795–807. [CrossRef]
30. Garcia-Alonso, V.; Titos, E.; Alcaraz-Quiles, J.; Rius, B.; Lopategi, A.; Lopez-Vicario, C.; Jakobsson, P.J.; Delgado, S.; Lozano, J.; Claria, J. Prostaglandin E2 Exerts Multiple Regulatory Actions on Human Obese Adipose Tissue Remodeling, Inflammation, Adaptive Thermogenesis and Lipolysis. *PLoS ONE* **2016**, *11*, e0153751. [CrossRef]
31. Hu, X.; Cifarelli, V.; Sun, S.; Kuda, O.; Abumrad, N.A.; Su, X. Major role of adipocyte prostaglandin E2 in lipolysis-induced macrophage recruitment. *J. Lipid Res.* **2016**, *57*, 663–673. [CrossRef] [PubMed]
32. Chan, P.C.; Liao, M.T.; Hsieh, P.S. The Dualistic Effect of COX-2-Mediated Signaling in Obesity and Insulin Resistance. *Int. J. Mol. Sci.* **2019**, *20*, 3115. [CrossRef] [PubMed]
33. Ceddia, R.P.; Downey, J.D.; Morrison, R.D.; Kraemer, M.P.; Davis, S.E.; Wu, J.; Lindsley, C.W.; Yin, H.; Daniels, J.S.; Breyer, R.M. The effect of the EP3 antagonist DG-041 on male mice with diet-induced obesity. *Prostaglandins Other Lipid Mediat.* **2019**, *144*, 106353. [CrossRef] [PubMed]
34. Schaid, M.D.; Wisinski, J.A.; Kimple, M.E. The EP3 Receptor/Gz Signaling Axis as a Therapeutic Target for Diabetes and Cardiovascular Disease. *AAPS J.* **2017**, *19*, 1276–1283. [CrossRef] [PubMed]
35. Santiago, E.; Martinez, M.P.; Climent, B.; Munoz, M.; Briones, A.M.; Salaices, M.; Garcia-Sacristan, A.; Rivera, L.; Prieto, D. Augmented oxidative stress and preserved vasoconstriction induced by hydrogen peroxide in coronary arteries in obesity: Role of COX-2. *Br. J. Pharmacol.* **2016**, *173*, 3176–3195. [CrossRef]

36. Yasui, M.; Tamura, Y.; Minami, M.; Higuchi, S.; Fujikawa, R.; Ikedo, T.; Nagata, M.; Arai, H.; Murayama, T.; Yokode, M. The Prostaglandin E2 Receptor EP4 Regulates Obesity-Related Inflammation and Insulin Sensitivity. *PLoS ONE* **2015**, *10*, e0136304. [CrossRef]
37. Yu, J.W.; Peng, J.; Zhang, X.Y.; Su, W.; Guan, Y.F. Role of prostaglandin E2 receptor EP4 in the regulation of adipogenesis and adipose metabolism. *Sheng Li Xue Bao* **2019**, *71*, 491–496.
38. Kimple, M.E.; Keller, M.P.; Rabaglia, M.R.; Pasker, R.L.; Neuman, J.C.; Truchan, N.A.; Brar, H.K.; Attie, A.D. Prostaglandin E-2 Receptor, EP3, Is Induced in Diabetic Islets and Negatively Regulates Glucose- and Hormone-Stimulated Insulin Secretion. *Diabetes* **2013**, *62*, 1904–1912. [CrossRef]
39. Samuchiwal, S.K.; Balestrieri, B.; Raff, H.; Boyce, J.A. Endogenous prostaglandin E2 amplifies IL-33 production by macrophages through an E prostanoid (EP)2/EP4-cAMP-EPAC-dependent pathway. *J. Biol. Chem.* **2017**, *292*, 8195–8206. [CrossRef]
40. Dozio, E.; Briganti, S.; Vianello, E.; Dogliotti, G.; Barassi, A.; Malavazos, A.E.; Ermetici, F.; Morricone, L.; Sigruener, A.; Schmitz, G.; et al. Epicardial adipose tissue inflammation is related to vitamin D deficiency in patients affected by coronary artery disease. *Nutr. Metab. Cardiovasc. Dis.* **2015**, *25*, 267–273. [CrossRef]
41. Coisne, A.; Ninni, S.; Ortmans, S.; Davin, L.; Kasprzak, K.; Longere, B.; Seunes, C.; Coppin, A.; Mouton, S.; Ridon, H.; et al. Epicardial fat amount is associated with the magnitude of left ventricular remodeling in aortic stenosis. *Int. J. Cardiovasc. Imaging* **2019**, *35*, 267–273. [CrossRef] [PubMed]
42. Klein, C.; Brunereau, J.; Lacroix, D.; Ninni, S.; Brigadeau, F.; Klug, D.; Longere, B.; Montaigne, D.; Pontana, F.; Coisne, A. Left atrial epicardial adipose tissue radiodensity is associated with electrophysiological properties of atrial myocardium in patients with atrial fibrillation. *Eur. Radiol.* **2019**, *29*, 3027–3035. [CrossRef] [PubMed]
43. Iacobellis, G.; Willens, H.J.; Barbaro, G.; Sharma, A.M. Threshold values of high-risk echocardiographic epicardial fat thickness. *Obesity (Silver Spring)* **2008**, *16*, 887–892. [CrossRef] [PubMed]

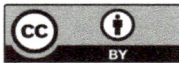

© 2020 by the authors. Licensee MDPI, Basel, Switzerland. This article is an open access article distributed under the terms and conditions of the Creative Commons Attribution (CC BY) license (http://creativecommons.org/licenses/by/4.0/).

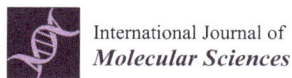

Review
Chemerin Isoforms and Activity in Obesity

Christa Buechler [1,*], Susanne Feder [1], Elisabeth M. Haberl [1] and Charalampos Aslanidis [2]

1. Department of Internal Medicine I, Regensburg University Hospital, 93053 Regensburg, Germany; susanne.feder@klinik.uni-regensburg.de (S.F.); haberl.elisabeth@gmx.de (E.M.H.)
2. Institute of Clinical Chemistry and Laboratory Medicine, Regensburg University Hospital, 93053 Regensburg, Germany; charalampos.aslanidis@klinik.uni-regensburg.de
* Correspondence: christa.buechler@klinik.uni-regensburg.de; Tel.: +49-941-944-7009

Received: 29 January 2019; Accepted: 28 February 2019; Published: 5 March 2019

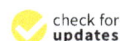

Abstract: Overweight and adiposity are risk factors for several diseases, like type 2 diabetes and cancer. White adipose tissue is a major source for adipokines, comprising a diverse group of proteins exerting various functions. Chemerin is one of these proteins whose systemic levels are increased in obesity. Chemerin is involved in different physiological and pathophysiological processes and it regulates adipogenesis, insulin sensitivity, and immune response, suggesting a vital role in metabolic health. The majority of serum chemerin is biologically inert. Different proteases are involved in the C-terminal processing of chemerin and generate diverse isoforms that vary in their activity. Distribution of chemerin variants was analyzed in adipose tissues and plasma of lean and obese humans and mice. The Tango bioassay, which is suitable to monitor the activation of the beta-arrestin 2 pathway, was used to determine the ex-vivo activation of chemerin receptors by systemic chemerin. Further, the expression of the chemerin receptors was analyzed in adipose tissue, liver, and skeletal muscle. Present investigations assume that increased systemic chemerin in human obesity is not accompanied by higher biologic activity. More research is needed to fully understand the pathways that control chemerin processing and chemerin signaling.

Keywords: proteolysis; Tango bioassay; biologic activity; chemerin receptors

---

1. Introduction

The protein chemerin is a chemoattractant for immune cells and it plays a role in adaptive and innate immunity [1,2]. Chemerin is also an adipokine that regulates angiogenesis, adipogenesis, and energy metabolism, which demonstrates a multifaceted function of this protein [3–6] (Figure 1). Positive correlations of systemic chemerin with obesity related phenotypes, such as insulin resistance, body mass index (BMI), and serum triglycerides, suggest a function of this adipokine in metabolic diseases [2]. Chemerin deficient mice had higher hepatic gluconeogenesis and increased skeletal muscle glucose uptake. In the null mice, the phosphorylation of protein kinase B (Akt) was improved in the muscle upon insulin injection. Of note, glucose stimulated insulin release of pancreatic beta-cells was impaired in the knock-out animals. Fat pad weight was not changed in the null mice, and serum leptin and adiponectin levels were also normal. Interestingly, there were less detectable adipose tissue macrophages. Although this suggests improved insulin sensitivity, insulin induced Akt phosphorylation was reduced in the fat tissue [7]. A separate study describes that the injection of recombinant chemerin reduced serum insulin and tissue glucose uptake in the obese mice but had no effect in the normal-weight animals [8]. In low density lipoprotein (LDL) receptor deficient mice, the overexpression of chemerin was found to induce insulin resistance in muscle, but not the liver or gonadal fat. There were no changes in body weight, levels of serum lipids, and severity of atherosclerosis [9].

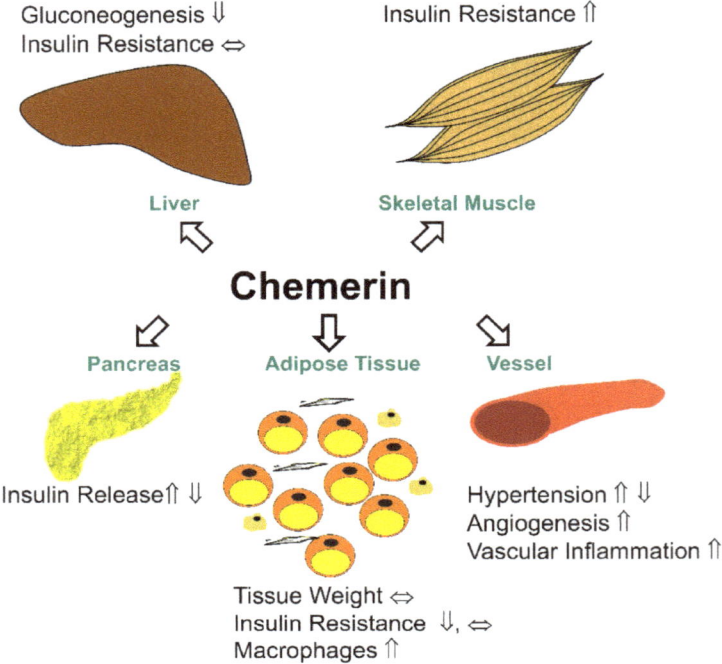

Figure 1. Effect of chemerin on the metabolic status of different organs (inconclusive results indicated by reverse arrows). Data published so far mostly agree that chemerin impairs skeletal muscle insulin response. This was not observed in the liver, here gluconeogenesis was enhanced in chemerin deficient mice. The function of chemerin on blood pressure was modified by gender. Chemerin further stimulated angiogenesis and vascular inflammation. Adipose tissue weight was not changed by chemerin. This adipokine may even improve insulin response of fat tissue although the number of adipose tissue resident macrophages was increased. Stimulatory and inhibitory effects of chemerin on glucose-induced release of insulin by pancreatic beta-cells was reported. Inconclusive findings may be partly explained by the different models studied.

Chemerin-stimulated angiogenesis was illustrated in-vitro and in-vivo [10]. Enhanced angiogenesis and increased endothelial-monocyte adhesion upon chemerin incubation indicate a proatherogenic role of this adipokine [11] (Figure 1).

Data on the role of chemerin in metabolic disease are not conclusive so far (Figure 1). Chemerin most likely impairs skeletal muscle insulin sensitivity, although it seems to have a modulatory role in the liver and adipose tissues. The overexpression of chemerin was shown to increase glucose induced insulin secretion, whereas the injection of recombinant protein blocked this process in the pancreatic beta-cell of mice [7,8].

Duration of chemerin signaling, the concentration of chemerin, cell type/tissue analyzed, chemerin processing, and chemerin receptor expression may vary in the different experiments. Pathological characteristics of the murine models used may further modify chemerin signaling [2].

The G protein-coupled receptor chemokine-like receptor 1 (CMKLR1) is one of the two described chemerin receptors with signaling activity so far. The second one is G protein-coupled receptor 1 (GPR1) [6,12,13]. Chemokine receptor-like 2 (CCRL2) is an atypical chemokine receptor that does most likely not exert any signaling activities [6,12,13]. CCRL2 is supposed to present chemerin to CMKLR1 and possibly to GPR1 [14]. Chemerin binds with low nanomolar affinity to all of these receptors [15]. The binding of chemerin to CMKLR1 activated the three Gαi subtypes and the two

Gαo isoforms. Chemerin stimulated the rise of intracellular calcium and the decline of cyclic AMP in CMKLR1 expressing CHO cells that are dependent on Gαi signaling [13]. None of the G-proteins were activated upon binding of chemerin to GPR1 or CCRL2 [15]. Nevertheless, the recruitment of beta-arrestin 1 and 2 was observed for both signaling competent receptors [15]. Chemerin further uses the RhoA and Rho-associated protein kinase-dependent pathway downstream of GPR1 and CMKLR1 to activate the transcriptional regulator serum-response factor [16].

Extracellular regulated kinase (ERK) 1/2 was phosphorylated upon chemerin treatment in various cells, including endothelial cells, adipocytes, and skeletal muscle cells. The activation of ERK1/2 at low, but not high chemerin concentration, was described in adipocytes [4,17,18]. Chemerin further activated p38 mitogen-activated protein kinase, Akt and phosphoinositide 3-kinase [2,19]. Short-time incubation with chemerin was shown to activate Akt in hepatocytes, whereas prolonged treatment up to two hours led to a decline of phosphorylated Akt in these cells [20]. Notably, one study reports that chemerin binding weakened the association of phosphatase and tensin homolog (PTEN) with CMKLR1. This enhanced the activity of PTEN and subsequently led to decreased Akt phosphorylation [20]. The activation of the protein kinase C by chemerin stimulated the internalization of CMKLR1. Blockage of this pathway enhanced calcium flux and ERK phosphorylation, showing that this mechanism terminates signaling via desensitization [21]. The nuclear factor kappa B (NFkB) pathway is activated by chemerin in skeletal muscles cells [18]. In adipocytes, the inhibition of chemerin signaling increased NFkB activity [22]. Chemerin thus activates various signaling pathways and the effects depend on incubation time and dose.

As an adipokine chemerin is released by adipocytes [23], but also hepatocytes produce considerable levels of the protein [24]. Serum chemerin is increased in overweight/obesity and correlations with obesity associated traits, like low grade inflammation, blood pressure, and insulin resistance, were identified in some but not all of the patient cohorts studied [1,25–30]. Hence, the associations of systemic chemerin levels with the metabolic syndrome are not fully resolved [1,25–30]. The serum chemerin levels are heritable with about 16% to 25% of variations being attributed to genetic factors. Polymorphisms in the gene encoding chemerin (retinoic acid receptor responder 2, *RARRES2*) were linked to increased systemic chemerin levels, visceral fat mass, and a higher incidence of the metabolic syndrome [31–34].

Positive correlations of systemic chemerin with inflammatory cytokines and C-reactive protein were described in chronic inflammatory diseases [35–37]. Chemerin has a role in the pathophysiology of rheumatoid arthritis, inflammatory bowel disease, psoriasis, and chronic renal disease [35–37]. More recent findings indicate a function of chemerin in cancer, and the pro- as well as anti-carcinogenic effects have been identified [38]. It was shown that chemerin suppressed hepatocellular carcinoma growth but enhanced squamous cell carcinoma migration [39,40].

Whether chemerin is a pro- or anti-inflammatory protein is still debated. Discordant results were obtained in cell culture studies and animal models [5,12]. Murine (m) Chem156, which is a highly active chemerin isoform, antagonized the activation of peritoneal macrophages that were triggered by lipopolysaccharide (LPS) or interferon gamma [41]. Anti-inflammatory effects of mChem156 were also described in a mouse model of acute lung inflammation induced by LPS [42]. In a colitis model, mChem156 aggravated inflammation and suppressed M2 polarization of macrophages [43].

Chemerin is secreted as an inactive precursor and it is activated through C-terminal processing by proteases. Thereby, different isoforms are generated, which have varying biological effects [5,12]. Chemerin derived C-terminal peptide chemerin 15 acted via CMKLR1 and suppressed inflammation [41]. The effects were already obvious at picomolar concentrations of the peptide demonstrating its potent activity [41].

This review article briefly describes the various C-terminal processing forms of chemerin. The expression of chemerin and its receptors, the distribution of chemerin isoforms, and analysis of chemerin bioactivity in obesity will be addressed in detail.

2. Expression of Chemerin and its Receptors in Different Tissues

2.1. Chemerin Expression in Adipose Tissues

Chemerin is most abundantly expressed in white adipose tissues, in the liver, and to a lesser extent in brown adipose tissue, the lung, skeletal muscles, the kidney, ovary, and the heart [2,25]. Serum chemerin levels are increased in obesity as a result of enhanced synthesis in fat tissues and possibly the liver [2]. The explants of adipose tissues from obese donors indeed released higher chemerin protein amounts than fat tissues that were obtained from lean individuals [18].

2.1.1. Expression of Chemerin in Human Tissues

Chemerin mRNA expression in subcutaneous and omental adipose tissues of patients was higher in obesity, and it decreased upon bariatric surgery evoked weight loss. Serum chemerin levels changed accordingly, indicating that adipose tissue is the main site controlling circulating protein levels in obesity [44]. The inflammatory factors tumor necrosis factor (TNF) and LPS enhanced chemerin production in adipocyte, thus demonstrating a close association between adipose tissue inflammation and chemerin synthesis [45–47]. Higher chemerin mRNA expression in visceral fat in obesity was related to the degree of inflammation, thereby confirming this relationship [46].

Another study described a negative correlation of chemerin mRNA levels in subcutaneous fat with circulating chemerin protein [48]. In obese patients with non-alcoholic fatty liver disease, neither subcutaneous nor visceral fat chemerin mRNA expression was associated with its systemic levels [49]. Studies so far mostly suppose that systemic chemerin concentrations are defined by its production in adipocytes. Whether this is regulated by transcriptional and/or posttranscriptional mechanisms has not been studied in detail.

2.1.2. Expression of Chemerin in Experimental Models

Whether chemerin expression is upregulated in obese adipose tissues was also analyzed in rodent models. In mesenteric fat of *Psammomys obesus*, a rodent animal model of obesity, chemerin mRNA expression was induced [25]. Female mice that were fed an atherogenic diet for eight weeks had increased chemerin protein in subcutaneous and visceral fat, and higher systemic chemerin levels than animals fed the control chow [45]. In epididymal fat of leptin deficient ob/ob and leptin receptor activity deficient db/db mice, such an induction was not observed when chemerin mRNA expression was measured [8]. In the db/db mice chemerin protein was two-fold higher when compared to the lean animals [8]. Chemerin protein was also strongly increased in the gonadal adipose tissue of male ob/ob mice. Injection of 0.5 µg leptin per gram body weight reduced chemerin protein levels in the white fat depot [50]. This indicates that leptin resistance, which accounts for metabolic disease in obese patients, may contribute to elevated chemerin protein [50,51]. In male rats that were fed a high fat diet for 12 weeks, gonadal adipose tissue chemerin protein levels were nevertheless similar to the respective controls [50].

Thus, studies in rodents mostly identified higher chemerin protein levels in obese adipose tissues. Chemerin mRNA and protein expression were analyzed in lean and obese fat and they were not concordantly regulated. Therefore, posttranscriptional processes seem to control cellular and eventually soluble chemerin protein levels.

2.2. Chemerin Receptor Expression in Adipose Tissues

The knock-down of chemerin or CMKLR1 in 3T3-L1 adipocyte cell line impaired adipogenesis. Further, these cells showed reduced expression of genes that are involved in glucose and lipid homeostasis [4]. Thus, chemerin–CMKLR1 signaling may enhance adipogenesis in obesity to allow for the storage of surplus lipids. However, when compared to studies measuring chemerin in obesity (see 2.1.), the expression of the respective receptors has been analyzed in less detail.

2.2.1. Expression of Chemerin Receptors in Human Tissues

One study showed that CMKLR1 expression was upregulated in visceral fat of obese patients. TNF induced chemerin in human adipocytes but it had no effect on CMKLR1 mRNA [18,46]. LPS was a strong inductor of chemerin in murine 3T3-L1 adipocytes, but it did not change the CMKLR1 protein [45]. This argues against a co-regulation of chemerin and CMKLR1 expression in adipocytes by inflammatory mediators that contribute to insulin resistance and metabolic disease in obesity [52,53]. CMKLR1 is expressed by macrophages and its induction in obese fat tissues may be related to the increased number of adipose tissue resident macrophages [54].

2.2.2. Expression of Chemerin Receptors in Experimental Models

An experimental model where female mice were fed an atherogenic diet for eight weeks showed higher CMKLR1 protein in subcutaneous and visceral fat [45]. In mesenteric adipose tissue of *Psammomys obesus*, CMKLR1 expression was also induced in obesity. This upregulation was, however, only seen in the fed state [25]. In epididymal adipose tissue of the ob/ob mice CMKLR1 protein levels were about five-fold higher when compared to lean wild type animals. The injection of 0.5 µg leptin per gram body weight reduced CMKLR1 protein level in this white fat depot [50]. An effect of leptin on CMKLR1 gene expression was, however, not observed in bovine adipocytes [55].

In contrast to the studies suggesting higher CMKLR1 in obese adipose tissue, further analysis in rats showed that the CMKLR1 protein was strongly reduced in the gonadal fat of male animals that were fed a high fat diet for 12 weeks [50]. CMKLR1 mRNA expression was also low in the epididymal fat of ob/ob and db/db mice [8].

Yet, whether CMKLR1 protein is indeed increased in obese fat tissue awaits clarification by additional studies. Adipocytes and stromal-vascular cells in adipose tissue express CMKLR1 [25,45], and immunohistochemical approaches have to identify the cell type specific regulation of CMKLR1 in obesity.

Adipose tissue GPR1 is primarily expressed in stromal-vascular cells [56]. Yet, the individual cells that present this receptor have not been described in detail. GPR1 mRNA was unchanged in gonadal fat of ob/ob and db/db mice when compared to lean animals [8]. GPR1 mRNA was also comparably abundant in epididymal fat of mice that were fed a control chow or a high fat diet [56]. The GPR1 protein has to be analyzed in future studies to confirm that GPR1 protein levels are indeed unchanged in obese adipose tissues.

To our knowledge, only one article regarding CCRL2 levels was published, showing that CCRL2 mRNA was significantly induced in the fat of db/db animals and tended to be higher in the leptin deficient mice [8].

2.3. Chemerin in the Liver

Chemerin and its receptors are expressed in the liver, but a detailed role of chemerin in hepatic function and metabolic liver diseases has not yet been explored [3]. Adeno-associated virus mediated overexpression of human chemerin in the liver of the LDL receptor knock-out mouse model led to increased systemic chemerin. This illustrates that hepatic chemerin synthesis may presumably contribute to its systemic levels. Chemerin surplus in these mice was associated with impaired insulin signaling in skeletal muscle, but not in the liver (Figure 1) [9]. Various hepatoprotective effects of recombinant mChem156 were identified in murine hepatocellular carcinoma models, but whether this isoform exists in the liver is still ambiguous [20,40].

2.3.1. Expression of Chemerin in Human Tissue

Human studies that have been published so far describe normal, lower, and higher chemerin mRNA expression in the liver. Doecke et al. analyzed chemerin mRNA in controls and patients with non-alcoholic fatty liver disease and described higher hepatic levels in the overweight [57]. In morbidly obese patients, hepatic chemerin mRNA showed a trend to be induced in those probands with a BMI > 40 kg/m^2 [58]. In a separate human study, such an association of hepatic chemerin mRNA levels with BMI was not reported [59]. Another investigation even showed reduced hepatic chemerin mRNA expression in obesity [60].

2.3.2. Expression of Chemerin in Experimental Models and in vitro Systems

In the db/db mice, hepatic chemerin mRNA, but not protein, was induced [8]. Similarly, chemerin mRNA was higher in the liver of mice that were fed a high fat diet, whereas cellular chemerin protein was not concomitantly upregulated [24]. Whether the hepatic release of chemerin protein in obesity is enhanced needs to be further analyzed. Leptin deficient ob/ob mice develop severe liver steatosis, whereas the hepatic chemerin mRNA and protein were not changed [8]. Separate investigations even report reduced hepatic chemerin levels in murine obesity [60].

Inflammatory cytokines, like TNF and LPS, are elevated in obesity and upregulated adipocyte chemerin [18,45,47]. These factors did not change chemerin expression in hepatocytes [24,47,57]. Leptin did not induce human hepatocyte chemerin levels [24].

Current data show that obesity is not necessarily associated with altered hepatic chemerin levels. For which reasons the different research groups identified normal, higher, and lower chemerin expression in the liver of overweight humans and mice is still an open question.

2.4. Chemerin Receptors in the Liver

Analysis of CMKLR1, CCRL2, and GPR1 in the liver of ob/ob and db/db mice revealed that only GPR1 mRNA was strongly decreased [8]. In mice that were fed a high fat diet hepatic CMKLR1 mRNA was found to be reduced [61]. Human studies described a positive or no association of hepatic CMKLR1 levels with BMI [57,62]. The CCRL2 mRNA levels were not different in normal-weight and overweight patients [63].

While CMKLR1 mRNA was found to be expressed in various liver cells, including hepatocytes, hepatic stellate cells, endothelial cells, and Kupffer cells, CCRL2 seems not to be expressed in hepatocytes [61,63]. The downregulation of CMKLR1 in Kupffer cells by a phosphatidyl inositol 3-kinase inhibitor improved hepatic insulin resistance and inflammation, suggesting that the chemerin–CMKLR1 signaling pathway contributes to metabolic disease in obesity by modulating the function of these immune cells [64]. Here, it has to be considered that resolvin E1 is a further ligand of CMKLR1, which is well described to have a function in the resolution of inflammation [65].

2.5. Chemerin and its Receptors in Skeletal Muscle

Analysis of chemerin, CMKLR1, CCRL2, and GPR1 in skeletal muscle of ob/ob and db/db mice revealed that CMKLR1 mRNA was strongly increased in both of the strains. Chemerin was only upregulated in the muscle of db/db mice [8]. GPR1 mRNA was markedly reduced in soleus muscle but not in the gastrocnemius muscle of mice that were fed a high fat diet [56].

Although chemerin induces skeletal muscle insulin resistance [18] (Figure 1), the expression of the corresponding receptors in muscle was not studied in detail. Analysis of chemerin and its receptors in skeletal muscle tissues of rodents and humans is needed to further understand the role of this adipokine in skeletal muscle insulin resistance.

3. Chemerin Isoforms and Activity in Adipose Tissue and Serum

3.1. C-terminal Processing and Activity of Chemerin Isoforms

The open reading frame of the human chemerin gene codes for a 163 amino acid protein. The secreted form is shorter by 20 amino acids due to the removal of the N-terminal signal peptide [2]. N-terminally cleaved chemerin with an intact C-terminus is traditionally named hChem163, although it only consists of 143 amino acids [19]. The number in the abbreviation thus corresponds to the respective amino acid position of the full-length protein. The analogous murine chemerin protein is one amino acid shorter and it is designated as mChem162. Human and murine chemerins are 64% identical with a similarity of 78% [6,66].

HChem163 and mChem162 need to be processed at their C-termini to become active proteins. Proteolytic cleavage by extracellular proteases at distinct C-terminal sites generates highly active, high active, moderate active, and inactive isoforms [2,66] (Figure 2). The similarity between human and murine chemerin suggests that protease cleavage sites are conserved between these two species [66]. Chemerin isoform bioactivity was mostly determined by chemotaxis assays and/or the analysis of intracellular calcium release. These assays revealed that hChem157 had the highest activity [2,13,67]. Analysis was undertaken with primary monocyte-derived dendritic cells and murine pre-B lymphoma L1.2 cells overexpressing human CMKLR1 [13,67].

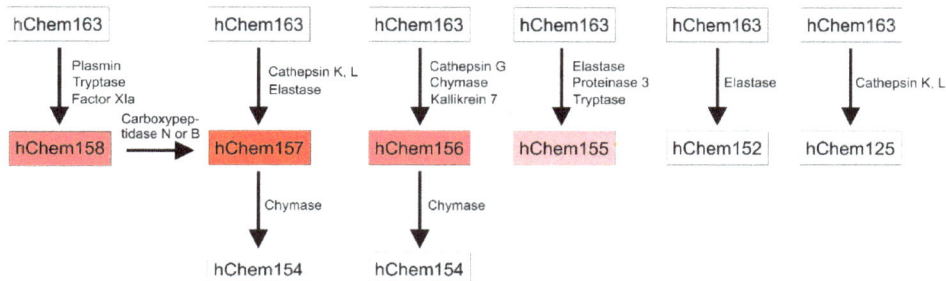

Figure 2. Processing of human chemerin. The proteases contributing to C-terminal processing of chemerin and the respective isoforms generated are shown. Inactive isoforms are in grey boxes, biologic active isoforms in red boxes. The intensity of the red color corresponds to the activity of the chemerin isoform (intense red: very active isoform). Activity has been mostly analyzed using Ca^{2+} flux and migration assays in chemokine-like receptor 1 (CMKLR1) expressing cells. Angiotensin converting enzyme converts hChem154 to hChem152. This is not shown in the figure. HChem154 is produced by different proteases and the enzymes upstream of angiotensin converting enzyme have not been identified yet.

HChem157 is produced by cathepsin K and L, and human leukocyte elastase cleavage of hChem163 [67,68] (Figure 2). HChem156 was as active as hChem157 when it was analyzed in a signal transduction assay using cells with CMKLR1 overexpression [69]. The analysis of Ca^{2+} mobilization using L1.2 cells stably expressing human CMKLR1 revealed that the shorter isoform was by far less active than hChem157 [70]. HChem156 originates from hChem163 by cathepsin G and chymase cleavage [70,71] (Figure 2). The serine protease kallikrein 7 also produced hChem156 from prochemerin, and it may contribute to chemerin activation in the skin [69]. HChem158 and hChem155 are low active isoforms. HChem158 was produced by plasmin, tryptase, and factor XIa cleavage [67,72] (Figure 2). HChem155 derives from hChem163 by elastase, proteinase 3, or tryptase mediated proteolysis [67,71]. Elastase, cathepsin K and L, and chymase also contribute to chemerin inactivation by further C-terminal processing [67,68,71] (Figure 2).

Angiotensin converting enzyme is a carboxypeptidase and it removes C-terminal dipeptidyl residues amongst others from angiotensin I to obtain the vasoconstrictor angiotensin II [73], thereby controlling blood pressure. This enzyme was shown to produce hChem152 from hChem154 [74]. Chemerin affects several pathways that control blood pressure, indicating a function of this adipokine herein [17,75] (Figure 1). Of note, systemic chemerin was increased in patients with hypertension indicating that this adipokines may increase blood pressure [76,77]. Surprisingly, hypertensive male rats with knock-out of chemerin had elevated mean and systolic blood pressure. In female rats, chemerin deficiency was associated with lower pressures, as one would have expected [78]. A second study using male rats observed decreased arterial blood pressure upon chemerin knock-down [79]. These studies show that chemerin has a causative function in blood pressure control, which is modified by gender. Analysis of chemerin isoform distribution in females and males and normo- and hypertensive patients may clarify the role of angiotensin converting enzyme mediated proteolysis of chemerin herein. Murine mChem156, which is a highly active isoform, increased blood pressure in male mice [75]. Whether this isoform is present in hypertension in biologically relevant concentrations needs to be elucidated.

Proteolytic cleavage sites for human chemerin, which are described above, are conserved in mice [66]. Here, mChem156 and mChem155 had nearly similar activities in Ca^{2+} mobilization and chemotaxis assays. A 15- to 20-fold lower potency was measured for mChem161 and mChem157 [66]. The authors of this paper failed to express recombinant mChem162, and mChem161 was detectable in the supernatants of the transfected cells. It was suggested that mChem161 had similar properties to mChem162. MChem154 did neither have chemoattractant properties nor did it induce Ca^{2+} release [66].

Activities of the various chemerin isoforms may deviate from the activity ranking that is described above in men and mice when biologic effects other than chemotaxis and Ca^{2+} influx are tested. For analysis of chemerin isoform activity, mostly cells with CMKLR1 overexpression were used [66,71]. These results may differ from chemerin induced GPR1 signaling that has been studied in less detail. Which of the receptors is more relevant for the biological and pathophysiological effects of chemerin is mostly unknown.

Processing of chemerin by various proteases produces different isoforms that differ in their activity. Short variants are mostly inactive and they may even antagonize the active isoforms [80]. This demonstrates that a complex regulatory network controls chemerin bioactivity. The analysis of total chemerin protein levels cannot provide appropriate information regarding its biologic activity.

There was even discrepancy when measuring total chemerin protein with a pan-chemerin ELISA or isoform specific ELISAs. The EC_{50} values (the concentration of antibodies showing half-maximal binding) of the human pan-chemerin ELISA were lower for hChem163, hChem158, and hChem155 when compared to hChem157. Thus, the analysis of samples with a low level of Chem157 using this pan-chemerin assay will underestimate the actual chemerin concentration [81]. EC_{50} values for the different murine chemerin isoforms vary by up to two-fold when using a commercial pan-chemerin ELISA kit. Using this assay to measure total chemerin will give too high values in samples that contain mChem155 and mChem154, and too low values when mChem162 and mChem157 are the abundant variants [66].

Chemerin isoforms in body fluids, cell supernatants, and tissues can be exactly defined by liquid chromatography/mass spectroscopy [81]. Isoform specific chemerin ELISAs have been established and they were used for the quantification of the individual human and murine variants [66,81]. The so-called Tango bioassay was developed to determine G protein-coupled receptor ligand induced beta-arrestin 2 recruitment [82] and it was applied to measure chemerin bioactivity in cell culture supernatants and plasma [47,83,84].

3.2. Quantification of Chemerin Activity with the Tango Bioassay

The Tango bioassay can quantitatively measure CMKLR1 and GPR1 beta-arrestin 2 activation [47]. In this analysis, human embryonic kidney (HEK) 293T cells that constitutively express a tobacco etch virus (TEV) protease fused to beta-arrestin 2 are used. Furthermore, these cells encode a reporter gene whose expression is induced by a transcriptional-transactivator (tTA). To test for the bioactivity of chemerin, the HEK293T cells are transfected with a plasmid encoding either CMKLR1 or GPR1. The C-terminus of these receptors carries a TEV N1a protease cleavage site and the tTA. Chemerin induces the recruitment of the beta-arrestin 2–protease fusion protein to GPR1-tTA or CMKLR1-tTA. The protease cleaves the TEV N1a site and it releases tTA, which passes into the nucleus. Here, tTA enhances the transcription of the respective reporter gene. By using appropriate standards, the biological activity of chemerin in different samples can be quantitatively determined. One has to keep in mind that only the beta-arrestin 2 dependent pathways are analyzed by these activity assays.

The human CMKLR1 based Tango bioassay revealed that murine chemerin activated this receptor. CMKLR1 activation was confirmed in murine adipocyte and hepatocyte conditioned media, demonstrating that both cell types produce bioactive chemerin [47]. TNF induced total chemerin protein in 3T3-L1 adipocytes and chemerin bioactivity in the supernatants was accordingly increased [47]. Mice that were injected with TNF had higher serum chemerin, which had a higher potency to activate CMKLR1 [47]. Therefore, the inflammatory cytokine TNF enhances chemerin production and concentrations of bioactive chemerin isoforms.

TNF is increased in obesity and it contributes to insulin resistance [85]. One may assume that low grade chronic inflammation in obesity may activate chemerin, which subsequently impairs skeletal muscle insulin resistance. However, recent research that is summarized in the next paragraphs did not report on higher chemerin activity in obesity.

3.3. Ex-vivo Analyzed Systemic Chemerin Activity in Human and Murine Obesity

Among the most widely used rodent models in obesity and type 2 diabetes research are the ob/ob mice and the db/db mice [86]. In both strains, the total serum chemerin protein and ex-vivo activation of CMKLR1 were about two-fold higher than in C57BL/6 controls [8]. A second study did not find higher CMKLR1 activity in the ob/ob mice [83]. The ob/ob mice in both of the studies were about three months old [8,83], excluding that different age contributed to this discordant findings. GPR1 activation was measured in the second study and it was found to rise in parallel to the total chemerin protein [83]. In mice that were fed a high fat diet for 14 weeks, CMKLR1 and GPR1 activities were induced. The ratio of bioactive chemerin to total chemerin was higher in the overweight animals with respect to CMKLR1 activation. This effect was not identified with regard to GPR1 activity [83]. This indicates that these receptors may vary in their affinity for distinct chemerin isoforms.

These experiments clearly show that chemerin bioactivity does not always correspond to total systemic chemerin protein levels, at least when measuring chemerin-induced beta-arrestin 2 recruitment [8,83].

To our knowledge, CMKLR1 activation was measured in only one study in human obesity. Here, the total circulating chemerin protein was detected by a pan-chemerin ELISA and ex-vivo CMKLR1 activity was determined with the beta-arrestin 2 Tango bioassay [84]. Obese females had higher total serum chemerin and unchanged CMKLR1 activation when compared to normal-weight women. Thus, the ratio of bioactive to total chemerin levels was significantly reduced in the obese [84]. This even reflects impaired chemerin activity, despite higher total systemic chemerin protein.

In this study, circulating chemerin protein and CMKLR1 activation were also investigated in the postprandial phase. Chemerin levels and ex-vivo CMKLR1 activation were similar in the fasted and the postprandial state [84]. This is in line with a previous analysis in a cohort of healthy individuals, where serum chemerin was similar in the fasted state, 1 h and 2 h after oral glucose uptake [87]. Impaired postprandial glucose and lipid clearance contribute to metabolic disease in obesity [88]. Current data principally argue against a function of chemerin herein.

3.4. Chemerin Isoforms in Serum

In human plasma, inactive, full-length chemerin (hChem163) was by far the most abundant form [81]. HChem157 was about 25-fold and hChem155 about 300-fold less present (Figure 3). The plasma levels of hChem157 were below the EC_{50} of about 1.2 +/- 0.7 nm, which was determined in the calcium mobilization assay using CMKLR1 expressing cells [80,81]. Type of diet, gender, and age were not associated with changes in chemerin isoform distribution, which was relatively invariable in lean volunteers during three years of follow up [81]. Systemic chemerin may thus reflect a reservoir of biologically inactive prochemerin that can be very quickly activated upon request.

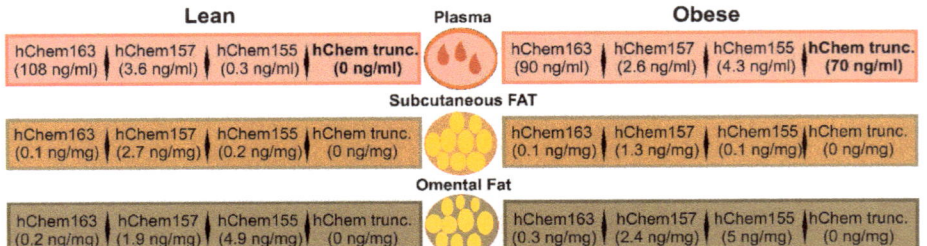

Figure 3. Chemerin isoform distribution in human obesity. The different chemerin isoforms identified in human plasma, subcutaneous and omental adipose tissues are shown. The concentrations analyzed by chemerin isoform-specific ELISAs in the tissues are given as ng chemerin/mg adipose tissue. Truncated (trunc.) isoforms are relatively short and they are most likely not biologically active. Comparison of the chemerin levels in the lean and the obese probands revealed that only the truncated forms in plasma are significantly induced in the latter.

Total chemerin protein that was analyzed by an ELISA supposed to measure all isoforms was higher in the overweight and the obese. The concentration of the chemerin isoforms hChem163, hChem157, and hChem155 was, however, not markedly changed in the overweight individuals or in obesity (Figure 3). So-called unattributed chemerin variants appeared in the plasma of the overweight and the obese. These chemerin forms were detected by commercially available chemerin ELISAs, but not by ELISAs that were designed to specifically measure hChem163, hChem157, or hChem155. These short variants had relatively large C-terminal truncations and hChem144 was significantly induced in the plasma of the obese [81]. The truncated chemerin variants were most likely biologically inactive, demonstrating that higher chemerin protein in obesity was not linked to increased chemerin bioactivity. Positive correlation of unattributed, truncated chemerin levels and elastase in blood suggests that this enzyme may participate in chemerin processing and inactivation. Because truncated forms of chemerin were not present in adipose tissues, proteolysis has to occur in the extracellular space and/or in blood [81].

In mice that were fed a high fat diet for 26 weeks (starting with six week old animals), the total plasma chemerin was increased and this was attributed to higher levels of inactive mChem162. Of note, 12 weeks high fat diet feeding raised mChem157 and mChem156 in plasma, and here, these two isoforms represented about 55% of systemic chemerin. Indeed, the levels of mChem157 and mChem156 were highest in the 12 week high fat diet fed mice when compared to animals that were fed a low fat diet for 12 or 26 weeks and the mice fed a high fat diet for 26 weeks. The authors of this work suggested that production of the highly active chemerin form coincides with the time of early adipogenesis that is promoted by chemerin [4,66]. The biologically modest-active mChem157 may be the source for mChem156 production, a hypothesis that has to be proven in future studies [66]. The levels of the isoforms mChem157 and mChem156 were similar in mice that were fed a low or a high fat diet for 26 weeks. MChem155 and mChem154 isoforms were not significantly different in the lean and the obese mice and when analyzed 12 or 26 weeks after starting the experiments [66]. ELISA only detected mChem154 at low levels in the older animals, while in the younger mice this isoform was not measured at all. MChem155, which was as active as mChem156, accounted for about 6.4–7.7% of total plasma chemerin, irrespective of age and diet [66].

The total chemerin protein levels and mChem162 were higher in the older mice, irrespective of the diet, while further isoforms were unchanged, showing that the aging of mice is associated with elevated levels of biologically inactive plasma chemerin [66].

3.5. Chemerin Isoforms in Adipose Tissues

Serum chemerin is supposed to be mainly derived from adipose tissues [1,2,8,47]. Unexpectedly, an analysis of chemerin isoforms in human subcutaneous and omental fat revealed that hChem163, which is the most prominent chemerin protein in the circulation, was not the dominant form in these tissues [81]. Indeed, in human subcutaneous adipose tissue, hChem157 represented about 90% of the three isoforms analyzed, which were hChem155, hChem157, and hChem163. In omental fat, about 80% of the chemerin isoforms was hChem155, while about 20% was hChem157 (Figure 3). HChem163 constituted approximately 1–2% of total omental fat chemerin protein [81] (Figure 3). The levels of the active hChem157 isoform in the fat depots were 1,000-fold higher than in plasma and by far sufficient to induce calcium mobilization in CMKLR1 expressing cells [80,81]. The total chemerin protein was more abundant in the omental fat depot, but it was unchanged in both adipose tissue depots in obesity. Truncated chemerin isoforms that were detected in plasma of the obese did not exist in the fat tissues [81] (Figure 3).

In murine epididymal adipose tissue of 18 week old mice, mChem155 was the predominant form, representing nearly 100% of total chemerin protein. This was completely changed when analyzing this fat depot 14 weeks later. Here, 85–91% was mChem162, approximately 5 to 10% was mChem154, while mChem155 was about 1–2%. MChem157 and mChem156 were not detected in the adipose tissues of the mice. High fat diet feeding for 12 or 26 weeks did neither affect total chemerin protein nor chemerin isoform distribution [66]. In this animal model, mChem155, but not mChem156, was the active chemerin isoform in the intraabdominal fat depot [66]. Chymase positive mast cells are localized in adipose tissues and this protease may generate mChem155 from prochemerin [70,89].

In the older mice, total chemerin protein in epididymal fat even declined in obesity, and it was negatively correlated with body weight, amount of fat, and plasma total chemerin protein [66]. Adipocytes differentiated from murine primary mesenchymal stem cells secreted chemerin and mChem152, -156, -158, -159, -160, -161, and -162 were detected in the supernatants [22]. Chemerin isoform abundance was, therefore, completely different in murine epididymal fat tissue and in-vitro differentiated murine adipocytes. This indicates that proteases that were produced by stromal-vascular cells contribute to chemerin processing in the fat depots.

Brown adipose tissue expressed about 15-fold lower levels of total chemerin protein when compared to epididymal fat of mice. While high fat diet feeding for 12 weeks did not change chemerin protein, it was induced in obesity when this diet was given 14 weeks longer [66].

Chemerin isoform distribution in adipose tissue was completely different from the variants that were found in the circulation. Prochemerin was released into the circulation, while further processed chemerin was present in fat tissues. Isoform distribution was not changed in obesity in mice and men. In murine fat tissue chemerin isoforms abundance was mostly affected by age and this may be related to the phase of life with increased adipogenesis [66,81].

4. Conclusions

Chemerin's importance in physiological and pathophysiological processes has been illustrated in numerous clinical and experimental studies. The role of chemerin is, however, incompletely understood. Systemic chemerin is increased in obese mice and humans, while its bioactivity is not concordantly changed. The signal transduction pathways and the physiologic function of GPR1 are mostly unstudied. The biologic activity of the chemerin isoforms binding to this receptor has not been characterized in detail. Chemerin processing seems to be changed in obesity. The respective proteases that are involved herein are still not defined. Synthetic chemerin-derived peptides that resemble the C-terminal amino acids of this adipokine reduce inflammation and enhance phagocytosis [41,90], and they may be used as therapeutic agents for the treatment of metabolic diseases and possibly further chronic inflammatory disorders.

Funding: Research of the authors related to chemerin is funded by the German Research Foundation, grant number BU 1141/7-1 and BU 1141/13-1.

Conflicts of Interest: The authors declare no conflict of interest.

References

1. Ernst, M.C.; Sinal, C.J. Chemerin: At the crossroads of inflammation and obesity. *Trends Endocrinol. Metab.* **2010**, *21*, 660–667. [CrossRef] [PubMed]
2. Rourke, J.L.; Dranse, H.J.; Sinal, C.J. Towards an integrative approach to understanding the role of chemerin in human health and disease. *Obes. Rev.* **2013**, *14*, 245–262. [CrossRef] [PubMed]
3. Buechler, C. Chemerin in Liver Diseases. *Endocrinol. Metab. Syndr.* **2014**, *3*, 144.
4. Goralski, K.B.; McCarthy, T.C.; Hanniman, E.A.; Zabel, B.A.; Butcher, E.C.; Parlee, S.D.; Muruganandan, S.; Sinal, C.J. Chemerin, a novel adipokine that regulates adipogenesis and adipocyte metabolism. *J. Biol. Chem.* **2007**, *282*, 28175–28188. [CrossRef] [PubMed]
5. Yoshimura, T.; Oppenheim, J.J. Chemerin reveals its chimeric nature. *J. Exp. Med.* **2008**, *205*, 2187–2190. [CrossRef] [PubMed]
6. Zabel, B.A.; Kwitniewski, M.; Banas, M.; Zabieglo, K.; Murzyn, K.; Cichy, J. Chemerin regulation and role in host defense. *Am. J. Clin. Exp. Immunol.* **2014**, *3*, 1–19. [PubMed]
7. Takahashi, M.; Okimura, Y.; Iguchi, G.; Nishizawa, H.; Yamamoto, M.; Suda, K.; Kitazawa, R.; Fujimoto, W.; Takahashi, K.; Zolotaryov, F.N.; et al. Chemerin regulates beta-cell function in mice. *Sci. Rep.* **2011**, *1*, 123. [CrossRef] [PubMed]
8. Ernst, M.C.; Issa, M.; Goralski, K.B.; Sinal, C.J. Chemerin exacerbates glucose intolerance in mouse models of obesity and diabetes. *Endocrinology* **2010**, *151*, 1998–2007. [CrossRef] [PubMed]
9. Becker, M.; Rabe, K.; Lebherz, C.; Zugwurst, J.; Goke, B.; Parhofer, K.G.; Lehrke, M.; Broedl, U.C. Expression of human chemerin induces insulin resistance in the skeletal muscle but does not affect weight, lipid levels, and atherosclerosis in LDL receptor knockout mice on high-fat diet. *Diabetes* **2010**, *59*, 2898–2903. [CrossRef] [PubMed]
10. Nakamura, N.; Naruse, K.; Kobayashi, Y.; Miyabe, M.; Saiki, T.; Enomoto, A.; Takahashi, M.; Matsubara, T. Chemerin promotes angiogenesis in vivo. *Physiol. Rep.* **2018**, *6*, e13962. [CrossRef] [PubMed]
11. Dimitriadis, G.K.; Kaur, J.; Adya, R.; Miras, A.D.; Mattu, H.S.; Hattersley, J.G.; Kaltsas, G.; Tan, B.K.; Randeva, H.S. Chemerin induces endothelial cell inflammation: Activation of nuclear factor-kappa beta and monocyte-endothelial adhesion. *Oncotarget* **2018**, *9*, 16678–16690. [CrossRef] [PubMed]
12. Bondue, B.; Wittamer, V.; Parmentier, M. Chemerin and its receptors in leukocyte trafficking, inflammation and metabolism. *Cytokine Growth Factor Rev.* **2011**, *22*, 331–338. [CrossRef] [PubMed]
13. Wittamer, V.; Franssen, J.D.; Vulcano, M.; Mirjolet, J.F.; Le Poul, E.; Migeotte, I.; Brezillon, S.; Tyldesley, R.; Blanpain, C.; Detheux, M.; et al. Specific recruitment of antigen-presenting cells by chemerin, a novel processed ligand from human inflammatory fluids. *J. Exp. Med.* **2003**, *198*, 977–985. [CrossRef] [PubMed]
14. Yoshimura, T.; Oppenheim, J.J. Chemokine-like receptor 1 (CMKLR1) and chemokine (C-C motif) receptor-like 2 (CCRL2); two multifunctional receptors with unusual properties. *Exp. Cell Res.* **2011**, *317*, 674–684. [CrossRef] [PubMed]
15. De Henau, O.; Degroot, G.N.; Imbault, V.; Robert, V.; De Poorter, C.; McHeik, S.; Gales, C.; Parmentier, M.; Springael, J.Y. Signaling Properties of Chemerin Receptors CMKLR1, GPR1 and CCRL2. *PLoS ONE* **2016**, *11*, e0164179. [CrossRef] [PubMed]
16. Rourke, J.L.; Dranse, H.J.; Sinal, C.J. CMKLR1 and GPR1 mediate chemerin signaling through the RhoA/ROCK pathway. *Mol. Cell. Endocrinol.* **2015**, *417*, 36–51. [CrossRef] [PubMed]
17. Kaur, J.; Adya, R.; Tan, B.K.; Chen, J.; Randeva, H.S. Identification of chemerin receptor (ChemR23) in human endothelial cells: Chemerin-induced endothelial angiogenesis. *Biochem. Biophys. Res. Commun.* **2010**, *391*, 1762–1768. [CrossRef] [PubMed]
18. Sell, H.; Laurencikiene, J.; Taube, A.; Eckardt, K.; Cramer, A.; Horrighs, A.; Arner, P.; Eckel, J. Chemerin is a novel adipocyte-derived factor inducing insulin resistance in primary human skeletal muscle cells. *Diabetes* **2009**, *58*, 2731–2740. [CrossRef] [PubMed]
19. Mattern, A.; Zellmann, T.; Beck-Sickinger, A.G. Processing, signaling, and physiological function of chemerin. *IUBMB Life* **2014**, *66*, 19–26. [CrossRef] [PubMed]

20. Li, J.J.; Yin, H.K.; Guan, D.X.; Zhao, J.S.; Feng, Y.X.; Deng, Y.Z.; Wang, X.; Li, N.; Wang, X.F.; Cheng, S.Q.; et al. Chemerin suppresses hepatocellular carcinoma metastasis through CMKLR1-PTEN-Akt axis. *Br. J. Cancer* **2018**, *118*, 1337–1348. [CrossRef] [PubMed]
21. Zhou, J.X.; Liao, D.; Zhang, S.; Cheng, N.; He, H.Q.; Ye, R.D. Chemerin C9 peptide induces receptor internalization through a clathrin-independent pathway. *Acta Pharmacol. Sin.* **2014**, *35*, 653–663. [CrossRef] [PubMed]
22. Dranse, H.J.; Muruganandan, S.; Fawcett, J.P.; Sinal, C.J. Adipocyte-secreted chemerin is processed to a variety of isoforms and influences MMP3 and chemokine secretion through an NFkB-dependent mechanism. *Mol. Cell. Endocrinol.* **2016**, *436*, 114–129. [CrossRef] [PubMed]
23. Bozaoglu, K.; Segal, D.; Shields, K.A.; Cummings, N.; Curran, J.E.; Comuzzie, A.G.; Mahaney, M.C.; Rainwater, D.L.; VandeBerg, J.L.; MacCluer, J.W.; et al. Chemerin is associated with metabolic syndrome phenotypes in a Mexican-American population. *J. Clin. Endocrinol. Metab.* **2009**, *94*, 3085–3088. [CrossRef] [PubMed]
24. Krautbauer, S.; Wanninger, J.; Eisinger, K.; Hader, Y.; Beck, M.; Kopp, A.; Schmid, A.; Weiss, T.S.; Dorn, C.; Buechler, C. Chemerin is highly expressed in hepatocytes and is induced in non-alcoholic steatohepatitis liver. *Exp. Mol. Pathol.* **2013**, *95*, 199–205. [CrossRef] [PubMed]
25. Bozaoglu, K.; Bolton, K.; McMillan, J.; Zimmet, P.; Jowett, J.; Collier, G.; Walder, K.; Segal, D. Chemerin is a novel adipokine associated with obesity and metabolic syndrome. *Endocrinology* **2007**, *148*, 4687–4694. [CrossRef] [PubMed]
26. Coimbra, S.; Brandao Proenca, J.; Santos-Silva, A.; Neuparth, M.J. Adiponectin, leptin, and chemerin in elderly patients with type 2 diabetes mellitus: A close linkage with obesity and length of the disease. *BioMed Res. Int.* **2014**, *2014*, 701915. [CrossRef] [PubMed]
27. Kukla, M.; Zwirska-Korczala, K.; Hartleb, M.; Waluga, M.; Chwist, A.; Kajor, M.; Ciupinska-Kajor, M.; Berdowska, A.; Wozniak-Grygiel, E.; Buldak, R. Serum chemerin and vaspin in non-alcoholic fatty liver disease. *Scand. J. Gastroenterol.* **2010**, *45*, 235–242. [CrossRef] [PubMed]
28. Stejskal, D.; Karpisek, M.; Hanulova, Z.; Svestak, M. Chemerin Is an Independent Marker of the Metabolic Syndrome in a Caucasian Population—A Pilot Study. *Biomed. Pap. Med. Fac. Univ. Palacky Olomouc Czech. Repub.* **2008**, *152*, 217–221. [CrossRef] [PubMed]
29. Weigert, J.; Neumeier, M.; Wanninger, J.; Filarsky, M.; Bauer, S.; Wiest, R.; Farkas, S.; Scherer, M.N.; Schaffler, A.; Aslanidis, C.; et al. Systemic chemerin is related to inflammation rather than obesity in type 2 diabetes. *Clin. Endocrinol.* **2010**, *72*, 342–348. [CrossRef] [PubMed]
30. Zhuang, X.H.; Sun, F.D.; Chen, S.H.; Liu, Y.T.; Liu, W.; Li, X.B.; Pan, Z.; Lou, N.J. Circulating chemerin levels are increased in first-degree relatives of type 2 diabetic patients. *Clin. Lab.* **2014**, *60*, 983–988. [CrossRef] [PubMed]
31. Bozaoglu, K.; Curran, J.E.; Stocker, C.J.; Zaibi, M.S.; Segal, D.; Konstantopoulos, N.; Morrison, S.; Carless, M.; Dyer, T.D.; Cole, S.A.; et al. Chemerin, a novel adipokine in the regulation of angiogenesis. *J. Clin. Endocrinol. Metab.* **2010**, *95*, 2476–2485. [CrossRef] [PubMed]
32. Er, L.K.; Wu, S.; Hsu, L.A.; Teng, M.S.; Sun, Y.C.; Ko, Y.L. Pleiotropic Associations of RARRES2 Gene Variants and Circulating Chemerin Levels: Potential Roles of Chemerin Involved in the Metabolic and Inflammation-Related Diseases. *Mediat. Inflamm.* **2018**, *2018*, 4670521. [CrossRef] [PubMed]
33. Mussig, K.; Staiger, H.; Machicao, F.; Thamer, C.; Machann, J.; Schick, F.; Claussen, C.D.; Stefan, N.; Fritsche, A.; Haring, H.U. RARRES2, encoding the novel adipokine chemerin, is a genetic determinant of disproportionate regional body fat distribution: A comparative magnetic resonance imaging study. *Metabolism* **2009**, *58*, 519–524. [CrossRef] [PubMed]
34. Tonjes, A.; Scholz, M.; Breitfeld, J.; Marzi, C.; Grallert, H.; Gross, A.; Ladenvall, C.; Schleinitz, D.; Krause, K.; Kirsten, H.; et al. Genome wide meta-analysis highlights the role of genetic variation in RARRES2 in the regulation of circulating serum chemerin. *PLoS Genet.* **2014**, *10*, e1004854. [CrossRef] [PubMed]
35. Buechler, C. Chemerin, a novel player in inflammatory bowel disease. *Cell. Mol. Immunol.* **2014**, *11*, 315–316. [CrossRef] [PubMed]
36. Fatima, S.S.; Rehman, R.; Baig, M.; Khan, T.A. New roles of the multidimensional adipokine: Chemerin. *Peptides* **2014**, *62*, 15–20. [CrossRef] [PubMed]
37. Mariani, F.; Roncucci, L. Chemerin/chemR23 axis in inflammation onset and resolution. *Inflamm. Res.* **2015**, *64*, 85–95. [CrossRef] [PubMed]

38. Shin, W.J.; Pachynski, R.K. Chemerin modulation of tumor growth: Potential clinical applications in cancer. *Discov. Med.* **2018**, *26*, 31–37. [PubMed]
39. Farsam, V.; Basu, A.; Gatzka, M.; Treiber, N.; Schneider, L.A.; Mulaw, M.A.; Lucas, T.; Kochanek, S.; Dummer, R.; Levesque, M.P.; et al. Senescent fibroblast-derived Chemerin promotes squamous cell carcinoma migration. *Oncotarget* **2016**, *7*, 83554–83569. [CrossRef] [PubMed]
40. Lin, Y.; Yang, X.; Liu, W.; Li, B.; Yin, W.; Shi, Y.; He, R. Chemerin has a protective role in hepatocellular carcinoma by inhibiting the expression of IL-6 and GM-CSF and MDSC accumulation. *Oncogene* **2017**, *36*, 3599–3608. [CrossRef] [PubMed]
41. Cash, J.L.; Hart, R.; Russ, A.; Dixon, J.P.; Colledge, W.H.; Doran, J.; Hendrick, A.G.; Carlton, M.B.; Greaves, D.R. Synthetic chemerin-derived peptides suppress inflammation through ChemR23. *J. Exp. Med.* **2008**, *205*, 767–775. [CrossRef] [PubMed]
42. Luangsay, S.; Wittamer, V.; Bondue, B.; De Henau, O.; Rouger, L.; Brait, M.; Franssen, J.D.; de Nadai, P.; Huaux, F.; Parmentier, M. Mouse ChemR23 is expressed in dendritic cell subsets and macrophages, and mediates an anti-inflammatory activity of chemerin in a lung disease model. *J. Immunol.* **2009**, *183*, 6489–6499. [CrossRef] [PubMed]
43. Lin, Y.; Yang, X.; Yue, W.; Xu, X.; Li, B.; Zou, L.; He, R. Chemerin aggravates DSS-induced colitis by suppressing M2 macrophage polarization. *Cell. Mol. Immunol.* **2014**, *11*, 355–366. [CrossRef] [PubMed]
44. Chakaroun, R.; Raschpichler, M.; Kloting, N.; Oberbach, A.; Flehmig, G.; Kern, M.; Schon, M.R.; Shang, E.; Lohmann, T.; Dressler, M.; et al. Effects of weight loss and exercise on chemerin serum concentrations and adipose tissue expression in human obesity. *Metabolism* **2012**, *61*, 706–714. [CrossRef] [PubMed]
45. Bauer, S.; Wanninger, J.; Schmidhofer, S.; Weigert, J.; Neumeier, M.; Dorn, C.; Hellerbrand, C.; Zimara, N.; Schaffler, A.; Aslanidis, C.; et al. Sterol regulatory element-binding protein 2 (SREBP2) activation after excess triglyceride storage induces Chemerin in hypertrophic adipocytes. *Endocrinology* **2011**, *152*, 26–35. [CrossRef] [PubMed]
46. Catalan, V.; Gomez-Ambrosi, J.; Rodriguez, A.; Ramirez, B.; Rotellar, F.; Valenti, V.; Silva, C.; Gil, M.J.; Salvador, J.; Fruhbeck, G. Increased levels of chemerin and its receptor, chemokine-like receptor-1, in obesity are related to inflammation: Tumor necrosis factor-α stimulates mRNA levels of chemerin in visceral adipocytes from obese patients. *Surg. Obes. Relat. Dis.* **2013**, *9*, 306–314. [CrossRef] [PubMed]
47. Parlee, S.D.; Ernst, M.C.; Muruganandan, S.; Sinal, C.J.; Goralski, K.B. Serum chemerin levels vary with time of day and are modified by obesity and tumor necrosis factor-α. *Endocrinology* **2010**, *151*, 2590–2602. [CrossRef] [PubMed]
48. Alfadda, A.A.; Sallam, R.M.; Chishti, M.A.; Moustafa, A.S.; Fatma, S.; Alomaim, W.S.; Al-Naami, M.Y.; Bassas, A.F.; Chrousos, G.P.; Jo, H. Differential patterns of serum concentration and adipose tissue expression of chemerin in obesity: Adipose depot specificity and gender dimorphism. *Mol. Cells* **2012**, *33*, 591–596. [CrossRef] [PubMed]
49. Wolfs, M.G.; Gruben, N.; Rensen, S.S.; Verdam, F.J.; Greve, J.W.; Driessen, A.; Wijmenga, C.; Buurman, W.A.; Franke, L.; Scheja, L.; et al. Determining the association between adipokine expression in multiple tissues and phenotypic features of non-alcoholic fatty liver disease in obesity. *Nutr. Diabetes* **2015**, *5*, e146. [CrossRef] [PubMed]
50. Sanchez-Rebordelo, E.; Cunarro, J.; Perez-Sieira, S.; Seoane, L.M.; Dieguez, C.; Nogueiras, R.; Tovar, S. Regulation of Chemerin and CMKLR1 Expression by Nutritional Status, Postnatal Development, and Gender. *Int. J. Mol. Sci.* **2018**, *19*, 2905. [CrossRef] [PubMed]
51. Friedman, J. The long road to leptin. *J. Clin. Investig.* **2016**, *126*, 4727–4734. [CrossRef] [PubMed]
52. Buechler, C.; Wanninger, J.; Neumeier, M. Adiponectin, a key adipokine in obesity related liver diseases. *World J. Gastroenterol.* **2011**, *17*, 2801–2811. [PubMed]
53. Sjoholm, A.; Nystrom, T. Inflammation and the etiology of type 2 diabetes. *Diabetes Metab. Res. Rev.* **2006**, *22*, 4–10. [CrossRef] [PubMed]
54. Russo, L.; Lumeng, C.N. Properties and functions of adipose tissue macrophages in obesity. *Immunology* **2018**, *155*, 407–417. [CrossRef] [PubMed]
55. Suzuki, Y.; Hong, Y.H.; Song, S.H.; Ardiyanti, A.; Kato, D.; So, K.H.; Katoh, K.; Roh, S.G. The Regulation of Chemerin and CMKLR1 Genes Expression by TNF-α, Adiponectin, and Chemerin Analog in Bovine Differentiated Adipocytes. *Asian-Australas. J. Anim. Sci.* **2012**, *25*, 1316–1321. [CrossRef] [PubMed]

56. Rourke, J.L.; Muruganandan, S.; Dranse, H.J.; McMullen, N.M.; Sinal, C.J. Gpr1 is an active chemerin receptor influencing glucose homeostasis in obese mice. *J. Endocrinol.* **2014**, *222*, 201–215. [CrossRef] [PubMed]
57. Docke, S.; Lock, J.F.; Birkenfeld, A.L.; Hoppe, S.; Lieske, S.; Rieger, A.; Raschzok, N.; Sauer, I.M.; Florian, S.; Osterhoff, M.A.; et al. Elevated hepatic chemerin gene expression in progressed human non-alcoholic fatty liver disease. *Eur. J. Endocrinol.* **2013**, *169*, 547–557. [CrossRef] [PubMed]
58. Kajor, M.; Kukla, M.; Waluga, M.; Liszka, L.; Dyaczynski, M.; Kowalski, G.; Zadlo, D.; Berdowska, A.; Chapula, M.; Kostrzab-Zdebel, A.; et al. Hepatic chemerin mRNA in morbidly obese patients with nonalcoholic fatty liver disease. *Pol. J. Pathol.* **2017**, *68*, 117–127. [CrossRef] [PubMed]
59. Pohl, R.; Haberl, E.M.; Rein-Fischboeck, L.; Zimny, S.; Neumann, M.; Aslanidis, C.; Schacherer, D.; Krautbauer, S.; Eisinger, K.; Weiss, T.S.; et al. Hepatic chemerin mRNA expression is reduced in human nonalcoholic steatohepatitis. *Eur. J. Clin. Investig.* **2017**, *47*, 7–18. [CrossRef] [PubMed]
60. Deng, Y.; Wang, H.; Lu, Y.; Liu, S.; Zhang, Q.; Huang, J.; Zhu, R.; Yang, J.; Zhang, R.; Zhang, D.; et al. Identification of Chemerin as a Novel FXR Target Gene Down-Regulated in the Progression of Nonalcoholic Steatohepatitis. *Endocrinology* **2013**, *154*, 1794–1801. [CrossRef] [PubMed]
61. Wanninger, J.; Bauer, S.; Eisinger, K.; Weiss, T.S.; Walter, R.; Hellerbrand, C.; Schaffler, A.; Higuchi, A.; Walsh, K.; Buechler, C. Adiponectin upregulates hepatocyte CMKLR1 which is reduced in human fatty liver. *Mol. Cell. Endocrinol.* **2012**, *349*, 248–254. [CrossRef] [PubMed]
62. Neumann, M.; Meier, E.M.; Rein-Fischboeck, L.; Krautbauer, S.; Eisinger, K.; Aslanidis, C.; Pohl, R.; Weiss, T.S.; Buechler, C. Chemokine-Like Receptor 1 mRNA Weakly Correlates with Non-Alcoholic Steatohepatitis Score in Male but Not Female Individuals. *Int. J. Mol. Sci.* **2016**, *17*, 1335. [CrossRef] [PubMed]
63. Zimny, S.; Pohl, R.; Rein-Fischboeck, L.; Haberl, E.M.; Krautbauer, S.; Weiss, T.S.; Buechler, C. Chemokine (CC-motif) receptor-like 2 mRNA is expressed in hepatic stellate cells and is positively associated with characteristics of non-alcoholic steatohepatitis in mice and men. *Exp. Mol. Pathol.* **2017**, *103*, 1–8. [CrossRef] [PubMed]
64. Zhang, W.; Liu, Y.; Wu, M.; Zhu, X.; Wang, T.; He, K.; Li, P.; Wu, X. PI3K inhibition protects mice from NAFLD by down-regulating CMKLR1 and NLRP3 in Kupffer cells. *J. Physiol. Biochem.* **2017**, *73*, 583–594. [CrossRef] [PubMed]
65. Herova, M.; Schmid, M.; Gemperle, C.; Hersberger, M. ChemR23, the Receptor for Chemerin and Resolvin E1, Is Expressed and Functional on M1 but Not on M2 Macrophages. *J. Immunol.* **2015**, *194*, 2330–2337. [CrossRef] [PubMed]
66. Zhao, L.; Yamaguchi, Y.; Shen, W.J.; Morser, J.; Leung, L.L.K. Dynamic and tissue-specific proteolytic processing of chemerin in obese mice. *PLoS ONE* **2018**, *13*, e0202780. [CrossRef] [PubMed]
67. Du, X.Y.; Zabel, B.A.; Myles, T.; Allen, S.J.; Handel, T.M.; Lee, P.P.; Butcher, E.C.; Leung, L.L. Regulation of chemerin bioactivity by plasma carboxypeptidase N, carboxypeptidase B (activated thrombin-activable fibrinolysis inhibitor), and platelets. *J. Biol. Chem.* **2009**, *284*, 751–758. [CrossRef] [PubMed]
68. Kulig, P.; Kantyka, T.; Zabel, B.A.; Banas, M.; Chyra, A.; Stefanska, A.; Tu, H.; Allen, S.J.; Handel, T.M.; Kozik, A.; et al. Regulation of chemerin chemoattractant and antibacterial activity by human cysteine cathepsins. *J. Immunol.* **2011**, *187*, 1403–1410. [CrossRef] [PubMed]
69. Schultz, S.; Saalbach, A.; Heiker, J.T.; Meier, R.; Zellmann, T.; Simon, J.C.; Beck-Sickinger, A.G. Proteolytic activation of prochemerin by kallikrein 7 breaks an ionic linkage and results in C-terminal rearrangement. *Biochem. J.* **2013**, *452*, 271–280. [CrossRef] [PubMed]
70. Zhao, L.; Yamaguchi, Y.; Ge, X.; Robinson, W.H.; Morser, J.; Leung, L.L.K. Chemerin 156F, generated by chymase cleavage of prochemerin, is elevated in joint fluids of arthritis patients. *Arthritis Res. Ther.* **2018**, *20*, 132. [CrossRef] [PubMed]
71. Guillabert, A.; Wittamer, V.; Bondue, B.; Godot, V.; Imbault, V.; Parmentier, M.; Communi, D. Role of neutrophil proteinase 3 and mast cell chymase in chemerin proteolytic regulation. *J. Leukoc. Biol.* **2008**, *84*, 1530–1538. [CrossRef] [PubMed]
72. Ge, X.; Yamaguchi, Y.; Zhao, L.; Bury, L.; Gresele, P.; Berube, C.; Leung, L.L.; Morser, J. Prochemerin cleavage by factor XIa links coagulation and inflammation. *Blood* **2018**, *131*, 353–364. [CrossRef] [PubMed]
73. Coates, D. The angiotensin converting enzyme (ACE). *Int. J. Biochem. Cell Biol.* **2003**, *35*, 769–773. [CrossRef]
74. John, H.; Hierer, J.; Haas, O.; Forssmann, W.G. Quantification of angiotensin-converting-enzyme-mediated degradation of human chemerin 145-154 in plasma by matrix-assisted laser desorption/ionization-time-of-flight mass spectrometry. *Anal. Biochem.* **2007**, *362*, 117–125. [CrossRef] [PubMed]

75. Kunimoto, H.; Kazama, K.; Takai, M.; Oda, M.; Okada, M.; Yamawaki, H. Chemerin promotes the proliferation and migration of vascular smooth muscle and increases mouse blood pressure. *Am. J. Physiol. Heart Circ. Physiol.* **2015**, *309*, H1017–H1028. [CrossRef] [PubMed]
76. Yang, M.; Yang, G.; Dong, J.; Liu, Y.; Zong, H.; Liu, H.; Boden, G.; Li, L. Elevated plasma levels of chemerin in newly diagnosed type 2 diabetes mellitus with hypertension. *J. Investig. Med.* **2010**, *58*, 883–886. [CrossRef] [PubMed]
77. Zylla, S.; Pietzner, M.; Kuhn, J.P.; Volzke, H.; Dorr, M.; Nauck, M.; Friedrich, N. Serum chemerin is associated with inflammatory and metabolic parameters-results of a population-based study. *Obesity* **2017**, *25*, 468–475. [CrossRef] [PubMed]
78. Watts, S.W.; Darios, E.S.; Mullick, A.E.; Garver, H.; Saunders, T.L.; Hughes, E.D.; Filipiak, W.E.; Zeidler, M.G.; McMullen, N.; Sinal, C.J.; et al. The chemerin knockout rat reveals chemerin dependence in female, but not male, experimental hypertension. *FASEB J.* **2018**, *32*, 3596–6614. [CrossRef] [PubMed]
79. Ferland, D.J.; Seitz, B.; Darios, E.S.; Thompson, J.M.; Yeh, S.T.; Mullick, A.E.; Watts, S.W. Whole-Body but Not Hepatic Knockdown of Chemerin by Antisense Oligonucleotide Decreases Blood Pressure in Rats. *J. Pharmacol. Exp. Ther.* **2018**, *365*, 212–218. [CrossRef] [PubMed]
80. Yamaguchi, Y.; Du, X.Y.; Zhao, L.; Morser, J.; Leung, L.L. Proteolytic cleavage of chemerin protein is necessary for activation to the active form, Chem157S, which functions as a signaling molecule in glioblastoma. *J. Biol. Chem.* **2011**, *286*, 39510–39519. [CrossRef] [PubMed]
81. Chang, S.S.; Eisenberg, D.; Zhao, L.; Adams, C.; Leib, R.; Morser, J.; Leung, L. Chemerin activation in human obesity. *Obesisty* **2016**, *24*, 1522–1529. [CrossRef] [PubMed]
82. Dogra, S.; Sona, C.; Kumar, A.; Yadav, P.N. Tango assay for ligand-induced GPCR-beta-arrestin2 interaction: Application in drug discovery. *Methods Cell Biol.* **2016**, *132*, 233–254. [PubMed]
83. Haberl, E.M.; Pohl, R.; Rein-Fischboeck, L.; Feder, S.; Eisinger, K.; Krautbauer, S.; Sinal, C.J.; Buechler, C. Ex vivo analysis of serum chemerin activity in murine models of obesity. *Cytokine* **2018**, *104*, 42–45. [CrossRef] [PubMed]
84. Toulany, J.; Parlee, S.D.; Sinal, C.J.; Slayter, K.; McNeil, S.; Goralski, K.B. CMKLR1 activation ex vivo does not increase proportionally to serum total chemerin in obese humans. *Endocr. Connect.* **2016**, *5*, 70–81. [CrossRef] [PubMed]
85. Hotamisligil, G.S.; Spiegelman, B.M. Tumor necrosis factor α: A key component of the obesity-diabetes link. *Diabetes* **1994**, *43*, 1271–1278. [CrossRef] [PubMed]
86. Wang, B.; Chandrasekera, P.C.; Pippin, J.J. Leptin- and leptin receptor-deficient rodent models: Relevance for human type 2 diabetes. *Curr. Diabetes Rev.* **2014**, *10*, 131–145. [CrossRef] [PubMed]
87. Bauer, S.; Bala, M.; Kopp, A.; Eisinger, K.; Schmid, A.; Schneider, S.; Neumeier, M.; Buechler, C. Adipocyte chemerin release is induced by insulin without being translated to higher levels in vivo. *Eur. J. Clin. Investig.* **2012**, *42*, 1213–1220. [CrossRef] [PubMed]
88. Pappas, C.; Kandaraki, E.A.; Tsirona, S.; Kountouras, D.; Kassi, G.; Diamanti-Kandarakis, E. Postprandial dysmetabolism: Too early or too late? *Hormones* **2016**, *15*, 321–344. [CrossRef] [PubMed]
89. Divoux, A.; Moutel, S.; Poitou, C.; Lacasa, D.; Veyrie, N.; Aissat, A.; Arock, M.; Guerre-Millo, M.; Clement, K. Mast cells in human adipose tissue: Link with morbid obesity, inflammatory status, and diabetes. *J. Clin. Endocrinol. Metab.* **2012**, *97*, E1677–E1685. [CrossRef] [PubMed]
90. Cash, J.L.; Christian, A.R.; Greaves, D.R. Chemerin peptides promote phagocytosis in a ChemR23- and Syk-dependent manner. *J. Immunol.* **2010**, *184*, 5315–5324. [CrossRef] [PubMed]

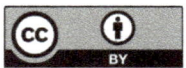

© 2019 by the authors. Licensee MDPI, Basel, Switzerland. This article is an open access article distributed under the terms and conditions of the Creative Commons Attribution (CC BY) license (http://creativecommons.org/licenses/by/4.0/).

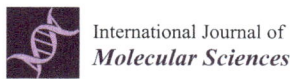

Review

More Than an Adipokine: The Complex Roles of Chemerin Signaling in Cancer

Kerry B. Goralski [1,2,3], Ashley E. Jackson [2], Brendan T. McKeown [2] and Christopher J. Sinal [2,*]

1. College of Pharmacy, Faculty of Health, Dalhousie University, Halifax, NS B3H 4R2, Canada; Kerry.Goralski@Dal.Ca
2. Department of Pharmacology, Faculty of Medicine, Dalhousie University, Halifax, NS B3H 4R2, Canada; a.jackson13@dal.ca (A.E.J.); Brendan.McKeown@Dal.Ca (B.T.M.)
3. Department of Pediatrics, Faculty of Medicine, Dalhousie University, Halifax, NS B3H 4R2, Canada
* Correspondence: Christopher.Sinal@dal.ca

Received: 14 August 2019; Accepted: 23 September 2019; Published: 26 September 2019

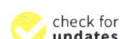

Abstract: Chemerin is widely recognized as an adipokine, with diverse biological roles in cellular differentiation and metabolism, as well as a leukocyte chemoattractant. Research investigating the role of chemerin in the obesity–cancer relationship has provided evidence both for pro- and anti-cancer effects. The tumor-promoting effects of chemerin primarily involve direct effects on migration, invasion, and metastasis as well as growth and proliferation of cancer cells. Chemerin can also promote tumor growth via the recruitment of tumor-supporting mesenchymal stromal cells and stimulation of angiogenesis pathways in endothelial cells. In contrast, the majority of evidence supports that the tumor-suppressing effects of chemerin are immune-mediated and result in a shift from immunosuppressive to immunogenic cell populations within the tumor microenvironment. Systemic chemerin and chemerin produced within the tumor microenvironment may contribute to these effects via signaling through CMKLR1 (chemerin$_1$), GPR1 (chemerin$_2$), and CCLR2 on target cells. As such, inhibition or activation of chemerin signaling could be beneficial as a therapeutic approach depending on the type of cancer. Additional studies are required to determine if obesity influences cancer initiation or progression through increased adipose tissue production of chemerin and/or altered chemerin processing that leads to changes in chemerin signaling in the tumor microenvironment.

Keywords: cancer; obesity; adipokine; chemerin; chemokine-like receptor 1; G protein-coupled receptor 1; C-C chemokine receptor-like 2

1. Obesity and Cancer

Overweight and obesity rates have increased steadily for several decades and at present are a major global health crisis of epidemic proportions [1]. Recent estimates indicate that approximately 1.5 billion adults are overweight, while a further 600 million are obese [1,2]. While the rise of obesity prevalence has slowed in some countries, it is predicted that global rates will continue to increase with time and thereby exacerbate the health impact of this disorder [3]. Obesity is directly linked to a decline in quality of life and overall reduced life-expectancy as well as being a major risk factor for several prevalent metabolic, cardiovascular, and malignant disorders. Among these, cancer continues to be a leading cause of death worldwide that is attributable to an estimated 14 million incident cases and 8 million deaths annually [2,3]. In addition to other well-established risk factors for cancer (e.g., genetics, tobacco use, ionizing radiation, environmental exposure), obesity is now recognized as a risk factor for several malignancies [4,5]. These include cancers of the digestive and secretory systems (e.g., colon, stomach, liver, esophagus, kidney, gallbladder), female and male reproductive systems (e.g., ovary, postmenopausal breast, endometrium, prostate), and hematological systems (e.g., non-Hodgkin's lymphoma, multiple myeloma, leukemia) [6–9]. Thus, with the increasing prevalence of obesity in our society, it is predicted that this disorder will soon surpass smoking as a leading significant preventable cause of cancer [10].

2. Role of Adipokines

While the linkage between obesity and cancer risk is an active area of investigation, the underlying biological mechanisms are not well understood. Moreover, many tumors develop in an adipocyte-rich environment. For example, adipocytes are a major cellular component of the mammary fat pad, and recent evidence indicates that these cells have dynamic interactions with cancer cells to modulate tumor growth and metastases [11,12]. Thus, local and ectopic fat depots may have an impact on cancer development that is not reflected or predicted by overall fat mass. The local and systemic alterations in physiology that are associated with obesity have the potential to impact cancer in many respects through direct effects on cancerous cells or indirect effects on the tumor microenvironment or immune function. As such, obesity can impact tumor initiation, metabolic reprogramming, angiogenesis, progression, and response to therapy variously.

Obesity is characterized not only by a generalized expansion of adipose, but also the development of a progressive metabolic and endocrine dysfunction characterized by profound alterations in the production of several factors including lipids, hormones, pro-inflammatory cytokines, and a suite of adipose derived-signaling molecules termed adipokines [13,14]. Adipokines are a heterogeneous group of peptides, mainly produced by adipose tissue, that fulfill critical regulatory roles in energy homeostasis and metabolic health [15,16]. Obesity-related alterations in the amounts and/or spectrum of adipokine release have been linked to metabolic disorders such as hyperlipidemia and type 2 diabetes and are increasingly recognized as a key factor linking obesity with cancer. For example, adiponectin is an adipokine with established pleiotropic roles in regulating insulin-sensitivity as well as lipid and glucose homeostasis [4]. Circulating levels of adiponectin are inversely correlated with adiposity and this is believed to contribute to the increased risk for obesity-related comorbidities such as type 2 diabetes and metabolic syndrome [4]. Lower levels of this adipokine have also been linked to an increased risk for several types of cancer [17,18]. In contrast to adiponectin, circulating levels of the adipokine leptin increase in proportion to fat mass. While different epidemiological studies have offered conflicting results regarding the impact of leptin on general cancer risk, a recent meta-analysis of 23 studies reported a positive association with breast cancer risk [19]. Moreover, overexpression of the receptor for leptin has been found in breast cancer and in particular for higher-grade tumors associated with metastasis and poor clinical prognosis [20–23].

3. Chemerin

Chemerin is a multifunctional secreted protein with established roles in energy metabolism, immune function, and fundamental cell processes such as differentiation, proliferation, and chemotaxis [24,25]. Consistent with its role as an adipokine, evidence from clinical and animal studies have firmly established that secretion and circulating levels of chemerin increase with adiposity and decline after bariatric surgery, diet, and exercise-based weight loss [26–35]. In addition to adipose tissue, chemerin is highly expressed in many other human tissues including the adrenals, liver, female reproductive organs, mammary tissue, and lung (Data Source: GTEx Analysis Release V7 (dbGaP, Accession phs000424.v7.p2, accessed on 29 July 2019)) as well as cell types such as intestinal epithelial cells, platelets, keratinocytes, synovial fibroblasts, and vascular endothelial cells [36–40]. Therefore, when assessing a role for this adipokine in cancer, the impact of chemerin produced locally within the affected tissue and/or tumor microenvironment must be considered in addition to systemic levels of circulating chemerin.

Chemerin is synthesized as pre-prochemerin, which requires N-terminal cleavage of a 19-amino acid signaling domain prior to its secretion as a 163-amino acid precursor (prochemerin) [37,41–44]. Subsequently, prochemerin undergoes extracellular proteolytic processing at the C-terminus exposing the active region and forming active chemerin [37,41,44]. In humans, prochemerin is processed to at least three active products; chemerin156, chemerin157, and chemerin158, all of which have been detected in biological fluids, including plasma and serum [42,45,46]. Further proteolytic events cleave active chemerin isoforms to shorter inactive or low activity proteins [35,47]. Chemerin is the endogenous ligand for two known cognate signaling receptors, chemokine-like receptor 1 (CMKLR1) and G protein-coupled receptor 1 (GPR1); herein these are referred to as chemerin receptor 1 (chemerin$_1$) and chemerin receptor 2 (chemerin$_2$) as established by the International Union of Basic and Clinical Pharmacology Committee on Receptor Nomenclature [48]. A third chemerin receptor, C-C chemokine receptor-like 2 (CCRL2), exhibits limited homology with chemerin$_1$ and chemerin$_2$ and is most closely related to the atypical chemokine receptor family [48]. Rather than directly mediating chemerin signaling, CCRL2 is thought to function as a chemerin membrane anchoring protein that increases local chemerin concentrations and presents the ligand to chemerin$_1$ or chemerin$_2$ expressing cells. [49,50] Depending upon the site of proteolytic cleavage and interaction with either of chemerin$_1$ or chemerin$_2$, the magnitude and nature of the biological effects of chemerin can vary dramatically (e.g., pro- versus anti-inflammatory) [24]. Chemerin has been shown to mediate the chemoattraction of several chemerin receptor-expressing leukocyte subsets that are often present in the tumor microenvironment, including dendritic cells, natural killer cells, and macrophages [42,51,52]. Therefore, chemerin signaling may play a role in cancer immunology through these mechanisms.

Circulating chemerin levels correlate positively with adiposity, and it is generally accepted that major peripheral white adipose depots, such as subcutaneous and visceral fat, are significant contributors to systemic chemerin levels. However, recent research indicates that locally-derived chemerin, produced either by tumors or by adipocytes in close proximity to the tumor, may have auto/paracrine effects that are distinct from the hormonal influence of systemic chemerin. The aim of this review is to summarize the evidence linking chemerin, and the cognate receptors, to the risk, mechanism, and prognosis of human cancer. Please note that this review provides complementary information to the paper by Treeck et al. [53] also published in this special issue.

4. Esophageal and Oral Cancers

Both systemic and tumor-localized chemerin levels are associated with pro-cancer effects in esophageal and oral carcinoma. Overexpression of chemerin has been demonstrated in oral squamous cell carcinoma (OSCC), squamous cell carcinoma of the oral tongue (SCCOT), and oesophageal squamous cancer (OSC) [54–56]. In a study of OSCC patients, increased circulating and salivary concentrations of both chemerin and the extracellular matrix remodeling enzyme matrix metalloproteinase-9 (MMP-9) were observed compared to patients with oral pre-malignant lesions (OPLs) and controls [54]. Table 1 summarizes the serum/plasma chemerin concentrations, as well as patient demographics (subject groups, numbers, age, sex, and BMI), for this and all other studies described in the present article. Furthermore, patients with pre-malignant lesions also displayed elevated levels of chemerin and MMP-9 when compared to healthy controls [54]. Similarly, several studies have reported increased expression of chemerin in SCCOT tissues compared to adjacent non-cancerous tissues and in OSC cancer-associated myofibroblasts (CAMs) compared to adjacent tissue myofibroblasts (ATMs) [55,57]. In SCCOT, overexpression of both chemerin mRNA and protein was correlated with a number of poor clinical indicators, including lymph node infiltration, microvessel density, tumor angiogenesis, and advanced clinical stage [54,55,58]. Furthermore, chemerin expression was greater in advanced-stage SCCOT tumors and thus, was linked to a poor prognosis [55].

Table 1. Summary of chemerin concentrations and tissue expression data.

Cancer Type	Demographics				Serum, Plasma, or Tissue Chemerin in ng/mL
	Group, n	Age in Years	Sex	BMI kg/m^2	
OSCC [54]	OSCC, 15 OPML, 15 Controls, 15	47.7 ± 14.1 42.3 ± 11.0 43.3 ± 11.8	M6/F9 M5/F10 M7/F8	22.8 ± 1.1 22.4 ± 1.1 22.7 ± 1.5	serum 655 ± 150 † 408 ± 85 * 187 ± 13
	OSCC, 15 OPML, 15 Controls, 15	47.7 ± 14.1 42.3 ± 11.0 43.3 ± 11.8	M6/F9 M5/F10 M7/F8	22.8 ± 1.1 22.4 ± 1.1 22.7 ± 1.5	salivary fluid 13.2 ± 3.8 † 9.1 ± 1.9 * 3.1 ± 0.7
Colorectal [59]	Patients, 41 Controls, 27	55 (32–75) 43 (18–64)	M28/F13 M15/F12	25.8 (16.2–35.5) 26.6 (21.5–45.8)	Serum 390 (250–630) 340 (270–480)
Colorectal [60]	Patients, 221	50 ± 9	62.1% F	16.5% > 30	plasma 148 (50–370)
Gastric [61]	Patients, 196 Controls, 196	44.4% ≥ 60 55.6% < 60	M112/F84 Matched	23.0 ± 3.1 23.4 ± 3.5	plasma 53.1 ± 19.0 * 31.3 ± 11.3
Colorectal [62]	Patients, 32 Controls, 20	57.6 ± 6.5 58.4 ± 7.2	M22/F10 M14/F6	25.8 ± 4.2 26.7 ± 5.3	serum 377.0 ± 80 * 87.8 ± 22.0
Colorectal [63]	Survivors, 110	56.3 ± 9.3	M55/F55	23.3 ± 3.1	serum 105 ± 14
Gastric [64]	Patients, 36 Controls, 40	47–83 31–68	M19/F17 M27/F13	non-obese	serum 42 * 28
HCC [65]	Patients, 44	71 (50–82)	M29/F15	22.5 (15.6–33.5)	serum 130 (80–312)
Thyroid [66]	BMI < 25, 51 BMI ≥ 25, 126	41.2 ± 11.9 55.4 ± 12.7	F51 M26/F100	21.8 ± 2.1 30.7 ± 4.1	serum 212 ± 47 229 ± 50 *
Breast [67]	Metastatic, 37 Non-Met, 80 All, 117	52.3 ± 11.8 51.7 ± 12.5 51.9 ± 12.2	F37 F80 F117	29.1 ± 5.5 28.6 ± 4.9 28.7 ± 5.1	serum 250 ± 59 261 ± 73 257 ± 69
CNS [46]	GBM, 12	N/A	N/A	N/A	CSF chem157S‡—0.2 ± 0.3 chem158K‡—5.1 ± 3.9 chem163S‡—3.0 ± 2.4
	ODC, 12	N/A	N/A	N/A	chem157S—0.7 ± 1.3 chem158K—3.8 ± 3.8 chem163S—2.9 ± 2.5
	NC CNS, 7	N/A	N/A	N/A	chem157S—1.0 ± 0.8 chem158K—6.3 ± 4.8 chem163S—5.5 ± 3.8
	Controls, 9	N/A	N/A	N/A	plasma chem157S—0.7 ± 0.8 chem158K—8.1 ± 2.9 chem163S—40 ± 7.9

Table 1. Cont.

Cancer Type	Demographics				Serum, Plasma, or Tissue Chemerin in ng/mL
	Group, n	Age in Years	Sex	BMI kg/m^2	
NSCLC [68]	Patients, 110	65.1	M91/F19	26.4	serum
	Controls, 110	65.0	M91/F19	27.7	245 *
					203
NSCLC [69]	Patients, 189	61.8 ± 11.2	M124/F65	NA	serum
	Controls, 120	62.6 ± 8.9	M69/F51		1.78 ± 0.57 *
					1.20 ± 0.23
Lung [70]	Patients, 42	56 (44–78)	M26/F16	N/A	plasma
	Controls, 31	48 (32–64)	M18/F13		1.97 ± 0.37 *
					1.11 ± 0.25
Pancreatic ductal [71]	Patients, 25	63.0 ± 9.8		24.5 (21.7–27.8)	serum
	Controls, 36	37.6 ± 6.4	M36	26.1 (24.2–29.5)	272 (221–314) *
					193 (173–214)
Prostate [72]	All patients, 74	67.1 ± 8.5	M74	27.9 ± 3.3	serum
	BPH, 66	61.5 ± 10.3	M66	27.3 ± 4.0	273 ± 29
	WD, 24	64.6 ± 8.5	M24	27.2 ± 3.6	268 ± 83
	MD, 28	66.7 ± 8.8	M28	28.0 ± 2.8	237 ± 72 +
	PD, 22	70.2 ± 7.5	M22	28.3 ± 3.4	274 ± 60 +
					313 ± 93 +
Prostate [73]	Non-obese, 25	68 (64–73)	M25	23.0 (21.5–24.3)	serum
	Obese, 37	64 (60–67)	M37	26.7 (25.7–27.6)	74.0 (59.4–88.1)
					75.0 (65.6–82.3)

Parentheses indicate the range of reported values. OSCC, oral squamous cell carcinoma; OPML, oral premalignant lesion; HCC, hepatocellular carcinoma; NSCLC, non-small cell lung cancer; GBM, malignant glioblastoma; ODC, oligodendrocytoma; NC CNS, non-cancer CNS disease; BPH, benign prostatic hyperplasia; WD, well differentiated prostate cancer (Gleason score ≤ 6); MD, moderately differentiated (Gleason 7); PD, poorly differentiated (Gleason ≥ 8). ‡ Number refers to the number of amino acids in the processed chemerin protein, † Significant compared to the other two groups; * significant compared to control group; + significant compared to other Gleason scores.

The mechanisms by which chemerin may contribute to esophageal tumor progression are multifaceted involving multiple cell types within the tumor microenvironment (Figure 1). One mechanism involves a paracrine interaction between chemerin-secreting CAMs and chemerin$_1$-expressing mesenchymal stromal cells (MSCs), leading to MSC migration into the tumor microenvironment (Figure 1, left). In in vitro transwell migration assays and transendothelial migration assays, chemerin stimulated the migration of MSCs via interactions with chemerin$_1$ but not chemerin$_2$ [57]. Notably, the effects on MSC migration were greater with conditioned media derived from esophageal CAMs versus that of ATMs [57]. These results were validated in an in vivo xenograft model, where BALB/c nu/nu mice injected S.C. with OE21 human esophageal carcinoma cells along with CAMs had more infiltrated MSCs than those mice injected with OE21 cells alone [57]. The in vivo homing of MSCs to the OE21 tumors was reduced by the chemerin$_1$ antagonist CCX832 confirming the effect was dependent on chemerin/chemerin$_1$ signaling. Evidence supported that chemerin/chemerin$_1$ signaling in the MSCs is relayed via protein kinase C (PKC) and subsequent phosphorylation and activation of protein kinases p42/44, p38 and JnkII, and matrix MMP-2 secretion, which contributes to the trans-endothelial migration of MSCs, potentially contributing to cancer progression [57]. The study by Kumar et al. went a step further by providing additional evidence for a contextual pro-cancer role for chemerin in these malignancies (Figure 1, right). Unlike with high concentrations of chemerin (20 ng/mL), low concentrations of chemerin (4 ng/mL) inhibited approximately 50% of chemerin/chemerin$_1$-mediated MSC migration through a 10-fold increase in the secretion of macrophage inhibitory factor (MIF) from MSCs [57]. The authors speculated that moderate levels of chemerin in normal tissue myofibroblasts (NTMs) would act to restrain MSC migration through the autoinhibitory action of MIF. However, in the tumor microenvironment, the MIF-inhibitory mechanism is released owing to higher chemerin concentrations in CAMs, increasing the capacity for recruiting MSCs to the tumor microenvironment [57].

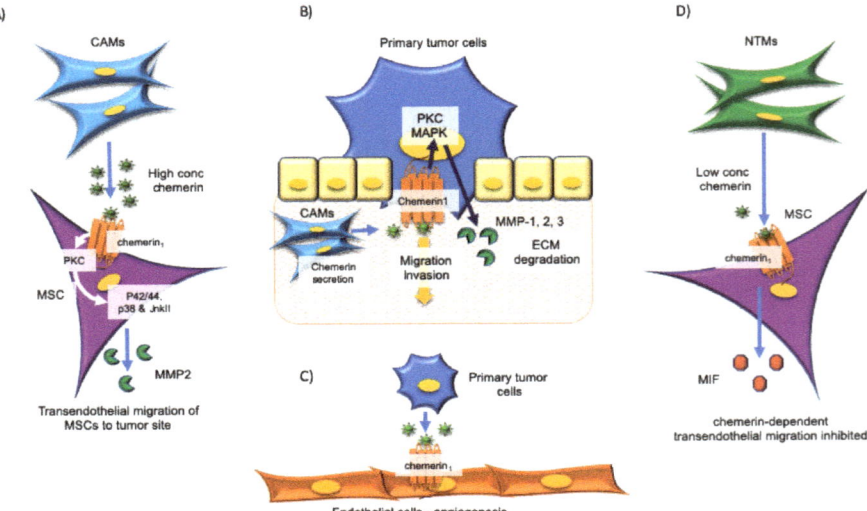

Figure 1. The mechanisms of tumor-promoting effects of chemerin in the esophageal carcinoma microenvironment. Chemerin is released from cancer-associated myofibroblasts (CAMs) and esophageal tumor cells and has autocrine and paracrine tumor-promoting effects in the esophageal carcinoma microenvironment. These include mediating mesenchymal stromal cell (MSC) transendothelial migration to the tumor site (**A**), tumor cell migration and invasion (**B**), and angiogenesis (**C**). In contrast, low chemerin concentrations inhibit MSC migration (**D**). ECM, extracellular matrix; MAPK, mitogen-activated protein kinase; MIF, macrophage inhibitory factor; MMP, matrix metalloproteinase; NTM, normal tissue myofibroblasts; PKC, protein kinase C.

A follow-up study by Kumar et al. expanded on this area of research by demonstrating paracrine interactions between chemerin-secreting CAMs and the chemerin$_1$-expressing esophageal cancer cell line OE21. Conditioned media from CAMs, more so than conditioned media from ATMs and NTMs, stimulated migration and Matrigel invasion of OE21 cells, which could be partially blocked by chemerin neutralization, siRNA knockdown of chemerin or chemerin$_1$, or pharmacological antagonism of chemerin$_1$ with CCX832 [56]. The invasion process was mediated through PKC- mitogen-activated protein kinase (MAPK) signaling but did not require phosphoinositide 3-kinase (PI3K) and led to MMP1, 2, and 3 secretion, which may facilitate invasion through extracellular matrix degradation (Figure 1, top-centre) [56].

Chemerin has previously been shown to stimulate angiogenesis [74,75]. Thus, interactions between tumor cell-secreted chemerin and chemerin$_1$-expressing endothelial cells leading to increased angiogenesis is another possible mechanism (Figure 1, bottom-centre). Supporting this idea, one study found that increased chemerin expression in SCCOT was strongly associated with increased microvessel density, an indicator of angiogenesis [55].

In the metaplasia–dysplasia–carcinoma sequence of Barrett's esophagus (BE) to high-grade dysplasia BE and esophageal carcinoma, a significant increase in myeloid dendritic cell (mDC) and plasmacytoid dendritic cell (pDC) density was observed that coincided with increased expression of their respective chemotactic factors, macrophage inflammatory protein-3 alpha (MIP3α), and chemerin in the same regions [76]. However, the metaplasia–dysplasia–carcinoma transition was also characterized by the infiltration of immune tolerogenic IL-10^{high} and IL-12^{low} mDCs, which stimulated the differentiation of immunosuppressive T regulatory (Treg) cells from naïve CD4$^+$ T cells [76]. Thus, while high tumor chemerin concentrations have an anti-tumoral effect in other cancers [52,77–79], these effects may be masked in the context of esophageal cancers because of an immune tolerogenic phenotype. Alternatively, chemerin could be contributing to the immune tolerogenic phenotype, but this remains to be determined experimentally.

5. Colorectal and Gastric Cancer

Similar to esophageal and oral cancers, the balance of clinical evidence indicates a positive association between serum chemerin concentrations and the risk for colorectal cancer [59,60,62,63] and gastric cancer as reviewed in greater detail by Treeck et al. [53] and originally reported by Wang et al. [64] and Zhang et al. [61] (Table 1). There is considerable variability among these studies with respect to reported absolute values for serum chemerin, possibly due to methodological differences. In spite of this variability, there is a consistent finding of elevated serum chemerin in gastric and colorectal cancer patients. There is also some uncertainty as to the linkage of chemerin to colorectal cancer owing to inherent differences (e.g., age) between the patient and control groups [59]. However, other studies have reported significantly higher circulating chemerin levels after considering potential confounds such as age, sex, BMI, waist circumference, and diet. For example, after adjusting for age and sex, Eichelmann et al. [60] reported an approximate 2-fold increase in overall risk for all colorectal cancers between the highest and lowest quartile of serum chemerin concentrations. This association was strongest for colon cancer (HR = 2.27) and specifically proximal colon cancer (HR 3.97) [60]. Consistent with these findings, Alkady et al. [62] reported that using a cut off of ≥ 161.5 ng/mL, serum chemerin had 100% sensitivity and 100% specificity for the presence of colorectal cancer. Increased serum chemerin was also found to correlate with general fatigue and other cancer-related symptoms in colorectal cancer patients [63]. Moreover, progressive increases in serum chemerin have been observed in patients with advanced stages of colorectal cancer [62]. Overall, these results support a cancer and stage-specific effect on serum chemerin concentrations. These studies are also in general agreement regarding the potential for the use of chemerin as a biomarker for colorectal cancer independent of inflammatory markers such as C-reactive peptide (CRP) [59,60,62].

In this issue, Treeck et al. [53], reported that high gastric tumor expression of chemerin, chemerin$_1$, and chemerin$_2$ were associated with shorter overall patient survival. Consistent with these findings, the results from several in vitro studies support a tumor-promoting role of chemerin signaling in gastric cancer (Figure 2). For example, Wang et al. [64] reported that exposure of human gastric cancer AGS or MKN28 cells to recombinant human chemerin promoted invasiveness in a dose-dependent fashion in Matrigel invasion assays. This was accompanied by increased expression of a panel of "pro-invasive" genes including *vascular endothelial growth factor (VEGF), Interleukin-6 (IL-6),* and *MMP-7* mRNA suggesting a mechanism whereby increased chemerin could increase the metastatic potential of gastric cancer cells [80–83]. When the invasion and gene expression assays were repeated in the presence of various MAPK inhibitors, the extracellular-related kinase (ERK) inhibitor UO126 most consistently blocked the effects of chemerin versus p38 and c-jUN N-terminal kinase (JNK) inhibitors, which were less effective. This suggested the effects of chemerin were primarily mediated by ERK signaling, a pathway with known involvement in the promotion of cell proliferation and migration [84]. However, there was no effect of chemerin on cell proliferation, a finding consistent with that of our research group which observed no effect of chemerin treatment on the proliferation or viability of AGS cells [85]. A new pathway for chemerin signaling through Gαi/o and RhoA/Rock was identified, which activates serum response factor regulated gene expression and chemotaxis of AGS cells [85]. It was postulated that these effects were chemerin$_2$ receptor-mediated, as AGS cells were found to express *chemerin$_2$* but not *chemerin$_1$*. In contrast, Kumar et al. detected both chemerin$_1$ and chemerin$_2$ proteins using immunohistochemistry in both primary gastric cancer cells and AGS cells [86]. Chemerin mRNA was not expressed in AGS cells [85] nor was secreted chemerin detected in the media of cultured

AGS cells [86]. However, chemerin was secreted by CAMs at concentrations sufficient to stimulate migration and morphological transformation of AGS cells [86] supporting a paracrine rather than autocrine mechanism of signaling. These effects of chemerin were inhibited by the putative chemerin receptor antagonists CCX832 and α-NETA [86]. Similarly, selective knockdown of either chemerin$_1$ or chemerin$_2$ resulted in inhibited migration and invasion in AGS cells, while simultaneous knockdown led to complete inhibition [86], supporting the functional signaling of chemerin$_1$ and chemerin$_2$ in AGS cells. These observations are consistent with clinical findings showing an increased risk for gastric cancer with increased serum chemerin. The study by Kumar et al. also uncovered the further complexity of chemerin signaling in gastric cancer by demonstrating that chemerin inhibited the secretion of tissue inhibitor of metalloproteinase 1 and 2 (TIMP -1/-2) via a PKC mediated pathway in AGS cells [86]. As TIMPs inhibit MMP activity, decreased secretion would be expected to increase metastatic and invasive potential [87]. Interestingly Treeck et al. reported that in contrast to chemerin$_1$ and chemerin$_2$, increased CCRL2 expression in gastric carcinoma was correlated with increased overall survival [53]. However, the mechanisms of this putative protective effect of CCRL2 remain unknown.

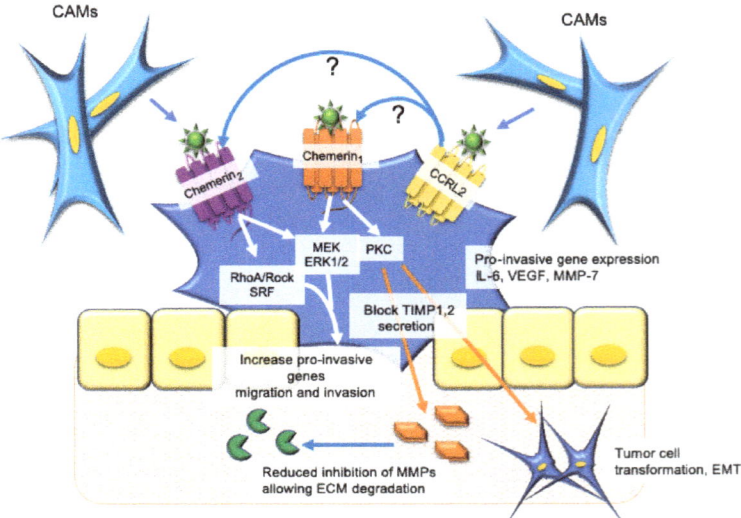

Figure 2. The mechanisms of tumor-promoting effects of chemerin in the gastric carcinoma microenvironment. Chemerin is released from cancer-associated myofibroblasts (CAMs) and acts on chemerin$_1$ and chemerin$_2$ receptors present on gastric carcinoma cells to activate several intracellular signaling pathways. Functionally this signaling leads to increased expression of pro-invasive genes, reduced secretion of tissue inhibitor of metalloproteinase 1, 2 (TIMP-1/2), and enhanced production of matrix metalloproteinases (MMPs) leading to migration and invasion of tumor cells and tumor cell transformation resembling an epithelial–to–mesenchymal transformation (EMT). It is unknown (?) how and if CCRL2-bound chemerin interacts with chemerin$_1$ and chemerin$_2$ to influence the tumor-promoting effects of chemerin signaling in gastric carcinoma. ECM, extracellular matrix; ERK1/2, extracellular-related kinase 1/2; IL-6, interleukin 6; MAPK, mitogen-activated protein kinase; PKC, protein kinase C; VEGF, vascular endothelial growth factor.

Expression of the non-signaling chemerin receptor, *CCRL2*, was reported to be reduced by about 2/3 in colorectal cancer patients versus disease-free controls [88]. Unlike chemerin, there was no correlation in *CCRL2* mRNA levels with colorectal cancer stage [88]. While CCRL2 expression was detectable in several colorectal cell lines (SW480, SW620, LS174T, Caco2), siRNA-mediated knockdown of *CCRL2* mRNA reduced proliferation, colony formation and migration only in LS174T cells [88].

When rat CC531 colorectal cancer cells were injected into the rat portal vein for liver colonization assays, the initial low *CCRL2* mRNA levels increased during initial colonization of the liver [88]. This suggests a linkage to tumor cell migration or invasion. Whether or not the increased CCRL2 facilitates chemerin interactions with chemerin$_1$ or chemerin$_2$ within this context remains to be determined.

6. Skin Cancer

In contrast to the aforementioned cancers, both melanoma and skin squamous cell carcinoma have been associated with decreased expression of chemerin mRNA and protein [52,89]. Available evidence suggests that this may promote skin cancer progression and tumor growth through a reduction in the recruitment of immune cells to the tumor microenvironment via chemerin-dependent mechanisms. Consistent with this, tumors with higher *chemerin* expression were associated with improved clinical outcomes in melanoma [52]. The same study found that an intratumoral injection of chemerin into a B16 transplantable mouse melanoma model resulted in reduced tumor growth [52]. The beneficial effects of chemerin in reducing melanoma progression appear to be mediated primarily through the recruitment of NK cells, and to a lesser extent, other immune effectors such as T and B cells to the tumor microenvironment [52]. In contrast, it was found that chemerin played little to no role in the activation of NK cells and had no discernible direct effects on melanoma cells [52].

Chemerin also appears to have an important role in regulating the ratio between beneficial and harmful immune cells in the tumor microenvironment (Figure 3). As the name suggests, myeloid-derived suppressor cells (MDSCs) originate from the myeloid-lineage and contribute to tumor progression via the suppression of appropriate immune responses [90]. MDSCs exert additional pro-cancer effects through the upregulation of angiogenic and metastatic factors in the tumor microenvironment [90]. Localized chemerin expression in melanoma was associated with an increase in the ratio of immune effectors (i.e., NK cells, T cells, and dendritic cells) to MDSCs in the tumor microenvironment, ultimately enhancing anti-tumor responses [52]. Additionally, pDCs play a significant role in melanoma and have been associated with poor clinical outcomes through the development of an immunosuppressive microenvironment [91]. Normally pDCs promote anti-viral immunity, but in melanoma, the suppression of type I interferon (IFN I) production by pDCs triggers immunosuppressive mechanisms including the recruitment of Treg cells to the tumor microenvironment [91]. Localized chemerin expression in melanoma has been demonstrated to decrease the presence of pDCs in the tumor microenvironment, ultimately inhibiting immune escape mechanisms [52].

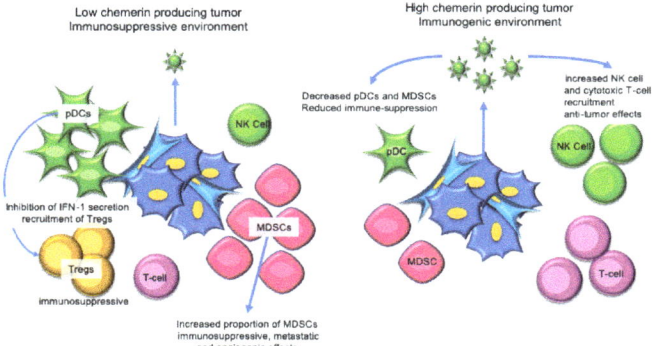

Figure 3. Chemerin has immune-mediated tumor-suppressive effects in melanoma. In low chemerin-producing melanoma tumors, there is an increased presence of myeloid-derived suppressor cells (MDSCs), plasmacytoid dendritic cells (pDCs), and regulatory T-cells (Tregs), which result in a tumor-promoting immunosuppressive environment. When melanomas produce higher amounts of chemerin, there is a switch to a tumor-suppressing immunogenic environment characterized by increased natural killer (NK) cell and cytotoxic T-cell infiltration and reduced infiltration of MDSCs and pDCs.

7. Hepatocellular Carcinoma

Similar to skin cancer, a number of studies support an anticancer role for chemerin in human hepatocellular carcinoma [77,78,92]. Collectively, these studies suggested that in certain hepatocellular carcinomas, hepatic chemerin production may be lowered, thus facilitating further advancement of the disease [77]. In contrast, increased serum chemerin concentrations have been associated with more favorable clinical characteristics, such as reduced tumor size, differentiation, and stage and indicate the potential value of chemerin as a prognostic factor for disease-free survival [78,92]. The clinical associations between chemerin signaling and hepatocellular carcinoma have been described in detail by Treeck et al. in this issue [53].

To explore the mechanisms underlying the clinical associations between chemerin signaling and hepatocellular carcinoma, Lin et al. and Li et al. utilized mouse models in which chemerin expression was manipulated in several complementary manners [77,92]. Mice injected in the left ventricle with chemerin-overexpressing portal vein tumor thrombus cells (PVTT-1-Che) only rarely developed metastatic foci, while those injected with control PVTT-1 cells consistently developed metastases at distant sites throughout the body [77]. Similarly, mice injected hepatically with PVTT-1-Che cells exhibited reduced liver tumor foci development, a 1.3-fold increase in survival (54 days versus 41 days) compared to mice injected with control PVTT-1 cells [77]. This lessening of metastasis and prolongation of survival was recapitulated by the intraventricular or intraperitoneal injection of recombinant chemerin to mice that also had an intraventricular or hepatic injection of control PVTT-1 cells [77]. Likewise, when implanted with Hepa1-6 tumor cells, chemerin knockout mice (chemerin$^{-/-}$) developed larger liver tumors, more frequent lung metastasis and showed significantly increased mortality as compared to the wild type mice [92]. Overexpression of chemerin in Hepa1-6 cells resulted in decreased mortality and decreased liver tumor growth compared to control Hepa1-6 cells injected into wild-type mice [92].

The study by Lin et al. supports that the hepatocellular protective effects of chemerin are immune-mediated involving a shift from tumor-infiltrating immunosuppressive and angiogenesis-stimulating MSDCs to tumor-suppressing interferon γ-secreting T cells (IFNγ^+T) (Figure 4). In support of this conclusion, Hepa1-6 tumors in chemerin$^{-/-}$ mice displayed increased proportions of MDSCs, tumor-associated macrophages (TAMs) and decreased IFNγ-expressing T-helper CD4$^+$ and cytotoxic CD8$^+$ T cells compared to Hepa1-6 tumors in wild-type mice [92]. Consistent with this result, chemerin-overexpression caused a shift from MDSCs to IFN-γ^+ T cells in the Hepa1-6 tumors [92]. An impairment but not a complete abolition of the hepatocellular carcinoma-inhibiting effect of chemerin was observed in T-cell and B-cell deficient Rag1-/- mice and CD8+ T cell-depleted mice confirming a partial role of CD8+ T cells in the antitumoral effects of chemerin [92]. There were no differences in Tregs or pDCs regardless of chemerin expression in the Hepa1-6 tumors [92]. Furthermore, there was no difference in tumor-infiltrating NK cells, which is consistent with the weak but significant positive correlation observed between human hepatocellular carcinoma chemerin expression levels and recruitment number of dendritic cells and NK cells to the tumor site [78,92]. A series of in vitro and in vivo experiments probed the cellular and molecular mechanisms of chemerin suppression of hepatocellular carcinoma progression. These studies identified that chemerin interacts with chemerin$_1$ and CCLR2 to inhibit nuclear factor kappa B (NF-κB) signaling in tumor cells and endothelial cells. This leads to reduced production and secretion of the pro-tumorigenic factors, granulocyte-macrophage colony-stimulating factor (GM-CSF) from tumor cells and IL-6 from hepatocytes, which in turn suppress the numbers of tumor-infiltrating MDSCs and allows for a restoration of T-cell immunity and reduced angiogenesis in the tumor microenvironment [92].

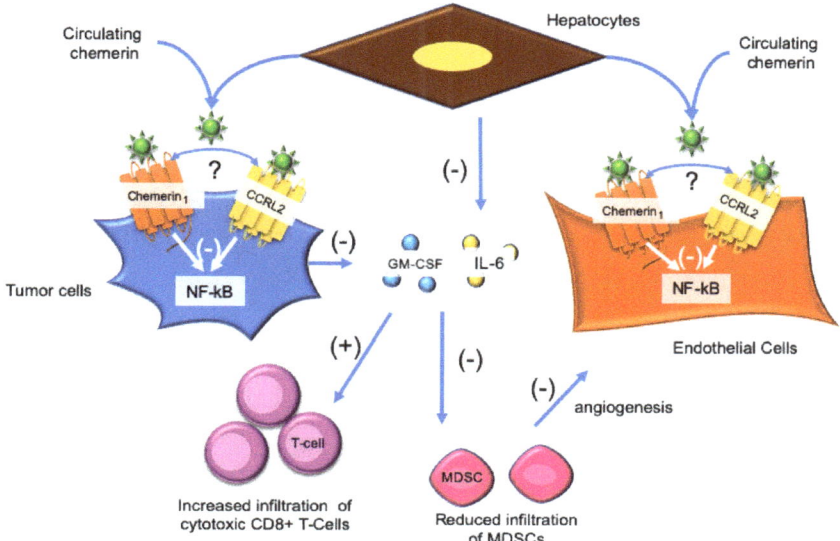

Figure 4. Chemerin has immune-mediated tumor-suppressive effects in hepatocellular carcinoma. Systemic or hepatocyte-secreted chemerin interacts with chemerin$_1$ and CCLR2 on hepatocellular carcinoma cells and endothelial cells to inhibit nuclear factor kappa B (NF-κB) signaling. By unknown mechanisms, this leads to reduced secretion of granulocyte-macrophage colony-stimulating factor (GM-CSF) from tumor cells and IL-6 from hepatocytes. In turn, this leads to reduced tumor infiltration of immunosuppressive and pro-angiogenic myeloid-derived suppressor cells (MDSCs) and increased infiltration of cytotoxic CD8+ T-cells. It is unknown (?) how and if CCRL2-bound chemerin interacts with chemerin$_1$. (−) = Reduction or suppression of a normal pathway and (+) Increase of a normal pathway.

Adding to the complexity of the actions of chemerin in this context, Li et al. demonstrated the protective effects of chemerin on the progression of hepatocellular carcinoma also involve autocrine effects of tumor cell-secreted chemerin [77]. These included a reduction in migration and invasion of multiple hepatocellular carcinoma cell lines in the presence of chemerin overexpression and a reversal of this effect with chemerin neutralizing antibodies [77]. In agreement with other studies, there was no impact of chemerin on hepatocellular carcinoma proliferation and apoptosis. Mechanistically, when chemerin concentrations were low, chemerin$_1$ physically interacted with the tumor suppressor phosphatase and tensin homolog (PTEN) as demonstrated by immunoprecipitation assays (Figure 5). This led to greater ubiquitination of PTEN, lowering its activity and suppressive effects on protein kinase B (AKT) activation. On the other hand, when chemerin concentrations were increased, the interaction between chemerin$_1$ and PTEN was disrupted, reducing PTEN ubiquitination and increasing its activity. In turn, AKT activation by phosphorylation was inhibited suppressing migration, invasion, and metastasis of hepatocellular carcinoma cells. Notably, in the study by Li et al., MMP-1 was increased along with AKT, whereas PTEN was decreased in metastatic foci of mice with PVTT control tumors. The opposite pattern was observed in metastatic foci of mice with PVTT-Che tumors. This suggested the antitumor effects of chemerin involve, in part, MPP-1 which is active in the promotion of tumor migration through proteolytic functions [87].

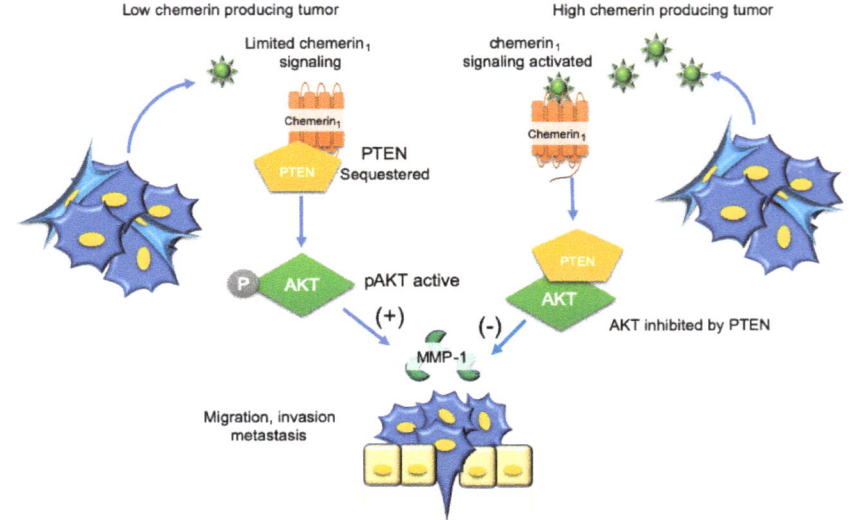

Figure 5. Hepatocellular carcinoma-derived chemerin inhibits tumor cell migration, invasion, and metastasis via an autocrine mechanism. When chemerin production by hepatocellular carcinoma is low (left) there is limited autocrine signaling through chemerin$_1$. This results in sequestering of the tumor suppressor phosphatase and tensin homolog (PTEN) through a direct physical interaction with chemerin$_1$, allowing for the activation of protein kinase B (AKT) and secretion of matrix metalloproteinase 1 (MMP-1), which is thought to facilitate migration, invasion, and metastasis. When chemerin production by hepatocellular carcinoma is high (right), chemerin$_1$ signaling is activated, the chemerin$_1$-PTEN complex is disrupted, allowing PTEN inhibition of AKT and blockade of migration, invasion, and metastasis of hepatocellular carcinoma. (+) = Activation, (−) inhibition.

A recent study by Sun et al. reported a modest inhibitory effect of chemerin on the proliferation of SMMC7721 human hepatoma cells but not QSG7701 immortalized human hepatic cells [93]. This appeared to be a result of S-phase cell cycle block involving reductions in p53, p27, and p21 proteins. Interestingly, the mechanism involved downregulation of iron transporters and regulatory proteins, including the divalent metal transporter, transferrin, transferrin receptors 1 and 2, iron regulatory proteins 1 and 2 and ferritin-H, and ferritin-L leading to decreased cellular iron concentrations [93]. Consistent with this, iron supplementation reversed the effects of chemerin on S-phase cell cycle block and p53, p27, and p21 proteins. The results of this study contrast with others that did not observe effects of chemerin on cell proliferation or apoptosis [77,92,93]. The reason for the discrepancy is not certain, but it could relate to the different cell lines used in the three studies. Furthermore, it is worth noting that the SMMC7721 and QSG7701 cells are potentially HeLa derivatives as they have been listed as being at risk for contamination [94,95].

Not all studies support a clear relationship between chemerin and hepatocellular carcinoma. For example, Imai et al. detected no significant difference in recurrence-free survival or disease-free survival between patients classified with having low (≤ 130.5 ng/mL) and high (> 130.5 ng/mL) serum chemerin concentration [65]. Furthermore, no association was found between serum chemerin and clinical stage of hepatocellular carcinoma in this study [65]. However, a correlation was observed between serum chemerin concentration and severity of liver disease suggesting that with advancing liver disease, hepatic chemerin production decreases and may increase the risk for further advancement of hepatocellular carcinoma [65]. Haberl et al. utilized a mouse model of low methionine-choline deficient diet-induced non-alcoholic steatohepatitis (NASH) compared to NASH with dimethylnitrosamine-induced hepatocarcinoma (NASH-HCC) to evaluate the function of chemerin in NASH-HCC. Hepatic and serum chemerin, as well as ex vivo activation of chemerin$_1$, did not differ in the two models. The authors concluded that tumors still develop despite high endogenous levels of serum and liver chemerin protein [96].

8. Adrenocortical Carcinoma

Adrenocortical carcinoma is a rare, aggressive form of cancer with poor prognosis [97]. Through microarray analysis to identify gene signatures of potential diagnostic value, a substantial downregulation of *chemerin* expression in adrenocortical carcinoma versus benign adrenal adenomas was discovered in two independent cohorts [98,99]. These findings have been replicated in additional independent sample cohorts, which also included a comparison to control non-cancerous adrenal tissue [79,100]. *Chemerin* expression was highest in control tissue, followed by an intermediate expression in the benign adrenal adenomas and lowest in the carcinomas. A positive correlation was observed for immunohistochemical detection of the chemerin protein in paired samples, providing evidence that reduced *chemerin* expression coincides with reduced chemerin protein [79]. The mechanism of reduced *chemerin* expression in adrenocortical carcinoma appears to be through repressive hypermethylation at 5 CpG sites, which could be reversed by the DNA-methyltransferase inhibitor decitabine [79].

Despite the significantly lower *chemerin* expression, a survival analysis of four independent data sets comparing subjects with the highest (top 50%) to lowest (bottom 50%) *chemerin* expression within adrenocortical carcinoma tissue revealed no significant difference [100]. Somewhat paradoxically, serum chemerin concentrations were increased in adrenocortical carcinoma subjects versus those with benign adenoma or healthy controls and were positively associated with longer overall survival [100]. To further assess the relationship between adrenal *chemerin* expression and serum chemerin concentrations, the researchers xenografted immunodeficient scid-γ mice with H295R adrenocortical carcinoma cells with and without human *chemerin* overexpression. The tumors, with higher *chemerin* expression, had higher serum human chemerin. Based on this result, the authors rationalized that since chemerin decreases in adrenocortical tumors, the increased serum chemerin concentration must be due to chemerin secretion from tissues other than the adrenals, but the exact tissues were not identified. Adipose tissue was ruled out as a contributor to increased serum chemerin for a number of reasons, but this was not confirmed experimentally [100]. Interestingly, mice transplanted with human *chemerin*-expressing H295R tumors had higher serum concentrations of human chemerin but proportionally lower mouse serum chemerin suggesting a type of negative regulatory feedback mechanism. The overall findings led the authors to reasonably postulate that the reduction in adrenal tumor chemerin concentrations could be an immune avoidance mechanism, but increased serum chemerin may counteract this in some individuals resulting in improved anti-tumor immune responses. While not tested in this study, it represents an interesting idea for a follow-up.

To evaluate the functional effects of chemerin in adrenocortical carcinoma, Li-Chittenden et al. performed a series of in vitro studies comparing the effects of transient human chemerin overexpression in H295R and SW13 adrenocortical carcinoma or HEK293 human embryonic kidney cells to exogenous chemerin treatment [79]. The effects of the transient transfection were cell-dependent and reduced the proliferation of the HEK293 cells and the cell invasion of the H295R cells but had no effect on proliferation or invasion of the SW13 cells. Furthermore, the transient transfection of the chemerin construct did not affect the migration of any of the cancer cell lines. Treatment with physiological levels of active chemerin had no impact on cell proliferation, invasion, or migration. The differential effects of chemerin overexpression versus exogenous treatment have also been observed with respect to adipocyte function [101]. While the exact mechanism is unknown, possibilities include differential post-translation processing of recombinant chemerin in a bacterial system versus in human cells, differential proteolytic processing of endogenous chemerin, or novel intracellular functions independent from chemerin$_1$ and chemerin$_2$ function. In support of the latter possibility, the cells tested in this study had barely detectable chemerin$_1$ [79]. However, no assessment of chemerin$_2$ levels was made. In further support of a direct tumor suppressive (rather than immune-mediated) effect of chemerin, H295R cells with stable expression of human chemerin had decreased colony formation and invasion in in vitro assays and formed smaller tumors when xenografted into the flanks immunodeficient T-cell deficient athymic nude and T, B, and NK-cell deficient and macrophage and dendritic cell-impaired NOD Scid γ mice. Further probing the tumor-suppressive mechanisms revealed that chemerin inhibits the Wnt/β catenin pathway, which is commonly activated in adrenocortical carcinoma and associated with higher tumor grades and decreased overall survival and disease-free survival (Figure 6) [102–104]. Thus, a reduction of chemerin in benign adrenal adenoma and adrenocortical carcinoma would be expected to lead to increased Wnt/β-catenin activity. Whether this plays a role in the initiation of adrenocortical carcinoma remains to be determined. The findings of Li-Chittenden et al. are consistent with previous studies in mesenchymal stem cells that showed chemerin$_1$ is a Wnt responsive gene that functions as a negative feedback regulator of the Wnt/β-catenin signaling pathway [105]. Thus, it would be interesting to determine if the low chemerin$_1$ expression is a factor that contributes to activation in Wnt/β-catenin activation in adrenocortical carcinoma. A second possible tumor-suppressive mechanism is through inhibition of p38 MAPK signaling.

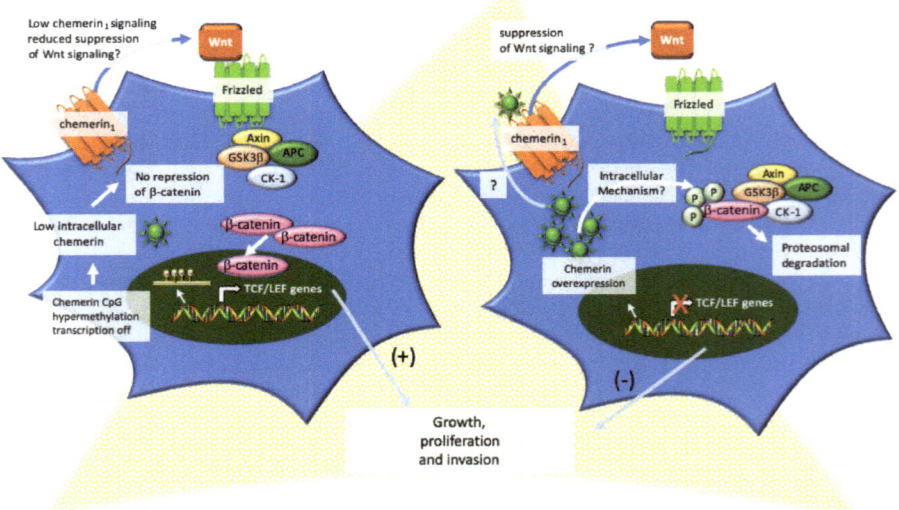

Figure 6. Endogenously derived chemerin mediates a tumor-suppressive effect through inhibition of Wnt/β-catenin signaling in adrenocortical carcinoma. In adrenocortical carcinoma, chemerin expression becomes suppressed due to CpG hypermethylation resulting in low intracellular chemerin concentrations. β-catenin accumulates and migrates to the nucleus where TCF/LEF genes are turned on mediating (+) cell growth, proliferation, and invasion. Based on the known feedback inhibition of chemerin$_1$ on Wnt/β-catenin signaling, it is also possible that low chemerin$_1$ expression could contribute to the activation of Wnt/β-catenin in adrenocortical carcinoma cells. When tumor chemerin production is increased, by unknown (?) intracellular mechanisms (and possibly autocrine signaling through chemerin$_1$), β-catenin is targeted for phosphorylation and proteasomal degradation reducing the expression of TCF/LEF genes and inhibiting (−) cell growth, proliferation, and invasion. APC, APC Regulator of Wnt Signaling Pathway; GSK3β, glycogen synthase kinase 3β; CK-1, casein kinase 1. (?) unknown or possible but unconfirmed mechanism.

9. Renal Carcinoma

An analysis of chemerin expression in RNA sequencing data available in the Cancer Genome Atlas (TCGA) and Genotype-Tissue Expression (GTEx) projects using the Gene Expression Profiling

Interactive Analysis (GEPIA) web server revealed that papillary renal cell carcinoma (pRCC) has significantly upregulated *chemerin* expression (Figure 7a) [106]. This is opposite to the majority of tumors that display decreased *chemerin*. While there is little information regarding the potential impact of elevated chemerin expression in renal carcinoma, a recent study sheds some light on the matter [107]. pRCC accounts for approximately 20% of all renal cancers. A unique feature of pRCC is the focal aggregation of foam cell macrophages inside the papillae. In the study by Krawczyk et al., foamy macrophages were histologically identified in 82% of pRCC tumors and the macrophages expressed cell surface markers CD689 and CD163 that are characteristic of the M2 anti-inflammatory phenotype [107]. The researchers hypothesized that the pRCC cells must secrete factors that recruit monocytes and contribute to their differentiation into foamy macrophages. Utilizing freshly isolated primary pRCC cultures, the prototypical monocyte chemoattract proteins were not detected in conditioned media. Rather the most abundant secreted cytokines/chemokines were chemerin, interleukin-8 (IL-8), and CXCL16. Confirming their hypothesis, these cytokines, alone or in combination, stimulated the migration of human monocytes in transwell chemotaxis assays. Furthermore, conditioned pRCC medium shifted macrophages from an M1 to M2 phenotype and promoted their lipid accumulation. Thus, it is possible that elevated chemerin expression in pRCC could contribute to monocyte recruitment and differentiation into lipid-containing foam cells. However, the exact role chemerin on pRCC tumor biology and the tumor microenvironment is not known. A GEPIA survival analysis conducted with data from TCGA and GTEx indicated the quartile of patients with the highest tumor *chemerin* expression had better overall survival than those in the lowest quartile (Figure 7b), providing preliminary support that the differential *chemerin* expression could be functionally important in pRCC [106].

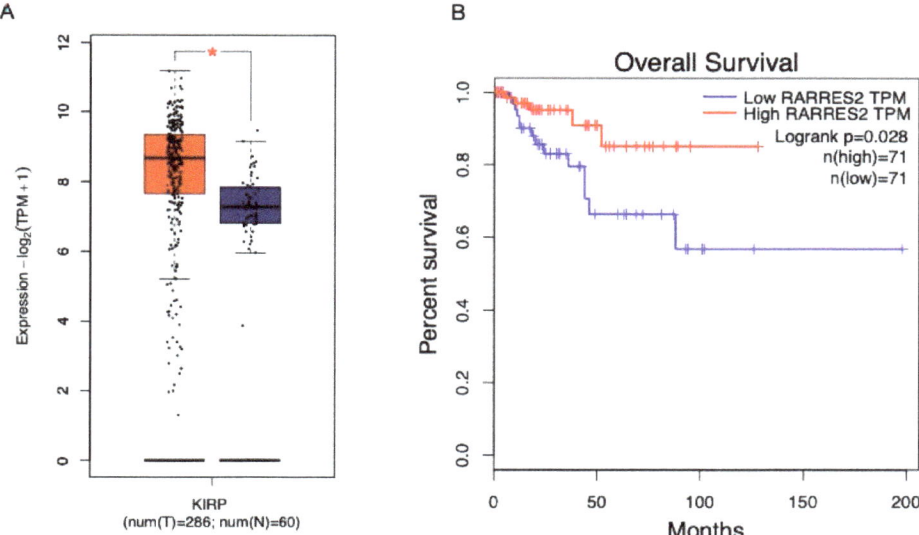

Figure 7. Chemerin expression is increased in papillary renal cell carcinoma (pRCC or KIRP) and is associated with higher overall survival. The Gene Expression Profiling Interactive Analysis (GEPIA) web server [106] was used for RNA sequencing expression analysis of *chemerin* in pRCC (red bar) and normal renal samples (blue bar) from the Cancer Genome Atlas (TCGA) and Genotype-Tissue Expression (GTEx) projects (**A**). The GEPIA web server survival analysis tool [106] was used to compare the overall survival of the quartile of pRCC patients with the highest *chemerin* expression (red line) versus the quartile of pRCC patients with the lowest *chemerin* expression (blue line) (**B**). * $p < 0.01$. TPM, transcripts per kilobase million.

10. Thyroid Cancer

Thyroid carcinoma is the most common of the endocrine cancers, typically affects women more than men, and is most often observed in the fourth and fifth decades of life. Thyroid cancer is an obesity-associated cancer with increased risk with increasing BMI and weight gain [6,108]. The mechanisms linking obesity to thyroid cancer are not completely understood, but there has been considerable interest in the role of adipocytokines. Recently, Warakomski et al. sought to evaluate the relationship between serum chemerin, IL-6, leptin, and adiponectin and papillary thyroid cancer [66]. Overweight or obese patients (BMI > 25 kg/m^2) did not have larger tumor sizes but were more often at an advanced clinical stage (II, III, or IV). While the overweight and obese subjects had higher preoperative serum chemerin (Table 1), there was no specific association between serum chemerin concentration and clinical stage. However, those subjects with higher leptin and IL-6 tended to have a more advanced clinical stage. While a direct association of chemerin with papillary thyroid cancer could not be determined in this study, there were a number of important limitations. First, the majority of study subjects (144) were diagnosed with stage I cancer, and thus, the sample size may have been too small for the advanced clinical stages to determine a relationship. Second, the study only evaluated serum chemerin concentration and did not perform any functional studies. GEPIA Analysis [106] of RNA sequencing data shows that *chemerin* and *chemerin$_1$* are expressed in thyroid tissue and significantly downregulated in thyroid cancer samples (Figure 8). *Chemerin$_2$* and *CCRL2* expression were lower and did not differ between tumor samples and normal thyroid tissue. It would be interesting for future studies to evaluate the relevance of *chemerin* and *chemerin$_1$* downregulation to thyroid tumor biology and if chemerin signaling has direct effects on thyroid cancer cells.

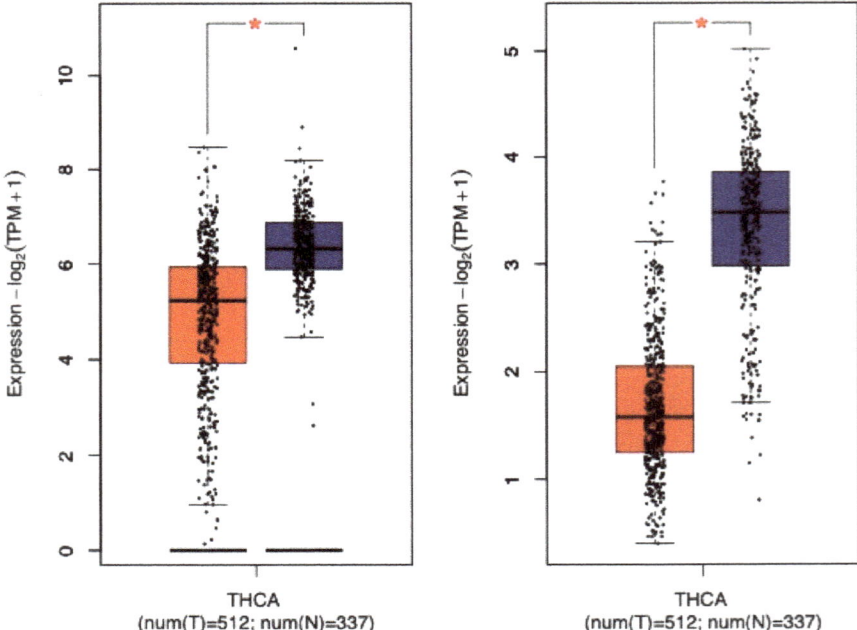

Figure 8. *Chemerin* and *chemerin$_1$* are decreased in thyroid carcinoma (THCA). The Gene Expression Profiling Interactive Analysis (GEPIA) web server [106] was used for RNA sequencing expression analysis of *chemerin* and *chemerin$_1$* in thyroid carcinoma (red bars) and normal renal samples (blue bars) from the Cancer Genome Atlas (TCGA) and Genotype-Tissue Expression (GTEx) projects. * $p < 0.01$. TPM, transcripts per kilobase million.

11. Breast Cancer

Studies of the relevance of chemerin to breast cancer have provided conflicting results. As reviewed in greater detail by Treeck et al. [53], and originally reported by El-Sagheer et al. [109], chemerin protein expression was higher in cancerous versus adjacent healthy tissues and in metastatic lymph nodes compared to non-metastatic malignant tissues. Tumour chemerin expression was also negatively correlated with estrogen and progesterone receptor levels as well as five-year-disease-free survival rates [109]. In contrast, Pachynski et al. [110] reported that increased *chemerin* expression promoted the recruitment of immune effector cells to the tumor microenvironment and thus, initiated anti-cancer effects. An analysis of several breast cancer databases revealed that *chemerin* expression was significantly downregulated in malignant breast tissue compared to adjacent healthy tissue and that low *chemerin* expression was associated with poorer survival outcomes [110]. Consistent with this, quantitative real-time PCR and in situ hybridization demonstrated significantly lower *chemerin* expression in invasive/infiltrating ductal carcinoma and invasive/infiltrating lobular carcinoma tissues versus healthy breast tissue samples [110]. These studies demonstrate an interesting finding that while *chemerin* expression is downregulated in breast cancer tissues, protein expression is upregulated. These findings suggest the potential for translational and post-translational regulatory mechanisms in breast cancer cells, which differentially affect chemerin mRNA and protein expression. Further research is required to determine the cause of the inverse relationship between these expression levels.

Pachynski et al. [110] also examined the impact of chemerin expression levels in the EMT6 murine model of mammary carcinoma. While lentiviral-induced expression of chemerin did not impact cell proliferation in vitro, tumors generated from high chemerin-secreting (HCS) EMT6 clones exhibited significantly lower growth compared to those derived from low chemerin-secreting (LCS) secreting or control EMT6 cells in an in vivo xenograft model [110]. Furthermore, there was a significant increase in the relative proportions of T cells, CD4+ T cells, and NK cells in the HCS-EMT6 tumors compared to controls, and this was associated with tumor suppression [110]. Depletion experiments indicated a critical role of NK cells and CD8+ T cells in the tumor suppression response to chemerin, while the depletion of CD4+ T regulatory cells enhanced tumor suppression [110]. Thus, a plausible mechanism by which chemerin may affect breast cancer progression is via the recruitment of immune cells to the tumor microenvironment. In contrast to the findings of Pachynski et al. [110], El-Sagheer et al. [109] suggested a potential for pro-tumorigenic effects via the influence on the breast cancer stem cell (BCSC) phenotype. It is well established that inflammatory cytokines can promote epithelial–to–mesenchymal transformation and angiogenesis, among other pro-cancer effects [111,112]. Notably, IL-6, a pro-inflammatory cytokine secreted by several immune cell types, has been shown to play a role in inducing the de-differentiation of malignant cells to BCSCs [111,113]. Although research is limited, it is believed that BCSCs contribute to tumor progression and poor prognosis in breast cancer patients [112,114]. The possibility that chemerin-mediated recruitment of immune effectors to the tumor microenvironment contributes to poor prognosis via the promotion of BCSC phenotype is an intriguing possibility that remains to be experimentally tested.

Akin et al. [67] reported correlations between serum chemerin concentrations and several clinical factors such as diabetes, age of diagnosis, BMI, hypertension, and menopause, but found no significant difference between serum chemerin levels in breast cancer patients with metastatic and non-metastatic cancer (Table 1). While these findings suggest that serum chemerin is not associated with breast cancer stage, an important limitation of this study was the lack of a control group without breast cancer. Thus, further studies are needed to determine if there is a relationship between chemerin levels and breast cancer, per se.

As reviewed in greater detail by Treeck et al. [53], and originally reported by Sarmadi et al., expression of the atypical chemokine receptor, CCRL2, has been observed in human malignant breast tissues samples, but not in adjacent non-cancerous tissues and exhibited no significant association with stage [115]. It has been hypothesized that due to the ability of CCRL2 to sequester chemerin and thereby limit its ability to act on signaling receptors, the upregulation of CCRL2 in malignant breast tissues may function as an immune evasion mechanism [115]. However, this idea conflicts with observations in hepatocellular carcinoma, where chemerin$_1$ and CCRL2 appear to act cooperatively in inhibiting infiltration of MDSCs into the tumor microenvironment [92].

12. Ovarian Cancer

In the seminal study that identified chemerin as a ligand for chemerin$_1$, chemerin was found to be abundant in ascitic fluid of ovarian cancer patients [42]. The authors suggested that chemerin signaling through chemerin$_1$ could be involved in diseases with a strong inflammatory component, such as autoimmune disorders and cancer [42]. While this study provided the first suggestion that chemerin could be involved in ovarian cancer, research in this area is very limited. As reviewed in greater detail by Treeck et al. [53], and reported originally by Hoffman et al. [116] and Reverchon et al. [117], experimental evidence exists for differential expression of chemerin and the cognate receptors, as well as the biological impact of this signaling pathway in several ovary cell types (normal and cancerous). However, further research is necessary to determine the impact on ovarian cancer development, progression, and the efficacy of hormonal therapies.

13. Central Nervous System Cancers

At present, investigation of the relevance of chemerin and the cognate receptors to cancers of the nervous system is very limited. Tummler et al. [118] reported that expression of chemerin$_1$, but not chemerin$_2$, was elevated (versus neural crest and benign neurofibroma cells) in tumors from patients with neuroblastoma, a pediatric cancer of the peripheral nervous system. Moreover, a significant correlation was found between high expression of chemerin$_1$, chemerin$_2$, or CCRL2 and a decrease in overall survival probability. Exogenous chemerin stimulated MAPK and Akt phosphorylation, increased calcium mobilization and MMP-2 secretion from neuroblastoma SK-N-AS cells, while treatment with the putative chemerin$_1$ inhibitor α-NETA reduced the viability and clonogenicity of these cells. Consistent with the latter, α-NETA impaired tumor growth in vivo in a murine SK-N-AS xenograft model. Taken together, these data provide evidence that chemerin/CMKLR1 signaling promotes neuroblastoma development through direct effects on tumor cells and the tumor microenvironment.

Zhao [46] reported that while the relatively inactive chemerin isoform chemerin163 is the major contributor (~80%) to total plasma chemerin, the majority (~55%) of cerebrospinal fluid chemerin is comprised of the bioactive isoforms chemerin158 and chemerin157. Silico analysis of published microarray datasets indicated that chemerin, but not *chemerin$_1$* or *CCRL2* mRNA levels were elevated in grade III and IV (malignant) tumors compared with grade II glioma [46]. Furthermore, treatment of human U-87 MG glioblastoma cells with chemerin157 triggered a dose-dependent transient increase of intracellular calcium levels. Taken together, these data reinforce the concept that anatomical locations can differ with respect to the spectrum of chemerin isoforms and indicate that glioblastoma cells both secrete and respond to chemerin. However, it is important to note that chemerin has not been linked to glioblastoma outcomes nor to biological effects that directly or indirectly promote the malignancy of glioblastoma cells.

14. Lung Cancer

Much of the research into the role of chemerin in lung cancer stems from clinical studies of patients with non-small cell lung carcinoma (NSCLC). Several clinical studies have reported that patients with lung cancer had higher circulating chemerin concentrations than controls and/or that serum chemerin concentrations were positively associated with several clinical parameters including stage, lymph node infiltration, and distant metastasis (Table 1) [68–70,119]. While higher serum chemerin concentrations are generally associated with pro-cancer effects in NSCLC, many findings point to a role of localized chemerin in promoting anti-cancer effects via the recruitment of NK cells to the tumor microenvironment [120,121]. Thus, a downregulation of chemerin secretion by tumor cells may promote immune evasion and consequently, poor clinical outcomes. Further empirical research is required to fill in the current gaps in the literature with respect to the causal effect of chemerin on lung cancer development and progression, as well as its effects on biological indicators of cancer such as proliferation, metastasis, and invasion. We refer the interested reader to the article by Treeck et al. [53] in this issue that provides a more complete assessment of chemerin in NSCLC.

15. Pancreatic Cancer

Patients that are positive for pancreatic ductal adenocarcinoma exhibit significantly higher plasma chemerin concentration than healthy volunteers (Table 1) [71]. Despite this marked difference between pancreatic cancer patients and healthy controls, this study found no significant correlation between cancer stage and plasma concentration of chemerin, nor any correlation between chemerin concentration and resectable versus unresectable tumors [71]. The authors proposed that chemerin concentration could be used as a biomarker for the presence of cancer, where a plasma concentration of >219.67 ng/mL showed 80% sensitivity and 83% specificity for the presence of disease [71].

16. Prostate Cancer

No significant difference in serum chemerin concentration was found between patients with prostate cancer and those with benign prostatic hyperplasia, however, differences were identified between cancer patients with different Gleason scores, a progressive measurement of prostate cancer aggressiveness as determined by tumor cell differentiation [72]. Serum chemerin concentration was observed to increase with Gleason score, where tumors with a score of ≥8, 7, and ≤6 were significantly different from one another [72]. There was also a positive correlation between the serum levels of chemerin and IL-6 [72]. Comparing non-obese to obese patients with prostate cancer who subsequently underwent radical prostatectomy, there was no significant difference found in serum chemerin concentration based on BMI prior to surgery (Table 1) [73]. Furthermore, serum chemerin was not found to be a predictive factor for advanced tumor stage in the overall population nor in patients with a BMI of > 25 kg/m^2 [73]. These latter findings argue against a role of adipose-derived chemerin in prostate cancer. However, while serum chemerin concentrations increased with Gleason score, the opposite effect was observed for *chemerin* expression in prostate tumor tissue [122]. Furthermore, *chemerin* was downregulated in prostate cancer as compared to benign prostate tissues, with greater downregulation observed in castration-resistant prostate cancers [123]. While chemerin$_1$ and chemerin$_2$ expression were not evaluated, CCRL2 mRNA and protein levels were reported to be increased in prostate cancer PC3 cells, and *CCRL2* expression increased in prostate cancer tissues versus prostate tissues from patients with benign prostatic hyperplasia [124]. However, the impact of these changes on chemerin signaling in tumor cells or the tumor microenvironment has not been evaluated.

17. Conclusions

Obesity is a major global health concern that has been linked to the development of many prevalent metabolic disorders such as type 2 diabetes, hyperlipidemia, and cardiovascular disease. There is also an increasing awareness that obesity represents a significant risk factor for the development of several malignancies. While our current understanding of the pathophysiological mechanisms linking obesity to cancer is evolving, growing interest has focused on the role of adipocyte-secreted signaling molecules as key mediators linking these disorders. Among these, circulating levels of the adipokine chemerin are well established to be directly related to adipose tissue mass and have been implicated in several obesity-related metabolic comorbidities. Altered levels of chemerin and the cognate receptors, chemerin$_1$, chemerin$_2$, and CCRL2 have also been identified in several cancer types and many of the fundamental biological activities (e.g., chemotaxis, proliferation, differentiation) of chemerin have the potential to affect tumorigenesis and tumor progression. These effects may be elicited through immune-independent mechanisms that directly impact the growth and tumorigenicity of cancer cells and/or immune-dependent effects that influence the composition of the tumor microenvironment.

At present, epidemiological studies have introduced the potential utility of this adipokine as a potential biomarker for several malignancies, and clinical and empirical evidence supports both pro-

and anti-cancer effects of chemerin. This suggests that the biological actions of chemerin with respect to cancer are highly contextual and dependent upon a number of factors that are important areas of further investigation. A fundamental issue in this regard is the large discrepancy (up to three orders of magnitude; see Table 1) in the reported values of serum/plasma chemerin concentration in the clinical literature—even among control populations. While this may reflect the inherent heterogeneity of the control populations, assay-dependent factors may also play a role. It is critical that methodologies are both reported in appropriate detail and rigorously validated with respect to sensitivity and specificity. Moreover, the overwhelming majority of studies have utilized methodologies that are unable to distinguish between chemerin isoforms and/or only test the actions of chemerin157. It will be important going forward to consider the actions of other known isoforms of chemerin as their relative abundance may differ depending upon anatomical location and their biological actions may be cell- and tissue-dependent. Similarly, most research to date has focused on chemerin$_1$-dependent actions of chemerin. Elucidation of the role of chemerin$_2$ and CCRL2 and the chemerin isoform-selectivity of these receptors in the context of cancer are priority areas for investigation. Moreover, while there has been considerable interest in the relationship of systemic concentrations of adipose-derived chemerin to cancer development and prognosis, comparatively little attention has been applied to the relevance of locally-derived chemerin secreted from cells located in the affected tissue or tumor microenvironment. This may be of particular importance to malignancies such as breast cancer where adipocytes are commonly found in close proximity to tumors and where evidence exists for an influence on tumor development and progression. Finally, most research regarding the impact of adipokines on cancer has focused on a single molecule. It is well known that the relative amounts and spectrum of adipokines is affected by adiposity and adipocyte function. Hence, while challenging, it will be important to apply a more holistic experimental approach to consider the interactions of multiple adipokines and consider synergistic and/or antagonistic effects in different tumor types and at different stages of tumor development.

Author Contributions: conceptualization, K.B.G., A.E.J., B.T.M., and C.J.S.; writing—original draft preparation, K.B.G., A.E.J., B.T.M., and C.J.S.; writing—review and editing, K.B.G., A.E.J., B.T.M., and C.J.S.

Funding: This research was funded by the Canadian Institutes of Health Research (C.J.S.; grant number 153419). B.T.M. is a trainee in the Cancer Research Training Program of the Beatrice Hunter Cancer Research Institute, with funds provided by the Terry Fox Research Institute. B.T.M. is supported by funds from the Natural Sciences and Engineering Research Council (Create grant number 510963).

Conflicts of Interest: The authors declare no conflict of interest.

Abbreviations

AKT	protein kinase B
APC	APC regulator of Wnt signaling pathway
ATM	adjacent tissue myofibroblast
BCSC	breast cancer stem cell
BE	Barrett's esophagus
BPH	benign prostatic hyperplasia
CA125	cancer antigen 125
CA 15-3	cancer antigen 15-3
CAM	cancer associated myofibroblast
CCRL2	C-C Chemokine Receptor-Like 2
CEA	carcinoembryonic antigen
chemerin$_1$	chemerin receptor 1
chemerin$_2$	chemerin receptor 2
CK-1	casein kinase 1
CMKLR1	Chemokine-Like Receptor 1
CRP	C-reactive peptide
CYFRA 21-1	cytokeratin 19 fragment 21-1
ECM	extracellular matrix
EMT	epithelial-to-mesenchymal transformation

ERK	extracellular-related kinase
GBM	malignant glioblastoma
GEPIA	Gene Expression Profiling Interactive Analysis
GM-CSF	granulocyte-macrophage colony-stimulating factor
GPR1	G Protein-coupled Receptor 1
GSK3β	glycogen synthase kinase 3β
GTEx	Genotype-Tissue Expression
HCC	hepatocellular carcinoma
HCS	high chemerin-secreting
hGC	human granulosa cells
IFN-I	type 1 interferon
IFNγ	interferon gamma
IFNγT	interferon γ-secreting T cells
IL-6	interleukin-6
IL-8	interleukin-8
JNK	c-jUN N-terminal kinase
KGN	human ovarian granulosa-like tumor
LCS	low chemerin-secreting
MAPK	mitogen-activated protein kinase
MD	moderately differentiated prostate cancer (Gleason 7)
mDC	myeloid dendritic cell
MDSC	myeloid-derived suppressor cells
MIF	macrophage inhibitory factor
MIP3α	macrophage inflammatory protein-3 alpha
MMP	matrix metalloproteinase
MSC	mesenchymal stromal cell
NASH	non-alcoholic steatohepatitis
NASH-HCC	non-alcoholic steatohepatitis with dimethylnitrosamine-induced hepatocarcinoma
NC CNS	non-cancer CNS disease
NF-κB	nuclear factor kappa B
NK	natural killer
NSCLC	non-small cell lung cancer
NTM	normal tissue myofibroblast
ODC	oligodendrocytoma
OPL	oral pre-malignant lesion
OSC	oesophageal squamous cancer
OSCC	oral squamous cell carcinoma
pRCC	papillary renal cell carcinoma
PD	poorly differentiated prostate cancer (Gleason ≥8)
pDC	plasmacytoid dendritic cell
PI3K	phosphoinositide 3-kinase
PKC	protein kinase C
PTEN	phosphatase and tensin homolog
PVTT-1	portal vein tumor thrombus cells
PVTT-1-Che	chemerin-overexpressing portal vein tumor thrombus cells
SCCOT	squamous cell carcinoma of the oral tongue
TAM	tumor associated macrophage
TCGA	The Cancer Genome Atlas
TIMP-1	tissue inhibitor of metalloproteinase 1
TIMP-2	tissue inhibitor of metalloproteinase 2
TME	tumor microenvironment
TNM	tumor-node-metastasis
TPM	transcripts per kilobase million
Treg	regulatory T cell
VEGF	vascular endothelial growth factor
WD	well differentiated prostate cancer (Gleason score ≤ 6)

References

1. Risk, N.C.D. Trends in adult body-mass index in 200 countries from 1975 to 2014: A pooled analysis of 1698 population-based measurement studies with 19.2 million participants. *Lancet* **2016**, *387*, 1377–1396. [CrossRef]
2. Ferlay, J.; Soerjomataram, I.; Dikshit, R.; Eser, S.; Mathers, C.; Rebelo, M.; Parkin, D.M.; Forman, D.; Bray, F. Cancer incidence and mortality worldwide: Sources, methods and major patterns in GLOBOCAN 2012. *Int. J. Cancer* **2015**, *136*, E359–E386. [CrossRef] [PubMed]
3. Bray, F.; Ferlay, J.; Soerjomataram, I.; Siegel, R.L.; Torre, L.A.; Jemal, A. Global cancer statistics 2018: GLOBOCAN estimates of incidence and mortality worldwide for 36 cancers in 185 countries. *CA Cancer J. Clin.* **2018**, *68*, 394–424. [CrossRef] [PubMed]
4. Dalamaga, M.; Diakopoulos, K.N.; Mantzoros, C.S. The role of adiponectin in cancer: A review of current evidence. *Endocr. Rev.* **2012**, *33*, 547–594. [CrossRef] [PubMed]
5. Vucenik, I.; Stains, J.P. Obesity and cancer risk: Evidence, mechanisms, and recommendations. *Ann. N. Y. Acad. Sci.* **2012**, *1271*, 37–43. [CrossRef] [PubMed]
6. Renehan, A.G.; Tyson, M.; Egger, M.; Heller, R.F.; Zwahlen, M. Body-mass index and incidence of cancer: A systematic review and meta-analysis of prospective observational studies. *Lancet* **2008**, *371*, 569–578. [CrossRef]
7. Arnold, M.; Pandeya, N.; Byrnes, G.; Renehan, P.A.G.; Stevens, G.A.; Ezzati, P.M.; Ferlay, J.; Miranda, J.J.; Romieu, I.; Dikshit, R.; et al. Global burden of cancer attributable to high body-mass index in 2012: A population-based study. *Lancet Oncol.* **2015**, *16*, 36–46. [CrossRef]
8. Lauby-Secretan, B.; Scoccianti, C.; Loomis, D.; Grosse, Y.; Bianchini, F.; Straif, K.; International Agency for Research on Cancer Handbook Working Group. Body Fatness and Cancer—Viewpoint of the IARC Working Group. *N. Engl. J. Med.* **2016**, *375*, 794–798. [CrossRef]
9. Steele, C.B.; Thomas, C.C.; Henley, S.J.; Massetti, G.M.; Galuska, D.A.; Agurs-Collins, T.; Puckett, M.; Richardson, L.C. Vital Signs: Trends in Incidence of Cancers Associated with Overweight and Obesity—United States, 2005–2014. *MMWR Morb. Mortal. Wkly. Rep.* **2017**, *66*, 1052–1058. [CrossRef]
10. Ligibel, J.A.; Alfano, C.M.; Courneya, K.S.; Demark-Wahnefried, W.; Burger, R.A.; Chlebowski, R.T.; Fabian, C.J.; Gucalp, A.; Hershman, D.L.; Hudson, M.M.; et al. American Society of Clinical Oncology position statement on obesity and cancer. *J. Clin. Oncol.* **2014**, *32*, 3568–3574. [CrossRef]
11. Choi, J.; Cha, Y.J.; Koo, J.S. Adipocyte biology in breast cancer: From silent bystander to active facilitator. *Prog. Lipid Res.* **2018**, *69*, 11–20. [CrossRef] [PubMed]
12. Sakurai, M.; Miki, Y.; Takagi, K.; Suzuki, T.; Ishida, T.; Ohuchi, N.; Sasano, H. Interaction with adipocyte stromal cells induces breast cancer malignancy via S100A7 upregulation in breast cancer microenvironment. *Breast Cancer Res.* **2017**, *19*, 70. [CrossRef] [PubMed]
13. Matafome, P.; Santos-Silva, D.; Sena, C.M.; Seica, R. Common mechanisms of dysfunctional adipose tissue and obesity-related cancers. *Diabetes Metab. Res. Rev.* **2013**, *29*, 285–295. [CrossRef] [PubMed]
14. Chi, J.; Wu, Z.; Choi, C.H.J.; Nguyen, L.; Tegegne, S.; Ackerman, S.E.; Crane, A.; Marchildon, F.; Tessier-Lavigne, M.; Cohen, P. Three-Dimensional Adipose Tissue Imaging Reveals Regional Variation in Beige Fat Biogenesis and PRDM16-Dependent Sympathetic Neurite Density. *Cell Metab.* **2018**, *27*, 226–236. [CrossRef] [PubMed]
15. Lau, W.B.; Ohashi, K.; Wang, Y.; Ogawa, H.; Murohara, T.; Ma, X.L.; Ouchi, N. Role of Adipokines in Cardiovascular Disease. *Circ. J.* **2017**, *81*, 920–928. [CrossRef]
16. Unamuno, X.; Gomez-Ambrosi, J.; Rodriguez, A.; Becerril, S.; Fruhbeck, G.; Catalan, V. Adipokine dysregulation and adipose tissue inflammation in human obesity. *Eur. J. Clin. Investig.* **2018**, *48*, e12997. [CrossRef] [PubMed]
17. Macis, D.; Guerrieri-Gonzaga, A.; Gandini, S. Circulating adiponectin and breast cancer risk: A systematic review and meta-analysis. *Int. J. Epidemiol.* **2014**, *43*, 1226–1236. [CrossRef]
18. Tworoger, S.S.; Eliassen, A.H.; Kelesidis, T.; Colditz, G.A.; Willett, W.C.; Mantzoros, C.S.; Hankinson, S.E. Plasma adiponectin concentrations and risk of incident breast cancer. *J. Clin. Endocrinol. Metab.* **2007**, *92*, 1510–1516. [CrossRef]

19. Pan, H.; Deng, L.L.; Cui, J.Q.; Shi, L.; Yang, Y.C.; Luo, J.H.; Qin, D.; Wang, L. Association between serum leptin levels and breast cancer risk: An updated systematic review and meta-analysis. *Medicine (Baltimore)* **2018**, *97*, e11345. [CrossRef]
20. Ishikawa, M.; Kitayama, J.; Nagawa, H. Enhanced expression of leptin and leptin receptor (OB-R) in human breast cancer. *Clin. Cancer Res.* **2004**, *10*, 4325–4331. [CrossRef]
21. Garofalo, C.; Koda, M.; Cascio, S.; Sulkowska, M.; Kanczuga-Koda, L.; Golaszewska, J.; Russo, A.; Sulkowski, S.; Surmacz, E. Increased expression of leptin and the leptin receptor as a marker of breast cancer progression: Possible role of obesity-related stimuli. *Clin. Cancer Res.* **2006**, *12*, 1447–1453. [CrossRef] [PubMed]
22. Jarde, T.; Caldefie-Chezet, F.; Damez, M.; Mishellany, F.; Penault-Llorca, F.; Guillot, J.; Vasson, M.P. Leptin and leptin receptor involvement in cancer development: A study on human primary breast carcinoma. *Oncol. Rep.* **2008**, *19*, 905–911. [CrossRef] [PubMed]
23. Miyoshi, Y.; Funahashi, T.; Tanaka, S.; Taguchi, T.; Tamaki, Y.; Shimomura, I.; Noguchi, S. High expression of leptin receptor mRNA in breast cancer tissue predicts poor prognosis for patients with high, but not low, serum leptin levels. *Int. J. Cancer* **2006**, *118*, 1414–1419. [CrossRef] [PubMed]
24. Rourke, J.L.; Dranse, H.J.; Sinal, C.J. Towards an integrative approach to understanding the role of chemerin in human health and disease. *Obes. Rev.* **2013**, *14*, 245–262. [CrossRef] [PubMed]
25. Helfer, G.; Wu, Q.F. Chemerin: A multifaceted adipokine involved in metabolic disorders. *J. Endocrinol.* **2018**, *238*, R79–R94. [CrossRef] [PubMed]
26. Toulany, J.; Parlee, S.D.; Sinal, C.J.; Slayter, K.; McNeil, S.; Goralski, K.B. CMKLR1 activation ex vivo does not increase proportionally to serum total chemerin in obese humans. *Endocr. Connect.* **2016**, *5*, 70–81. [CrossRef] [PubMed]
27. Parlee, S.D.; Wang, Y.; Poirier, P.; Lapointe, M.; Martin, J.; Bastien, M.; Cianflone, K.; Goralski, K.B. Biliopancreatic diversion with duodenal switch modifies plasma chemerin in early and late post-operative periods. *Obesity* **2015**, *23*, 1201–1208. [CrossRef] [PubMed]
28. Bozaoglu, K.; Bolton, K.; McMillan, J.; Zimmet, P.; Jowett, J.; Collier, G.; Walder, K.; Segal, D. Chemerin is a novel adipokine associated with obesity and metabolic syndrome. *Endocrinology* **2007**, *148*, 4687–4694. [CrossRef] [PubMed]
29. Ernst, M.C.; Haidl, I.D.; Zuniga, L.A.; Dranse, H.J.; Rourke, J.L.; Zabel, B.A.; Butcher, E.C.; Sinal, C.J. Disruption of the chemokine-like receptor-1 (CMKLR1) gene is associated with reduced adiposity and glucose intolerance. *Endocrinology* **2012**, *153*, 672–682. [CrossRef]
30. Ernst, M.C.; Issa, M.; Goralski, K.B.; Sinal, C.J. Chemerin exacerbates glucose intolerance in mouse models of obesity and diabetes. *Endocrinology* **2010**, *151*, 1998–2007. [CrossRef]
31. Parlee, S.D.; Ernst, M.C.; Muruganandan, S.; Sinal, C.J.; Goralski, K.B. Serum chemerin levels vary with time of day and are modified by obesity and tumor necrosis factor-{alpha}. *Endocrinology* **2010**, *151*, 2590–2602. [CrossRef] [PubMed]
32. Ress, C.; Tschoner, A.; Engl, J.; Klaus, A.; Tilg, H.; Ebenbichler, C.F.; Patsch, J.R.; Kaser, S. Effect of bariatric surgery on circulating chemerin levels. *Eur. J. Clin. Investig.* **2010**, *40*, 277–280. [CrossRef] [PubMed]
33. Sell, H.; Divoux, A.; Poitou, C.; Basdevant, A.; Bouillot, J.L.; Bedossa, P.; Tordjman, J.; Eckel, J.; Clement, K. Chemerin correlates with markers for fatty liver in morbidly obese patients and strongly decreases after weight loss induced by bariatric surgery. *J. Clin. Endocrinol. Metab.* **2010**, *95*, 2892–2896. [CrossRef] [PubMed]
34. van Herpen, N.A.; Sell, H.; Eckel, J.; Schrauwen, P.; Mensink, R.P. Prolonged fasting and the effects on biomarkers of inflammation and on adipokines in healthy lean men. *Horm. Metab. Res.* **2013**, *45*, 378–382. [CrossRef] [PubMed]
35. Chang, S.S.; Eisenberg, D.; Zhao, L.; Adams, C.; Leib, R.; Morser, J.; Leung, L. Chemerin activation in human obesity. *Obesity* **2016**, *24*, 1522–1529. [CrossRef] [PubMed]
36. Banas, M.; Zabieglo, K.; Kasetty, G.; Kapinska-Mrowiecka, M.; Borowczyk, J.; Drukala, J.; Murzyn, K.; Zabel, B.A.; Butcher, E.C.; Schroeder, J.M.; et al. Chemerin is an antimicrobial agent in human epidermis. *PLoS ONE* **2013**, *8*, e58709. [CrossRef]
37. Du, X.Y.; Zabel, B.A.; Myles, T.; Allen, S.J.; Handel, T.M.; Lee, P.P.; Butcher, E.C.; Leung, L.L. Regulation of chemerin bioactivity by plasma carboxypeptidase N, carboxypeptidase B (activated thrombin-activable fibrinolysis inhibitor), and platelets. *J. Biol. Chem.* **2009**, *284*, 751–758. [CrossRef]

38. Eisinger, K.; Bauer, S.; Schaffler, A.; Walter, R.; Neumann, E.; Buechler, C.; Muller-Ladner, U.; Frommer, K.W. Chemerin induces CCL2 and TLR4 in synovial fibroblasts of patients with rheumatoid arthritis and osteoarthritis. *Exp. Mol. Pathol.* **2012**, *92*, 90–96. [CrossRef]
39. Lande, R.; Gafa, V.; Serafini, B.; Giacomini, E.; Visconti, A.; Remoli, M.E.; Severa, M.; Parmentier, M.; Ristori, G.; Salvetti, M.; et al. Plasmacytoid dendritic cells in multiple sclerosis: Intracerebral recruitment and impaired maturation in response to interferon-beta. *J. Neuropathol. Exp. Neurol.* **2008**, *67*, 388–401. [CrossRef]
40. Maheshwari, A.; Kurundkar, A.R.; Shaik, S.S.; Kelly, D.R.; Hartman, Y.; Zhang, W.; Dimmitt, R.; Saeed, S.; Randolph, D.A.; Aprahamian, C.; et al. Epithelial cells in fetal intestine produce chemerin to recruit macrophages. *Am. J. Physiol. Gastrointest. Liver Physiol.* **2009**, *297*, G1–G10. [CrossRef]
41. Wittamer, V.; Bondue, B.; Guillabert, A.; Vassart, G.; Parmentier, M.; Communi, D. Neutrophil-mediated maturation of chemerin: A link between innate and adaptive immunity. *J. Immunol.* **2005**, *175*, 487–493. [CrossRef] [PubMed]
42. Wittamer, V.; Franssen, J.D.; Vulcano, M.; Mirjolet, J.F.; Le Poul, E.; Migeotte, I.; Brezillon, S.; Tyldesley, R.; Blanpain, C.; Detheux, M.; et al. Specific recruitment of antigen-presenting cells by chemerin, a novel processed ligand from human inflammatory fluids. *J. Exp. Med.* **2003**, *198*, 977–985. [CrossRef] [PubMed]
43. Yamaguchi, Y.; Du, X.Y.; Zhao, L.; Morser, J.; Leung, L.L. Proteolytic cleavage of chemerin protein is necessary for activation to the active form, Chem157S, which functions as a signaling molecule in glioblastoma. *J. Biol. Chem.* **2011**, *286*, 39510–39519. [CrossRef] [PubMed]
44. Zabel, B.A.; Allen, S.J.; Kulig, P.; Allen, J.A.; Cichy, J.; Handel, T.M.; Butcher, E.C. Chemerin activation by serine proteases of the coagulation, fibrinolytic, and inflammatory cascades. *J. Biol. Chem.* **2005**, *280*, 34661–34666. [CrossRef] [PubMed]
45. Meder, W.; Wendland, M.; Busmann, A.; Kutzleb, C.; Spodsberg, N.; John, H.; Richter, R.; Schleuder, D.; Meyer, M.; Forssmann, W.G. Characterization of human circulating TIG2 as a ligand for the orphan receptor ChemR23. *FEBS Lett.* **2003**, *555*, 495–499. [CrossRef]
46. Zhao, L.; Yamaguchi, Y.; Sharif, S.; Du, X.Y.; Song, J.J.; Lee, D.M.; Recht, L.D.; Robinson, W.H.; Morser, J.; Leung, L.L. Chemerin158K protein is the dominant chemerin isoform in synovial and cerebrospinal fluids but not in plasma. *J. Biol. Chem.* **2011**, *286*, 39520–39527. [CrossRef]
47. Guillabert, A.; Wittamer, V.; Bondue, B.; Godot, V.; Imbault, V.; Parmentier, M.; Communi, D. Role of neutrophil proteinase 3 and mast cell chymase in chemerin proteolytic regulation. *J. Leukoc. Biol.* **2008**, *84*, 1530–1538. [CrossRef]
48. Kennedy, A.J.; Davenport, A.P. International Union of Basic and Clinical Pharmacology CIII: Chemerin Receptors CMKLR1 (Chemerin1) and GPR1 (Chemerin2) Nomenclature, Pharmacology, and Function. *Pharmacol. Rev.* **2018**, *70*, 174–196. [CrossRef]
49. Mazzotti, C.; Gagliostro, V.; Bosisio, D.; Del Prete, A.; Tiberio, L.; Thelen, M.; Sozzani, S. The Atypical Receptor CCRL2 (C-C Chemokine Receptor-Like 2) Does Not Act As a Decoy Receptor in Endothelial Cells. *Front. Immunol.* **2017**, *8*, 1233. [CrossRef]
50. Monnier, J.; Lewen, S.; O'Hara, E.; Huang, K.; Tu, H.; Butcher, E.C.; Zabel, B.A. Expression, regulation, and function of atypical chemerin receptor CCRL2 on endothelial cells. *J. Immunol.* **2012**, *189*, 956–967. [CrossRef]
51. Parolini, S.; Santoro, A.; Marcenaro, E.; Luini, W.; Massardi, L.; Facchetti, F.; Communi, D.; Parmentier, M.; Majorana, A.; Sironi, M.; et al. The role of chemerin in the colocalization of NK and dendritic cell subsets into inflamed tissues. *Blood* **2007**, *109*, 3625–3632. [CrossRef] [PubMed]
52. Pachynski, R.K.; Zabel, B.A.; Kohrt, H.E.; Tejeda, N.M.; Monnier, J.; Swanson, C.D.; Holzer, A.K.; Gentles, A.J.; Sperinde, G.V.; Edalati, A.; et al. The chemoattractant chemerin suppresses melanoma by recruiting natural killer cell antitumor defenses. *J. Exp. Med.* **2012**, *209*, 1427–1435. [CrossRef] [PubMed]
53. Treeck, O.; Buechler, C.; Ortmann, O. Chemerin and Cancer. *Int. J. Mol. Sci.* **2019**, *20*, 3750. [CrossRef] [PubMed]
54. Ghallab, N.A.; Shaker, O.G. Serum and salivary levels of chemerin and MMP-9 in oral squamous cell carcinoma and oral premalignant lesions. *Clin. Oral Investig.* **2017**, *21*, 937–947. [CrossRef] [PubMed]
55. Wang, N.; Wang, Q.J.; Feng, Y.Y.; Shang, W.; Cai, M. Overexpression of chemerin was associated with tumor angiogenesis and poor clinical outcome in squamous cell carcinoma of the oral tongue. *Clin. Oral Investig.* **2014**, *18*, 997–1004. [CrossRef] [PubMed]

56. Kumar, J.D.; Kandola, S.; Tiszlavicz, L.; Reisz, Z.; Dockray, G.J.; Varro, A. The role of chemerin and ChemR23 in stimulating the invasion of squamous oesophageal cancer cells. *Br. J. Cancer* **2016**, *114*, 1152–1159. [CrossRef] [PubMed]
57. Kumar, J.D.; Holmberg, C.; Kandola, S.; Steele, I.; Hegyi, P.; Tiszlavicz, L.; Jenkins, R.; Beynon, R.J.; Peeney, D.; Giger, O.T.; et al. Increased expression of chemerin in squamous esophageal cancer myofibroblasts and role in recruitment of mesenchymal stromal cells. *PLoS ONE* **2014**, *9*, e104877. [CrossRef] [PubMed]
58. Cabia, B.; Andrade, S.; Carreira, M.C.; Casanueva, F.F.; Crujeiras, A.B. A role for novel adipose tissue-secreted factors in obesity-related carcinogenesis. *Obes. Rev.* **2016**, *17*, 361–376. [CrossRef] [PubMed]
59. Erdogan, S.; Yilmaz, F.M.; Yazici, O.; Yozgat, A.; Sezer, S.; Ozdemir, N.; Uysal, S.; Purnak, T. Inflammation and chemerin in colorectal cancer. *Tumor Biol.* **2016**, *37*, 6337–6342. [CrossRef] [PubMed]
60. Eichelmann, F.; Schulze, M.B.; Wittenbecher, C.; Menzel, J.; Weikert, C.; di Giuseppe, R.; Biemann, R.; Isermann, B.; Fritche, A.; Boeing, H.; et al. Association of Chemerin Plasma Concentration With Risk of Colorectal Cancer. *JAMA Netw. Open* **2019**, *2*, e190896. [CrossRef] [PubMed]
61. Zhang, J.; Jin, H.-C.; Zhu, A.-K.; Ying, R.-C.; Wei, W.; Zhang, F.-J. Prognostic significance of plasma chemerin levels in patients with gastric cancer. *Peptides* **2014**, *61*, 7–11. [CrossRef] [PubMed]
62. Alkady, M.M.; Abdel-Messeih, P.L.; Nosseir, N.M. Assessment of serum levels of the adipocytokine chemerin in colorectal cancer patients. *J. Med. Biochem.* **2018**, *37*, 313–319. [CrossRef] [PubMed]
63. Lee, J.-Y.; Lee, M.-K.; Kim, N.-K.; Chu, S.-H.; Lee, D.-C.; Lee, H.-S.; Lee, J.-W.; Jeon, J.Y. Serum chemerin levels are independently associated with quality of life in colorectal cancer survivors: A pilot study. *PLoS ONE* **2017**, *12*, e0176929. [CrossRef] [PubMed]
64. Wang, C.; Wu, W.K.K.; Liu, X.; To, K.-F.; Chen, G.G.; Yu, J.; Ng, E.K.W. Increased serum chemerin level promotes cellular invasiveness in gastric cancer: A clinical and experimental study. *Peptides* **2014**, *51*, 131–138. [CrossRef] [PubMed]
65. Imai, K.; Takai, K.; Hanai, T.; Shiraki, M.; Suzuki, Y.; Hayashi, H.; Naiki, T.; Nishigaki, Y.; Tomita, E.; Shimizu, M.; et al. Impact of serum chemerin levels on liver functional reserves and platelet counts in patients with hepatocellular carcinoma. *Int. J. Mol. Sci.* **2014**, *15*, 11294–11306. [CrossRef]
66. Warakomski, J.; Romuk, E.; Jarzab, B.; Krajewska, J.; Sieminska, L. Concentrations of Selected Adipokines, Interleukin-6, and Vitamin D in Patients with Papillary Thyroid Carcinoma in Respect to Thyroid Cancer Stages. *Int. J. Endocrinol.* **2018**, *2018*, 4921803. [CrossRef] [PubMed]
67. Akin, S.; Akin, S.; Gedik, E.; Haznedaroglu, E.; Dogan, A.L.; Altundag, M.K. Serum Chemerin Level in Breast Cancer. *Int. J. Hematol. Oncol.* **2017**, *27*. [CrossRef]
68. Sotiropoulos, G.P.; Dalamaga, M.; Antonakos, G.; Marinou, I.; Vogiatzakis, E.; Kotopouli, M.; Karampela, I.; Christodoulatos, G.S.; Lekka, A.; Papavassiliou, A.G. Chemerin as a biomarker at the intersection of inflammation, chemotaxis, coagulation, fibrinolysis and metabolism in resectable non-small cell lung cancer. *Lung Cancer* **2018**, *125*, 291–299. [CrossRef]
69. Xu, C.H.; Yang, Y.; Wang, Y.C.; Yan, J.; Qian, L.H. Prognostic significance of serum chemerin levels in patients with non-small cell lung cancer. *Oncotarget* **2017**, *8*, 22483–22489. [CrossRef]
70. Qu, X.; Han, L.; Wang, S.; Zhang, Q.; Yang, C.; Xu, S.; Zhang, L. Detection of Chemerin and It's Clinical Significance in Peripheral Blood of Patients with Lung Cancer. *Zhongguo Fei Ai Za Zhi* **2009**, *12*, 1174–1177. [CrossRef]
71. Kiczmer, P.; Szydło, B.e.; Seńkowska, A.P.; Jopek, J.; Wiewióra, M.; Peicuch, J.; Ostrowska, Z.; Świętochowska, E.b. Serum omentin-1 and chemerin concentrations in pancreatic cancer and chronic panreatitis. *Folia Med. Crac.* **2018**, *58*, 77–87.
72. Siemińska, L.; Borowski, A.; Marek, B.; Nowak, M.; Kajdaniuk, D.; Warakomski, J.; Kos-Kudła, B. Serum concentrations of adipokines in men with prostate cancer and benign prostate hyperplasia. *Endokrynol. Pol.* **2018**, *69*, 120–127. [PubMed]
73. Kang, M.; Byun, S.-S.; Lee, S.E.; Hong, S.K. Clinical significance of serum adipokines according to body mass index in patients with clinically localized prostate cancer undergoing radical porstatectomy. *World J. Mens Health* **2018**, *36*, 57–65. [CrossRef] [PubMed]
74. Kaur, J.; Adya, R.; Tan, B.K.; Chen, J.; Randeva, H.S. Identification of chemerin receptor (ChemR23) in human endothelial cells: Chemerin-induced endothelial angiogenesis. *Biochem. Biophys. Res. Commun.* **2010**, *391*, 1762–1768. [CrossRef] [PubMed]

75. Bozaoglu, K.; Curran, J.E.; Stocker, C.J.; Zaibi, M.S.; Segal, D.; Konstantopoulos, N.; Morrison, S.; Carless, M.; Dyer, T.D.; Cole, S.A.; et al. Chemerin, a novel adipokine in the regulation of angiogenesis. *J. Clin. Endocrinol. Metab.* **2010**, *95*, 2476–2485. [CrossRef] [PubMed]
76. Somja, J.; Demoulin, S.; Roncarati, P.; Herfs, M.; Bletard, N.; Delvenne, P.; Hubert, P. Dendritic cells in Barrett's esophagus carcinogenesis: An inadequate microenvironment for antitumor immunity? *Am. J. Pathol.* **2013**, *182*, 2168–2179. [CrossRef] [PubMed]
77. Li, J.J.; Yin, H.K.; Guan, D.X.; Zhao, J.S.; Feng, Y.X.; Deng, Y.Z.; Wang, X.; Li, N.; Wang, X.F.; Cheng, S.Q.; et al. Chemerin suppresses hepatocellular carcinoma metastasis through CMKLR1-PTEN-Akt axis. *Br. J. Cancer* **2018**, *118*, 1337–1348. [CrossRef] [PubMed]
78. Lin, W.; Chen, Y.L.; Jiang, L.; Chen, J.K. Reduced expression of chemerin is associated with a poor prognosis and a lowed infiltration of both dendritic cells and natural killer cells in human hepatocellular carcinoma. *Clin. Lab.* **2011**, *57*, 879–885.
79. Liu-Chittenden, Y.; Jain, M.; Gaskins, K.; Wang, S.; Merino, M.J.; Kotian, S.; Kumar Gara, S.; Davis, S.; Zhang, L.; Kebebew, E. RARRES2 functions as a tumor suppressor by promoting beta-catenin phosphorylation/degradation and inhibiting p38 phosphorylation in adrenocortical carcinoma. *Oncogene* **2017**, *36*, 3541–3552. [CrossRef]
80. Adachi, Y.; Yamamoto, H.; Itoh, F.; Hinoda, Y.; Okada, Y.; Imai, K. Contribution of matrilysin (MMP-7) to the cetastatic pathway of human colorectal cancers. *Gut* **1999**, *45*, 252–258. [CrossRef]
81. Ashizawa, T.; Okada, R.; Suzuki, Y.; Takagi, M.; Yamazaki, T.; Sumi, T.; Aoki, T.; Ohnuma, S.; Aoki, T. Clinical significance of interleukin-6 (IL-6) in the spread of gastric cancer: Role of IL-6 as a prognostic factor. *Gastric Cancer* **2005**, *8*, 124–131. [CrossRef] [PubMed]
82. Nakamura, N.; Naruse, K.; Kobayashi, Y.; Miyade, M.; Saiki, T.; Enomoto, A.; Takahashi, M.; Matsubara, T. Chemerin promotes angiogenesis in vivo. *Physiol. Rep.* **2018**, *6*, e13962. [CrossRef] [PubMed]
83. Yang, L.P.; Fu, L.C.; Guo, H.; Xie, L.X. Expression of vascular endothelial growth factor c correlates with lymphatic vessel density and prognosis in human gastroesophageal junction carcinoma. *Onkologie* **2012**, *35*, 88–93. [CrossRef] [PubMed]
84. Krishna, M.; Narang, H. The complexity of mitogen-activated protein kinases (MAPKs) made simple. *Cell. Mol. Life Sci.* **2008**, *65*, 3525–3544. [CrossRef] [PubMed]
85. Rourke, J.L.; Dranse, H.J.; Sinal, C.J. CMKLR1 and GPR1 mediate chemerin signaling through the RhoA/ROCK pathway. *Mol. Cell. Endocrinol.* **2015**, *417*, 36–51. [CrossRef] [PubMed]
86. Kumar, J.D.; Aolymat, I.; Tiszlavicz, L.; Reisz, Z.; Garalla, H.M.; Beynon, R.; Simpson, D.; Dockray, G.J.; Varro, A. Chemerin acts via CMKLR1 and GPR1 to stimulate migration and invasion of gastric cancer cells: Putative role of decreased TIMP-1 and TIMP-2. *Oncotarget* **2019**, *10*, 98–112. [CrossRef] [PubMed]
87. Egeblad, M.; Werb, Z. New functions for the matrix metalloproteinases in cancer progression. *Nat. Rev. Cancer* **2002**, *2*, 161–174. [CrossRef] [PubMed]
88. Akram, I.G.; Georges, R.; Hielscher, T.; Adwan, H.; Berger, M.R. The chemokines CCR1 and CCRL2 have a role in colorectal cancer liver metastasis. *Tumor Biol.* **2016**, *37*, 2461–2471. [CrossRef] [PubMed]
89. Zheng, Y.; Luo, S.; Wang, G.; Peng, Z.; Zeng, W.; Tan, S.; Xi, Y.; Fan, J. Downregulation of tazarotene induced gene-2 (TIG2) in skin squamous cell carcinoma. *Eur. J. Dermatol.* **2008**, *18*, 638–641. [CrossRef]
90. Gabrilovich, D.I. Myeloid-Derived Suppressor Cells. *Cancer Immunol. Res.* **2017**, *5*, 3–8. [CrossRef]
91. Di Domizio, J.; Demaria, O.; Gilliet, M. Plasmacytoid dendritic cells in melanoma: Can we revert bad into good? *J. Investig. Dermatol.* **2014**, *134*, 1797–1800. [CrossRef] [PubMed]
92. Lin, Y.; Yang, X.; Liu, W.; Li, B.; Yin, W.; Shi, Y.; He, R. Chemerin has a protective role in hepatocellular carcinoma by inhibiting the expression of IL-6 and GM-CSF and MDSC accumulation. *Oncogene* **2017**, *36*, 3599–3608. [CrossRef]
93. Sun, P.; Wang, S.; Wang, J.; Sun, J.; Peng, M.; Shi, P. The involvement of iron in chemerin induced cell cycle arrest in human hepatic carcinoma SMMC7721 cells. *Metallomics* **2018**, *10*, 838–845. [CrossRef] [PubMed]
94. Rebouissou, S.; Zucman-Rossi, J.; Moreau, R.; Qiu, Z.; Hui, L. Note of caution: Contaminations of hepatocellular cell lines. *J. Hepatol.* **2017**, *67*, 896–897. [CrossRef] [PubMed]
95. Ye, F.; Chen, C.; Qin, J.; Liu, J.; Zheng, C. Genetic profiling reveals an alarming rate of cross-contamination among human cell lines used in China. *FASEB J.* **2015**, *39*, 4268–4272. [CrossRef]
96. Haberl, E.M.; Pohl, R.; Rein-Fischboeck, L.; Feder, S.; Sinal, C.J.; Buechler, C. Chemerin in a mouse model of non-alcoholic steatohepatitis and hepatocarcinogenesis. *Anticancer Res.* **2018**, *38*, 2649–2657. [PubMed]

97. Ayala-Ramirez, M.; Jasim, S.; Feng, L.; Ejaz, S.; Deniz, F.; Busaidy, N.; Waguespack, S.G.; Naing, A.; Sircar, K.; Wood, C.G.; et al. Adrenocortical carcinoma: Clinical outcomes and prognosis of 330 patients at a tertiary care center. *Eur. J. Endocrinol.* **2013**, *169*, 891–899. [CrossRef]
98. Fernandez-Ranvier, G.G.; Weng, J.; Yeh, R.F.; Khanafshar, E.; Suh, I.; Barker, C.; Duh, Q.Y.; Clark, O.H.; Kebebew, E. Identification of biomarkers of adrenocortical carcinoma using genomewide gene expression profiling. *Arch. Surg.* **2008**, *143*, 841–846; discussion 846. [CrossRef]
99. Velazquez-Fernandez, D.; Laurell, C.; Geli, J.; Hoog, A.; Odeberg, J.; Kjellman, M.; Lundeberg, J.; Hamberger, B.; Nilsson, P.; Backdahl, M. Expression profiling of adrenocortical neoplasms suggests a molecular signature of malignancy. *Surgery* **2005**, *138*, 1087–1094. [CrossRef]
100. Liu-Chittenden, Y.; Patel, D.; Gaskins, K.; Giordano, T.J.; Assie, G.; Bertherat, J.; Kebebew, E. Serum RARRES2 Is a Prognostic Marker in Patients With Adrenocortical Carcinoma. *J. Clin. Endocrinol. Metab.* **2016**, *101*, 3345–3352. [CrossRef]
101. Dranse, H.J.; Muruganandan, S.; Fawcett, J.P.; Sinal, C.J. Adipocyte-secreted chemerin is processed to a variety of isoforms and influences MMP3 and chemokine secretion through an NFkB-dependent mechanism. *Mol. Cell. Endocrinol.* **2016**, *436*, 114–129. [CrossRef] [PubMed]
102. Gaujoux, S.; Grabar, S.; Fassnacht, M.; Ragazzon, B.; Launay, P.; Libe, R.; Chokri, I.; Audebourg, A.; Royer, B.; Sbiera, S.; et al. beta-catenin activation is associated with specific clinical and pathologic characteristics and a poor outcome in adrenocortical carcinoma. *Clin. Cancer Res.* **2011**, *17*, 328–336. [CrossRef] [PubMed]
103. Tissier, F.; Cavard, C.; Groussin, L.; Perlemoine, K.; Fumey, G.; Hagnere, A.M.; Rene-Corail, F.; Jullian, E.; Gicquel, C.; Bertagna, X.; et al. Mutations of beta-catenin in adrenocortical tumors: Activation of the Wnt signaling pathway is a frequent event in both benign and malignant adrenocortical tumors. *Cancer Res.* **2005**, *65*, 7622–7627. [CrossRef] [PubMed]
104. Zheng, S.; Cherniack, A.D.; Dewal, N.; Moffitt, R.A.; Danilova, L.; Murray, B.A.; Lerario, A.M.; Else, T.; Knijnenburg, T.A.; Ciriello, G.; et al. Comprehensive Pan-Genomic Characterization of Adrenocortical Carcinoma. *Cancer Cell* **2016**, *29*, 723–736. [CrossRef] [PubMed]
105. Muruganandan, S.; Govindarajan, R.; McMullen, N.M.; Sinal, C.J. Chemokine-Like Receptor 1 Is a Novel Wnt Target Gene that Regulates Mesenchymal Stem Cell Differentiation. *Stem Cells* **2017**, *35*, 711–724. [CrossRef] [PubMed]
106. Tang, Z.; Kang, B.; Li, C.; Chen, T.; Zhang, Z. GEPIA2: An enhanced web server for large-scale expression profiling and interactive analysis. *Nucleic Acids Res.* **2019**, *47*, W556–W560. [CrossRef]
107. Krawczyk, K.M.; Nilsson, H.; Allaoui, R.; Lindgren, D.; Arvidsson, M.; Leandersson, K.; Johansson, M.E. Papillary renal cell carcinoma-derived chemerin, IL-8, and CXCL16 promote monocyte recruitment and differentiation into foam-cell macrophages. *Lab. Investig.* **2017**, *97*, 1296–1305. [CrossRef]
108. Kwon, H.; Han, K.D.; Park, C.Y. Weight change is significantly associated with risk of thyroid cancer: A nationwide population-based cohort study. *Sci. Rep.* **2019**, *9*, 1546. [CrossRef]
109. El-Sagheer, G.; Gayyed, M.; Ahmad, A.; Abd El-Fattah, A.; Mohamed, M. Expression of chemerin correlates with a poor prognosis in female breast cancer patients. *Breast Cancer (Dove Med. Press)* **2018**, *10*, 169–176. [CrossRef]
110. Pachynski, R.K.; Wang, P.; Salazar, N.; Zheng, Y.; Nease, L.; Rosalez, J.; Leong, W.I.; Virdi, G.; Rennier, K.; Shin, W.J.; et al. Chemerin Suppresses Breast Cancer Growth by Recruiting Immune Effector Cells Into the Tumor Microenvironment. *Front. Immunol.* **2019**, *10*, 983. [CrossRef]
111. Boyle, S.T.; Kochetkova, M. Breast cancer stem cells and the immune system: Promotion, evasion and therapy. *J. Mammary Gland Biol. Neoplasia* **2014**, *19*, 203–211. [CrossRef] [PubMed]
112. Jeong, Y.J.; Oh, H.K.; Park, S.H.; Bong, J.G. Association between inflammation and cancer stem cell phenotype in breast cancer. *Oncol. Lett.* **2018**, *15*, 2380–2386. [CrossRef] [PubMed]
113. Tanaka, T.; Narazaki, M.; Kishimoto, T. IL-6 in inflammation, immunity, and disease. *Cold Spring Harb. Perspect. Biol.* **2014**, *6*, a016295. [CrossRef] [PubMed]
114. Iqbal, J.; Chong, P.Y.; Tan, P.H. Breast cancer stem cells: An update. *J. Clin. Pathol.* **2013**, *66*, 485–490. [CrossRef] [PubMed]
115. Sarmadi, P.; Tunali, G.; Esendagli-Yilmaz, G.; Yilmaz, K.B.; Esendagli, G. CRAM-A indicates IFN-gamma-associated inflammatory response in breast cancer. *Mol. Immunol.* **2015**, *68*, 692–698. [CrossRef] [PubMed]

116. Hoffmann, M.; Rak, A.; Ptak, A. Bisphenol A and its derivatives decrease expression of chemerin, which reverses its stimulatory action in ovarian cancer cells. *Toxicol. Lett.* **2018**, *291*, 61–69. [CrossRef] [PubMed]
117. Reverchon, M.; Cornuau, M.; Rame, C.; Guerif, F.; Royere, D.; Dupont, J. Chemerin inhibits IGF-1-induced progesterone and estradiol secretion in human granulosa cells. *Hum. Reprod.* **2012**, *27*, 1790–1800. [CrossRef] [PubMed]
118. Tummler, C.; Snapkov, I.; Wickstrom, M.; Moens, U.; Ljungblad, L.; Maria Elfman, L.H.; Winberg, J.O.; Kogner, P.; Johnsen, J.I.; Sveinbjornsson, B. Inhibition of chemerin/CMKLR1 axis in neuroblastoma cells reduces clonogenicity and cell viability in vitro and impairs tumor growth in vivo. *Oncotarget* **2017**, *8*, 95135–95151. [CrossRef] [PubMed]
119. Ntikoudi, E.; Kiagia, M.; Boura, P.; Syrigos, K.N. Hormones of adipose tissue and their biologic role in lung cancer. *Cancer Treat. Rev.* **2014**, *40*, 22–30. [CrossRef] [PubMed]
120. Wu, J.; Lanier, L.L. Natural killer cells and cancer. *Adv. Cancer Res.* **2003**, *90*, 127–156.
121. Zhao, S.; Li, C.; Ye, Y.B.; Peng, F.; Chen, Q. Expression of Chemerin Correlates With a Favorable Prognosis in Patients With Non-Small Cell Lung Cancer. *Labmedicine* **2011**, *42*, 553–557. [CrossRef]
122. Stamey, T.A.; Warrington, J.A.; Caldwell, M.C.; Chen, Z.; Fan, Z.; Mahadevappa, M.; McNeal, J.E.; Nolley, R.; Zhang, Z. Molecular genetic profiling of Gleason grade 4/5 prostate cnacers compared to benign prostatic hyperplasia. *J. Urol.* **2001**, *166*, 2171–2177. [CrossRef]
123. Lin, P.-C.; Giannopoulou, E.G.; Park, K.; Mosquera, J.M.; Sboner, A.; Tewari, A.K.; Garraway, L.A.; Beltran, H.; Rubin, M.A.; Elemento, O. Epigenomic alterations in localized and advanced prostate cancer. *Neoplasia* **2013**, *15*, 373–383. [CrossRef] [PubMed]
124. Reyes, N.; Benedetti, I.; Rebollo, J.; Correa, O.; Geliebter, J. Atypical chemokine receptor CCRL2 is overexpressed in prostate cancer cells. *J. Biomed. Res.* **2019**, *33*, 17–23.

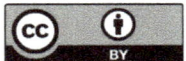

© 2019 by the authors. Licensee MDPI, Basel, Switzerland. This article is an open access article distributed under the terms and conditions of the Creative Commons Attribution (CC BY) license (http://creativecommons.org/licenses/by/4.0/).

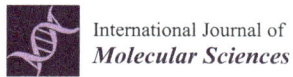

Review

Chemerin and Cancer

Oliver Treeck [1,*], Christa Buechler [2] and Olaf Ortmann [1]

[1] Department of Obstetrics and Gynecology, University Medical Center Regensburg, 93053 Regensburg, Germany
[2] Department of Internal Medicine I, University Medical Center Regensburg, 93053 Regensburg, Germany
* Correspondence: otreeck@caritasstjosef.de

Received: 2 July 2019; Accepted: 30 July 2019; Published: 31 July 2019

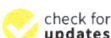

Abstract: Chemerin is a multifunctional adipokine with established roles in inflammation, adipogenesis and glucose homeostasis. Increasing evidence suggest an important function of chemerin in cancer. Chemerin's main cellular receptors, chemokine-like receptor 1 (CMKLR1), G-protein coupled receptor 1 (GPR1) and C-C chemokine receptor-like 2 (CCRL2) are expressed in most normal and tumor tissues. Chemerin's role in cancer is considered controversial, since it is able to exert both anti-tumoral and tumor-promoting effects, which are mediated by different mechanisms like recruiting innate immune defenses or activation of endothelial angiogenesis. For this review article, original research articles on the role of chemerin and its receptors in cancer were considered, which are listed in the PubMed database. Additionally, we included meta-analyses of publicly accessible DNA microarray data to elucidate the association of expression of chemerin and its receptors in tumor tissues with patients' survival.

Keywords: adipokine; chemerin; leukocyte; cancer

---

1. Chemerin—A Multifunctional Cytokine and Adipokine

Chemerin, also known as retinoic acid receptor responder 2 (RARRES2), is expressed ubiquitously, but is most abundant in adipose tissue and the liver. Human chemerin is a 163 amino acid protein whose 20 amino acid N-terminal signal sequence is removed prior to secretion of the biologic inactive prochemerin into the bloodstream. Chemotactic active forms are produced by C-terminal processing. Extracellular serine and cysteine proteases generate different chemerin isoforms with chemerin 157 being the most active variant [1,2]. The biologic activities of chemerin isoforms are primarily mediated by two receptors, chemokine-like receptor 1 (CMKLR1) and G protein-coupled receptor 1 (GPR1) [3]. Chemerin similarly binds and activates both receptors, which triggers different cellular responses. Whereas activation of CMKLR1 leads to strong calcium mobilization and ERK1/2 phosphorylation, chemerin binding to GPR1 only leads to weak activation of both signaling mechanisms [4]. C-C motif chemokine receptor like 2 (CCRL2) is an additional chemerin receptor without known downstream signaling, which is thought to affect local activity of chemerin by presenting it to CMKLR1 and GPR1 [2].

Chemerin is a chemoattractant protein and its role in inflammation was studied in detail. In experimental pancreatitis chemerin infusion prior to disease induction reduces NF-κB signaling and thus exerts anti-inflammatory activities [5]. Chemerin activates NF-κB and up-regulates expression of adhesion molecules in endothelial cells thus enhancing monocyte adhesion and development of atherosclerosis [6]. In diabetic nephropathy chemerin activates the p38 MAPK pathway and thereby contributes to inflammation and renal injury [7]. In allergic asthma chemerin is shown to inhibit CCL2 secretion and subsequent recruitment of inflammatory dendritic cells [8]. Chemerin may be regarded as an immunoregulatory protein, and dependent on the context, acts as an anti-inflammatory or pro-inflammatory mediator.

Circulating chemerin is increased in obesity and may contribute to adiposity-related dyslipidemia, low-grade inflammation, hypertension and insulin resistance. Chemerin activation of CMKLR1 and GPR1 is not induced in parallel and short, inactive isoforms are elevated in the obese [9]. Detailed evaluation of chemerin processing and the activities of the different isoforms are essential to clarify the function of chemerin in obesity and its related comorbidities.

Chemerin protein levels are elevated in hypertensive patients, and experimental studies support a causative role of chemerin in the control of blood pressure [1]. Angiotensin-I-converting enzyme (ACE) cleaves angiotensin I to produce angiotensin II, a physiological regulator of blood pressure. Inhibition of ACE exerts antihypertensive effects and lowers serum and renal chemerin protein [10]. ACE removes two C-terminal amino acids from the decapeptide chemerin 145–154 indicating a function in chemerin processing [11]. Future work that evaluates the role of particularly the short isoforms of chemerin will help to establish the function of this chemokine in blood pressure control.

In the tightly controlled glucose metabolism, chemerin was shown to regulate glucose-induced insulin release and insulin-stimulated glucose uptake in skeletal muscle, but did not contribute to peripheral insulin resistance in general. Chemerin dose, duration of treatment, type of experimental model and the tissues/cell types analyzed seem to affect chemerin signaling [1,2]. Considering processing of chemerin to different isoforms, which vary in their biological effects and modulation of chemerin activity by the expression levels of its receptors, it is reasonable to postulate a complex association of chemerin with traits of the metabolic syndrome [1,2].

Adipose tissue growth in obesity includes adipocyte hyperplasia and hypertrophy [12]. Chemerin and CMKLR1 have been demonstrated to play a fundamental function in clonal expansion during early adipogenesis [13]. Knock-down of chemerin or CMKLR1 impairs 3T3-L1 cell adipogenesis [14]. Peroxisome proliferator-activated receptor γ (PPARγ) is a crucial regulator of adipogenesis and also elevates chemerin levels [13]. Chemerin release is strongly induced in hypertrophic adipocytes and this seems to contribute to higher systemic levels in the obese [15].

Recent studies suggested that chemerin plays an important role in cancer. Chemerin was found reduced or upregulated in cancer tissues and protective as well as promoting effects on carcinogenesis were identified. Thus similar to its role in inflammation, where chemerin acts as a pro- and anti-inflammatory factor, its effect in cancer depends on the disease context [16].

2. Chemerin and Cancer

2.1. Molecular Mechanisms Underlying the Role of Chemerin in Cancer

2.1.1. Chemerin and Leukocyte Recruitment

Chemerin is an important chemoattractant inducing immunocyte recruitment by its receptors CMKLR1, GPR1 and CCRL2, leading to suppression of tumor growth. Activation of chemoattractant receptors triggers arrest, diapedesis and infiltration of specialized immune cells into the tumor microenvironment, regulating the growth and survival of cancer. Anti-tumoral effector immune cells can slow down the growth of malignancies, like immunostimulatory DC, NK cells and cytotoxic T cells. On the other hand, cancer cells can escape anti-tumoral immune responses in order to survive by different mechanisms like the recruitment of immunosuppressive regulatory T cells or myeloid-derived suppressor cells (MDSC), which are able to inhibit cytotoxic anti-tumor responses. The balance between pro- and anti-tumoral leukocytes finally determines tumor progression [17].

Chemerin receptors are expressed in normal and cancer tissues and on various immune cells. In an early study, CMKLR1 was found in human blood to be expressed by plasmacytoid dendritic cells (pDCs) only, but not in monocytes, neutrophils, eosinophils, lymphocytes or myeloid DCs [18]. A conflicting study identified CMKLR1 protein not only in all human pDCs, but also in about 40% of myeloid DCs, and reported expression of this receptor in mature DCs [19]. LPS and interferon (IFN)-γ were reported to enhance CMKLR1 transcription in macrophages. These inflammatory stimuli induced monocytes to differentiate to the so-called M1 macrophages. M1 but not M2 macrophages were chemotactic to chemerin [20]. Chemerin affects local inflammatory processes, which are characterized by the induction of pro-inflammatory as well as anti-inflammatory and pro-resolving factors, and thereby can accelerate its resolution [21].

Chemerin has been shown to promote pDC migration [18]. This subset of dendritic cells produces type I interferons and has a function in innate and adaptive immune response and cancer. In cancer, pDCs were reported to exert a decreased or absent IFN-α production and contribute to the establishment of an immunosuppressive tumor microenvironment [22]. Chemerin further was shown to promote chemotaxis of macrophages and monocyte derived immature dendritic cells generated by granulocyte macrophage colony stimulating factor (GM–CSF) and IL-13 [23]. A separate study found that chemerin attracted pDC but not mDC (derived from monocytes stimulated with GM–CSF and IL-4) [18]. Mature DCs can activate resting NK cells, which in turn either kill or enable maturation of immature DCs. Chemerin attracts NK cells and mediates co-localization of NK cells with pDC and mDC [24].

In a melanoma model, chemerin transfected cancer cells exhibited a growth inhibitory immune cell distribution in the tumor microenvironment, which was characterized by a higher number of NK and T cells and a relative decline of MDSC and pDCs. In vivo experiments showed that chemerin-expressing mouse B16F0 melanoma grew significantly more slowly than control tumors. Importantly, these tumor suppressive effects were specifically mediated by NK cells, as only NK cell depletion abrogated the effect, and required host expression of CMKLR1, as chemerin-expressing tumors showed accelerated growth in CMKLR1-negative mice [25]. With regard to adrenocortical carcinoma (ACC), studies report that chemerin is down-regulated in malignant tumors compared to benign or normal tissue [26,27]. These studies also report that increased chemerin serum levels were associated with better overall survival, and proposed that tumors may downregulate chemerin to escape immune defenses while host systems may up-regulate chemerin to activate immune responses. Supporting this hypothesis, mouse xenograft models confirmed that the increased serum chemerin levels do not result from expression in tumor tissue, but result of host secretion suggesting an important role of chemerin in host-mediated leukocyte recruitment [27]. Other studies showed that chemerin is expressed in endothelial cells being triggered by inflammatory cytokines, which resulted in increased dendritic cell transmigration mediated by CMKLR1 [28]. In mouse models chemerin has also been observed to suppress M2 macrophage polarization, but to increase the production of pro-inflammatory cytokines such as IFN-γ [29].

In conclusion, an important mechanism by which chemerin exerts anti-tumoral effects is recruiting growth inhibitory immune cells like NK cells to the tumor microenvironment. Tumor cells in turn are reported to reduce chemerin expression to escape immune defense [30].

2.1.2. Intracellular Signaling of Chemerin Receptors

Expression of chemerin and its receptors has been detected in all tumor types tested, but their expression levels vary between different cancer entities and individual patients (Supplemental Figure S1) [31]. Using the GEPIA server analyzing RNAseq data of 9736 tumors and 8587 normal samples of the TCGA and GTEx projects revealed chemerin mRNA expression to be down-regulated in 23 of 31 cancer entities (74.2%), but to be up-regulated in eight of 31 cancer types tested (25.8%; Supplemental Figure S2) [32]. Chemerin has been reported to activate both tumor-promoting and -suppressing intracellular pathways in a receptor- and context-specific manner. Chemerin binding to CMKLR1, but not to GPR1 or CCRL2, strongly increases intracellular calcium concentration, decreases cyclic AMP levels and induces the phosphorylation of p42-p44 MAP kinases, through the Gi class of G proteins [4,23]. Binding of chemerin to CMKLR1 or GPR1 led to recruitment of β-arrestin 1 and 2 [4]. Arrestin binding to the receptors blocks further G protein-mediated signaling, targets receptors for internalization and redirects signaling to alternative G protein-independent pathways, such as β-arrestin signaling [33]. Binding of β-arrestin 1 or β-arrestin 2 exerts opposite effects in cancer progression by interacting with different signaling pathways, which may depend on the tumor microenvironment [34]. While β-arrestin 1 is reported to act tumor-promoting via interaction with c-Src [35], β-arrestin 2 has been shown to inhibit cancer growth and angiogenesis [36]. Chemerin receptor CCRL2 is considered to exert no specific downstream signaling activities, but to present chemerin to CMKLR1 and possibly to GPR1 [23,37,38]. A recent study reported that chemerin activates the transcriptional regulator serum-response factor (SRF) by binding to CMKLR1 and GPR1 through a RhoA and rho-associated protein kinase (ROCK)-dependent pathway [3]. SRF is a transcription factor, which has important roles in tumor progression [39,40]. Chemerin-triggered activation of SRF might be an important molecular mechanism underlying the role of chemerin in cancer. Induction of SRF by chemerin activated its target gene early growth response-1 (EGR1), a transcription factor, which has been suggested to be a tumor suppressor due to its growth inhibitory and pro-apoptotic effects [3,41,42]. Various studies report chemerin-triggered activation of c-FOS via CMKLR1 and SRF [3,43,44]. While c-FOS has been initially demonstrated to act as an oncogene, which is associated with tumor progression and decreased survival of cancer patients [45], recent studies also discovered a tumor-suppressing and pro-apoptotic function of c-FOS in various cancer types including ovarian cancer, hepatocellular carcinoma or prostate cancer and has been shown to be associated with increased survival in ovarian cancer [46–50]. Furthermore, a recent study demonstrated that chemerin suppresses hepatocellular carcinoma (HCC) metastasis through upregulation of expression and phosphatase activity of tumor suppressor PTEN by interfering with PTEN-CMKLR1 interaction, resulting in decreased p-Akt levels, also leading to suppressed migration, invasion and metastasis of HCC cells in vitro. Positive correlation between chemerin and PTEN were also observed in HCC clinical samples [51]. In vivo xenograft mouse models on adrenocortical cancer cells demonstrated that chemerin can decrease the levels of phosphorylated p38 MAPK and β-catenin and was suggested to act as a tumor suppressor [26]. Since the tumor-promoting role of Wnt/β-catenin and MAPK pathway activities is well established [52,53], chemerin might mediate tumor inhibition by reducing Wnt/β-catenin and MAPK pathway activity in adrenocortical carcinoma and, potentially, other cancer types.

In contrast, phosphorylation of p38 and ERK1/2 MAP kinases was reported to be elevated in gastric cancer cells after treatment with chemerin in vitro, leading to increased invasiveness of these cells and up-regulation of vascular endothelial growth factor (VEGF) and matrix metalloproteinase 7 (MMP-7) [54]. Given that MAPK pathways are known to enhance tumor progression and invasion in various cancer types, several other studies support the finding that chemerin may stimulate tumor growth via these mechanisms in gastric cancers [55,56]. Chemerin-triggered activation of MMP-7 expression is considered to be an important molecular mechanism underlying the increased invasiveness of gastric cancer cells, as this protease facilitates tumor cell invasion by degradation of extracellular matrix components, E-cadherin and integrins [57]. Chemerin-triggered activation of MMP expression and invasion of cancer cells has been reported in a variety of studies, including ones on squamous esophageal cancer and neuroblastoma [58,59], supporting the hypothesis that MMP activation is a mechanism underlying a tumor-promoting effect of chemerin in some tumor types.

In conclusion, with regard to intracellular chemerin receptor signaling, convincing evidence both for anti-tumoral actions (activation of PTEN, EGR1 and β-arrestin 2 and inhibition of β-catenin and MAPK activity) and tumor-promoting effects of chemerin (activation of MMP expression, p38 and ERK1/2 MAPK activity and of β-arrestin 1), were reported in different tumor types. Chemerin receptors are able to activate distinct signaling pathways, and chemerin seems to differentially regulate intracellular pathways depending on the tumor type. Thus, more effort is necessary to elucidate the role of chemerin receptor signaling in different cancer entities (Figure 1).

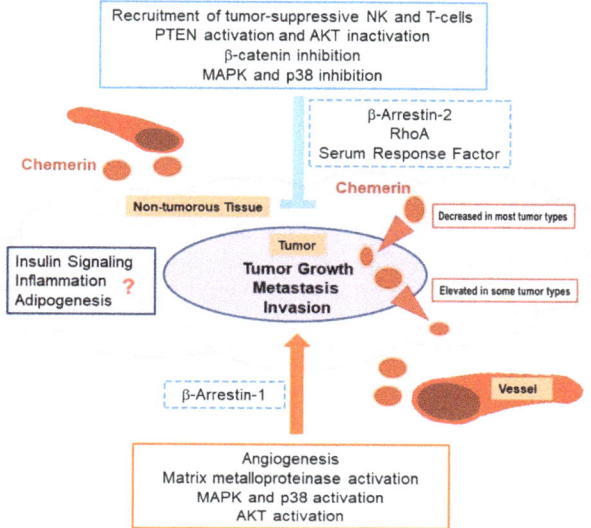

Figure 1. Anti-tumoral and cancer-promoting effects of chemerin. Anti-tumoral activities of chemerin, which are dominant in most cancer entities, include inhibition of MAPK, β-catenin and AKT where the latter is achieved by PTEN activation. These actions partially are mediated via the β2-arrestin and RhoA/serum response factor induced signaling. Both pathways are activated by chemerin binding to GPR1 and CMKLR1. In contrast, tumor-promoting effects are mediated by activation of matrix metalloproteinases, MAPK, p38 and AKT with involvement of β-arrestin-1. Angiogenesis is partly enhanced via these pathways. In about $\frac{3}{4}$ of the tumor types tested, chemerin expression is reduced in cancer tissue when compared to non-tumorous tissues, whereas in about $\frac{1}{4}$ of cancer entities chemerin expression is elevated. Insulin resistance, inflammation and adipogenesis are influenced by chemerin and may also contribute to tumor growth. Impact of these factors was not studied in detail so far.

2.1.3. Chemerin and Angiogenesis

The observed up-regulation of VEGF by chemerin leads to another important mechanism, which might cause a tumor-promoting effect of this adipokine, the activation of angiogenesis. Angiogenesis plays a central role in tumor growth, since solid cancers cannot grow beyond a limited size without an adequate blood supply. VEGF is considered as a key factor of angiogenesis, activating both migration and mitosis of endothelial cells and MMP expression. In a recent study, chemerin was demonstrated to be potently angiogenic via binding to CMKLR1 present on endothelial cells, and dose-dependently induced MMP-2 and MMP-9 activity in these cells [60]. These results were supported by a study observing the same effect of chemerin on angiogenesis and even more demonstrated that chemerin mediated the formation of blood vessels to a similar extent as VEGF [61]. Another recent study reported chemerin-triggered angiogenesis in mice. Chemerin also stimulated the differentiation of human umbilical vein endothelium cells (HUVECs) into capillary-like structures, promoted their proliferation, and functioned as a chemoattractant in migration assays. Chemerin promoted angiogenesis by phosphorylation of Akt and p42/44 extracellular signal-regulated kinase (ERK). Knockdown of chemerin receptor CMKLR1, but not of CCRL2, completely inhibited the chemerin-induced migration and angiogenesis of HUVECs, which indicated that chemerin promoted the migration and angiogenic activities mainly through CMKLR1 [62]. Taken together, convincing data clearly suggest that chemerin induces endothelial angiogenesis, and thereby is able to promote tumor growth.

2.2. Expression of Chemerin and its Receptors and Cancer Survival

2.2.1. Breast Cancer

The role of chemerin in breast cancer has been only addressed by a very limited number of studies. A recent study including 117 breast cancer patients reported that serum chemerin levels did not significantly differ between early or advanced-stage breast cancer [63]. Chemerin and its receptors have been shown to be expressed in breast cancer tissue by means of immunohistochemistry (IHC) or DNA microarray analysis [64]. In a recent study demonstrating CCRL2 expression in breast cancer by means of IHC, increased amounts of CCRL2 were found in breast tumor tissues with high immune cell infiltration. Its expression was upregulated in the presence of pro-inflammatory cytokines, IL-1β, TNF-α, IL-6 and especially IFN-γ [65]. With regard to chemerin expression in breast cancer tissue, a small study including 53 patients [66] detected a significantly higher expression of chemerin in malignant tissue than in the corresponding normal breast tissue ($p = 0.001$). Moreover, its expression was significantly higher in metastatic lymph nodes than in the primary tumor ($p = 0.01$). Chemerin expression was found to be weakly associated with tumor size ($r = 0.235, p = 0.03$), lymph node metastasis ($r = 0.265, p = 0.045$), distant metastasis ($r = 0.267, p = 0.02$) and showed good association with tumor grading, ($r = 0.421, p = 0.004$). Kaplan–Meier survival analysis revealed that patients with higher chemerin expression had worse overall survival in comparison to those with a lower chemerin expression, ($p = 0.001$). In contrast to this study on a small patients´ collective, in a metaanalysis of publicly available DNA microarray data of 3951 breast cancer patients, chemerin expression was observed to be significantly lower in breast cancer tissue than in a normal breast ($p = 2.17 \times 10^{-7}$) and use of Kaplan–Meier plotter software [64] revealed that high chemerin expression in breast cancer tissue did not affect overall survival (OS), but turned out to negatively affect relapse-free survival (RFS; $p = 0.015$; Figure 2). In contrast, high CMKLR1 expression, which did not significantly differ between normal and tumorigenic breast, had robust beneficial effects on RFS of breast cancer patients, but did not affect OS. Chemerin receptor GPR1 was found to be up-regulated in cancer tissue ($p = 0.002$), and high expression of GPR1 also led to prolonged RFS ($p = 0.00082$), but did not affect OS of breast cancer patients. Tissue expression of CCRL2 chemerin receptor, which was similar in normal and malignant breast tissue, neither affected RFS nor OS of women with breast cancer.

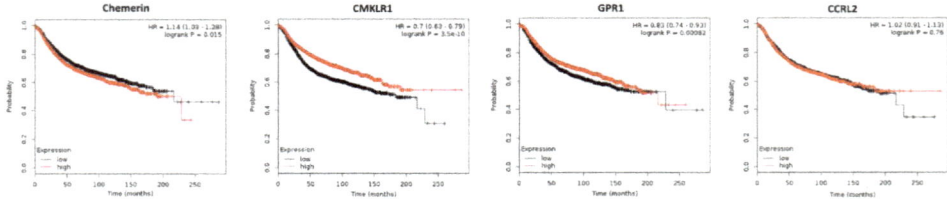

Figure 2. Kaplan–Meier diagrams showing the relapse-free survival (RFS) of 3951 breast cancer patients depending on expression of chemerin and its receptors CMKLR, GPR1 and CCRL2 in tumor tissue, based on a metaanalysis of DNA microarray data (http://kmplot.com/analysis/) [64].

In conclusion, with regard to tumor expression of chemerin receptors, this adipokine is suggested to exert a tumor-suppressive role in breast cancer via binding to CMKLR1 and GPR1. DNA microarray data from 3951 breast cancer patients demonstrated that high mRNA expression of chemerin receptors CMKLR1 and GPR1 in tumor tissue was strongly associated with a longer RFS of breast cancer patients, whereas tissue expression of chemerin slightly decreased RFS and CCRL2 did not significantly affect patients' survival. Given that tumor expression of chemerin is not the major source of this adipokine, the effects of CMKLR1 and GPR1 on survival in this context must be considered to be most relevant, as they bind chemerin from all sources and have been shown to exert intracellular downstream signaling, in contrast to CCRL2. The small IHC-based study including 53 patients mentioned above, which came to conflicting results, was judged to be less significant. The fact that the OS was not significantly affected in this 3951 patients collective might be due to the reported tumor-promoting effects of chemerin like activation of endothelial angiogenesis. However, further studies correlating chemerin serum levels and activity with survival are needed as well as further attempts to integrate the anti-tumoral and proposed tumor-promoting effects of this adipokine on survival of breast cancer patients.

2.2.2. Ovarian Cancer

High levels of active chemerin have been found in a large proportion of ascitic fluids of ovarian carcinomas [67]. Bioactive chemerin and its receptor CMKLR1 have also been detected in human granulosa cells [68]. A recent study demonstrated expression of CMKLR1 in a granulosa cell tumor cell line to be higher than in epithelial cancer cells, whereas chemerin expression and secretion were lower. Treatment with chemerin in vitro was reported not to affect growth of ovarian non-cancer and cancer cell lines [69]. Using an obesity mouse model, the chemerin/CMKLR1 system was observed to be upregulated in the serum, ovaries and granulosa cells and was associated with apoptotic ovarian follicles, oxidative stress and apoptosis biomarkers. Further in vitro experiments confirmed the apoptotic effect of chemerin on granulosa cells [70]. No publications are available examining the effect of serum chemerin or its tumor expression on ovarian cancer growth. However, analyzing publicly available DNA microarray data of 1656 ovarian cancer patients revealed a lower chemerin expression in ovarian cancer tissue than in normal ovary ($p = 0.018$), and using the Kaplan–Meier plotter software revealed that high chemerin expression negatively affected both OS ($p = 5.8 \times 10^{-5}$) and progression-free survival (PFS; $p = 0.00024$) of ovarian cancer patients [64,71]. In contrast, higher expression of chemerin receptor CMKLR1 had a beneficial effect both on OS ($p = 0.05$; Figure 3) and on PFS ($p = 0.0009$). GPR1, which was down-regulated in ovarian cancer tissue ($p = 0.006$), had no significant effect on OS or on PFS of ovarian cancer patients. Expression of CCRL2, which was similar in normal and cancer tissue, also did not affect OS or PFS of ovarian cancer patients (Figure 3 and data not shown).

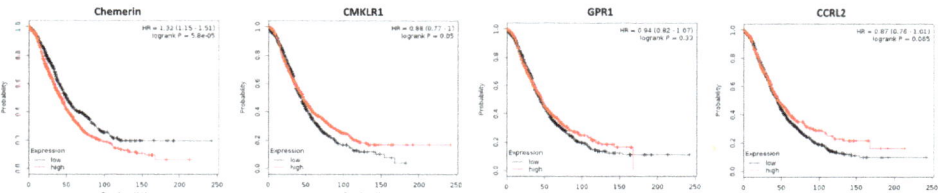

Figure 3. Kaplan–Meier diagrams showing the overall survival (OS) of 1656 ovarian cancer patients depending on expression of chemerin and its receptors CMKLR1, GPR1 and CCRL2 in tumor tissue, based on a metaanalysis of DNA microarray data (http://kmplot.com/analysis/) [71].

In conclusion, with regard to tumor expression of chemerin receptors, this adipokine is suggested to exert a tumor-suppressive role in ovarian cancer via binding to CMKLR1 and CCRL2. The observation that chemerin was able to induce apoptosis in ovarian follicles via CMKLR1 raises the question, whether the same effect could be present in ovarian cancer. The results of DNA microarray analyses of 1656 ovarian cancer patients, demonstrating a significantly decreased survival of patients with high chemerin tumor expression, seemed not to support this hypothesis, but it has to be considered that tumor tissue is only a minor source of chemerin. The prolonged OS of patients with high expression of CMKLR1 and CCRL2 clearly suggested an anti-tumoral effect of serum chemerin being activated in ovarian cancer tissue. However, further studies, particularly on serum chemerin levels, on protein expression of its receptors in ovarian cancer tissue and considering the reported tumor-promoting angiogenic effects of this adipokine, are required to further elucidate the role of chemerin in ovarian cancer.

2.2.3. Non-Small-Cell Lung Cancer (NSCLC)

Circulating chemerin has been reported to be elevated and to exert adverse effects in non-small-cell lung cancer (NSCLC) patients. In a recent case-control study including 220 patients and controls, NSCLC cases exhibited significantly elevated serum chemerin levels compared to controls. In NSCLC cases, chemerin was positively associated with tumor and inflammatory biomarkers, number of infiltrated lymph nodes and NSCLC stage. Serum chemerin was found to be independently associated with NSCLC [72]. These results were supported by another large study reporting elevated levels of circulating chemerin in NSCLC patients, and higher levels of chemerin being associated with advanced TNM stage, lymph node metastasis and distant metastasis. Further analyses revealed that the higher serum chemerin patients had a shorter OS and PFS compared with lower chemerin patients and identified serum chemerin to be an independent risk factor for the prognosis of NSCLC patients [73]. Increased chemerin serum levels in NSCLC patients were also reported in a smaller study, which could not find any association with clinicopathological parameters [74]. A recent study analyzing chemerin expression in NSCLC tissue by IHC in 108 patients observed a decreased expression of this adipokine in about half of the tested patients. Chemerin expression was significantly correlated with the histological grade and the infiltration of NK cells. NSCLC patients with a lower chemerin expression had poorer survival rates than those with a higher expression. Multi-variable Cox regression analysis suggested expression of chemerin to be an independent predictor of a better prognosis for patients with NSCLC [75].

Analyzing publicly available DNA microarray data of 1926 NSCLC patients revealed that chemerin expression was significantly down-regulated in lung cancer tissue when compared to normal lung ($p = 0.0009$), supporting the results of the study mentioned above [76]. However, in contrast to this study, the use of Kaplan–Meier plotter software on these data revealed that high chemerin expression did not affect OS nor time to first progression (FP; Figure 4 and data not shown). CMKLR1, which was found to be up-regulated in cancer tissue ($p = 0.005$), positively affected OS of NSCLC patients ($p = 3.5 \times 10^{-6}$), but not FP. Expression of GPR1 was down-regulated in NSCLC tissue ($p = 7.25 \times 10^{-9}$) and did not affect patients' OS or FP. Elevated expression of CCRL2 was found to have a positive effect on OS and FP of NSCLC patients ($p = 0.0002$ or $p = 0.016$, respectively; Figure 4 and data not shown).

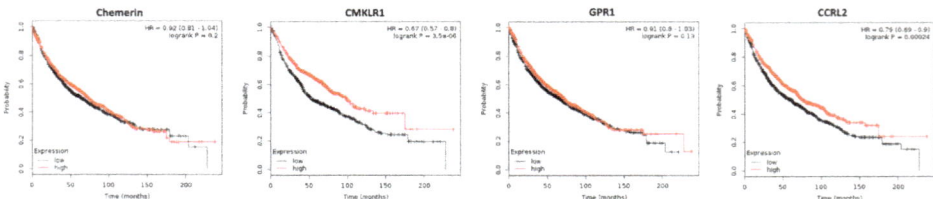

Figure 4. Kaplan–Meier diagrams showing the overall survival (OS) of 1926 patients with non-small-cell lung cancer (NSCLC) depending on expression of chemerin and its receptors CMKLR1, GPR1 and CCRL2 in NSCLC tissue, based on a metaanalysis of DNA microarray data (http://kmplot.com/analysis/) [76].

Importantly, a study performing a genome-wide scan of 307,260 single-nucleotide polymorphisms (SNPs) in 327 advanced-stage NSCLC patients revealed that only a CMKLR1 SNP was significantly associated with overall survival [77].

In conclusion, chemerin serum levels have been reported to be elevated in NSCLC patients, to exert adverse effects on survival and to be an independent risk factor of prognosis of NSCLC patients. In contrast, gene expression analysis of 1926 NSCLC patients revealed that tumor expression of this adipokine did not affect survival. In conflict with the above mentioned studies reporting adverse effects of serum chemerin, the metaanalysis of DNA microarray data demonstrated tumor expression of CMKLR1 and CCRL2 to exert significant beneficial effects on the OS of NSCLC patients, a fact that was supported for CMKLR1 by SNP analyses. To address this controversy, further studies are needed examining chemerin receptor activation in tumor tissue and their expression on the protein level to validate the role of chemerin receptors in NSCLC. It also has to be examined to what extent chemerin-triggered endothelial angiogenesis might contribute to the reported adverse effects of serum chemerin in this cancer entity.

2.2.4. Gastric Cancer

Two recent studies demonstrated elevated chemerin serum levels in patients with gastric cancer, which were associated with tumor progression. In the first study, the increase of serum chemerin levels was shown to be associated with elevated cellular invasiveness, advanced clinical stages and non-intestinal type of gastric cancer [54]. These observations were supported by a second study reporting increased levels of circulating chemerin in gastric cancer patients, which also identified this adipokine as an independent predictor for five-year mortality (odds ratio (OR), 2.718; $p = 0.005$) and adverse event (OR, 2.982; $p = 0.003$) of gastric cancer. High plasma chemerin levels also were observed as an independent predictor for shorter OS and RFS and were suggested to be a potential prognostic biomarker in gastric cancer survival [78]. Chemerin receptors CMKLR1 and GPR1 have been recently reported to be expressed in gastric cancer tissue, as assessed by IHC. In a gastric cancer cell line, chemerin stimulated both, cellular migration and invasion, in a CMKLR1- and GPR1-dependent manner [79]. In line with these studies, the analysis of publicly available DNA microarray data of 876 gastric cancer patients by means of the Kaplan–Meier plotter software [80] demonstrated that high chemerin tumor expression reduced OS of gastric cancer patients ($p = 0.0059$; Figure 5) and also higher tissue expression of CMKLR1 and GPR1 significantly decreased OS of gastric cancer patients ($p = 0.0085$ or $p = 1.7 \times 10^{-7}$, respectively). In contrast, elevated expression of CCRL2 increased OS of these patients ($p = 4.2 \times 10^{-10}$).

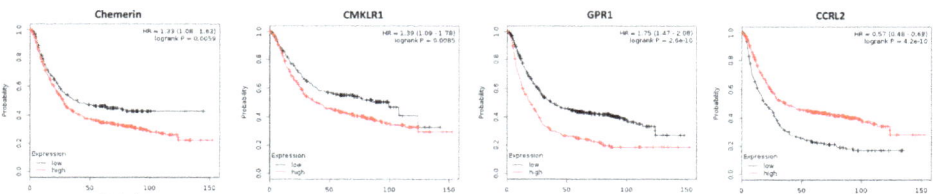

Figure 5. Kaplan–Meier diagrams showing the overall survival (OS) of 876 patients with gastric cancer depending on expression of chemerin and its receptors CMKLR1, GPR1 and CCRL2 in gastric cancer tissue, based on a metaanalysis of DNA microarray data (http://kmplot.com/analysis/) [80].

In conclusion, all present publications and gene expression data clearly suggest a tumor-promoting effect of chemerin in gastric cancer. Both high chemerin serum levels and tumor expression were associated with shorter OS of gastric cancer patients. Chemerin receptors CMKLR1 and GPR1 induced migration and invasion of gastric cancer cells in vitro and were associated with a significantly decreased OS of gastric cancer patients. Thus, serum chemerin levels and tumor expression of CMKLR1 and GPR1 might have the potential to act as prognostic biomarkers in gastric cancer survival. However, further studies are needed to examine chemerin receptor expression on the protein level, their activation and to elucidate the mechanisms underlying the divergent effect of CCRL2.

2.2.5. Hepatocellular Carcinoma

Hepatocellular carcinoma (HCC) is linked to inflammation and immunosuppression. Chemerin is highly expressed in the liver and implicated in the regulation of inflammation. However, the role of chemerin in HCC remains unclear. A recent study reported that chemerin was significantly decreased in blood and tumor tissues of HCC patients, and low tumor chemerin expression was associated with a bad prognosis [81]. Accordingly, two further studies suggested an anti-tumoral effect of chemerin in HCC. The first one also reported chemerin to be decreased in HCC tissue, and lower chemerin expression positively correlated with tumor size and the infiltration of DC and NK cells. Survival analysis indicated that HCC patients with lower chemerin expression had poorer survival than those with higher expression ($p < 0.001$). Multivariable Cox regression analysis revealed that the chemerin expression level was an independent factor for prognosis (HR 3.034, $p = 0.047$) [82]. In line with this study, decreased tumor expression of chemerin was also found to be associated with a poor prognosis of HCC patients in a second study. Additionally, administration of chemerin effectively suppressed extrahepatic and intrahepatic metastases of HCC cells, resulting in prolonged survival of tumor-bearing nude mice [51].

Supporting the mentioned studies suggesting a tumor-suppressive role of chemerin, the metaanalysis of publicly available gene expression data of 364 patients with HCC by means of the Kaplan–Meier plotter software [83] revealed that high chemerin expression in cancer tissue significantly increased patients' OS ($p = 0.00027$) and progression-free survival (PFS; $p = 0.012$). Higher expression of CMKLR1 did not significantly affect OS of HCC patients, but increased their PFS ($p = 0.0017$). Tumor expression of GPR1 or CCRL2 did not significantly alter OS or PFS of patients with HCC (Figure 6 and data not shown).

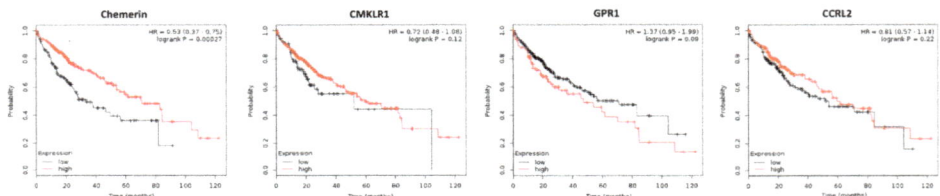

Figure 6. Kaplan–Meier diagrams showing the overall survival (OS) of 364 patients with hepatocellular carcinoma (HCC) depending on expression of chemerin and its receptors CMKLR1, GPR1 and CCRL2 in tumor tissue, based on a metaanalysis of DNA microarray data (http://kmplot.com/analysis/) [83].

In conclusion, the majority of the present data clearly suggest an anti-tumoral role of chemerin in HCC. However, further studies are needed to elucidate the relationship of serum chemerin levels and cancer survival, to examine chemerin receptor activation and their tumor expression on the protein level.

2.2.6. Other Cancer Types

In adrenocortical carcinoma (ACC), chemerin has been suggested to act as a tumor-suppressor. In a genome-wide gene expression study on 85 patients, chemerin expression was found to be strongly down-regulated in adrenocortical carcinoma when compared to benign tumors and was suggested to have an excellent diagnostic accuracy for distinguishing benign from malignant adrenocortical tumors [84]. Another study reported decreased tumor chemerin gene expression, but increased serum levels of this adipokine as compared with patients with benign adrenocortical tumors. Higher serum chemerin levels were associated with improved overall survival [27]. The decreased chemerin expression in ACC was demonstrated to be the result of chemerin gene CpG hypermethylation. In contrast, chemerin overexpression in ACC cell lines not only reduced cell proliferation, cell invasion and tumorigenicity in vitro, but also inhibited tumor growth in vivo in immunodeficient mouse xenograft models [26].

In acute myeloid leukemia (AML), a recent study also suggests a tumor-suppressing role of chemerin, demonstrating that chemerin was down-regulated in the bone marrow mononuclear cells of AML patients compared to that of healthy controls. In patients with AML, low chemerin expression correlated with poorer overall survival. It was shown that chemerin was independently able to prognosticate AML patients, and high chemerin expression was associated with positive prognosis [85]. Chemerin receptor CCRL2 was reported to be overexpressed in AML cells and was suggested to be a potential therapeutic target [86].

In melanoma, chemerin was shown to inhibit tumor growth by eliciting antitumor responses and altering the tumor microenvironment in favor of growth inhibition. Chemerin was found to be down-regulated in melanoma and high chemerin mRNA expression in tumors correlated with improved outcome in human melanoma. The anti-tumoral effect of chemerin was associated with increased recruitment of NK cells and was CMKLR1-dependent [25].

Further research is needed to elucidate the role of chemerin in cancer, particularly with regard to cancer entities not mentioned here.

3. Conclusions

Chemerin is a pleiotropic protein, which has been demonstrated to affect tumor growth, being able to exert both anti-tumoral and tumor-promoting effects. The majority of present data report down-regulation of chemerin in cancer tissue and suggest a tumor-suppressing role of chemerin in most cancer entities, being mediated by recruiting innate immune defenses and by growth-inhibitory downstream signaling by chemerin receptors CMKLR1 and GPR1. However, this anti-tumoral effect seems to be tissue-specific, since e.g., in gastric cancer, all available data suggest a tumor-promoting role of chemerin, which is mediated by different receptor signal transduction. Although the activating effect of this protein on endothelial angiogenesis is an important mechanism promoting tumor growth, it does not seem to significantly affect the beneficial role of chemerin. Association of tumor expression of chemerin receptors on patients' survival was observed in most cancer entities. Further studies are needed to elucidate the role of this protein in different cancer types and to what extent therapeutic modulation of chemerin might be an option for cancer therapy.

Supplementary Materials: Supplementary materials can be found at http://www.mdpi.com/1422-0067/20/15/3750/s1. Figure S1. Tumor tissue expression of chemerin and its receptors as assessed by means of RNA-seq shown as median FPKM (number Fragments Per Kilobase of exon per Million reads), generated by The Cancer Genome Atlas (TCGA). Data are from the open-access database (www.proteinatlas.org) [31]. The links to the single genes are: https://www.proteinatlas.org/ENSG00000106538-RARRES2/pathology, https://www.proteinatlas.org/ENSG00000174600-CMKLR1/pathology, https://www.proteinatlas.org/ENSG00000183671-GPR1/pathology and https://www.proteinatlas.org/ENSG00000121797-CCRL2/pathology. Figure S2. Comparison of chemerin mRNA expression in normal and tumor tissues using GEPIA, a newly developed interactive web server for analyzing the RNA sequencing expression data of 9736 tumors and 8587 normal samples from the TCGA and the GTEx projects [32]. (http://gepia.cancer-pku.cn/detail.php?gene=RARRES2). Values are expressed in transcripts per million (TPM). Abbreviations: ACC Adrenocortical carcinoma, BLCA Bladder Urothelial Carcinoma, BRCA Breast invasive carcinoma, CESC Cervical squamous cell carcinoma and endocervical adenocarcinoma, CHOL Cholangio carcinoma, COAD Colon adenocarcinoma, DLBC Lymphoid Neoplasm Diffuse Large B-cell Lymphoma, ESCA Esophageal carcinoma, GBM Glioblastoma multiforme, HNSC Head and Neck squamous cell carcinoma, KICH Kidney Chromophobe, KIRC Kidney renal clear cell carcinoma, KIRP Kidney renal papillary cell carcinoma, LAML Acute Myeloid Leukemia, LGG Brain Lower Grade Glioma LIHC Liver hepatocellular carcinoma, LUAD Lung adenocarcinoma, LUSC Lung squamous cell carcinoma, MESO Mesothelioma, OV Ovarian serous cystadenocarcinoma, PAAD Pancreatic adenocarcinoma, PCPG Pheochromocytoma and Paraganglioma, PRAD Prostate adenocarcinoma, READ Rectum adenocarcinoma, SARC Sarcoma, SKCM Skin Cutaneous Melanoma, STAD Stomach adenocarcinoma, TGCT Testicular Germ Cell Tumors, THCA Thyroid carcinoma, THYM Thymoma, UCEC Uterine Corpus Endometrial Carcinoma, UCS Uterine Carcinosarcoma. UVM Uveal Melanoma.

Funding: Research of C.B. was funded by the German Research Foundation, grant number BU 1141/13-1.

Conflicts of Interest: The authors declare no conflict of interest.

References

1. Buechler, C.; Feder, S.; Haberl, E.M.; Aslanidis, C. Chemerin isoforms and activity in obesity. *Int. J. Mol. Sci.* **2019**, *20*, 1128. [CrossRef]
2. Rourke, J.L.; Dranse, H.J.; Sinal, C.J. Towards an integrative approach to understanding the role of chemerin in human health and disease. *Obes. Rev. Off. J. Int. Assoc. Study Obes.* **2013**, *14*, 245–262. [CrossRef]
3. Rourke, J.L.; Dranse, H.J.; Sinal, C.J. CMKLR1 and GPR1 mediate chemerin signaling through the RhoA/ROCK pathway. *Mol. Cell. Endocrinol.* **2015**, *417*, 36–51. [CrossRef]

4. Henau, O. de; Degroot, G.N.; Imbault, V.; Robert, V.; Poorter, C. de; Mcheik, S.; Galés, C.; Parmentier, M.; Springael, J.Y. Signaling properties of chemerin receptors CMKLR1, GPR1 and CCRL2. *PLoS ONE* **2016**, *11*, e0164179. [CrossRef]
5. Jaworek, J.; Szklarczyk, J.; Kot, M.; Góralska, M.; Jaworek, A.; Bonior, J.; Leja-Szpak, A.; Nawrot-Porąbka, K.; Link-Lenczowski, P.; Ceranowicz, P.; et al. Chemerin alleviates acute pancreatitis in the rat thorough modulation of NF-κB signal. *Pancreatol. Off. J. Int. Assoc. Pancreatol.* **2019**, *19*, 401–408. [CrossRef]
6. Dimitriadis, G.K.; Kaur, J.; Adya, R.; Miras, A.D.; Mattu, H.S.; Hattersley, J.G.; Kaltsas, G.; Tan, B.K.; Randeva, H.S. Chemerin induces endothelial cell inflammation: Activation of nuclear factor-kappa β and monocyte-endothelial adhesion. *Oncotarget* **2018**, *9*, 16678–16690. [CrossRef]
7. Shang, J.; Wang, L.; Zhang, Y.; Zhang, S.; Ning, L.; Zhao, J.; Cheng, G.; Liu, D.; Xiao, J.; Zhao, Z. Chemerin/ChemR23 axis promotes inflammation of glomerular endothelial cells in diabetic nephropathy. *J. Cell. Mol. Med.* **2019**, *23*, 3417–3428. [CrossRef]
8. Zhao, L.; Yang, W.; Yang, X.; Lin, Y.; Lv, J.; Dou, X.; Luo, Q.; Dong, J.; Chen, Z.; Chu, Y.; et al. Chemerin suppresses murine allergic asthma by inhibiting CCL2 production and subsequent airway recruitment of inflammatory dendritic cells. *Allergy* **2014**, *69*, 763–774. [CrossRef]
9. Chang, S.S.; Eisenberg, D.; Zhao, L.; Adams, C.; Leib, R.; Morser, J.; Leung, L. Chemerin activation in human obesity. *Obesity* **2016**, *24*, 1522–1529. [CrossRef]
10. Huang, H.; Hu, L.; Lin, J.; Zhu, X.; Cui, W.; Xu, W. Effect of fosinopril on chemerin and VEGF expression in diabetic nephropathy rats. *Int. J. Clin. Exp. Pathol.* **2015**, *8*, 11470–11474.
11. John, H.; Hierer, J.; Haas, O.; Forssmann, W.G. Quantification of angiotensin-converting-enzyme-mediated degradation of human chemerin 145–154 in plasma by matrix-assisted laser desorption/ionization-time-of-flight mass spectrometry. *Anal. Biochem.* **2007**, *362*, 117–125. [CrossRef]
12. Buechler, C.; Wanninger, J.; Neumeier, M. Adiponectin, a key adipokine in obesity related liver diseases. *World J. Gastroenterol.* **2011**, *17*, 2801–2811.
13. Muruganandan, S.; Parlee, S.D.; Rourke, J.L.; Ernst, M.C.; Goralski, K.B.; Sinal, C.J. Chemerin, a novel peroxisome proliferator-activated receptor gamma (PPARgamma) target gene that promotes mesenchymal stem cell adipogenesis. *J. Biol. Chem.* **2011**, *286*, 23982–23995. [CrossRef]
14. Goralski, K.B.; Mc Carthy, T.C.; Hanniman, E.A.; Zabel, B.A.; Butcher, E.C.; Parlee, S.D.; Muruganandan, S.; Sinal, C.J. Chemerin, a novel adipokine that regulates adipogenesis and adipocyte metabolism. *J. Biol. Chem.* **2007**, *282*, 28175–28188. [CrossRef]
15. Bauer, S.; Wanninger, J.; Schmidhofer, S.; Weigert, J.; Neumeier, M.; Dorn, C.; Hellerbrand, C.; Zimara, N.; Schäffler, A.; Aslanidis, C.; et al. Sterol regulatory element-binding protein 2 (SREBP2) activation after excess triglyceride storage induces chemerin in hypertrophic adipocytes. *Endocrinology* **2011**, *152*, 26–35. [CrossRef]
16. Shin, W.J.; Pachynski, R.K. Chemerin modulation of tumor growth: Potential clinical applications in cancer. *Discov. Med.* **2018**, *26*, 31–37.
17. Galon, J.; Angell, H.K.; Bedognetti, D.; Marincola, F.M. The continuum of cancer immunosurveillance: Prognostic, predictive, and mechanistic signatures. *Immunity* **2013**, *39*, 11–26. [CrossRef]
18. Zabel, B.A.; Silverio, A.M.; Butcher, E.C. Chemokine-like receptor 1 expression and chemerin-directed chemotaxis distinguish plasmacytoid from myeloid dendritic cells in human blood. *J. Immunol.* **2005**, *174*, 244–251. [CrossRef]
19. Vermi, W.; Riboldi, E.; Wittamer, V.; Gentili, F.; Luini, W.; Marrelli, S.; Vecchi, A.; Franssen, J.D.; Communi, D.; Massardi, L.; et al. Role of ChemR23 in directing the migration of myeloid and plasmacytoid dendritic cells to lymphoid organs and inflamed skin. *J. Exp. Med.* **2005**, *201*, 509–515. [CrossRef]
20. Herová, M.; Schmid, M.; Gemperle, C.; Hersberger, M. ChemR23, the receptor for chemerin and resolvin E1, is expressed and functional on M1 but not on M2 macrophages. *J. Immunol.* **2015**, *194*, 2330–2337. [CrossRef]
21. Buechler, C.; Pohl, R.; Aslanidis, C. Pro-resolving molecules-new approaches to treat sepsis? *Int. J. Mol. Sci.* **2017**, *18*, 476. [CrossRef]
22. Mitchell, D.; Chintala, S.; Dey, M. Plasmacytoid dendritic cell in immunity and cancer. *J. Neuroimmunol.* **2018**, *322*, 63–73. [CrossRef]
23. Wittamer, V.; Franssen, J.D.; Vulcano, M.; Mirjolet, J.F.; Le Poul, E.; Migeotte, I.; Brézillon, S.; Tyldesley, R.; Blanpain, C.; Detheux, M.; et al. Specific recruitment of antigen-presenting cells by chemerin, a novel processed ligand from human inflammatory fluids. *J. Exp. Med.* **2003**, *198*, 977–985. [CrossRef]
24. Parolini, S.; Santoro, A.; Marcenaro, E.; Luini, W.; Massardi, L.; Facchetti, F.; Communi, D.; Parmentier, M.; Majorana, A.; Sironi, M.; et al. The role of chemerin in the colocalization of NK and dendritic cell subsets into inflamed tissues. *Blood* **2007**, *109*, 3625–3632. [CrossRef]

25. Pachynski, R.K.; Zabel, B.A.; Kohrt, H.E.; Tejeda, N.M.; Monnier, J.; Swanson, C.D.; Holzer, A.K.; Gentles, A.J.; Sperinde, G.V.; Edalati, A.; et al. The chemoattractant chemerin suppresses melanoma by recruiting natural killer cell antitumor defenses. *J. Exp. Med.* **2012**, *209*, 1427–1435. [CrossRef]
26. Liu-Chittenden, Y.; Jain, M.; Gaskins, K.; Wang, S.; Merino, M.J.; Kotian, S.; Kumar Gara, S.; Davis, S.; Zhang, L.; Kebebew, E. RARRES2 functions as a tumor suppressor by promoting β-catenin phosphorylation/degradation and inhibiting p38 phosphorylation in adrenocortical carcinoma. *Oncogene* **2017**, *36*, 3541–3552. [CrossRef]
27. Liu-Chittenden, Y.; Patel, D.; Gaskins, K.; Giordano, T.J.; Assie, G.; Bertherat, J.; Kebebew, E. Serum RARRES2 is a prognostic marker in patients with adrenocortical carcinoma. *J. Clin. Endocrinol. Metab.* **2016**, *101*, 3345–3352. [CrossRef]
28. Gonzalvo-Feo, S.; Del Prete, A.; Pruenster, M.; Salvi, V.; Wang, L.; Sironi, M.; Bierschenk, S.; Sperandio, M.; Vecchi, A.; Sozzani, S. Endothelial cell-derived chemerin promotes dendritic cell transmigration. *J. Immunol.* **2014**, *192*, 2366–2373. [CrossRef]
29. Lin, Y.; Yang, X.; Yue, W.; Xu, X.; Li, B.; Zou, L.; He, R. Chemerin aggravates DSS-induced colitis by suppressing M2 macrophage polarization. *Cell. Mol. Immunol.* **2014**, *11*, 355–366. [CrossRef]
30. Shin, W.J.; Zabel, B.A.; Pachynski, R.K. Mechanisms and functions of chemerin in cancer: Potential roles in therapeutic intervention. *Front. Immunol.* **2018**, *9*, 2772. [CrossRef]
31. Uhlen, M.; Zhang, C.; Lee, S.; Sjöstedt, E.; Fagerberg, L.; Bidkhori, G.; Benfeitas, R.; Arif, M.; Liu, Z.; Edfors, F.; et al. A pathology atlas of the human cancer transcriptome. *Science* **2017**, *357*. [CrossRef]
32. Tang, Z.; Li, C.; Kang, B.; Gao, G.; Li, C.; Zhang, Z. GEPIA: A web server for cancer and normal gene expression profiling and interactive analyses. *Nucleic Acids Res.* **2017**, *45*, W98–W102. [CrossRef]
33. Cahill, T.J.; Thomsen, A.R.B.; Tarrasch, J.T.; Plouffe, B.; Nguyen, A.H.; Yang, F.; Huang, L.Y.; Kahsai, A.W.; Bassoni, D.L.; Gavino, B.J.; et al. Distinct conformations of GPCR-β-arrestin complexes mediate desensitization, signaling, and endocytosis. *Proc. Natl. Acad. Sci. USA* **2017**, *114*, 2562–2567. [CrossRef]
34. Song, Q.; Ji, Q.; Li, Q. The role and mechanism of β-arrestins in cancer invasion and metastasis (Review). *Int. J. Mol. Med.* **2018**, *41*, 631–639. [CrossRef]
35. Buchanan, F.G.; Gorden, D.L.; Matta, P.; Shi, Q.; Matrisian, L.M.; DuBois, R.N. Role of β-arrestin 1 in the metastatic progression of colorectal cancer. *Proc. Natl. Acad. Sci. USA* **2006**, *103*, 1492–1497. [CrossRef]
36. Raghuwanshi, S.K.; Nasser, M.W.; Chen, X.; Strieter, R.M.; Richardson, R.M. Depletion of β-arrestin-2 promotes tumor growth and angiogenesis in a murine model of lung cancer. *J. Immunol.* **2008**, *180*, 5699–5706. [CrossRef]
37. Bondue, B.; Wittamer, V.; Parmentier, M. Chemerin and its receptors in leukocyte trafficking, inflammation and metabolism. *Cytokine Growth Factor Rev.* **2011**, *22*, 331–338. [CrossRef]
38. Yoshimura, T.; Oppenheim, J.J. Chemokine-like receptor 1 (CMKLR1) and chemokine (C-C motif) receptor-like 2 (CCRL2); two multifunctional receptors with unusual properties. *Exp. Cell Res.* **2011**, *317*, 674–684. [CrossRef]
39. Yin, J.; Lv, X.; Hu, S.; Zhao, X.; Liu, Q.; Xie, H. Overexpression of serum response factor is correlated with poor prognosis in patients with gastric cancer. *Hum. Pathol.* **2019**, *85*, 10–17. [CrossRef]
40. O'Hurley, G.; Prencipe, M.; Lundon, D.; O'Neill, A.; Boyce, S.; O'Grady, A.; Gallagher, W.M.; Morrissey, C.; Kay, E.W.; Watson, R.W.G. The analysis of serum response factor expression in bone and soft tissue prostate cancer metastases. *Prostate* **2014**, *74*, 306–313. [CrossRef]
41. Nair, P.; Muthukkumar, S.; Sells, S.F.; Han, S.S.; Sukhatme, V.P.; Rangnekar, V.M. Early growth response-1-dependent apoptosis is mediated by p53. *J. Biol. Chem.* **1997**, *272*, 20131–20138. [CrossRef]
42. Krones-Herzig, A.; Adamson, E.; Mercola, D. Early growth response 1 protein, an upstream gatekeeper of the p53 tumor suppressor, controls replicative senescence. *Proc. Natl. Acad. Sci. USA* **2003**, *100*, 3233–3238. [CrossRef]
43. Muruganandan, S.; Dranse, H.J.; Rourke, J.L.; McMullen, N.M.; Sinal, C.J. Chemerin neutralization blocks hematopoietic stem cell osteoclastogenesis. *Stem Cells* **2013**, *31*, 2172–2182. [CrossRef]
44. Li, L.; Huang, C.; Zhang, X.; Wang, J.; Ma, P.; Liu, Y.; Xiao, T.; Zabel, B.A.; Zhang, J.V. Chemerin-derived peptide C-20 suppressed gonadal steroidogenesis. *Am. J. Reprod. Immunol.* **2014**, *71*, 265–277. [CrossRef]
45. Guo, J.C.; Li, J.; Zhao, Y.P.; Zhou, L.; Cui, Q.C.; Zhou, W.X.; Zhang, T.P.; You, L. Expression of c-fos was associated with clinicopathologic characteristics and prognosis in pancreatic cancer. *PLoS ONE* **2015**, *10*, e0120332. [CrossRef]
46. Mahner, S.; Baasch, C.; Schwarz, J.; Hein, S.; Wölber, L.; Jänicke, F.; Milde-Langosch, K. C-Fos expression is a molecular predictor of progression and survival in epithelial ovarian carcinoma. *Br. J. Cancer* **2008**, *99*, 1269–1275. [CrossRef]

47. Oliveira-Ferrer, L.; Rößler, K.; Haustein, V.; Schröder, C.; Wicklein, D.; Maltseva, D.; Khaustova, N.; Samatov, T.; Tonevitsky, A.; Mahner, S.; et al. c-FOS suppresses ovarian cancer progression by changing adhesion. *Br. J. Cancer* **2014**, *110*, 753–763. [CrossRef]
48. Teng, C.S. Protooncogenes as mediators of apoptosis. *Int. Rev. Cytol.* **2000**, *197*, 137–202.
49. Mikula, M.; Gotzmann, J.; Fischer, A.N.M.; Wolschek, M.F.; Thallinger, C.; Schulte-Hermann, R.; Beug, H.; Mikulits, W. The proto-oncoprotein c-Fos negatively regulates hepatocellular tumorigenesis. *Oncogene* **2003**, *22*, 6725–6738. [CrossRef]
50. Zhang, X.; Zhang, L.; Yang, H.; Huang, X.; Otu, H.; Libermann, T.A.; DeWolf, W.C.; Khosravi-Far, R.; Olumi, A.F. c-Fos as a proapoptotic agent in TRAIL-induced apoptosis in prostate cancer cells. *Cancer Res.* **2007**, *67*, 9425–9434. [CrossRef]
51. Li, J.J.; Yin, H.K.; Guan, D.X.; Zhao, J.S.; Feng, Y.X.; Deng, Y.Z.; Wang, X.; Li, N.; Wang, X.F.; Cheng, S.Q.; et al. Chemerin suppresses hepatocellular carcinoma metastasis through CMKLR1-PTEN-Akt axis. *Br. J. Cancer* **2018**, *118*, 1337–1348. [CrossRef]
52. Krishnamurthy, N.; Kurzrock, R. Targeting the Wnt/β-catenin pathway in cancer: Update on effectors and inhibitors. *Cancer Treat. Rev.* **2018**, *62*, 50–60. [CrossRef]
53. Burotto, M.; Chiou, V.L.; Lee, J.M.; Kohn, E.C. The MAPK pathway across different malignancies: A new perspective. *Cancer* **2014**, *120*, 3446–3456. [CrossRef]
54. Wang, C.; Wu, W.K.K.; Liu, X.; To, K.F.; Chen, G.G.; Yu, J.; Ng, E.K.W. Increased serum chemerin level promotes cellular invasiveness in gastric cancer: A clinical and experimental study. *Peptides* **2014**, *51*, 131–138. [CrossRef]
55. Graziosi, L.; Mencarelli, A.; Santorelli, C.; Renga, B.; Cipriani, S.; Cavazzoni, E.; Palladino, G.; Laufer, S.; Burnet, M.; Donini, A.; et al. Mechanistic role of p38 MAPK in gastric cancer dissemination in a rodent model peritoneal metastasis. *Eur. J. Pharmacol.* **2012**, *674*, 143–152. [CrossRef]
56. Fujimori, Y.; Inokuchi, M.; Takagi, Y.; Kato, K.; Kojima, K.; Sugihara, K. Prognostic value of RKIP and p-ERK in gastric cancer. *J. Exp. Clin. Cancer Res. CR* **2012**, *31*, 30. [CrossRef]
57. Rémy, L.; Trespeuch, C. Matrilysine 1 et pathologie cancéreuse. *Med. Sci. M/S* **2005**, *21*, 498–502.
58. Kumar, J.D.; Kandola, S.; Tiszlavicz, L.; Reisz, Z.; Dockray, G.J.; Varro, A. The role of chemerin and ChemR23 in stimulating the invasion of squamous oesophageal cancer cells. *Br. J. Cancer* **2016**, *114*, 1152–1159. [CrossRef]
59. Tümmler, C.; Snapkov, I.; Wickström, M.; Moens, U.; Ljungblad, L.; Maria Elfman, L.H.; Winberg, J.O.; Kogner, P.; Johnsen, J.I.; Sveinbjørnsson, B. Inhibition of chemerin/CMKLR1 axis in neuroblastoma cells reduces clonogenicity and cell viability in vitro and impairs tumor growth in vivo. *Oncotarget* **2017**, *8*, 95135–95151. [CrossRef]
60. Kaur, J.; Adya, R.; Tan, B.K.; Chen, J.; Randeva, H.S. Identification of chemerin receptor (ChemR23) in human endothelial cells: Chemerin-induced endothelial angiogenesis. *Biochem. Biophys. Res. Commun.* **2010**, *391*, 1762–1768. [CrossRef]
61. Bozaoglu, K.; Curran, J.E.; Stocker, C.J.; Zaibi, M.S.; Segal, D.; Konstantopoulos, N.; Morrison, S.; Carless, M.; Dyer, T.D.; Cole, S.A.; et al. Chemerin, a novel adipokine in the regulation of angiogenesis. *J. Clin. Endocrinol. Metab.* **2010**, *95*, 2476–2485. [CrossRef]
62. Nakamura, N.; Naruse, K.; Kobayashi, Y.; Miyabe, M.; Saiki, T.; Enomoto, A.; Takahashi, M.; Matsubara, T. Chemerin promotes angiogenesis in vivo. *Physiol. Rep.* **2018**, *6*, e13962. [CrossRef]
63. Serkan, A.; Safak, A.; Emre, G.; Elif, H.; Ayse, L.D.; Mustafa, K.A. Serum chemerin level in breast cancer. *Int. J. Hematol. Oncol.* **2019**, 127–132.
64. Györffy, B.; Lanczky, A.; Eklund, A.C.; Denkert, C.; Budczies, J.; Li, Q.; Szallasi, Z. An online survival analysis tool to rapidly assess the effect of 22,277 genes on breast cancer prognosis using microarray data of 1809 patients. *Breast Cancer Res. Treat.* **2010**, *123*, 725–731. [CrossRef]
65. Sarmadi, P.; Tunali, G.; Esendagli-Yilmaz, G.; Yilmaz, K.B.; Esendagli, G. CRAM-A indicates IFN-γ-associated inflammatory response in breast cancer. *Mol. Immunol.* **2015**, *68*, 692–698. [CrossRef]
66. El-Sagheer, G.; Gayyed, M.; Ahmad, A.; Abd El-Fattah, A.; Mohamed, M. Expression of chemerin correlates with a poor prognosis in female breast cancer patients. *Breast Cancer* **2018**, *10*, 169–176. [CrossRef]
67. Schutyser, E.; Struyf, S.; Proost, P.; Opdenakker, G.; Laureys, G.; Verhasselt, B.; Peperstraete, L.; van de Putte, I.; Saccani, A.; Allavena, P.; et al. Identification of biologically active chemokine isoforms from ascitic fluid and elevated levels of CCL18/pulmonary and activation-regulated chemokine in ovarian carcinoma. *J. Biol. Chem.* **2002**, *277*, 24584–24593. [CrossRef]
68. Reverchon, M.; Cornuau, M.; Ramé, C.; Guerif, F.; Royère, D.; Dupont, J. Chemerin inhibits IGF-1-induced progesterone and estradiol secretion in human granulosa cells. *Hum. Reprod.* **2012**, *27*, 1790–1800. [CrossRef]

69. Hoffmann, M.; Rak, A.; Ptak, A. Bisphenol A and its derivatives decrease expression of chemerin, which reverses its stimulatory action in ovarian cancer cells. *Toxicol. Lett.* **2018**, *291*, 61–69. [CrossRef]
70. Yao, J.; Li, Z.; Fu, Y.; Wu, R.; Wang, Y.; Liu, C.; Yang, L.; Zhang, H. Involvement of obesity-associated upregulation of chemerin/chemokine-like receptor 1 in oxidative stress and apoptosis in ovaries and granulosa cells. *Biochem. Biophys. Res. Commun.* **2019**, *510*, 449–455. [CrossRef]
71. Gyorffy, B.; Lánczky, A.; Szállási, Z. Implementing an online tool for genome-wide validation of survival-associated biomarkers in ovarian-cancer using microarray data from 1287 patients. *Endocr. Relat. Cancer* **2012**, *19*, 197–208. [CrossRef] [PubMed]
72. Sotiropoulos, G.P.; Dalamaga, M.; Antonakos, G.; Marinou, I.; Vogiatzakis, E.; Kotopouli, M.; Karampela, I.; Christodoulatos, G.S.; Lekka, A.; Papavassiliou, A.G. Chemerin as a biomarker at the intersection of inflammation, chemotaxis, coagulation, fibrinolysis and metabolism in resectable non-small cell lung cancer. *Lung Cancer* **2018**, *125*, 291–299. [CrossRef] [PubMed]
73. Xu, C.H.; Yang, Y.; Wang, Y.C.; Yan, J.; Qian, L.H. Prognostic significance of serum chemerin levels in patients with non-small cell lung cancer. *Oncotarget* **2017**, *8*, 22483–22489. [CrossRef] [PubMed]
74. Qu, X.; Han, L.; Wang, S.; Zhang, Q.; Yang, C.; Xu, S.; Zhang, L. Detection of chemerin and it's clinical significance in peripheral blood of patients with lung cancer. *Chin. J. Lung Cancer* **2009**, *12*, 1174–1177.
75. Zhao, S.; Li, C.; Ye, J.B.; Peng, F.; Chen, Q. Expression of chemerin correlates with a favorable prognosis in patients with non-small cell lung cancer. *Lab. Med.* **2011**, *42*, 553–557. [CrossRef]
76. Győrffy, B.; Surowiak, P.; Budczies, J.; Lánczky, A. Online survival analysis software to assess the prognostic value of biomarkers using transcriptomic data in non-small-cell lung cancer. *PLoS ONE* **2013**, *8*, e82241. [CrossRef] [PubMed]
77. Wu, X.; Ye, Y.; Rosell, R.; Amos, C.I.; Stewart, D.J.; Hildebrandt, M.A.T.; Roth, J.A.; Minna, J.D.; Gu, J.; Lin, J.; et al. Genome-wide association study of survival in non-small cell lung cancer patients receiving platinum-based chemotherapy. *J. Natl. Cancer Inst.* **2011**, *103*, 817–825. [CrossRef] [PubMed]
78. Zhang, J.; Jin, H.C.; Zhu, A.K.; Ying, R.C.; Wei, W.; Zhang, F.J. Prognostic significance of plasma chemerin levels in patients with gastric cancer. *Peptides* **2014**, *61*, 7–11. [CrossRef]
79. Kumari, N.; Dwarakanath, B.S.; Das, A.; Bhatt, A.N. Role of interleukin-6 in cancer progression and therapeutic resistance. *Tumor Biol. J. Int. Soc. Oncodevelop. Biol. Med.* **2016**, *37*, 11553–11572. [CrossRef] [PubMed]
80. Szász, A.M.; Lánczky, A.; Nagy, Á.; Förster, S.; Hark, K.; Green, J.E.; Boussioutas, A.; Busuttil, R.; Szabó, A.; Győrffy, B. Cross-validation of survival associated biomarkers in gastric cancer using transcriptomic data of 1065 patients. *Oncotarget* **2016**, *7*, 49322–49333. [CrossRef]
81. Lin, Y.; Yang, X.; Liu, W.; Li, B.; Yin, W.; Shi, Y.; He, R. Chemerin has a protective role in hepatocellular carcinoma by inhibiting the expression of IL-6 and GM-CSF and MDSC accumulation. *Oncogene* **2017**, *36*, 3599–3608. [CrossRef] [PubMed]
82. Lin, W.; Chen, Y.L.; Jiang, L.; Chen, J.K. Reduced expression of chemerin is associated with a poor prognosis and a lowed infiltration of both dendritic cells and natural killer cells in human hepatocellular carcinoma. *Clin. Lab.* **2011**, *57*, 879–885. [PubMed]
83. Menyhárt, O.; Nagy, A.; Győrffy, B. Determining consistent prognostic biomarkers of overall survival and vascular invasion in hepatocellular carcinoma. *R. Soc. Open Sci.* **2018**, 181006–181010.
84. Fernandez-Ranvier, G.G.; Weng, J.; Yeh, R.F.; Khanafshar, E.; Suh, I.; Barker, C.; Duh, Q.Y.; Clark, O.H.; Kebebew, E. Identification of biomarkers of adrenocortical carcinoma using genomewide gene expression profiling. *Arch. Surg.* **2008**, *143*, 841–846. [CrossRef]
85. Zhang, J.; Zhou, J.; Tang, X.; Zhou, L.Y.; Zhai, L.L.; Vanessa, M.E.D.; Yi, J.; Yi, Y.Y.; Lin, J.; Qian, J.; et al. Reduced expression of chemerin is associated with poor clinical outcome in acute myeloid leukemia. *Oncotarget* **2017**, *8*, 92536–92544. [CrossRef]
86. Maiga, A.; Lemieux, S.; Pabst, C.; Lavallée, V.P.; Bouvier, M.; Sauvageau, G.; Hébert, J. Transcriptome analysis of G protein-coupled receptors in distinct genetic subgroups of acute myeloid leukemia: Identification of potential disease-specific targets. *Blood Cancer J.* **2016**, *6*, e431. [CrossRef] [PubMed]

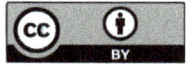

© 2019 by the authors. Licensee MDPI, Basel, Switzerland. This article is an open access article distributed under the terms and conditions of the Creative Commons Attribution (CC BY) license (http://creativecommons.org/licenses/by/4.0/).

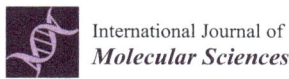

Article

Serum Chemerin Does Not Differentiate Colorectal Liver Metastases from Hepatocellular Carcinoma

Susanne Feder [1], Arne Kandulski [1], Doris Schacherer [1], Thomas S. Weiss [2] and Christa Buechler [1,*]

[1] Department of Internal Medicine I, Regensburg University Hospital, 93053 Regensburg, Germany
[2] Children's University Hospital (KUNO), Regensburg University Hospital, 93053 Regensburg, Germany
* Correspondence: christa.buechler@klinik.uni-regensburg.de; Tel.: +49-941-944-7009

Received: 31 July 2019; Accepted: 10 August 2019; Published: 12 August 2019

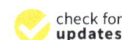

Abstract: The chemoattractant adipokine chemerin is related to the metabolic syndrome, which is a risk factor for different cancers. Recent studies provide evidence that chemerin is an important molecule in colorectal cancer (CRC) and hepatocellular carcinoma (HCC). Serum chemerin is high in CRC patients and low in HCC patients and may serve as a differential diagnostic marker for HCC and liver metastases from CRC. To this end, serum chemerin was measured in 36 patients with CRC metastases, 32 patients with HCC and 49 non-tumor patients by ELISA. Chemerin serum protein levels were, however, similar in the three cohorts. Serum chemerin was higher in hypertensive than normotensive tumor patients but not controls. Cancer patients with hypercholesterolemia or hyperuricemia also had increased serum chemerin. When patients with these comorbidities were excluded from the calculation, chemerin was higher in CRC than HCC patients but did not differ from controls. Chemerin did not correlate with the tumor markers carcinoembryonic antigen, carbohydrate antigen 19-9 and alpha-fetoprotein in both cohorts and was not changed with tumor-node-metastasis stage in HCC. Chemerin was not associated with hepatic fat, liver inflammation and fibrosis. To conclude, systemic chemerin did not discriminate between CRC metastases and HCC. Comorbidities among tumor patients were linked with elevated systemic chemerin.

Keywords: alpha-fetoprotein; liver steatosis; hypertension

1. Introduction

Colorectal cancer (CRC) is the third most prevalent cancer worldwide and a leading cause of tumor-related mortality. The liver is a common site for CRC metastasis [1,2]. Hepatocellular carcinoma (HCC) typically develops in the cirrhotic liver, but about 20% arise in the non-cirrhotic liver [3]. Discrimination between secondary hepatocarcinoma and HCC may be challenging in those patients. Clinically it is, however, highly relevant to distinguish primary and metastatic liver tumors. First, there are different therapies for patients with CRC metastases and HCC. Second, it is important to identify the primary tumor in metastatic disease [4], therefore biomarkers may be helpful in early diagnosis. Carcinoembryonic antigen (CEA) is already clinically used as diagnostic and prognostic marker in CRC [5], and systemic levels were indeed higher in secondary than primary liver tumors. Sensitivity of serum CEA for CRC metastases was 88% and 25% for HCC [1]. Cancer antigen 19-9 (CA19-9) had a 16% sensitivity for colon cancer and a 7.7% sensitivity for HCC and could be used as an additional prognostic tool [2,6]. Alpha-fetoprotein (AFP) is a diagnostic biomarker for HCC with a low sensitivity and specificity, and thus cannot differentiate between HCC and CRC metastases [1].

Recent studies described a role of chemerin in CRC pathophysiology and diagnosis [7–9]. Chemerin is a chemoattractant protein most abundant in adipocytes and hepatocytes [10]. Chemerin is released from the cells as a biological inert molecule, which is activated by C-terminal proteolysis.

Chemerin attracts immune cells such as macrophages and natural killer cells [11]. Moreover, chemerin regulates adipogenesis, angiogenesis and glucose metabolism [12]. Chemerin expression was reduced in a variety of cancers, and was also low in colon adenomas [13].

High plasma chemerin predicted a greater risk of CRC. Notably, this association was still significant when CRC risk factors such as age, body mass index and dietary habits were considered [8]. A second study detected higher chemerin in patients with CRC compared to healthy controls. Here, serum chemerin positively correlated with tumor-node-metastasis (TNM) stage [7]. In colon cancer patients, chemerin was increased though it was not associated with TNM classification [9]. Sytemic chemerin was further positively related to the number of adenomas in patients with colorectal adenomas [14].

Chemerin also plays a role in hepatocellular carcinoma (HCC) and low expression in the tumor was an independent prognostic factor [15]. Similarly, circulating chemerin levels were about 20-fold reduced in HCC patients [16]. Chemerin was not related to HCC prognosis [17]. Negative correlations of chemerin with Child–Pugh score, alanine aminotransferase and bilirubin demonstrated a close and negative association of serum chemerin with hepatic function in patients with liver cirrhosis [17,18]. In contrast, chronic hepatitis C patients had higher serum chemerin compared to controls, which was surprisingly negatively correlated with biopsy proven necro-inflammation [19]. Likewise, chemerin was high in men with alcohol abuse [20]. In patients with non-alcoholic steatohepatitis (NASH) serum chemerin was either induced or normal [21]. Decline of serum chemerin thus happens particularly in patients with severely impaired liver function and possibly HCC.

Obesity, hyperglycemia, dyslipidemia and hypertension are components of the metabolic syndrome, and all of them were linked with the development of cancers [22]. Patients with non-alcoholic fatty liver disease (NAFLD) have a higher risk for gastrointestinal tumors and the underlying factor is most likely the close relationship between NAFLD and traits of the metabolic syndrome [23].

Of note, circulating chemerin was positively associated with all of the components of the metabolic syndrome [10,24,25]. Therefore, chemerin's association with CRC may in part stem from the relationship between CRC and features of the metabolic syndrome [7,8,10,14,24,25]. Metabolic diseases also contribute to HCC development [22]. Whether chemerin correlates with traits of the metabolic syndrome in patients with cancers is, however, not well studied.

The liver is a common site of metastases from tumors arising in the gastrointestinal tract [26]. Here, we suggested that chemerin in serum may be appropriate to discriminate between colorectal liver metastases and HCC. A further aim was to identify associations of chemerin levels with components of the metabolic syndrome in patients with cancers.

2. Results

2.1. Association of Chemerin with Gender, Age and BMI

Serum chemerin was measured in 32 HCC, 36 CRC patients and 49 controls by ELISA (Table 1). Controls were patients which came to the hospital because of mostly epigastric or stomach pain but without any cancers [27,28]. HCC patients had higher bilirubin and aminotransferase activities than CRC patients in accordance with previous studies [29]. Levels of γ-glutamyltransferase were also increased in HCC patients (Table 1). Control cohort had lower aminotransferase activities than the group of HCC patients (Table 1). There were fewer female patients in the HCC compared to the control group (Table 1).

Chemerin was comparable in male and female tumor patients in the whole cohort ($p = 0.354$) and in the individual subgroups ($p = 0.976$ for controls, $p = 0.540$ for CRC and $p = 0.511$ for HCC). Levels neither correlated with age ($r = 0.20$, $p = 0.10$) nor BMI ($r = -0.27$, $p = 0.83$) in the tumor patients. This was also the case when the two cohorts of cancer patients were analyzed separately (CRC: age: $r = 0.06$, $p = 0.73$; BMI $r = 0.09$, $p = 0.61$; HCC: age: $r = 0.30$, $p = 0.10$; BMI $r = -0.49$, $p = 0.79$). In the controls chemerin positively correlated with age ($r = 0.368$, $p = 0.009$) but not with BMI ($r = 0.059$, $p = 0.688$).

Table 1. Characteristics of the study group.

Parameter	HCC (32 Patients)	CRC (36 Patients)	Controls (49 Patients)	p-Value
Male/Female	27/5	24/12	24/25	#*
Age (years)	63.5 (33.0–85.0)	67.0 (36.0–79.0)[35]	58.0 (21.0–88.0)	
BMI (kg/m^2)	27.2 (19.7–44.6)[31]	26.6 (16.3–45.4)	26.2 (20.3–39.7)	
Prothrombin Time (%)	30.8 (26.7–307.0)[30]	28.8 (25.2–39.0)[35]	n.d.	
Bilirubin (mg/dl)	0.6 (0.2–2.5)[31]	0.5 (0.1–1.0)[35]	0.5 (0.2–1.9)	*
ALT (U/l)	49.5 (17.0–378)[30]	28.0 (10.0–81.0)[34]	20.0 (12.0–44.0)	**;#***
AST (U/l)	36.0 (14.0–502.0)[31]	20.5 (11.0–165.0)[34]	28.0 (20.0–48.0)	*; #*
GGT (U/l)	105 (25–807)[27]	53 (19–590)[33]	n.d.	**
T2D	15	6	9	**; #**
HC	3	8	8	
HT	18	16	18	
HU	4	3	n.d.	
Tumor Grade: G1/G2/G3	5/20/4[29]	1/23/1[25]		
Primary Tumor T1/T2/T3/T4	13/9/9/1	7/20/3/0[30]		
Vascular Invasion No/yes	20/12	24/2[26]		
TNM Stage IA/IB/IIA/IIB/III/IV	14/8/7/2/1/0	1/4/13/9/1/1/2[31]		

Median values and range, or number of patients per subgroup are shown. Uppercase numbers refer to the patients where this laboratory value / feature was known when data were unavailable for the whole cohort. Reference values for ALT and AST: < 35 U/L for females and < 50 U/L for males, for bilirubin: 0.2–1.4 mg/dL, for GGT: < 40 U/L for females and < 60 U/l for males, for prothrombin time: < 70%. Abbreviations: Alanine aminotransferase, ALT, aspartate aminotransferase, AST; body mass index, BMI; colorectal cancer, CRC; γ-glutamyltransferase, GGT; hepatocellular carcinoma, HCC; hypercholesterolemia, HC; hypertension, HT; hyperuricemia, HU; not documented, n.d.; tumor-node-metastasis, TNM; type 2 diabetes, T2D. The respective p-values are listed in the last column of the table. * $p < 0.05$, ** $p < 0.01$ for comparison of CRC and HCC, #* $p < 0.05$, #** $p < 0.01$ and #*** $p < 0.001$ for comparison of controls and HCC patients.

2.2. Chemerin, CEA and CA19-9 in HCC and CRC Patients

Chemerin levels were similar in controls, HCC and CRC patients (Figure 1A). The tumor marker alpha-fetoprotein (AFP; known from 25 HCC patients and 15 CRC patients) did not differ between the two cohorts of tumor patients ($p = 0.07$). CEA (known from 20 HCC patients and 32 CRC patients) and CA19-9 (known from 19 HCC patients and 31 CRC patients) were higher in CRC patients (Figure 1B,C).

Chemerin did not correlate with AFP ($r = -0.20$, $p = 0.22$), CEA ($r = 0.08$, $p = 0.57$) and CA19-9 ($r = 0.15$, $p = 0.31$) in the cancer patients of the whole cohort and when both groups were analyzed separately (CRC: AFP $r = -0.08$, $p = 0.77$, CEA $r = 0.18$, $p = 0.34$ and CA19-9 $r = 0.31$, $p = 0.09$; HCC: AFP $r = -0.15$ $p = 0.48$, CEA $r = -0.19$, $p = 0.41$ and CA19-9 $r = -0.42$, $p = 0.07$). In the HCC group chemerin was not associated with tumor size ($r = 0.271$, $p = 0.13$), grade ($r = 0.044$, $p = 0.82$) or tumor-node-metastasis (TNM) stage (Figure 1D). Patients without vascular invasion had serum chemerin similar to those with this development (Figure 1E).

For the CRC cohort, serum was collected shortly before hepatic resection of the metastases whereas primary tumor was diagnosed up to six years earlier. Therefore, associations of serum chemerin with tumor stage and grade of CRC were not calculated. In the CRC group, 13 patients received neoadjuvant chemotherapy before liver resection which was, however, not associated with changes in chemerin levels (Figure 1F).

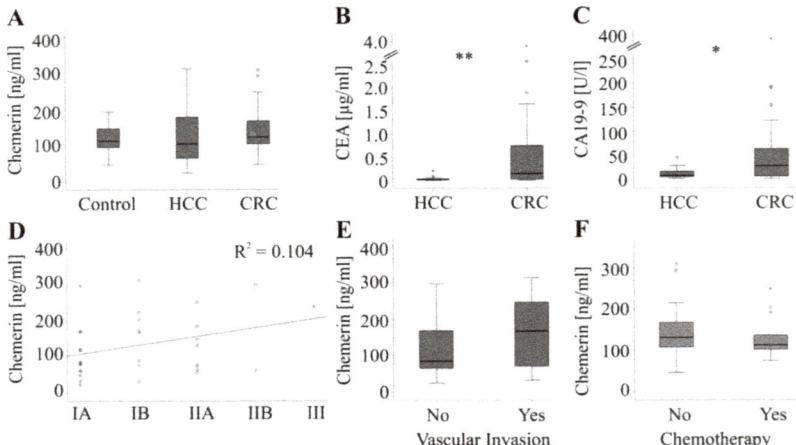

Figure 1. Chemerin and tumor markers. (**A**) Chemerin in serum of 49 controls, 32 patients with hepatocellular carcinoma (HCC) and 36 patients with colorectal carcinoma (CRC). (**B**) CEA in 20 HCC and 32 CRC patients. (**C**) CA19-9 in 19 HCC and 31 CRC patients. (**D**) Correlation of chemerin with TNM stage in HCC patients (TNM stage: IA/IB/IIA/IIB/III, number of patients 14/8/7/2/1). (**E**) Chemerin in 20 HCC patients without and 12 HCC patients with vascular invasion. (**F**) Chemerin in 13 CRC patients with and 23 CRC patients without chemotherapy. * $p < 0.05$, ** $p < 0.01$.

2.3. Association of Chemerin with Type 2 Diabetes, Hypertension, Hypercholesterolemia and Hyperuricemia

Circulating chemerin is associated with traits of the metabolic syndrome and some studies described higher levels in type 2 diabetes patients [12,24,30,31]. Chemerin was, however, not increased in those 21 cancer patients with type 2 diabetes compared to patients without this disease (Figure 2A). Chemerin was not changed in the 15 type 2 diabetic HCC patients and the 6 CRC patients when both cohorts were analyzed separately ($p = 0.25$ for HCC and $p = 0.47$ for CRC patients). Likewise, the 9 type 2 diabetes patients of the control group did not have high chemerin serum levels ($p = 0.09$). It should be noted that there were more type 2 diabetic patients in the HCC cohort than in the CRC and control group (Table 1).

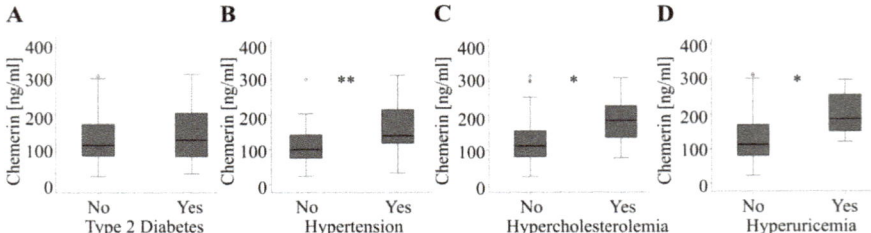

Figure 2. Serum chemerin and comorbidities in tumor patients. (**A**) Chemerin in 21 patients with and 47 patients without type 2 diabetes. (**B**) Chemerin in 34 patients with and 34 patients without hypertension. (**C**) Chemerin in 11 patients with and 57 patients without hypercholesterolemia. (**D**) Chemerin in seven patients with and 61 patients without hyperuricemia. * $p < 0.05$, ** $p < 0.01$.

Chemerin further regulated blood pressure, and was induced in hypertension [12]. Accordingly, chemerin was higher in the 34 patients with arterial hypertension (Figure 2B). In the HCC subgroup, the 18 hypertensive patients had higher chemerin than the 14 normotensive patients ($p = 0.02$). Moreover, chemerin was elevated in the 16 hypertensive CRC patients when compared to the 20 normotensive patients ($p = 0.03$). Although chemerin positively correlated with systolic blood pressure in the control group ($r = 0.337$, $p = 0.02$) serum levels were not induced in the 18 hypertensive patients ($p = 0.36$).

In addition, hypercholesterolaemic (11 patients) and hyperuricaemic cancer patients (seven patients) had elevated systemic chemerin levels (Figure 2C,D). Again, in the control group chemerin was not changed in the eight patients with hypercholesterolaemia ($p = 0.65$). Distribution of hypercholesterolaemia was comparable in the three groups of patients. Hyperuricemia was only documented in the tumor patients with similar prevalence for CRC and HCC patients (Table 1).

In the HCC group hypercholesterolaemia was diagnosed in three patients and hyperuricaemia in four patients. In the CRC cohort eight patients were hypercholesterolaemic and three were hyperuricaemic. The low number of patients suffering from hypercholesterolaemia and hyperuricaemia in the subgroups may be the reason chemerin changes were not significant (HCC: $p = 0.13$ for hypercholesterolaemia and $p = 0.12$ for hyperuricaemia; CRC: $p = 0.15$ for hypercholesterolaemia and $p = 0.06$ for hyperuricaemia).

The strong association of serum chemerin with comorbidities led us to individually analyze serum chemerin in patients suffering from hypertension, hypercholesterolemia or hyperuricemia and patients, which did not have these comorbidities. In the latter cohort chemerin ($p = 0.01$) and CEA ($p = 0.02$) were higher in CRC patients whereas AFP ($p = 0.03$) was reduced (Figure 3A,B). In the patients suffering from these comorbidities chemerin was similar in both cohorts. CA19-9 ($p = 0.008$) was induced in CRC patients and AST ($p < 0.001$), ALT ($p = 0.001$) and GGT ($p = 0.003$) were lower than in the HCC patients (Figure 3C,D). Above all, chemerin did not differ between patients with liver tumors and non-tumorous controls in both subgroups (Figure 3A,C).

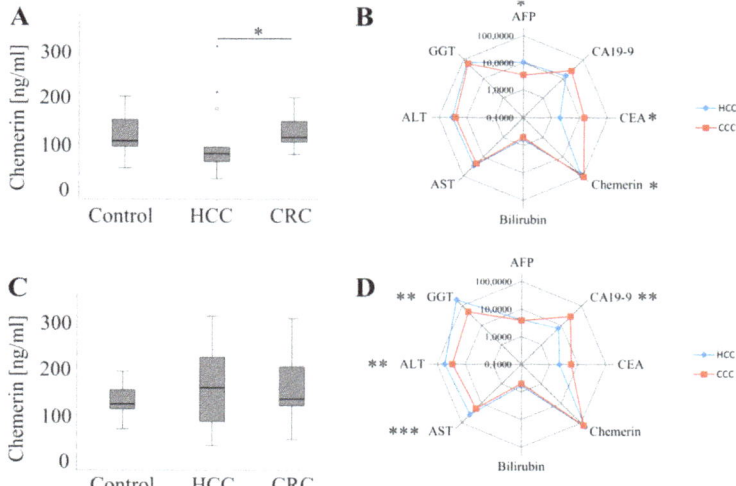

Figure 3. Serum chemerin and comorbidities. (**A**) Chemerin in 27 controls, 14 HCC and 18 CRC patients not suffering from hypertension, hypercholesterolemia or hyperuricemia. (**B**) Spider diagram presentation of chemerin, carcinoembryonic antigen (CEA), cancer antigen 19-9 (CA19-9), alpha-fetoprotein (AFP), γ-glutamyltransferase (GGT), alanine aminotransferase (ALT), aspartate aminotransferase (AST) and bilirubin in the serum of HCC and CRC patients described in A. The spider diagram shows the respective median values on a logarithmic scale. (**C**) Chemerin in 22 controls, 18 HCC and 18 CRC patients suffering from hypertension, hypercholesterolemia or hyperuricemia. (**D**) Spider diagram presentation of chemerin, CEA, CA19-9, AFP, GGT, ALT, AST and bilirubin in the serum of HCC and CRC patients described in C. The spider diagram shows the respective median values on a logarithmic scale. * $p < 0.05$, ** $p < 0.01$, *** $p < 0.001$.

2.4. Association of Chemerin with Liver Dysfunction

So far, the association of chemerin with hepatic injury was not resolved [21]. In the control group serum chemerin did not correlate with alanine aminotransferase, aspartate aminotransferase or bilirubin (Table 2). In the tumor patients, serum chemerin was not associated with alanine aminotransferase, aspartate aminotransferase, γ-glutamyltransferase or prothrombin time in the whole cohort, and when CRC and HCC patients were analyzed separately (Table 2). Negative correlations with bilirubin were identified in the whole cohort (Figure 4A and Table 2) and in CRC patients (Table 2).

Table 2. Correlation of serum chemerin with markers of liver function.

Correlation of Chemerin with:	HCC	CRC	All Tumor Patients	Controls
Prothrombin Time (%)	$r = -0.103$ $p = 0.587$	$r = -0.262$ $p = 0.128$	$r = -0.172$ $p = 0.170$	n.d.
Bilirubin (mg/dL)	$r = -0.316$ $p = 0.083$	**$r = -0.477$** **$p = 0.004$**	**$r = -0.386$** **$p = 0.001$**	$r = -0.930$ $p = 0.540$
ALT (U/L)	$r = -0.103$ $p = 0.590$	$r = -0.186$ $p = 0.292$	$r = -0.174$ $p = 0.169$	$r = -0.182$ $p = 0.215$
AST (U/L)	$r = 0.100$ $p = 0.593$	$r = -0.267$ $p = 0.127$	$r = -0.070$ $p = 0.577$	$r = -0.196$ $p = 0.181$
GGT (U/L)	$r = 0.145$ $p = 0.469$	$r = -0.298$ $p = 0.092$	$r = -0.087$ $p = 0.511$	n.d.

Correlation coefficient and p-values for the association of chemerin with prothrombin time, bilirubin, alanine aminotransferase (ALT), aspartate aminotransferase (AST) and γ-glutamyltransferase (GGT) are listed for the whole cohort, HCC and CRC patients and controls. Significant correlations are marked in bold. Not defined, n.d.

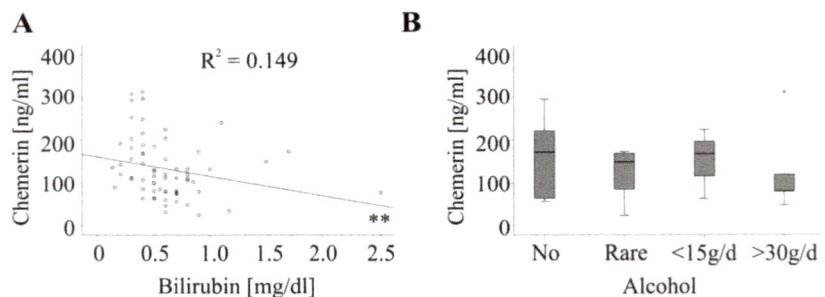

Figure 4. Serum chemerin, bilirubin and alcohol. (**A**) Correlation of chemerin with bilirubin in 31 HCC and 35 CRC patients. (**B**) Chemerin in HCC patients stratified for alcohol intake (No alcohol: 11 patients; Rare: 5 patients; <15 g/d: 3 patients; > 30 g/d 5 patients). ** $p < 0.01$.

Chemerin was further not related to alcohol intake which was documented for 24 HCC patients (11 patients did not consume alcohol, five patients rarely drank alcohol, three patients daily had alcohol but less than 15 g and five patients daily had more than 30 g) (Figure 4B).

We additionally evaluated potential associations of serum chemerin with histologic liver abnormalities. In the HCC cohort 16 patients had liver steatosis, 18 had liver inflammation and 23 liver fibrosis. In the CRC group, hepatic steatosis was confirmed by histology in 17 patients, hepatitis in 13 and liver fibrosis in 17 patients. All of these features were comparable in the cohorts. Serum chemerin was, however, not related to any of these traits. Accordingly, serum chemerin did not change with extent of steatosis, inflammation or fibrosis in the whole study group (Figure 5A–C) and when both cohorts were analyzed separately (HCC: $p = 0.71$ for steatosis, $p = 0.31$ for inflammation and $p = 0.75$ for fibrosis; CRC: $p = 0.77$ for steatosis, $p = 0.44$ for inflammation and $p = 0.05$ for fibrosis It is important to note that in the group of tumor patients there was only one patient in the following subgroups: steatosis grade 3, inflammation grade 2 and fibrosis grade 2. Therefore, statistical test is not valid. Chemerin was, however, comparable in patients having no, grade 1 and grade 2 hepatic steatosis. Levels in patients without and grade 1 hepatic inflammation were also comparable. Chemerin in patients without, grade 1 and grade 4 hepatic fibrosis did also not differ. It is thus admissible to conclude that serum chemerin is not associated with hepatic features of liver injury.

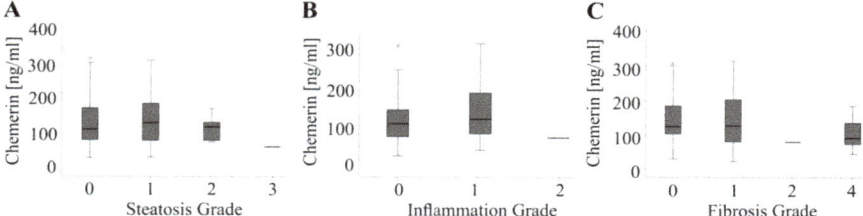

Figure 5. Serum chemerin and liver injury in cancer patients. (**A**) Chemerin in patients stratified for hepatic steatosis (25 patients: no steatosis; 27 patients grade 1; 5 patients grade 2 and 1 patients grade 3; Steatosis grade of 10 patients was not known) (**B**) Chemerin in patients stratified for hepatic inflammation (28 patients: no inflammation; 29 patients grade 1 and 1 patient grade 2. Inflammation grade of 9 patients was not known). (**C**) Chemerin in patients stratified for hepatic fibrosis (28 patients: no fibrosis; 25 patients grade 1; 1 patient grade 2 and 14 patients grade 4). Number of patients in some subgroups was 1 and statistical test is not reliable for these subgroups.

3. Discussion

This study showed that serum chemerin did not discriminate patients with CRC metastases from HCC patients or controls. Moreover, chemerin levels were not changed with hepatic steatosis, inflammation or fibrosis. TNM stage in HCC patients was not correlated with serum chemerin.

Elevated circulating chemerin in CRC patients was described in recent studies [7,9]. In patients with adenomas serum chemerin was nearly 50% higher than in healthy controls [14]. Chemerin concentration of CRC patients was about 15% increased in one CRC cohort whereas the second analysis reported a more than four-fold induction compared to healthy controls [7,9]. In the present study groups, chemerin serum levels did not differ between CRC patients with liver metastases and patients without tumors. This suggests that chemerin is not solely raised in CRC patients but is high in patients suffering from different diseases. Indeed, higher chemerin was described in psoriasis, inflammatory bowel disease, coronary artery stenosis, obstructive sleep apnea syndrome and chronic obstructive pulmonary disease [32–36]. Therefore, high chemerin may be related to inflammatory processes rather than being a specific marker of CRC. Moreover, chemerin expression was reduced in colon adenomas [13] and may be low in CRC. Therefore, it is unlikely that increased serum chemerin levels do result from the tumor tissue [37]. Serum chemerin comes from adipose tissues and the relationship between fat depots and CRC in tumor patients warrants further investigation.

The mechanisms that contribute to higher serum chemerin in different diseases are presently unknown. Inflammation increased adipocyte chemerin production whereas hepatic synthesis was not changed [21,38,39]. Elevated serum chemerin in obesity did not result in enhanced activation of the chemerin receptor CMKLR1 [40]. Accordingly, C-terminal truncated chemerin isoforms were identified in human obesity [41]. These short variants cannot activate the chemerin receptor [12]. Future work has to examine the factors that influence serum chemerin protein levels and activity in health and disease.

In the tumor patients, serum chemerin was induced in those with hypertension, hypercholesterolemia and hyperuricemia. Accordingly, chemerin was elevated in hypertensive and dyslipidemic patients in different studies [30,42]. Above all, hypertensive or hypercholesterolaemic controls enrolled in the present study did not have higher serum chemerin levels. Notably, a positive correlation of serum chemerin with systolic blood pressure existed in the control cohort. Distribution of these comorbidities was similar between the three cohorts, and thus higher chemerin should have been identified in all groups. This suggests that comorbidity associated induction of chemerin was stronger in tumor patients than controls. Because there were only few patients in some of the subgroups, future studies are needed to validate this suggestion.

Moreover, chemerin did not decline in HCC patients when compared to the non-tumor controls. Chemerin could not discriminate CRC and HCC. HCC patients more often had type 2 diabetes albeit the prevalence of further comorbidities was comparable in both groups. Type 2 diabetes was not linked to higher chemerin in accordance with previous studies [30,42]. Notably, when HCC and CRC patients without hypertension, hyperuricemia or dyslipidemia were compared, chemerin was lower in HCC. In this subgroup besides chemerin, AFP and CEA also differed with the first being higher and the second being lower in HCC. When only patients suffering from these comorbidities were analyzed chemerin was similar in HCC and CRC. Here, transferases were induced in HCC indicating exaggerated liver injury in HCC patients with these complications. Moreover, CA19-9 was higher in the CRC patients.

In the cancer patients, tumor markers CEA and CA19-9 were higher in CRC compared to HCC patients in accordance with previous studies [1,2]. Although tumor markers were not related to comorbidities CEA was only increased in CRC patients without comorbidities, whereas CA19-9 was higher in the CRC patients with secondary complication. Specificities of these markers were thus changed in the two subgroups and future studies have to find out whether this is relevant in the clinical routine. Above all, this analysis showed that chemerin cannot be recommended as a clinical biomarker to discriminate between primary and secondary liver tumors.

A further unresolved issue is whether serum chemerin is a marker of liver injury [21]. In HCC patients chemerin negatively correlated with Child–Pugh score, alanine aminotransferase and bilirubin, and positively with prothrombin time [17]. Associations of chemerin with aminotransferases and bilirubin were not identified in patients with liver cirrhosis [43]. In the cohort studied herein, serum chemerin was negatively correlated with bilirubin in CRC patients whereas associations with further markers of liver health such as aminotransferases and prothrombin time were not identified in any cohort. In addition, chemerin did not change in patients with higher grade of steatosis, inflammation and fibrosis. Limitation of this analysis is that there was only one patient in some of the subgroups and present findings have to be confirmed in the future. Altogether, these preliminary data exclude a strong relation between serum chemerin and liver function.

In line with this suggestion, serum chemerin was not changed in non-alcoholic fatty liver disease (NAFLD) patients with increasing steatosis, inflammation and fibrosis grades [44]. A separate study identified a trend to raised serum chemerin in morbidly obese NAFLD patients with a higher degree of liver steatosis [45]. In a similar patient cohort elevated chemerin was reported in patients with portal inflammation and fibrosis [46]. In chronic hepatitis C serum chemerin was even negatively correlated with necro-inflammatory grade [19].

Serum chemerin was, however, reduced in patients with decompensated liver cirrhosis when compared to patients with compensated disease [43]. Here, a negative correlation with Quick prothrombin time was identified [43]. Coagulation was normal in the patients enrolled in the present study, and all patients had compensated liver cirrhosis. Therefore, a decline of serum chemerin is an indicator of severe liver dysfunction [43], whereas levels are quite normal in patients with compensated disease.

Moreover, chemerin did not correlate with AFP, tumor number or size in a recent study [17]. In the present cohort, chemerin was not associated with AFP, tumor size, grading, TNM stage or vascular invasion. Based on these results it is unlikely that serum chemerin may become a robust biomarker of hepatic injury and HCC.

4. Materials and Methods

4.1. Patients

Details of the cohorts are summarized in Table 1. Prospective collection of serum of the CRC patients was done from January 2012 to June 2015. Prospective collection of serum of the HCC patients was done from May 2012 to May 2015. Inclusion criteria were histologically confirmed HCC or CRC metastases and age above 18 years. Exclusion criteria was pregnancy.

Liver was histologically examined and scoring was done as suggested by Kleiner et al. [47]. TNM stages were calculated as described [48]. Experiments complied with the guidelines of the charitable state controlled foundation Human Tissue and Cell Research. Each patient signed a written informed consent. The study was approved by the ethical committee of the Regensburg University Hospital (Ethikkommission an der Universität Regensburg) (approval code 15-101-0052, approved on 26 March 2015).

Serum of patients without tumors was obtained from January to June 2008. The cohort included outdoor patients and hospitalized patients who were referred to the interdisciplinary ultrasound department of the University Hospital and was used in previous studies to analyze chemerin and soluble CD163 in serum of controls and patients with non-alcoholic fatty liver disease (NAFLD) [27,28]. Both factors were not changed in the patients with NAFLD [27,28]. The study cohort initially included 56 patients and serum of 49 patients was available for the present study. Patients with hepatobiliary diseases, malignancies, ascites, drugs that cause hepatic steatosis, inflammatory bowel disease, infection with the human immunodeficiency virus, chronic alcohol and drug abuse, familial hyperlipidemia and acute medical conditions with confounding effect on laboratory values, were excluded from the study. All participants signed a form of written consent, and the study was approved by the local Ethics Committee. Aliquots of the sera were stored at −80 °C and freeze-thaw cycles were avoided. It is important to note that serum storage time differed for up to 7 years. This is a limitation of our study. There was no difference in serum chemerin of patients with CRC collected in 2012 (6 patients) and 2015 (10 patients; $p = 0.1$). This suggests that a four year storage period at −80 °C did not grossly affect serum chemerin levels. Chemerin levels may decline during 7 year storage but this effect may be rather small.

4.2. Chemerin ELISA

Chemerin ELISA was purchased from R&D Systems (Wiesbaden, Germany) and performed as recommended by the distributor. The plate reader used was the iMark^{TM} Microplate Absorbance Reader (Bio-Rad, Munich, Germany). Absorbance was measured at 450 nm, with the correction wavelength set at 540 nm. Serum was diluted 1:500 fold before analysis.

4.3. Laboratory Values

Laboratory values such as bilirubin and tumor markers were routinely measured in the Institute for Clinical Chemistry and Laboratory Medicine, University Hospital Regensburg. Total bilirubin was determined using the Dimension Vista® Flex® reagent cartridge TBIL (Siemens Healthcare Diagnostics Inc , Berkeley, CA, USA). Unconjugated bilirubin was solubilized in a caffeine/benzoate/acetate/ethylene diamine tetraacetic acid mixture. Conjugated bilirubin is soluble in aqueous solvents like water. Solublized bilirubin in serum was coupled with diazotized sulfanilic acid. Thereby diazo-bilirubin was produced. This red chromophore absorbs at 540 nm and was measured by the use of a bichromatic endpoint technique (540 nm, 700 nm).

The ADVIA Centaur® AFP-Assay (Siemens Healthcare GmbH, Erlangen, Germany) and the ADVIA Centaur CEA Assay are sandwich immunoassays with chemiluminescent detection. Two different antigen specific antibodies, a polyclonal rabbit and a monoclonal murine antibody, are used in the assay. ADVIA Centaur® CA 19-9 Assay is a sandwich immunoassay using the same monoclonal antibody in the solid phase and the Lite-reagent.

4.4. Statistics

Data are shown as box plots and here the median values, lower and upper quartiles and the range of the values are given. Statistical tests used were Mann–Whitney U Test (to test for significant differences between two independent groups), Spearman correlation (non-parametric correlation analysis), one-way Anova with post-hoc Bonferroni (for comparison of three groups) or Kruskall–Wallis test (for comparison of more than three groups where one of the groups had only 1 patient) (SPSS Statistics 25.0 program, International Business Machines Corporation, Armonk, New York, USA). Chi-square test was used to analyze gender and comorbidity distribution. A value of $p < 0.05$ was regarded as significant. Outliners—greater than 1.5 times the interquartile range—are given as circles, and outliners—greater than 3.0 times the interquartile range—are given as stars.

5. Conclusions

Serum chemerin does not discriminate HCC from CRC metastases. Equally important is that levels were neither related to measures of liver injury nor to TNM stage of HCC patients. Chemerin was induced in tumor patients with comorbidities (hypertension, hypercholesterolemia, hyperuricemia), which has to be considered in future clinical studies.

Author Contributions: Conceptualization, C.B., T.S.W., A.K.; methodology, S.F.; software, formal analysis, S.F., C.B.; resources, T.S.W., D.S.; writing- original draft preparation, C.B.; writing- review and editing, C.B., S.F., A.K., D.S., T.S.W.

Funding: This research was funded by the German Research Foundation, grant number BU 1141/13-1.

Acknowledgments: The excellent technical assistance of Elena Underberg is greatly acknowledged.

Conflicts of Interest: The authors declare no conflicts of interest.

Abbreviations

ALT	alanine aminotransferase
AFP	alpha-fetoprotein
AST	aspartate aminotransferase
BMI	body mass index
CA19-9	cancer antigen 19-9
CEA	carcinoembryonic antigen
CRC	colorectal cancer
GGT	γ-glutamyltransferase
HCC	hepatocellular carcinoma
NAFLD	non-alcoholic fatty liver disease
NASH	non-alcoholic steatohepatitis
TNM	tumor-node-metastasis

References

1. Abdel-Hamid, N.M.; Abouzied, M.M.; Nazmy, M.H.; Fawzy, M.A.; Gerges, A.S. A suggested guiding panel of seromarkers for efficient discrimination between primary and secondary human hepatocarcinoma. *Tumour Biol.* **2016**, *37*, 2539–2546. [CrossRef] [PubMed]
2. Attallah, A.M.; Al-Ghawalby, N.A.; Aziz, A.A.; El-Sayed, E.A.; Tabll, A.A.; El-Waseef, A.M. Clinical value of serum CEA, CA 19-9, CA 242 and AFP in diagnosis of gastrointestinal tract cancer. *Int. J. Cancer Res.* **2006**, *2*, 50–56.
3. Desai, A.; Sandhu, S.; Lai, J.P.; Sandhu, D.S. Hepatocellular carcinoma in non-cirrhotic liver: A comprehensive review. *World J. Hepatol.* **2019**, *11*, 1–18. [CrossRef]
4. Gozde, A.E.I. Evaluation of Hepatocellular Carcinomas and Liver Metastases—How Far can we Go with Diffusion Weighted Imaging? *J. Nucl. Med. Radiat. Ther.* **2017**, *8*, 1–4.

5. Campos-da-Paz, M.; Dorea, J.G.; Galdino, A.S.; Lacava, Z.G.M.; de Fatima Menezes Almeida Santos, M. Carcinoembryonic Antigen (CEA) and Hepatic Metastasis in Colorectal Cancer: Update on Biomarker for Clinical and Biotechnological Approaches. *Recent Pat. Biotechnol.* **2018**, *12*, 269–279. [CrossRef] [PubMed]
6. Shin, J.K.; Kim, H.C.; Lee, W.Y.; Yun, S.H.; Cho, Y.B.; Huh, J.W.; Park, Y.A.; Chun, H.K. High preoperative serum CA 19-9 levels can predict poor oncologic outcomes in colorectal cancer patients on propensity score analysis. *Ann. Surg. Treat. Res.* **2019**, *96*, 107–115. [CrossRef]
7. Alkady, M.M.; Abdel-Messeih, P.L.; Nosseir, N.M. Assessment of Serum Levels of the Adipocytokine Chemerin in Colorectal Cancer Patients. *J. Med. Biochem.* **2018**, *37*, 313–319. [CrossRef] [PubMed]
8. Eichelmann, F.; Schulze, M.B.; Wittenbecher, C.; Menzel, J.; Weikert, C.; di Giuseppe, R.; Biemann, R.; Isermann, B.; Fritsche, A.; Boeing, H.; et al. Association of Chemerin Plasma Concentration With Risk of Colorectal Cancer. *JAMA Netw. Open* **2019**, *2*, e190896. [CrossRef]
9. Erdogan, S.; Yilmaz, F.M.; Yazici, O.; Yozgat, A.; Sezer, S.; Ozdemir, N.; Uysal, S.; Purnak, T.; Sendur, M.A.; Ozaslan, E. Inflammation and chemerin in colorectal cancer. *Tumour Biol.* **2016**, *37*, 6337–6342. [CrossRef]
10. Ernst, M.C.; Sinal, C.J. Chemerin: At the crossroads of inflammation and obesity. *Trends Endocrinol. Metab.* **2010**, *21*, 660–667. [CrossRef] [PubMed]
11. Parolini, S.; Santoro, A.; Marcenaro, E.; Luini, W.; Massardi, L.; Facchetti, F.; Communi, D.; Parmentier, M.; Majorana, A.; Sironi, M.; et al. The role of chemerin in the colocalization of NK and dendritic cell subsets into inflamed tissues. *Blood* **2007**, *109*, 3625–3632. [CrossRef]
12. Buechler, C.; Feder, S.; Haberl, E.M.; Aslanidis, C. Chemerin Isoforms and Activity in Obesity. *Int. J. Mol. Sci.* **2019**, *20*, 1128. [CrossRef]
13. Pachynski, R.K.; Zabel, B.A.; Kohrt, H.E.; Tejeda, N.M.; Monnier, J.; Swanson, C.D.; Holzer, A.K.; Gentles, A.J.; Sperinde, G.V.; Edalati, A.; et al. The chemoattractant chemerin suppresses melanoma by recruiting natural killer cell antitumor defenses. *J. Exp. Med.* **2012**, *209*, 1427–1435. [CrossRef]
14. Yagi, M.; Sasaki, Y.; Abe, Y.; Yaoita, T.; Sakuta, K.; Mizumoto, N.; Shoji, M.; Onozato, Y.; Kon, T.; Nishise, S.; et al. Association between High Levels of Circulating Chemerin and Colorectal Adenoma in Men. *Digestion* **2019**, 1–8. [CrossRef]
15. Lin, W.; Chen, Y.L.; Jiang, L.; Chen, J.K. Reduced expression of chemerin is associated with a poor prognosis and a lowed infiltration of both dendritic cells and natural killer cells in human hepatocellular carcinoma. *Clin. Lab.* **2011**, *57*, 879–885.
16. Lin, Y.; Yang, X.; Liu, W.; Li, B.; Yin, W.; Shi, Y.; He, R. Chemerin has a protective role in hepatocellular carcinoma by inhibiting the expression of IL-6 and GM-CSF and MDSC accumulation. *Oncogene* **2017**, *36*, 3599–3608. [CrossRef]
17. Imai, K.; Takai, K.; Hanai, T.; Shiraki, M.; Suzuki, Y.; Hayashi, H.; Naiki, T.; Nishigaki, Y.; Tomita, E.; Shimizu, M.; et al. Impact of serum chemerin levels on liver functional reserves and platelet counts in patients with hepatocellular carcinoma. *Int. J. Mol. Sci.* **2014**, *15*, 11294–11306. [CrossRef]
18. Buechler, C.; Haberl, E.M.; Rein-Fischboeck, L.; Aslanidis, C. Adipokines in Liver Cirrhosis. *Int J Mol. Sci.* **2017**, *18*, 1392. [CrossRef]
19. Kukla, M.; Zwirska-Korczala, K.; Gabriel, A.; Waluga, M.; Warakomska, I.; Szczygiel, B.; Berdowska, A.; Mazur, W.; Wozniak-Grygiel, E.; Kryczka, W. Chemerin, vaspin and insulin resistance in chronic hepatitis C. *J. Viral. Hepat.* **2010**, *17*, 661–667. [CrossRef]
20. Ren, R.Z.; Zhang, X.; Xu, J.; Zhang, H.Q.; Yu, C.X.; Cao, M.F.; Gao, L.; Guan, Q.B.; Zhao, J.J. Chronic ethanol consumption increases the levels of chemerin in the serum and adipose tissue of humans and rats. *Acta Pharm. Sin.* **2012**, *33*, 652–659. [CrossRef]
21. Buechler, C. Chemerin in Liver Diseases. *Endocrinol. Metab. Syndr.* **2014**, *3*, 1–6.
22. Uzunlulu, M.; Telci Caklili, O.; Oguz, A. Association between Metabolic Syndrome and Cancer. *Ann. Nutr. Metab.* **2016**, *68*, 173–179. [CrossRef]
23. Sanna, C.; Rosso, C.; Marietti, M.; Bugianesi, E. Non-Alcoholic Fatty Liver Disease and Extra-Hepatic Cancers. *Int J. Mol. Sci.* **2016**, *17*, 717. [CrossRef]
24. Bozaoglu, K.; Bolton, K.; McMillan, J.; Zimmet, P.; Jowett, J.; Collier, G.; Walder, K.; Segal, D. Chemerin is a novel adipokine associated with obesity and metabolic syndrome. *Endocrinology* **2007**, *148*, 4687–4694. [CrossRef]

25. Zylla, S.; Pietzner, M.; Kuhn, J.P.; Volzke, H.; Dorr, M.; Nauck, M.; Friedrich, N. Serum chemerin is associated with inflammatory and metabolic parameters-results of a population-based study. *Obesty* **2017**, *25*, 468–475. [CrossRef]
26. Milette, S.; Sicklick, J.K.; Lowy, A.M.; Brodt, P. Molecular Pathways: Targeting the Microenvironment of Liver Metastases. *Clin. Cancer Res.* **2017**, *23*, 6390–6399. [CrossRef]
27. Bauer, S.; Weiss, T.S.; Wiest, R.; Schacherer, D.; Hellerbrand, C.; Farkas, S.; Scherer, M.N.; Ritter, M.; Schmitz, G.; Schaffler, A.; et al. Soluble CD163 is not increased in visceral fat and steatotic liver and is even suppressed by free fatty acids in vitro. *Exp. Mol. Pathol.* **2011**, *91*, 733–739. [CrossRef]
28. Pohl, R.; Haberl, E.M.; Rein-Fischboeck, L.; Zimny, S.; Neumann, M.; Aslanidis, C.; Schacherer, D.; Krautbauer, S.; Eisinger, K.; Weiss, T.S.; et al. Hepatic chemerin mRNA expression is reduced in human nonalcoholic steatohepatitis. *Eur. J. Clin. Invest.* **2017**, *47*, 7–18. [CrossRef]
29. Yamashita, S.; Sakamoto, Y.; Yamamoto, S.; Takemura, N.; Omichi, K.; Shinkawa, H.; Mori, K.; Kaneko, J.; Akamatsu, N.; Arita, J.; et al. Efficacy of Preoperative Portal Vein Embolization Among Patients with Hepatocellular Carcinoma, Biliary Tract Cancer, and Colorectal Liver Metastases: A Comparative Study Based on Single-Center Experience of 319 Cases. *Ann. Surg. Oncol.* **2017**, *24*, 1557–1568. [CrossRef]
30. Rourke, J.L.; Dranse, H.J.; Sinal, C.J. Towards an integrative approach to understanding the role of chemerin in human health and disease. *Obes Rev.* **2013**, *14*, 245–262. [CrossRef]
31. Weigert, J.; Neumeier, M.; Wanninger, J.; Filarsky, M.; Bauer, S.; Wiest, R.; Farkas, S.; Scherer, M.N.; Schaffler, A.; Aslanidis, C.; et al. Systemic chemerin is related to inflammation rather than obesity in type 2 diabetes. *Clin. Endocrinol.* **2010**, *72*, 342–348. [CrossRef]
32. Boyuk, B.; Guzel, E.C.; Atalay, H.; Guzel, S.; Mutlu, L.C.; Kucukyalcin, V. Relationship between plasma chemerin levels and disease severity in COPD patients. *Clin. Respir. J.* **2015**, *9*, 468–474. [CrossRef]
33. Gisondi, P.; Lora, V.; Bonauguri, C.; Russo, A.; Lippi, G.; Girolomoni, G. Serum chemerin is increased in patients with chronic plaque psoriasis and normalizes following treatment with infliximab. *Br. J. Derm.* **2013**, *168*, 749–755. [CrossRef]
34. Weigert, J.; Obermeier, F.; Neumeier, M.; Wanninger, J.; Filarsky, M.; Bauer, S.; Aslanidis, C.; Rogler, G.; Ott, C.; Schaffler, A.; et al. Circulating levels of chemerin and adiponectin are higher in ulcerative colitis and chemerin is elevated in Crohn's disease. *Inflamm. Bowel Dis.* **2010**, *16*, 630–637. [CrossRef]
35. Motawi, T.M.K.; Mahdy, S.G.; El-Sawalhi, M.M.; Ali, E.N.; El-Telbany, R.F.A. Serum levels of chemerin, apelin, vaspin, and omentin-1 in obese type 2 diabetic Egyptian patients with coronary artery stenosis. *Can. J. Physiol. Pharm.* **2018**, *96*, 38–44. [CrossRef]
36. Feng, X.; Li, P.; Zhou, C.; Jia, X.; Kang, J. Elevated levels of serum chemerin in patients with obstructive sleep apnea syndrome. *Biomarkers* **2012**, *17*, 248–253. [CrossRef]
37. Liu-Chittenden, Y.; Patel, D.; Gaskins, K.; Giordano, T.J.; Assie, G.; Bertherat, J.; Kebebew, E. Serum RARRES2 Is a Prognostic Marker in Patients With Adrenocortical Carcinoma. *J. Clin. Endocrinol. Metab.* **2016**, *101*, 3345–3352. [CrossRef]
38. Parlee, S.D.; Ernst, M.C.; Muruganandan, S.; Sinal, C.J.; Goralski, K.B. Serum chemerin levels vary with time of day and are modified by obesity and tumor necrosis factor-alpha. *Endocrinology* **2010**, *151*, 2590–2602. [CrossRef]
39. Bauer, S.; Wanninger, J.; Schmidhofer, S.; Weigert, J.; Neumeier, M.; Dorn, C.; Hellerbrand, C.; Zimara, N.; Schaffler, A.; Aslanidis, C.; et al. Sterol regulatory element-binding protein 2 (SREBP2) activation after excess triglyceride storage induces Chemerin in hypertrophic adipocytes. *Endocrinology* **2011**, *152*, 26–35. [CrossRef]
40. Toulany, J.; Parlee, S.D.; Sinal, C.J.; Slayter, K.; McNeil, S.; Goralski, K.B. CMKLR1 activation ex vivo does not increase proportionally to serum total chemerin in obese humans. *Endocr Connect.* **2016**, *5*, 70–81. [CrossRef]
41. Chang, S.S.; Eisenberg, D.; Zhao, L.; Adams, C.; Leib, R.; Morser, J.; Leung, L. Chemerin activation in human obesity. *Obesity* **2016**, *24*, 1522–1529. [CrossRef]
42. Mattern, A.; Zellmann, T.; Beck-Sickinger, A.G. Processing, signaling, and physiological function of chemerin. *IUBMB Life* **2014**, *66*, 19–26. [CrossRef]
43. Eisinger, K.; Krautbauer, S.; Wiest, R.; Weiss, T.S.; Buechler, C. Reduced serum chemerin in patients with more severe liver cirrhosis. *Exp. Mol. Pathol.* **2015**, *98*, 208–213. [CrossRef]
44. Kukla, M.; Zwirska-Korczala, K.; Hartleb, M.; Waluga, M.; Chwist, A.; Kajor, M.; Ciupinska-Kajor, M.; Berdowska, A.; Wozniak-Grygiel, E.; Buldak, R. Serum chemerin and vaspin in non-alcoholic fatty liver disease. *Scand. J. Gastroenterol.* **2010**, *45*, 235–242. [CrossRef]

45. Kajor, M.; Kukla, M.; Waluga, M.; Liszka, L.; Dyaczynski, M.; Kowalski, G.; Zadlo, D.; Berdowska, A.; Chapula, M.; Kostrzab-Zdebel, A.; et al. Hepatic chemerin mRNA in morbidly obese patients with nonalcoholic fatty liver disease. *Pol. J. Pathol.* **2017**, *68*, 117–127. [CrossRef]
46. Sell, H.; Divoux, A.; Poitou, C.; Basdevant, A.; Bouillot, J.L.; Bedossa, P.; Tordjman, J.; Eckel, J.; Clement, K. Chemerin correlates with markers for fatty liver in morbidly obese patients and strongly decreases after weight loss induced by bariatric surgery. *J. Clin. Endocrinol. Metab.* **2010**, *95*, 2892–2896. [CrossRef]
47. Kleiner, D.E.; Brunt, E.M.; Van Natta, M.; Behling, C.; Contos, M.J.; Cummings, O.W.; Ferrell, L.D.; Liu, Y.C.; Torbenson, M.S.; Unalp-Arida, A.; et al. Design and validation of a histological scoring system for nonalcoholic fatty liver disease. *Hepatology* **2005**, *41*, 1313–1321. [CrossRef]
48. Kinoshita, A.; Onoda, H.; Fushiya, N.; Koike, K.; Nishino, H.; Tajiri, H. Staging systems for hepatocellular carcinoma: Current status and future perspectives. *World J. Hepatol.* **2015**, *7*, 406–424. [CrossRef]

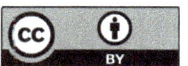

© 2019 by the authors. Licensee MDPI, Basel, Switzerland. This article is an open access article distributed under the terms and conditions of the Creative Commons Attribution (CC BY) license (http://creativecommons.org/licenses/by/4.0/).

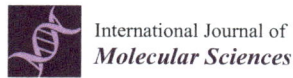

Review

Involvement of Novel Adipokines, Chemerin, Visfatin, Resistin and Apelin in Reproductive Functions in Normal and Pathological Conditions in Humans and Animal Models

Anthony Estienne [1,2,3,4,†], Alice Bongrani [1,2,3,4,†], Maxime Reverchon [5], Christelle Ramé [1,2,3,4], Pierre-Henri Ducluzeau [1,2,3,4,6], Pascal Froment [1,2,3,4] and Joëlle Dupont [1,2,3,4,*]

1. INRA UMR 85 Physiologie de la Reproduction et des Comportements, F-37380 Nouzilly, France
2. CNRS UMR 7247 Physiologie de la Reproduction et des Comportements, F-37380 Nouzilly, France
3. Université François Rabelais de Tours F-37041 Tours, France
4. IFCE, F-37380 Nouzilly, France
5. SYSAAF-Syndicat des Sélectionneurs Avicoles et Aquacoles Français, Centre INRA Val de Loire, F-37380 Nouzilly, France
6. Internal Medicine Department, Unit of Endocrinology, CHRU Tours, F-37044 Tours, France
* Correspondence: joelle.dupont@inra.fr; Tel.: +33-2-4742-7789
† Equal contribution.

Received: 2 August 2019; Accepted: 6 September 2019; Published: 9 September 2019

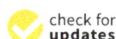

Abstract: It is well known that adipokines are endocrine factors that are mainly secreted by white adipose tissue. Their central role in energy metabolism is currently accepted. More recently, their involvement in fertility regulation and the development of some reproductive disorders has been suggested. Data concerning the role of leptin and adiponectin, the two most studied adipokines, in the control of the reproductive axis are consistent. In recent years, interest has grown about some novel adipokines, chemerin, visfatin, resistin and apelin, which have been found to be strongly associated with obesity and insulin-resistance. Here, we will review their expression and role in male and female reproduction in humans and animal models. According to accumulating evidence, they could regulate the secretion of GnRH (Gonadotropin-Releasing Hormone), gonadotropins and steroids. Furthermore, their expression and that of their receptors (if known), has been demonstrated in the human and animal hypothalamo-pituitary-gonadal axis. Like leptin and adiponectin, these novel adipokines could thus represent metabolic sensors that are able to regulate reproductive functions according to energy balance changes. Therefore, after investigating their role in normal fertility, we will also discuss their possible involvement in some reproductive troubles known to be associated with features of metabolic syndrome, such as polycystic ovary syndrome, gestational diabetes mellitus, preeclampsia and intra-uterine growth retardation in women, and sperm abnormalities and testicular pathologies in men.

Keywords: ovary; testis; adipose tissue; polycystic ovary syndrome; preeclempsia; gestational diabetes; testicular pathologies

---

1. Introduction

Nowadays, it is well known that there is a close link between metabolism and reproductive function [1,2]. Adipose tissue is now considered as an endocrine organ that could influence fertility through the hormonal secretion of adipokines, which are cytokines involved in various physiological processes [3–5]. Those biologically active proteins are considered the main regulators of whole body energy homeostasis [3,6–8]. Many reviews have already described and discussed the crucial roles of leptin and adiponectin in different physiological processes including reproduction [9–14]. So, here we focused on four novel adipokines named chemerin, visfatin, resistin and apelin that have been also identified and recognised as important regulators of energy metabolism [15–18]. Moreover, several studies have highlighted their involvement in reproductive functions, in normal or pathological contexts [19–22]. In this present review, we will discuss the structure of these adipokines and their roles in the male and female reproductive tract in human and animal models, with a discussion of their involvement in several female and male reproductive pathologies including polycystic ovary syndrome and gestational diseases (gestational diabetes mellitus, preeclampsia and intra-uterine growth retardation) and sperm abnormalities and testicular pathologies, respectively.

2. Structure of Adipokine Genes and Proteins

2.1. Chemerin

Chemerin was identified in 2003 as the product of the *rarres2* (retinoic acid receptor responder 2) gene, which is located on chromosome 7 in humans and is composed of 5 coding exons with a full length of 1618 bp [23,24]. Expression of this gene is up-regulated by the synthetic retinoid tazarotene and occurs in a wide variety of tissues [23,24]. This gene encodes a 163 amino acid protein (16 kDa) secreted in an inactive form as prochemerin, with the secreted form being 20 amino acids shorter due to the cleavage of the C-terminus by inflammatory and coagulation serine proteases [25] (Figure 1). The cleavage of the signal peptide results in the release of an inactive precursor (chemerin-S163) into the extracellular media. The precursor requires further extracellular C-terminal cleavages at various sites to generate active and deactivated chemerins. For example, the proteolytic cleavage by plasmin, elastase and cathepsin G activates chemerin and generates various isoforms (chemerin-K158, -S157 and -F156, respectively) (Figure 1). Further cleavage of bioactive chemerin by chymase produces chemerin-F154 and terminates its activity [26]. Thus, several isoforms of chemerin have been identified that are dependent on processing by various serine and cysteine proteases (Figure 1). The role of these various forms is still unclear. Chemerin mRNA is detected in a wide range of different tissues in various species including humans, rodents, bovine and poultry [27]. In humans, it is most abundantly expressed in white adipose tissues, the liver and the placenta, and to a lesser extent in brown adipose tissue, the lungs, skeletal muscles, kidneys, ovaries, and the heart [28]. Chemerin is a cytokine described as an important regulator of several physiological processes such as blood pressure control, immune system regulation, angiogenesis and inflammation [26]. It was first discovered in human inflammatory fluids as a potential ligand of an orphan G protein-coupled receptor related to chemokine receptors called ChemR23 or CMKLR1 (Chemokine-Like Receptor 1, cf. paragraph 3.1).

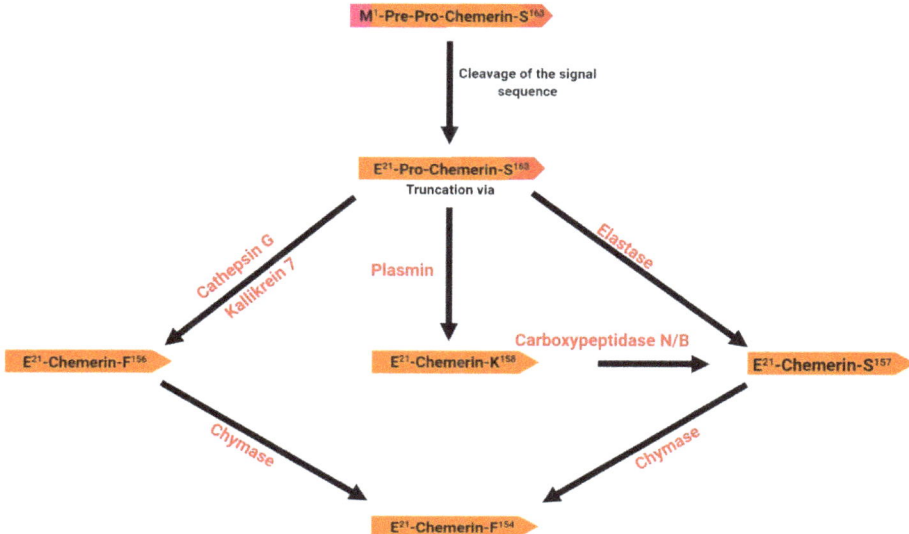

Figure 1. Structure and specific forms of human chemerin. The initial preprochemerin and its different products are processed by different proteases related to inflammation. The signal peptide (purple) is cleaved prior to secretion. Then, the C-terminus is cleaved by different proteases giving several active isoforms such as chemerin F^{156}, chemerin S^{157} and chemerin K^{158}.

2.2. Visfatin

Visfatin/NAMPT (nicotinamide phosphoribosyltransferase) was originally cloned in 1994 as a cytokine named pre-B-cell colony enhancing factor (PBEF) from a human peripheral blood lymphocyte cDNA library [29]. The mRNA for *PBEF* is 2.4 kb long and codes for a 52-kDa secreted protein. The 3′ untranslated region is 69% AT and contains multiple TATT motifs. There are two atypical polyadenylation signals, AATAAA, located upstream of the 3′ end. The protein lacks a typical signal sequence for secretion. Human PBEF has ubiquitous expression, although it is predominantly expressed in the human bone marrow, liver, and muscles [29]. In 2001, a study identified the gene *nadV*; its presence allows nicotinamide adenine dinucleotide (NAD)-independent growth of the Gram-negative bacteria *Haemophilus influenza* and *Actinobacillus pleuropneumoniae*. The authors found *NadV* to have significant sequence homology to *PBEF*, thereby suggesting a novel role for PBEF in NAD biosynthesis [30]. Indeed, in 2002 the murine homologue of PBEF was found to be an enzyme catalysing the reaction between nicotinamide and 5-phosphoribosyl-1-pyrophosphate to yield nicotinamide mononucleotide (NMN), an intermediate in the biosynthesis of NAD [31]. The crystal structure of a dimeric PBEF, now called NAMPT, in the presence and absence of NMN further underscores NAMPT as an important enzyme in NAD biosynthesis [32] (Figure 2). At the same time, visfatin has been identified as a cytokine hormone and an enzyme involved in metabolic (obesity, type II diabetes) and immune disorders [33]. In humans, visfatin plasma concentrations are positively correlated with measures of obesity [34]. In mammals, visfatin or NAMPT exists as two forms, the intra- and extracellular forms, iNAMPT and eNAMPT, respectively [35] (Figure 2). In mice, the protein expression of iNAMPT is highest in brown adipose tissue (BAT), and the liver and kidneys, at intermediate levels in the heart, low in white adipose tissue (WAT), and the lungs, spleen, testis, and skeletal muscle, and under detectable levels in the pancreas and brain [35]. While the function of iNAMPT has been firmly established as an NAD biosynthetic enzyme and having an important role in sirtuin activation in mitochondria, the function of eNAMPT is controversial. eNAMPT is released by a number of normal cell types, such as adipocytes, hepatocytes, myocytes, pancreatic cells, neurons and immune cells [35,36]. Moreover, it has been shown that eNAMPT is released under pathological conditions by cancer cells and that it could be used as a marker for cancer development [37–39].

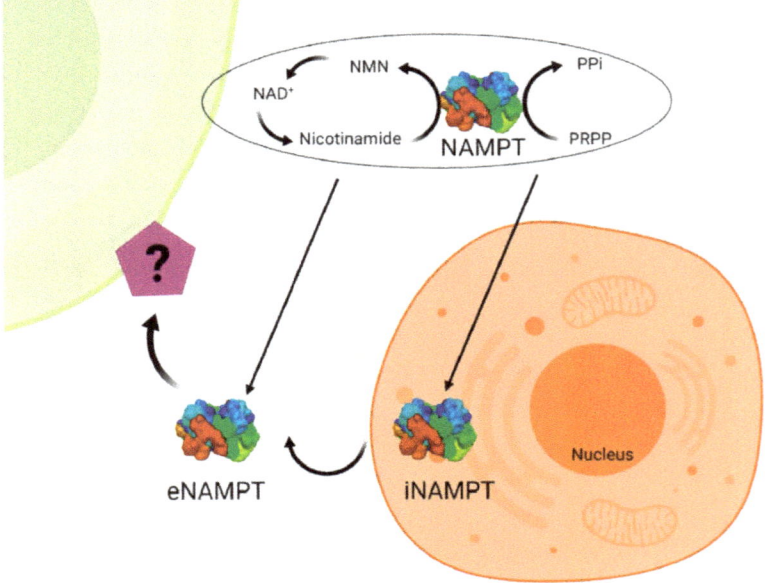

Figure 2. Structure and specific forms of human visfatin. Human visfatin can be found under the intra-cellular form of nicotinamide phosphoribosyltransferase (iNAMPT) having an enzymatic role to produce NAD+ (nicotinamide adenine dinucleotide), and under the extracellular form (eNAMPT) with the same role. Visfatin acts also as a cytokine that could act on target cells. NAMPT catalyzes the reaction between nicotinamide and 5-phosphoribosyl-1-pyrophosphate (PRPP) to yield nicotinamide mononucleotide (NMN), an intermediate in the biosynthesis of NAD+.

2.3. Resistin

Resistin (Retn) is a pro-inflammatory adipokine that was first identified in mice about 20 years ago, where it was identified as "adipose-tissue-specific secretory factor" (ADSF) [40], "found in the inflammatory zone 3" (FIZZ3) [41] and eventually renamed "resistin" (or "resistance to insulin") due to its ability to resist the action of insulin [42]. The gene coding for human resistin is located on chromosome 19p13.2 and spans 1369 bp, with three introns and four exons [43]. Resistin is a 108-amino acid propeptide, which includes a signal peptide, a variable region, and a conserved C-terminus [42] (Figure 3). Resistin (12.5 kDa) circulates in human blood as a dimeric protein consisting of two 92-amino acid polypeptides that are linked by a disulphide bridge and forms high- and low-molecular weight complexes (Figure 3). Indeed, a common feature of resistin is the existence of a motif (10–11 cysteine-rich) at the carboxyl terminus that could support the globular domain of the resistin monomer via the formation of 5 disulphide bridges [44,45] (Figure 3). Disulphide and non-disulphide bonds also play an important role in the formation of dimer, trimer, and hexamer forms of circulating resistin. In mice, the *Retn* gene is almost exclusively expressed in white adipocytes and blood cells [42], whereas peripheral blood mononuclear cells (PBMCs), macrophages, and bone marrow cells are the primary source of circulating resistin in humans [46]. In rodents, resistin represents a clear pathogenic factor in the severity of insulin resistance (IR) [42]. However, in humans, despite initially being proposed as the potential link between obesity and diabetes [47], this adipokine does not represent a major determinant of IR. Indeed,

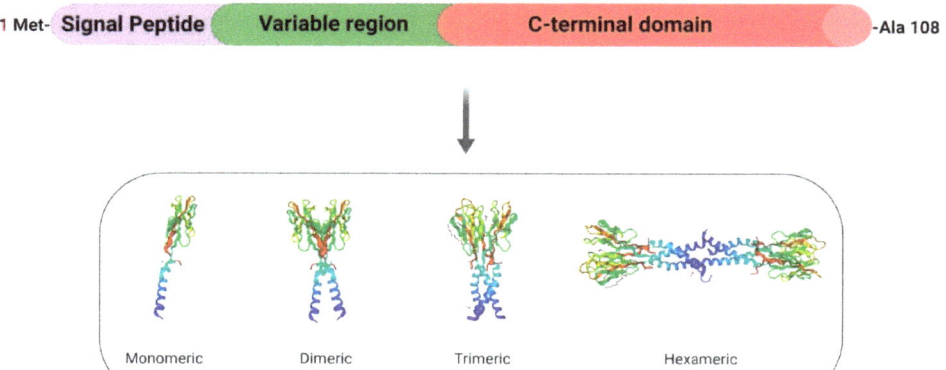

Figure 3. Structure and specific forms of human resistin. Human resistin is composed by a signal peptide (purple), a variable region (green) and a C-terminal domain. Resistin can be found under the monomeric form and can form dimeric and trimeric proteins thanks to disulfide bridges. Then, disulfide and non-disulfide bridges can be involved in the formation of the hexameric protein.

2.4. Apelin

APJ, now known as apelin receptor, was considered as an orphan G protein-coupled receptor. In 1998, a Japanese team purified a peptide that is able to bind the APJ orphan receptor, named apelin, from bovine stomach extracts [48]. Apelin is widely expressed in various types of tissues and organs such as the central nervous system and peripheral tissues, including the hypothalamus, adipose tissue, skeletal muscle, digestive system and the ovary [49–52]. The human apelin gene is found on chromosome Xq25-q26.1. The apelin gene sequence contains an intron of around 6kb in length with recognised intron/exon boundaries interrupting the ORF (Open Reading Frame) at the position encoding Gly22. Similar to the rat preproapelin cDNA, the reported start codon for human preproapelin does not appear to conform to the Kozak consensus sequence, again due to the presence of an adenosine immediately following the start codon. The cDNA of apelin encodes a 77-amino-acid preproprotein (Figure 4). The N-terminal sections of bovine and human proteins are rich in hydrophobic amino acids, indicating that these represent secretory signal sequences. The amino acid sequence of the isolated bovine peptide corresponds to the deduced sequence of the bovine preproprotein from position 42 to position 58. These results suggest that apelin is one of the processing products derived from the C-terminal portion of the preproprotein [48]. To date, the main active forms of apelin are apelin-13, -17 and 36 and the pyroglutaminated isoform of apelin-13 (Pyr(1)-apelin 13), which is characterised by a higher resistance to degradation [53] (Figure 4). In the heart, the described predominant form is the Pyr(1)-apelin-13 [54]. Pyr(1)-apelin-13, apelin-13 and apelin-36 have comparable efficacy and potency in human cardiovascular tissues [54], whereas apelin-17 appears to be the most efficient in promoting apelin receptor internalisation [55]. The rat, bovine and human preproapelin sequences for the last 23 C-terminal amino acids share a sequence homology of 100% [48].

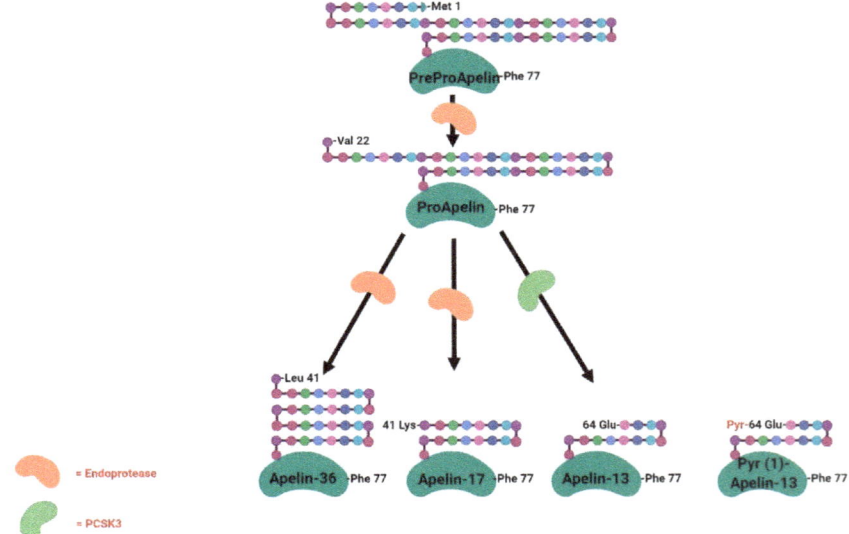

Figure 4. Structure and specific forms of human apelin. Human apelin is first of all found under the preproapelin form (77 amino acids) that will be cleaved by endopeptidases acting on basic amino-acid-rich regions giving the proapelin (55 amino-acids) and then the other tissue-dependent active isoforms (36, 17, 13 and Pyr-13 amino-acids). PCSK3 (proprotein convertase subtilisin/kexin 3) is involved in the cleavage of proapelin to apelin-13.

3. Adipokines Receptors and Signalling Pathways

3.1. Chemerin

The first chemerin receptor identified was CMKLR1, originally named ChemR23. It has been described as an orphan G protein-coupled receptor and was cloned to identify novel chemotactic factor receptors [56]. Subsequently, it has been found to be expressed in monocyte-derived dendritic cells and macrophages and as a co-receptor for SIV (Simian Immunodeficiency Virus) and some primary HIV-1 (Human Immunodeficiency Virus-1) strains, and is known as ChemR23 [57]. A second receptor, named LPS (LipoPolySaccharide) inducible C-C chemokine receptor-related gene (L-CCR), has been discovered in mouse macrophage activation [58] and its orthologue in human, firstly named as Human Chemokine Receptor (HCR), have been identified in a human neutrophil cDNA library [59]. Firstly, this receptor was considered as an orphan receptor. A third receptor named G Protein Receptor 1 (GPR1), has also been identified as an orphan receptor in humans and rodents, and is involved in peptide transmission in brain functioning [60]. Also, besides CMKLR1, orphan receptors GPR1 and CCRL2 have been identified by in vitro assays as spare receptors for chemerin (Figure 5, [61,62]. Those three receptors are protein G-coupled receptors with seven-transmembrane domains. The expression of CMKLR1 mRNA was detected in a wide variety of tissues such as haematopoietic tissues [24,56,63], adipocytes [64], endothelial cells [65], osteoclasts [66] and ovarian cells [67]. CCRL2 has been found to be expressed in cell types such as macrophages [68], mast cells [62], lung epithelial cells [69] and the ovary [67]. Contrary to CMKLR1 and CCRL2, GPR1 expression has not been found in immune cells but has been reported in central nervous system cells [60,70], murine brown adipose tissue, white adipose tissue, and skeletal muscle. GPR1 is mainly expressed in vascular cells in white adipose tissue [16]. Chemerin binding to CMKLR1 enhances leukocyte chemotaxis [71]. Chemerin binding to CCRL2 does not mediate cell signalling, but might present chemerin to nearby CMKLR1-positive cells to promote its function and play a key role in immune responses, inflammation, and other physiological processes

(Figure 5, [62]. GPR1 is an active receptor of chemerin and could regulate glucose homeostasis in the development of obesity because glucose intolerance was found to be increased in Gpr1-knockout mice fed a high-fat diet compared to wild-type (WT) mice. Within the mice ovary, it has been shown that chemerin/GPR1 signalling regulates progesterone secretion during the processes of follicular development, corpus luteum formation, and PGF2α-induced luteolysis [72].

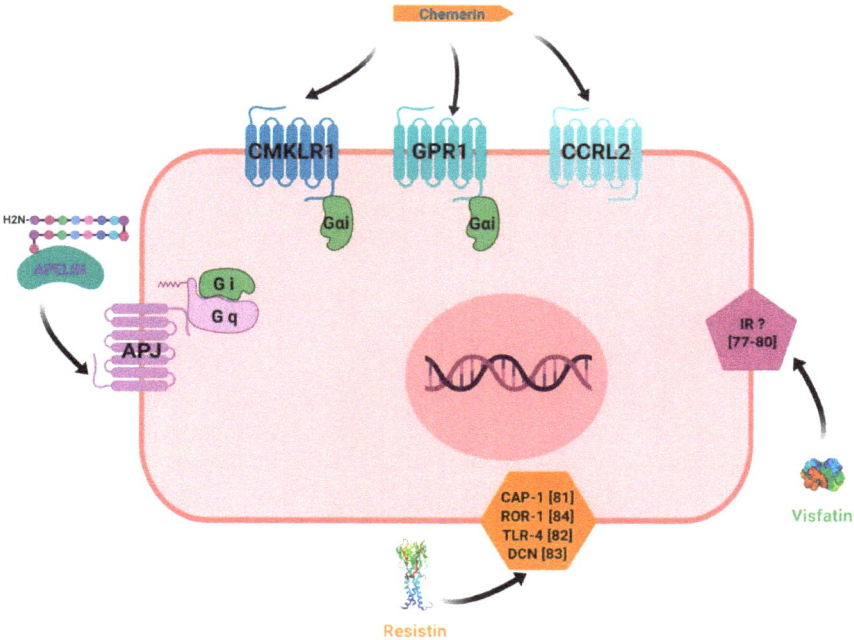

Figure 5. Receptors used by chemerin, visfatin, resistin and apelin for their signaling pathways. chemerin can bind three different receptors that are CMKLR1, GPR1 and CCRL2. CMKLR1 and GPR1 are coupled with intracellular Gαi proteins. The last receptor doesn't have any active signaling pathway identified until now suggesting a putative role of co-receptor for CCRL2. Apelin has its own receptor called APJ coupled with intracellular Gq and Gαi proteins. Resistin could bind receptors such as CAP-1, ROR-1 and TLR-4 but it has to be confirmed. No receptor for visfatin has been identified until now.

Chemerin binding to CMKLR1 activates the three Gαi subtypes and the two Gαo isoforms (Figure 5). Chemerin stimulates the increase in intracellular calcium and a decrease of cyclic AMP in CMKLR1-expressing CHO cells that are dependent on Gαi signalling [24]. It further uses the RhoA- and Rho-associated protein kinase-dependent pathway downstream of GPR1 and CMKLR1 to activate the transcriptional regulator serum-response factor [73]. Mitogen-activated protein kinase ERK1/2 is phosphorylated upon chemerin treatment in various cells, including endothelial cells, adipocytes, and skeletal muscle cells. The activation of ERK1/2 at low, but not high, chemerin concentrations was described in adipocytes [65,74]. Chemerin further activated p38 mitogen-activated protein kinase, Akt and phosphoinositide 3-kinase [26]. Short periods of incubation with chemerin were shown to activate Akt in hepatocytes, whereas prolonged treatment of up to two hours led to a decline in phosphorylated Akt in these cells [75]. The same study reports that chemerin binding weakened the association of phosphatase and tensin homolog (PTEN) with CMKLR1. This enhanced the activity of PTEN and subsequently led to decreased Akt phosphorylation. The nuclear factor kappa B (NFkB) pathway is activated by chemerin in skeletal muscles cells [76]. Chemerin thus activates various signalling pathways, with effects that are dependent on incubation time and dose.

3.2. Visfatin

The receptor of visfatin is still unknown (Figure 5) and the exact cellular mechanism of extracellular visfatin (eNAMPT) remains unclear, even though various authors have implicated intracellular insulin receptor signalling pathways in the action of visfatin [77–80].

3.3. Resistin

Like visfatin, the receptor of resistin remains unknown and the molecular mechanism of resistin action is unclear. However, recent reports have suggested potential receptors for resistin (Figure 5). In humans, there are two putative resistin receptors: adenylyl cyclase-associated protein 1 (CAP 1) [81] and toll-like receptor 4 (TLR4) [82]. Studies have involved the use of an isoform of decorin (DCN) [83], as this is supposed to be a receptor of resistin. Moreover, mouse receptor tyrosine kinase-like orphan receptor 1 (ROR1) has been identified as a putative receptor for resistin [84]. It is well known that resistin activates signalling pathways in different tissues such as Akt, MAPK (Mitogen-Activated Protein Kinases, ERK1/2 and p38), Stat-3 (signal transducer and activator of transcription 3) and PPAR gamma (PPARγ).

3.4. Apelin

Apelin receptor (APJ) was first identified in 1993 as a class A (rhodopsin-like) orphan G protein-coupled receptor which shows high homology with the angiotensin II (AngII) receptor [85]. The gene encoding APJ is intronless and is known as *APLNR* in humans. The *APLNR* gene encodes a 380-amino acid protein and is located on chromosome 11q12 [85]. The promoter of the rat APLNR gene does not include a TATA box, but contains a potential CAAT box at −1257 bp and a number of activator protein 1 and specificity protein 1 (Sp1) motifs [86]. There are two transcriptional start sites at −247 and −210 bp [86]. The protein structure of APJ is typical of a GPCR (G protein-coupled receptor), containing seven hydrophobic transmembrane domains, with consensus sites for phosphorylation by protein kinase A (PKA), palmitoylation and glycosylation (Figure 5, [85]. The apelin system is able to activate a high number of signalling pathways through various G proteins. Apelin-13 and apelin-36 activate the phosphorylation of ERK1/2 in Chinese hamster ovary (CHO) cells stably expressing mouse APJ [87]. The phosphorylation, and thus activation, of Akt has been shown to be a downstream effector of apelin signalling; this was first shown to occur via a PTX-sensitive G-protein and PKC [87]. The same study showed that Apelin induces the dual phosphorylation of the S6 ribosomal protein kinase (p70S6K) in human umbilical vein endothelial cells (HUVECs), where apelin promotes cell proliferation via PTX-sensitive, ERK1/2-, mammalian target of rapamycin (mTOR)-, and Akt-dependent intracellular cascades. In the absence of ligands, the apelin receptor is also able to heterodimerise with other GPCRs and activate signalling pathways.

4. Adipokines and Reproductive Functions at the Hypothalamo-Pituitary Level in Non-Pathological Conditions

4.1. Chemerin

In the hypothalamus, the expression of chemerin and its receptors was observed within the tanycytes and ependymal cells (Figure 6), with increased expression reported for long (LD) versus short (SD) photoperiods, pointing to a physiological role. [88]. In the pituitary, *RARRES2* gene expression has been found in baboons and chimpanzees [89] (Figure 7). Furthermore, in rats, chemerin administration (8 and 16 μg/kg) decreased both food intake and body weight compared to vehicle, possibly associated with a significant increase in serotonin synthesis and release, in the hypothalamus [90]. These results suggest an important role of chemerin in hypothalamus–pituitary function especially in feeding behaviour; however, interactions between chemerin and the central nervous system involved in reproduction need further investigation. No in vivo or in vitro studies have investigated the effect of chemerin on pituitary cells.

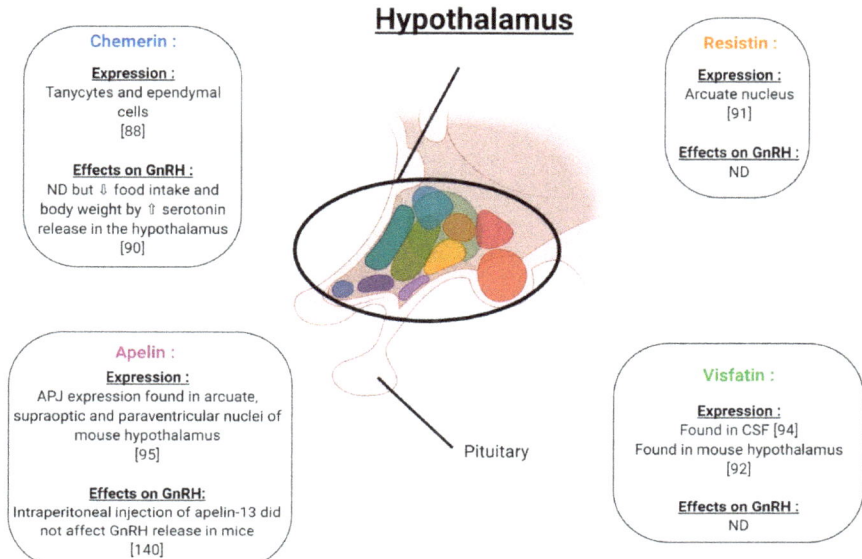

Figure 6. Expression and effects on GnRH (Gonadotropin-Releasing Hormone) release of chemerin, visfatin, resistin and apelin in hypothalamus. ⇧ Increase/stimulation. ⇩ Decrease/inhibition. ND: not determined. CSF: cerebrospinal fluid.

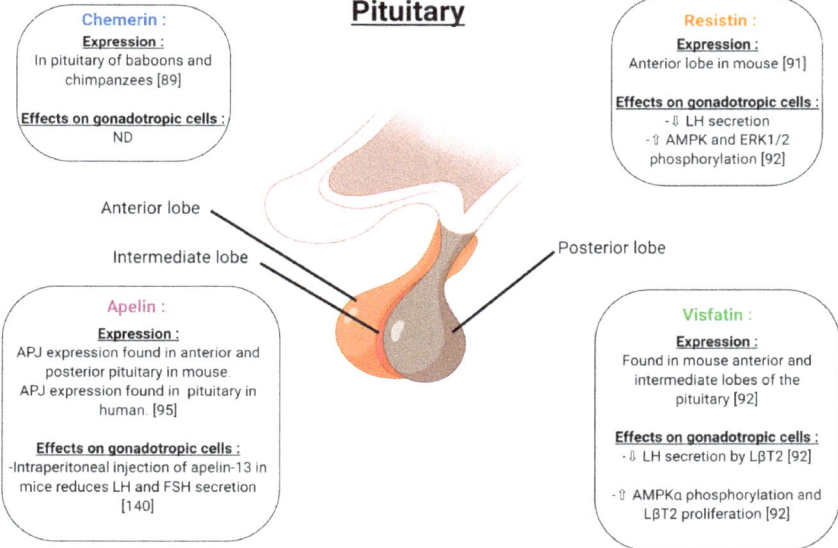

Figure 7. Expression and effects on gonadotropic cells of chemerin, visfatin, resistin and apelin in pituitary. ⇧ Increase/stimulation. ⇩ Decrease/inhibition. ND: not determined.

4.2. Resistin

In rodents, resistin is expressed in the hypothalamus in a region responsible for energy balance [91] (Figure 6). Maillard et al. (2017) showed staining by immunohistochemistry of resistin in the anterior lobe of the mouse pituitary (Figure 7). Resistin 1 and 10 ng/mL decreased LH (Luteinizing Hormone) secreted by LβT2 cells. Furthermore, a 0.01; 0.1 and 1 ng/mL resistin concentration significantly decreased mouse pituitary cell LH secretion, but 10 ng/mL resistin did not significantly affect LH release [92] (Figure 7). Thus, the effect of resistin on pituitary cells seems to be dependent on the concentration. In LβT2 mouse cells, resistin (1 ng/mL) increased phosphorylation in the AMPK and ERK1/2 signalling pathways (Figure 7). Furthermore, resistin has been shown to be regulated by gonadotrophins from the pituitary [93]. All of these data suggest a potential role of resistin in the hypothalamo-pituitary axis.

4.3. Visfatin

Visfatin has been found in the cerebrospinal fluid but its origin is not known [94]. Visfatin is present in the mouse brain, hypothalamic area (Figure 6) and pituitary, as well as in LβT2 mouse gonadotrophin cells [92]. By immunohistochemistry, visfatin was localised in the anterior and intermediate lobes of the pituitary and seems to be co-localised with βLH (Figure 7). In LβT2 cells, LH secretion was decreased by visfatin stimulation from 0.1 to 10 ng/mL, whereas visfatin did not affect LH secretion in the primary mouse pituitary cells [92]. Thus, visfatin could play a regulatory role at the hypothalamo-pituitary level.

4.4. Apelin

Apelin receptor (APJ) has been characterised in the mouse central nervous system by immunohistochemistry (Figure 6). APJ was localised in hypothalamic nuclei, such as arcuate, supraoptic and paraventricular nuclei, and in the anterior pituitary, implying potential roles in the control of reproduction [95]. These brain regions are known to be the central control points of energy utilisation and reproductive behaviour. The intraperitoneal injection of apelin-13 in mice reduced LH, FSH (Follicle Stimulating Hormone) and testosterone serum levels and showed negative effects on the reproductive function (Figure 7). However, in these mice, no measurement of GnRH release was performed. Based on these results, the authors suggested that the inhibitory effect of apelin on testosterone levels was due to a direct action of apelin on gonadotropic cells [96–98].

5. Adipokines and Reproductive Functions at the Gonad Level in Non-Pathological Conditions

5.1. Ovary

5.1.1. Chemerin

Under normal physiological conditions, chemerin and CMKLR1 have been shown to be expressed in the mouse ovary [74]. Another study went further, demonstrating that the chemerin system is expressed within the human ovary at mRNA and protein levels, but also has a functional role in ovarian physiology (Figure 8). This study showed that chemerin and its receptor CMKLR1 are present and active in human granulosa cells. Chemerin reduces IGF-1 (Insulin Like Growth Factor 1)-induced steroidogenesis and cell proliferation through a decrease in the activation of IGF-1R signalling pathways in primary human granulosa cells (hGCs) [67]. Chemerin also inhibits FSH-induced mRNA and protein expression of aromatase and p450scc in rodent granulosa cells [99,100] (Figure 8). In bovine species, chemerin and its three receptors CMKLR1, GPR1 and CCRL2 are expressed within the ovary and recombinant chemerin decreases in vitro steroidogenesis and cholesterol synthesis at the basal level as well as after IGF-1 and/or FSH induction [101] (Figure 8). This down-regulation is associated with a reduction in protein levels of STAR (Steroid Acute Regulatory protein), cytochrome P450 family 19 subfamilies A member 1, and 3-Hydroxy-3-Methylglutaryl-CoA Reductase and the phosphorylation of MAPK ERK1/2, which is dependent on CMKLR1. Moreover, human recombinant chemerin also inhibits bovine oocyte maturation at the germinal vesicle stage and decreases MAPK ERK1/2 phosphorylation in oocytes and cumulus cells [101] (Figure 8). In avian species, it has also been demonstrated that chemerin and its three receptors are expressed in the hen ovary and that chemerin plasma concentration is positively correlated with egg hatchability [102]. Chemerin and its receptors are also expressed in turkeys, more particularly in the theca and granulosa cells, with higher levels in theca cells. Moreover, this study showed that chemerin plasma concentrations decreased during the laying period [103]. All of these data suggest that chemerin could be a key hormone linking reproductive and metabolic functions.

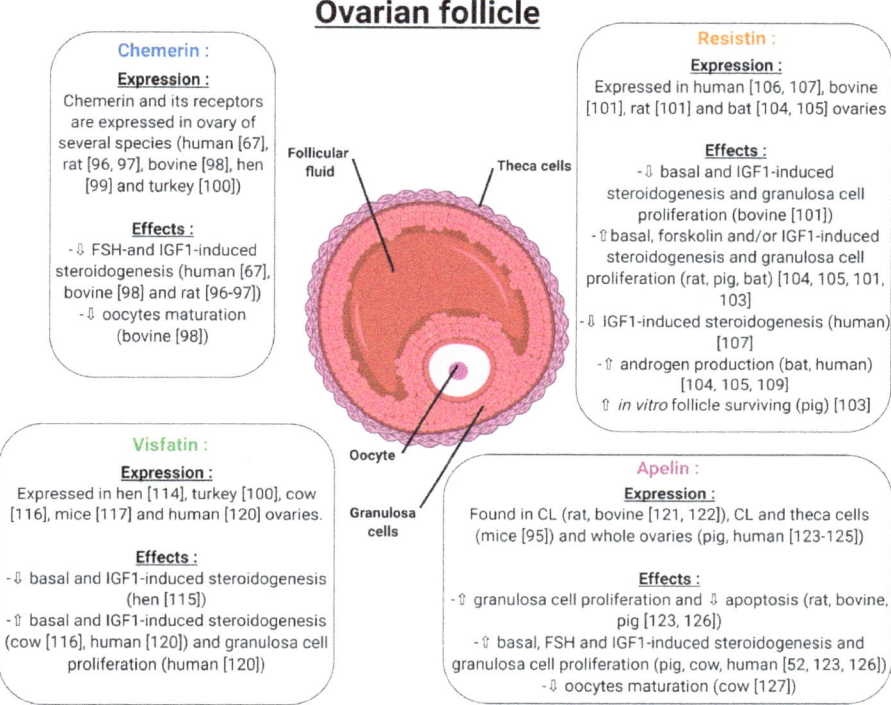

Figure 8. Expression and effects of chemerin, visfatin, resistin and apelin on the ovarian follicle. ⇧ Increase/stimulation. ⇩ Decrease/inhibition.

5.1.2. Resistin

Resistin has been shown to be expressed within the ovaries of rodent and bovine species [104]. More precisely, resistin is expressed by theca cells, luteinised granulosa cells of the corpus luteum and oocytes, but its expression is very weak in granulosa cells. By contrast, in bovine species, resistin is expressed by granulosa cells of growing follicles, with its expression decreasing in the corpus luteum and being almost undetectable in oocytes (Figure 8). Furthermore, in these cells, the authors observed that recombinant resistin can modulate steroidogenesis and proliferation in a basal state or in response to IGF-1 in vitro [104] (Figure 8). Another study showed that resistin inhibits steroidogenesis of undifferentiated (small follicles) granulosa cells and mitogenesis of differentiated (large follicle) granulosa cells [105]. These results highlighted a huge species difference between rat and bovine species in terms of resistin expression and its effects [104]. In a porcine model, resistin is expressed by theca cells, but also and more abundantly in granulosa cells of growing follicles (Figure 8). In these cells, resistin supports the survival of in vitro cultured porcine follicles (Figure 8). It also has a positive effect on steroidogenesis and mitosis on ovarian cells [106]. In the greater Asiatic yellow bat (*Scotophilus heathii*), resistin is expressed in the ovary, more precisely by the theca cells, as in rats, with an increase in expression around the ovulation period. Moreover, recombinant resistin alone on cultured bat granulosa cells preferentially stimulates progesterone secretion. Furthermore, resistin increases androgenic action in the ovary [107,108].

In humans, resistin expression has been demonstrated in luteinised granulosa cells recovered after follicle punction in a programme of in vitro fertilisation [109,110]. In 2009, a study demonstrated that ovarian hormones did not have any effects on resistin concentrations in serum [111]. However, resistin itself influences in vitro ovarian functions. Indeed, Munir et al. demonstrated that resistin enhances mRNA expression and the activity of 17alpha-hydroxylase in human theca cells in the presence of forskolin and insulin [112] (Figure 8). This finding confirms the results obtained in rat testes, where resistin increases testosterone secretion in a dose-dependent manner [93]. In contrast, Reverchon et al. showed that resistin decreases IGF-1-induced steroidogenesis in primary human granulosa cells. These effects were confirmed by Messini et al. in response to FSH [113]. Despite its negative effect on the regulation of ovarian steroidogenesis [110,114] (Figure 8), resistin does not seem to play a key role in human ovarian physiology. Indeed, its levels in follicular fluid have been repeatedly found to be lower than in plasma [110,115], suggesting that human granulosa cells, while expressing resistin protein [110], are unlikely to secrete it into follicular fluid or the circulation. Varnagy et al. showed that resistin levels in follicular fluid were a positive predictor of oocyte and embryo number, indicating a beneficial effect of this adipokine on the outcome of in vitro fertilisation procedures [116]. However, this finding has not been confirmed by other authors, who concluded that resistin cannot play a significant role in the maturation and development of oocytes [115,117]. This discrepancy could be explained by the number of patients and also by the experimental design.

5.1.3. Visfatin

In the chicken model, this adipokine is widely expressed in a lot of tissues, in a sex-dependent manner (Figure 8). It has been found in hen ovaries at both the mRNA and protein levels [118], and an in vitro study has shown that visfatin inhibits progesterone production in granulosa cells through STAR and HSD3B at basal level or after IGF-1 stimulation [119]. Still in birds, visfatin is expressed mainly by theca cells and more weakly by granulosa cells of turkey follicles. During a laying cycle, its concentration in serum significantly decreases in the same model [103]. In cows, visfatin is expressed within the ovary in theca, granulosa, cumulus cells and oocytes. Contrary to the chicken model, visfatin increases in vitro steroidogenesis and potentialises IGF-1 effects by increasing STAR and HSD3B expression, as well as E2 and P4 secretion [120] (Figure 8). In mice, visfatin is also expressed within the ovary and more precisely in stromal cells, endothelial cells, granulosa cells and cumulus cells. Its main production comes from granulosa cells and increases during follicular growth. The administration of visfatin during ovulation induction in aged female mice improves the developmental competency of oocytes [121] (Figure 8). Furthermore, Shen et al. found a significant positive correlation between visfatin concentration in follicular fluid and the number of retrieved oocytes in women [122], confirming a possible positive role of this adipokine in female reproductive function. However, visfatin concentration in follicular fluid has been shown to be similar [122] or lower [123] than in serum, and no correlation was found between visfatin plasma and follicular fluid levels [122]. Hence, circulating visfatin concentration does not seem to contribute significantly to visfatin concentration in follicular fluid [122] which could, therefore, be independently and differently regulated at the ovarian level. In humans, visfatin is expressed in granulosa cells, but also in cumulus cells and oocytes, and less abundantly in theca cells. Moreover, recombinant human visfatin increases cell proliferation and E2 and P4 production by luteinized human granulosa cells [124]. Thus, as in bovine species and mice, visfatin has a positive effect on steroidogenesis in human granulosa cells [124].

5.1.4. Apelin

Apelin and APJ have been detected by in situ hybridisation in the corpus luteum (CL) of the rat ovary [125]. In mice, the apelin system is found in the corpus luteum but also in theca cells of follicles, showing a species difference between mice and rats [95]. In bovine species, this adipokine is also expressed in the early and mid-luteal stages of the corpus luteum to then decline during the regression phase. More precisely, apelin was localised in the smooth muscle cells of intraluteal arterioles, and responded to PGF2-alpha at the periphery of CL in cows [126]. In porcine species, the expression of apelin and APJ increased with ovarian follicular growth [127]. In humans, apelin and its receptor are expressed by granulosa, cumulus, and theca cells with a putative weak expression in oocytes (Figure 8). Even if plasma apelin levels are largely dependent on the assay, apelin concentration in follicular fluid seems to be higher than in plasma [128,129]. It can thus be speculated that follicular apelin is partly derived by granulosa cell production and regulates the function of granulosa cells in a paracrine and/or autocrine manner. Indeed, although mice lacking apelin or APJ genes are viable and fertile [52], some in vitro evidence suggests a potential role of apelin in the control of ovarian function. Indeed, it enhances progesterone and oestradiol secretion in human and porcine granulosa cells [52,96,127] (Figure 8). In primary human granulosa cells, Apelin-13 and Apelin-17 isoforms are both able to increase basal and IGF-1-induced progesterone and oestradiol secretion, which was associated with an increase in HSD3B protein concentration and AKT and MAPK ERK1/2 phosphorylation [52]. Apelin also improves rat, bovine and porcine granulosa cell proliferation [127], and seems to be involved in the regulation of bovine corpus luteum luteolysis processes [126] and oocyte maturation [97]. Notably, apelin has been suggested to be implicated in bovine follicular atresia [96] and, in different animal species, both the mRNA and protein levels of apelin and APJ changed during follicular growth with the highest expression in large follicles [127]. In bovine species, apelin exerts a negative effect on in vitro oocyte maturation through blocking of the meiotic progression at the germinal vesicle stage [97] (Figure 8).

In summary, chemerin and the apelin system, resistin and visfatin are expressed in the ovary of various species. The effects of these adipokines mainly studied in vitro are dependent on the species but also on the dose used, experimental design and probably on the methodological uncertainties. In primary human granulosa cells, chemerin and resistin inhibit in vitro steroidogenesis induced by IGF-1, whereas visfatin and apelin improve it (Figure 9).

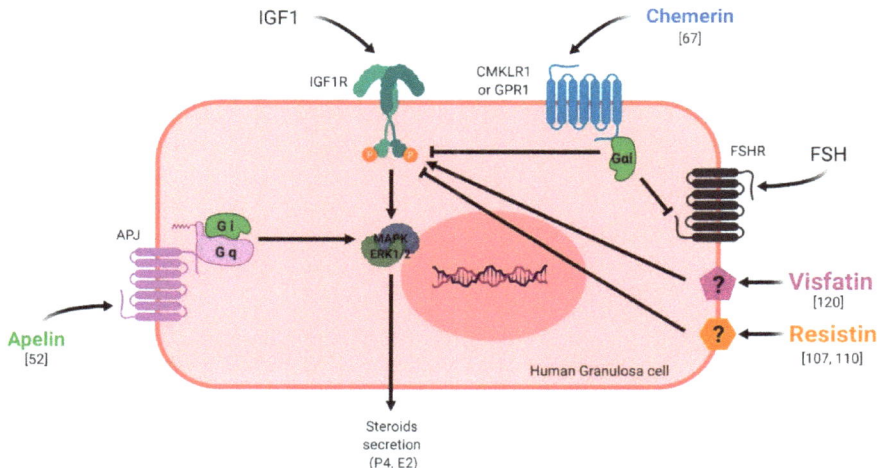

Figure 9. Effects of chemerin, visfatin, resistin and apelin on steroidogenesis in vitro in primary human granulosa cells. Chemerin and resistin are known to inhibit IGF-1 (Insulin Like Growth Factor 1)-induced steroidogenesis whereas visfatin and apelin exert stimulatory effects.

5.2. Testis

Recent reports have pointed to an emerging role of adipokine in male reproductive functions. Indeed, it has been shown that obesity is positively correlated with defective spermatogenesis, especially in developed countries where semen quality is seriously lowered. Furthermore, obesity is associated with decreased testosterone concentrations and sperm motility [98]; however, the action by which testosterone production is reduced remains unclear. The link between obesity, adipokine and male fertility problems needs to be elucidated. The effect of adiponectin and leptin in male fertility has already been described [19]. In this section, we will focus on the role of other novel adipokines (chemerin, apelin, visfatin, resistin) in male reproductive functions.

5.2.1. Chemerin

Chemerin and its three receptors CMKLR1, GPR1 and CCRL2 are expressed in rat and human male reproductive tracts. [130,131]. Chemerin, CMKLR1 and GPR1 proteins are specifically localised in Leydig cells of the human and rat testis [132] (Figure 10). In rat primary Leydig cell cultures, chemerin suppressed the testosterone production induced by human chorionic gonadotropin (hGC, [133]) (Figure 10). This is associated with an inhibition of gene and protein expression of the 3β-hydroxysteroid dehydrogenase and MAPK ERK1/2 phosphorylation [133]. The C-20 chemerin derived peptide presents similar effects to chemerin, suggesting that this peptide can present similar functions as the different peptide forms of chemerin [130]. In mice deleted for CMKLR1 (CMKLR1−/−), the plasma testosterone level is lower compared to in wild-type animals [134]. Furthermore, in cultured Leydig cells isolated from CMKLR1−/− mice, gene expression of *HSD3B*, *STAR*, *P450scc*, *Sf1*, *Gata4* and *Insl3* was significantly decreased compared to wild-type mice. All of these data suggest that chemerin plays an important role in male steroidogenesis, as in females. In humans, chemerin is present in seminal plasma at lower concentrations than in human blood plasma [135]. Obesity is associated with reduced sperm motility and lower testosterone serum levels, and it is known that chemerin secretion is increased in the case of obesity, suggesting that chemerin could have a negative effect on sperm motility/maturation in the epididymis through direct effects on spermatozoa or indirect effects during epidydimal maturation.

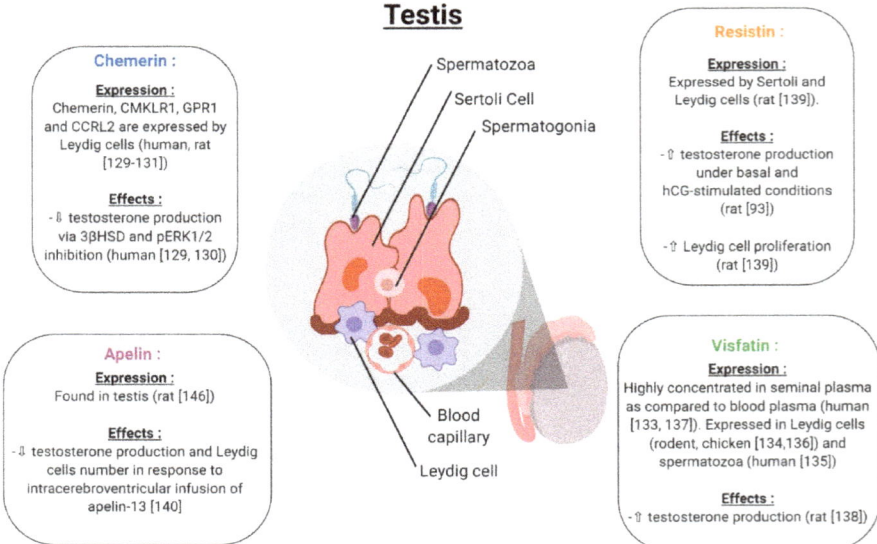

Figure 10. Expression and effects of chemerin, visfatin, resistin and apelin on testicular function. ⇧ Increase/stimulation. ⇩ Decrease/inhibition.

5.2.2. Visfatin

Visfatin is present in rodent and human testes [136,137]. It is also expressed in pre-pubertal and adult chicken testes, and more particularly in the nucleus of sertoli cells, and Leydig cells [138] (Figure 10). In humans, visfatin concentrations in seminal plasma is higher than in blood plasma [139] suggesting local production or by the male annex glands. Moreover, visfatin is present in the human spermatozoa and is regulated in a maturation-dependent manner [137]. In rats, visfatin increased testosterone production through Ras1 kinase from in vitro cultured Leydig cells [140] (Figure 10). Moreover, Jeremy et al. showed that visfatin protein expression in the rodent testis is decreased by a D-galactose treatment which induces aging [136]. The visfatin expression is specifically decreased in Leydig cells and decreases serum testosterone levels. These data suggest an important role of visfatin in testicular aging by regulating spermatogenesis and steroidogenesis [136].

5.2.3. Resistin

Resistin has been found to be expressed in the testis and seminiferous tubules of rats, and especially in Sertoli and Leydig cells. Resistin is equally expressed in mouse Leydig cell lines (MA-10 and TM3) [141]. In rat Leydig cells, in vitro stimulation with resistin increased both basal and human chorionic gonadotropin (hCG)-stimulated testosterone production [93] (Figure 10). Roumaud et al. cited that exposure to a low resistin concentration (10 ng/mL = obesity physiological concentration) increases Leydig cell proliferation [141]. These data suggest that resistin could positively regulate Leydig cell steroidogenesis and proliferation.

5.2.4. Apelin

Apelin is found in the rat testis [142]. Only one study showed that the intracerebroventricular infusion of apelin-13 in male rats significantly reduced serum testosterone levels compared to the control group [143] (Figure 10). Histological analyses demonstrated a reduction in the number of Leydig cells, suggesting that apelin may play a role in the central regulation and decrease testosterone release by suppressing LH secretion (Figure 10).

6. Adipokines and Pregnancy

6.1. Adipokines and Uterus

Chemerin was first identified in normal human myometrial cells and fibroidic cells by microarray and real-time quantitative polymerase chain reaction (RT–qPCR) [144]. Later, it was demonstrated that chemerin is expressed in human primary cultures of stromal cells and extravillous trophoblast cells from pregnant women. Moreover, data indicate that chemerin is up-regulated during decidualisation and might contribute to natural killer (NK) cell accumulation and vascular remodelling during early pregnancy [145]. In the human and rat myometrium, visfatin had similar dose-dependent effects on the inhibition of both spontaneous and oxytocin-induced contractions of pregnant rat and human myometrial tissue in vitro [146]. In the mouse model, visfatin is also expressed by the uterus and its expression varies during the sexual cycle. Indeed, it appeared that E2 and P4 regulate visfatin expression explaining variations during sexual cycle expression in mice uterus [113].

Only one study has demonstrated that resistin is expressed within the uterus, by showing that this adipokine is expressed in the ovine uterus and that its expression varies according to the nutritional status of the animal, an observation that strengthens the link between nutritional status and reproductive activity [147]. First evidence of apelin expression in the uterus appeared in 2001 in a study showing the purification of the apelin-36 isoform by gel filtration chromatography from uterine tissue extracts from rats [148]. As in rats, apelin and its receptor appear to be expressed in the mouse uterus [95]. In humans, an in vitro study brought evidence that apelin had inhibitory effects on uterine contractility by down-regulating spontaneous and oxytocin-induced contractions in the human myometrium [149]. Similar results have since been found in rats [150].

6.2. Adipokines and Placenta

Acting as a chemoattractant, chemerin has been hypothesised to play a role in placentation. Indeed, this adipokine is produced by the rat placenta during gestation and has also been found to be expressed in human placenta. Chemerin plays a role in placentation by regulating NK cell accumulation and endothelial cell morphogenesis during early pregnancy, along with the expression of this adipokine in stromal cells and extravillous trophoblast cells; however, this expression remains low compared to that in the liver and adipose tissues [145,151]. It has also been found to be expressed within the umbilical cord, playing a protective role by regulating umbilical vein endothelial cell-induced nitric oxide signalling in preeclampsia [152]. Finally, the chemerin/GPR1 system has been found to be expressed in mice and human placenta with a putative role as a feedback mechanism that could regulate the carbohydrate balance during pregnancy [153].

Visfatin has been immunolocalised throughout gestation in the amniotic epithelium and mesenchymal cells as well as the chorionic cytotrophoblast and parietal decidua. This adipokine is constitutively expressed by the foetal membranes during pregnancy. It increased the expression of IL-6 and IL-8 and may be important in both normal spontaneous labour and infection-induced preterm labour [154]. It has also been linked with the initiation of normal labour with a role at the end of the signalling cascade. Indeed, a previous study demonstrated that visfatin activates pro-inflammatory cytokine release and phospholipid metabolism in the human placenta via activation of the NF-κB pathway, leading to normal labour [155,156]. Its production has also been linked to the equilibrium and homeostasis of amniotic fluid by regulating its reabsorption by the amniotic fluid through stimulation of VEGFR2 ((Vascular endothelial growth factor receptor 2) expression in the placenta [157]. In vitro, the PPAR-γ signalling pathway has been linked to the regulation of visfatin by IL-6 in BeWo (Placental cell line cell), providing a novel insight into the roles of visfatin in trophoblastic cells [158].

In a rat model, resistin expression has been demonstrated in the placenta under normal conditions [159]. First evidence of its expression in the human placenta was provided by Yura et al. in 2003 [160] with a study showing that this adipokine is produced by the placenta with a maximum at full-term pregnancy. Resistin mRNA and protein are also localised to the syncytiotrophoblast and EVTs in early gestation and the syncytiotrophoblast in late gestation [160]. Maternal serum levels in the first and second trimesters are relatively constant and comparable to values in non-pregnant women. However, resistin levels and placental mRNA expression are increased by the third trimester [161]. Because adipose resistin expression remains unchanged during pregnancy, placental production is likely a major source of resistin in the maternal circulation. Such changes in resistin levels could contribute to the decrease in insulin sensitivity during the latter half of pregnancy, which is beneficial for the rapid growth of the foetus [162]. In the human placenta, resistin could affect glucose-uptake, presumably by decreasing the cell surface glucose transporter [163].

The apelin system is also expressed within the human placenta under normal conditions [164]. In rats, apelin expression is lower than in the brain, with a localisation of the protein in the perivascular smooth muscle [165]. In the same species, in cases of induced hypertension by nitric oxide treatment, the apelin receptor, but not apelin itself, is up-regulated in the placenta. The authors of this study concluded that this suggests that the apelinergic system may control foetal growth and cardiovascular functions in utero [133]. In humans again, labour down-regulates apelin expression in foetal membranes. Furthermore, a role of apelin in the regulation of pro-inflammatory and pro-labour mediators, like interleukin (IL)-1β-induced IL-6, IL-8 release and cyclooxygenase-2, is suggested in foetal membranes [166]. Moreover, apelin controls foetal and neonatal glucose homeostasis and is altered by foetal growth restriction induced by maternal under-nutrition [167]. Finally, apelin seems to be implicated in trophoblastic amino acid transport by stimulating amino acid uptake by the placenta [168].

7. Adipokines and Female Reproductive Pathologies

7.1. Polycystic Ovary Syndrome

Polycystic ovary syndrome (PCOS) is a very common endocrinopathy affecting 6% to 13% of women of reproductive age and one of the leading causes of female poor fertility [169]. According to recommendations in 2018 from the international evidence-based guidelines, its diagnosis requires the presence of at least two of the following criteria: oligo/anovulation, hyperandrogenism and polycystic ovary morphology on ultrasound (corresponding to a follicle number per ovary >20 and/or an ovarian volume >10 mL on either ovary) [170]. Despite its high prevalence and relevant impact on female health, the aetiology of PCOS, and notably the causal relationship between reproductive and metabolic features, has not yet been fully elucidated. Typically, PCOS is associated with visceral obesity [171] and an original adipose tissue dysfunction, possibly due to an in utero androgen hyperexposure, which is supposed to play a key role in determining both insulin-resistance (IR) and altered androgen metabolism characterising this syndrome [172]. Indeed, 50 to 90% of PCOS females have IR to a significantly greater extent than age- and body mass index (BMI)-matched control women [173] and present a significantly increased risk of developing type 2 diabetes [174]. Hyperinsulinaemia derived from insulin-resistant states would further stimulate the intrinsically increased androgen biosynthesis, characterising theca cells of PCOS ovaries [175]. In turn, androgen excess, observed in 60 to 80% of women suffering from PCOS [176] and further exacerbated by abdominal obesity, might play a crucial role in preferentially determining the expansion of visceral adipose tissue, contributing to IR and thus creating a vicious cycle ([172].

7.1.1. Chemerin

Chemerin has been discovered as a novel adipokine associated with obesity and metabolic syndrome in 2007 [64]. Its strong interaction with insulin metabolism is evident. Indeed, insulin profoundly enhances chemerin secretion from adipose tissue [177], while chemerin has been demonstrated to modulate insulin signalling and glucose disposal in in vitro and animal studies [178], inducing an insulin-resistant state in both adipocytes and skeletal muscle [142].

Independently from insulin and obesity, the existence of a correlation between Chemerin and PCOS has repeatedly been evoked [179]. Serum and ovarian levels of chemerin have been shown to be elevated in a dihydrotestosterone (DHT)-induced rat PCOS model [99] and, despite some discordant data [180], most of the authors report higher plasma chemerin concentrations in PCOS women [177,181–183] (Figure 11). These patients also seem to present increased chemerin expression in the subcutaneous and omental adipose tissue [177] (Figure 11); very recently, Wang et al. demonstrated that chemerin follicular fluid concentration and its mRNA levels in granulosa cells were higher in PCOS normal-weight patients than in controls [184] (Figure 11), a finding that we have confirmed subsequently in our laboratory (Bongrani et al., in press).

Interestingly, circulating chemerin levels were greater in PCOS hyperandrogenic women compared to the euandrogenic ones [180] and positively correlated with free androgen index [180] and total testosterone levels [184]. Furthermore, in DHT-treated rats, CMKLR1 gene deletion protected against the negative effects of chronic androgen treatment on progesterone secretion, cycling and ovulation [185]. As testosterone treatment has been demonstrated to up-regulate the expression of chemerin and its receptors in vitro [184], Lima et al. suggested that negative androgen effects on ovary could be partly mediated by this adipokine [186] (Figure 12). Indeed, hyperandrogenism would increase ovarian chemerin, which, in turn, functions as a chemoattractant ligand for blood monocytes expressing CMKLR1. Inflammatory monocyte-derived CMKLR1+ M1 macrophages, attracted to chemerin-rich ovarian follicles, would induce granulosa cell apoptosis contributing to the antral follicular growth arrest associated with the hyperandrogenic pro-inflammatory state characteristic of PCOS [186] (Figure 12). It is noteworthy that elevated chemerin levels in the DHT-induced rat PCOS model were positively related to increased granulosa cell apoptosis [19] and that women presenting higher chemerin concentrations in follicular fluid had significantly fewer oocytes and lower high-quality embryo rates [184], suggesting that chemerin could actually be involved in folliculogenesis disruption at the origin of PCOS [19] (Figure 12).

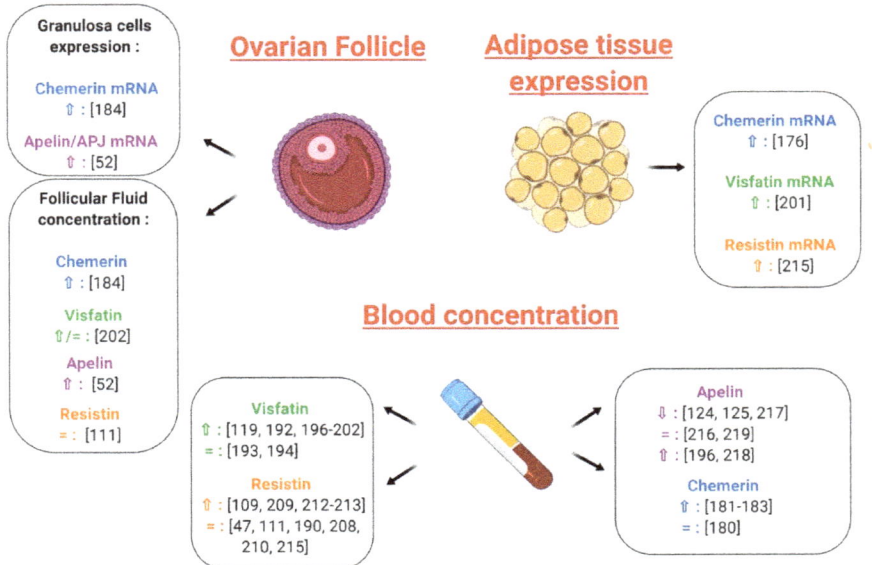

Figure 11. Effects of chemerin, visfatin, resistin and apelin on ovarian physiology, plasma and adipose tissue in polycystic ovarian syndrome (PCOS) as compared to control patients. ⇧ Increase/stimulation. ⇩ Decrease/inhibition.

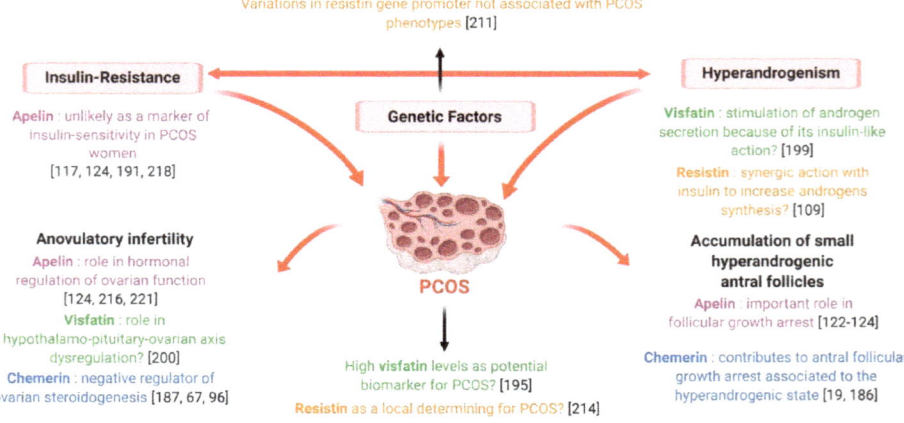

Figure 12. Description of PCOS syndrome and possible involvement of chemerin, visfatin, resistin and apelin in this syndrome.

As described in paragraph 5.1, the expression of chemerin and its receptors in human ovarian cells has been largely demonstrated [67] and the role of the chemerin/CMKLR1 pathway in follicle function and steroidogenesis has repeatedly been evoked [185]. Indeed, chemerin acts as an important negative regulator of ovarian steroidogenesis, inhibiting the IGF-1-induced secretion of progesterone and oestradiol in human granulosa cells [67] and suppressing the FSH-induced expression of aromatase and P450scc in cultured rat pre-antral follicles and granulosa cells [99,187]. Remarkably, chemerin concentration has been shown to be higher in follicular fluid than in plasma [67] and, in contrast to serum chemerin, the rise of follicular chemerin in women with PCOS has been demonstrated to be independent of changes in adiposity [186]. Thus, chemerin regulation at the ovarian level seems to be different from the systemic one, suggesting that this adipokine could play a paracrine and/or autocrine regulatory role in the ovary. Moreover, by negatively affecting steroidogenesis and participating in androgen induction of antral follicle growth arrest, chemerin seems to be strongly involved in the pathogenesis of anovulatory infertility characterising PCOS patients [186] (Figure 12).

7.1.2. Visfatin

Despite some conflicting results [188–190], a recent meta-analysis revealed that plasma visfatin levels are significantly increased in subjects presenting overweight/obesity, IR, metabolic syndrome and cardiovascular diseases [191], with visfatin expression seeming to be modulated by some insulin-sensitising agents. Indeed, 3 month-treatment with metformin in PCOS women resulted in a significant decrease in serum visfatin concentration [192]. Although two studies failed to highlight a significant difference between PCOS and healthy women [193,194] (Figure 11), most of the authors, and particularly the recent Sun et al. meta-analysis [195], found significantly higher plasma visfatin levels in PCOS patients [123,192,196–202] (Figure 11). Similarly, in PCOS women, visfatin expression in adipose tissue was increased independent of BMI [201] (Figure 11) and visfatin concentrations in follicular fluid were similar [123] or higher [202] in comparison with BMI-matched normally ovulatory women (Figure 11). Interestingly, the adipose tissue of PCOS women is characterised by an up-regulating alteration of lipolysis due to a selective increase in the function of protein-kinase A hormone-sensitive lipase complex [203] and 50% higher responsiveness to norepinephrine then healthy adipose tissue [203]. Since visfatin seems to be released during the lysis of fat cells rather than being secreted [204], the increased visfatin concentrations observed in PCOS women are possibly derived from this up-regulated lipolysis [123]. Visfatin is also known to display pro-inflammatory properties and immune functions [78,205] and, within adipose tissue, it has been demonstrated to be secreted not only by adipocytes, but also by inflammatory cells, such as macrophages [199]. As PCOS is characterised by low-grade inflammation, this could additionally explain its association with higher visfatin levels.

Interestingly, Panidis et al. found a positive correlation between circulating visfatin and plasma LH, evoking a possible role of this adipokine in the hypothalamo-pituitary-ovarian axis dysregulation observed in PCOS [200] (Figure 12). It is also noteworthy that serum visfatin levels have been found to be significantly higher in PCOS hyperandrogenic women than in the euandrogenic ones [193] and in PCOS hirsute adolescents when compared with non-hirsute patients [194]. Furthermore, despite some discordant results [123,195], a positive association between circulating visfatin and markers of hyperandrogenism has repeatedly been highlighted [193,194,198,200], even independent from insulin-sensitivity and other confounding factors [199]. As previously described, visfatin exerts an insulin-mimetic action and insulin can stimulate theca cell androgen synthesis, notably in IR-related hyperinsulinaemic conditions [193]. Thus, visfatin could be implicated in PCOS pathogenesis by influencing ovarian androgen secretion because of its insulin-like action [199] (Figure 12).

In conclusion, whether visfatin plays a role in the physiopathology of PCOS remains a matter of debate and further studies are needed to elucidate its significance. However, high visfatin levels seem to be an intrinsic characteristic of PCOS, suggesting that this adipokine could be a potential biomarker for this syndrome [195].

7.1.3. Resistin

Interestingly, in a randomised placebo-controlled study involving overweight women suffering from PCOS, circulating levels of resistin were significantly decreased by the insulin-sensitising agent rosiglitazone [206]. However, although a significant correlation between plasma resistin and IR or type 2 diabetes has been reported [207], most of the studies do not confirm the existence of such an association [47,115,208–210] (Figure 11). In particular, Panidis et al. showed that plasma resistin levels did not differ between PCOS and control normal-weight women, even though the former were more insulin-resistant. Furthermore, after stepwise multiple regression analysis, circulating resistin was not associated with any parameter independent of BMI, suggesting that it correlated with IR as a consequence of obesity itself rather than as an independent causative factor [47] (Figure 11).

As discussed above, resistin involvement in human female reproduction is known. However, at present, the existence of an association between resistin and PCOS is largely debated. Indeed, variations in the resistin gene promoter were not associated with PCOS phenotypes [211] (Figure 12) and data concerning plasma resistin levels in PCOS women are inconsistent. While some authors pointed out significantly higher resistin concentrations in the plasma of PCOS patients [112,209,212,213] (Figure 11), no difference between PCOS and healthy women has been reported by several others [47,115,190,208,210,214] (Figure 11). Similarly, resistin concentrations in follicular fluid did not differ between normal-weight PCOS and healthy women [115] (Figure 11). On the contrary, resistin mRNA levels in adipocytes have been found to be twice as high in PCOS patients compared to controls [214] (Figure 11) and significantly decreased after laparoscopic ovarian electrocautery [215], suggesting that, although systemic resistin does not seem to be actively involved in PCOS pathogenesis, it may act as a local determining factor for this syndrome [47,214] (Figure 12).

Remarkably, in humans, Seow et al. found greater mRNA resistin levels in the adipocytes of PCOS women presenting higher serum testosterone levels [214] (Figure 11) and the study of Munir et al. showed that circulating resistin in the PCOS group, but not in controls, was positively correlated with plasma testosterone [112]. Thus, it has been suggested that some important differences in polycystic ovaries may facilitate the responsiveness of theca cells to resistin, which may synergise with insulin to increase androgen synthesis [112].

In conclusion, in light of the data collected so far, resistin does not seem to be a major determining factor in PCOS pathogenesis. However, its role in ovarian theca cells and, notably, in androgen production deserves to be further investigated.

7.1.4. Apelin

Data about the existence of an association between circulating apelin and IR in PCOS are still inconsistent. Indeed, plasma apelin levels have been found to correlate negatively [216], but also positively [196] with HOMA-IR (Homeostatic Model Assessment for Insulin Resistance), and most studies have excluded the existence of any significant association between this adipokine and IR [128,191,217,218]. It is therefore unlikely that apelin could represent a marker of insulin-sensitivity in women with PCOS.

In our laboratory, we repeatedly found that apelin concentration in follicular fluid and levels of apelin and its receptor APJ mRNA in granulosa cells are higher in PCOS patients than in healthy controls [52] (Figure 11). More conflicting data are, however, available for circulating apelin in PCOS women, with an almost equal number of authors reporting significantly lower [128,129,217], higher [196,218] or unchanged [216,219] levels compared to control women (Figure 11).

Interestingly, in our laboratory we recently demonstrated that, independent of PCOS diagnosis, apelin and APJ expression in granulosa cells and follicular fluid is increased in women presenting a high number of ovarian small antral follicles resulting from the failure in selection of a dominant follicle (Bongrani et al., in press). Hence, according to these data, apelin could be significantly involved in PCOS pathogenesis, markedly contributing to the arrest of follicular development (Figure 12). It is currently admitted that folliculogenesis disruption observed in PCOS is derived from an increased responsiveness of small follicles to FSH in terms of oestradiol and progesterone synthesis, inducing a premature responsiveness to LH [220]. As a consequence, PCOS anovulatory women present higher LH and oestradiol levels, as well as lower FSH concentrations, than those in the normal early follicular phase [220]. Interestingly, in rats, apelin is expressed in the arcuate supraoptic and paraventricular hypothalamic nuclei and suppresses LH, FSH and prolactin secretion [221]. Furthermore, in women with PCOS a negative correlation between plasma apelin and LH levels has repeatedly been found [128,216

(Figure 12), strongly suggesting a role of this adipokine in the hormonal regulation of ovarian function, especially with regard to follicular development.

In conclusion, current knowledge strongly supports the involvement of apelin in follicular growth arrest and hypothalamus-pituitary-ovary axis perturbations at the origin of ovulatory dysfunction typically associated with PCOS, encouraging further studies about the role of this adipokine in reproductive function.

7.2. Gestational Diseases

During pregnancy, the placenta secretes cytokines, including TNF-alpha, IL-6 and IL-1β, and increases both their local and systemic levels, which is believed to be important in determining foetal allograft fate [222]. As described in paragraph 6.3, several adipokines, such as adiponectin, leptin, resistin, visfatin and apelin, are also secreted by the placenta [223] and have been implicated in metabolic adaptations to normal gestation, as well as in preeclampsia and other complications of pregnancy [224]. Moreover, some of these molecules are postulated to play a significant role in creating a favourable environment for implantation and placental development [222]. In contrast to adiponectin and leptin, studies about the regulation of chemerin, visfatin, resistin and apelin in gestational diabetes, preeclampsia and intrauterine growth restriction are limited. Furthermore, data are mostly descriptive, not allowing clarification of the physiological significance of the dysregulation of these novel adipokines in pregnancy complications.

7.2.1. Gestational Diabetes Mellitus

Gestational diabetes mellitus (GDM) is defined as a carbohydrate intolerance first detected in pregnancy, which affects approximately 14% of pregnancies worldwide (International Diabetes Federation. IDF Diabetes Atlas, 8th ed. Brussels, Belgium, 2017). It poses serious risks for the mother and developing foetus. Moreover, although it usually resolves following delivery, in the long-term, women with a past history of GDM and babies born of GDM pregnancies are at an increased risk of obesity, type 2 diabetes mellitus and cardiovascular diseases [225]. Pregnancy is a unique condition characterised by transient physiological IR, which progresses with advancing gestation, aimed at facilitating delivery of nutrients to the foetus. In fact, slightly elevated glycaemia makes glucose available to be transported across the placenta to fuel foetal growth. IR also promotes endogenous hepatic glucose production and lipolysis in adipose tissue, resulting in a further increase in blood glucose and free fatty acid concentrations [225]. Pregnant women compensate for these changes through hypertrophy and hyperplasia of pancreatic β-cells, as well as increased glucose-stimulated insulin secretion [226]. Failure of this compensatory response gives raise to maternal hyperglycaemia or GDM [227]. Thus, GDM is usually the result of β-cell dysfunction on a background of chronic IR during pregnancy. IR is mainly attributed to placental hormones and increased maternal adiposity, although the underlying mechanisms are not fully understood [223]. Recently, several new potential mediators of IR have been identified and, among these, adipokines seem to play a key role [223].

Chemerin

Chemerin has been suggested to constitute an insulin-sensitising factor which may counteract IR [228]. Contrary to normal pregnancy, which is associated with increased plasma chemerin levels that decrease post-partum, Hare et al. showed that circulating chemerin was reduced in GDM women and did not change with the normalisation of glucose tolerance following delivery [228] (Figure 13). However, a recent meta-analysis by Zhou et al., evaluating 11 studies carried out between 2010 and 2017 and including a total of 742 GDM patients and 840 normal pregnant women [229], reported that the overall levels of plasma chemerin in GDM women were significantly increased when compared with healthy pregnant ones and that this difference was more evident in the second- than in the third-trimester. The authors thus concluded that chemerin may play a powerful role in the pathophysiology of GDM by increasing IR and promoting subclinical inflammation [229] (Figure 13).

These results are, however, contradicted by a previous review, evaluating various adipokines in GDM, which demonstrated that adiponectin, leptin and TNF-alpha are more likely than chemerin, resistin and visfatin to play a role in the pathogenic mechanism of GDM [230] (Figure 13). Finally, no difference in chemerin levels, either in the early third trimester or at delivery, was reported between healthy and GDM women by Van Poppel et al. [231] (Figure 13). They instead demonstrated that, compared to infants from healthy mothers, newborns from GDM patients had higher chemerin levels in arterial but not venous cord blood, probably reflecting a higher pro-inflammatory status in the foetus of pregnancies complicated by GDM [231]. In summary, although chemerin seems to contribute to the increasing IR and subclinical inflammation that is characteristic of GDM, at present, data concerning its role in the physiopathology of this pregnancy complication are still controversial and do not allow a unique conclusion.

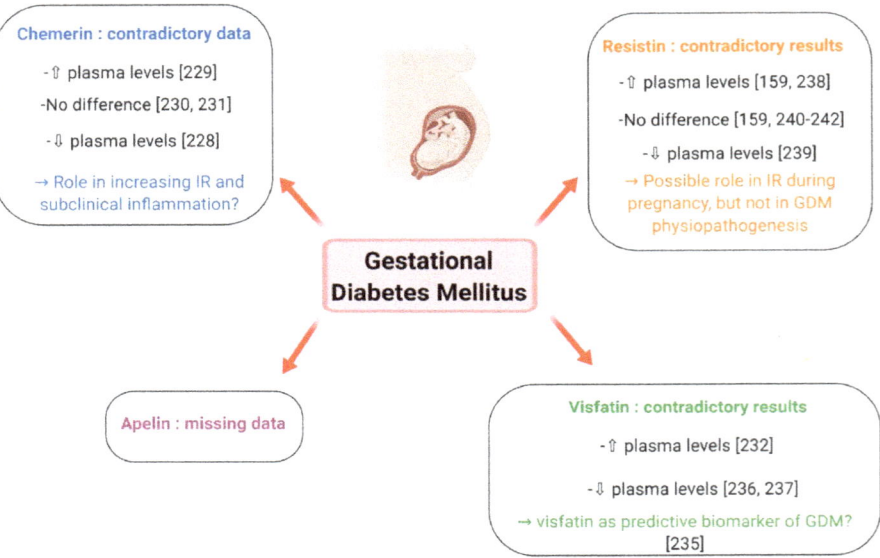

Figure 13. Putative involvement of plasma levels of chemerin, visfatin, resistin and apelin in gestational diabetes mellitus. ⇧ Increase/stimulation. ⇩ Decrease/inhibition.

Visfatin

Visfatin promotes adipogenesis and exerts insulino-mimetic effects [223]. In normal pregnancy, it may improve insulin sensitivity during the second and third trimesters and its up-regulation in the IR state during gestation may be part of a physiological feedback mechanism to improve insulin signalling [223]. However, there are huge discrepancies in reports about visfatin levels in pregnancies complicated by GDM. Higher serum visfatin levels in GDM women compared to normal glucose tolerance controls were observed in a nested case-control study, but no relationship with fasting plasma glucose, insulin, IR or BMI could be obtained [232] (Figure 13). On the contrary, two cross-sectional studies found that, in women with GDM, circulating visfatin was positively correlated with fasting and post-glucose load insulin in the third trimester [233], and that GDM was independently associated with increased maternal plasma visfatin concentrations [234]. Subsequently, Ferreira et al. reported increased levels of visfatin in the first trimester of women who later developed GDM, suggesting that this adipokine could be a biomarker of this pregnancy complication [235] (Figure 13). However, many other studies reported lower visfatin levels in GDM patients [236,237] (Figure 13). Differences in study design, including the number of patients, gestational age and BMI, may contribute to explain the different results between studies. In conclusion, further research is still needed to clarify the relationship between visfatin and obesity and any causal association with IR and GDM. In particular, prospective studies are required to evaluate whether visfatin can be predictive of GDM.

Resistin

The role of resistin in managing glucose homeostasis remains unclear, as most studies have failed to show a correlation between plasma resistin levels and insulin sensitivity in humans [223]. Resistin is expressed in the human placenta and, in normal pregnancy, it is up-regulated in the third trimester, possibly contributing to the decrease in insulin sensitivity [160]. In GDM, the studies available so far did not give unique results. Circulating resistin has been shown to be elevated in women with GDM compared to normal pregnancies [161,238] (Figure 13). Nevertheless, Kuzmicki et al. could not demonstrate an independent relationship between serum resistin concentration and insulin levels or IR [238]. Contrary to these results, another study found lower resistin levels in GDM patients in comparison with euglycaemic controls [239] (Figure 13) and most case-control studies reported no difference in circulating resistin levels in women with and without GDM [162,240] (Figure 13), a finding further confirmed in a large prospective study [241] (Figure 13) and in a recent meta-analysis [242] (Figure 13). Moreover, no difference was reported in resistin release from placental and subcutaneous adipose tissue obtained from normal pregnant subjects and GDM women [243]. Collectively, current data suggest that resistin may mediate IR during pregnancy, but it is unlikely to have a central role in glucose homeostasis and the development of GDM.

Apelin

Apelin is known to be an adipokine implicated in glucose homeostasis, and is found to be increased in obese and T2DM individuals [240]. Although its presence has been documented in human placental tissue [164], very few studies have addressed the expression of apelin in human pregnancy. An increase in apelin fat mRNA expression was observed only in early gestation, suggesting that apelin is not associated with hyperinsulinaemia of late pregnancy, but rather related to adipose tissue accumulation [223]. In GDM, cross-sectional studies of circulating apelin have contradictory results, including unchanged and increased levels [230] (Figure 13). Moreover, no association between plasma apelin concentration or apelin/APJ mRNA expression and GDM or the indices of IR was noted in a study involving 101 GDM patients and 101 women with normal glucose tolerance between 24 and 32 weeks of gestation and 20 GDM and 16 healthy controls at term [244]. In light of these data, it seems thus unlikely that apelin is directly involved in GDM physiopathogenesis.

7.2.2. Preeclampsia

Preeclampsia (PE) is a pregnancy complication affecting 4.6% of pregnant women worldwide [245] and a major contributor to foetal, neonatal and maternal morbidity and mortality [246]. It may develop from 20 weeks of gestation up to 6 weeks postpartum [246] and is characterised by the de novo development of arterial hypertension associated with one of the following features: proteinuria, maternal organ impairment (comprising renal insufficiency, hepatic cytolysis, neurological complication or haematological disorder like thrombocytopenia or haemolysis) and uteroplacental dysfunction, including foetal growth restriction [247]. Indeed, PE is associated with small-for gestational age (SGA) neonates in 10–25% of cases [248]. The pathophysiology of PE has not yet been fully elucidated, but abnormal placentation and imbalance between angiogenic and anti-angiogenic factors (including VEGF, PlGF (Placental growth factor), soluble fms-like tyrosine kinase 1 and endoglin) appear to be major contributors [222]. Initial incomplete trophoblast invasion and abnormal uterine spiral artery remodelling induce uteroplacental ischemia. This is followed by the release of placental factors, such as inflammatory cytokines and reactive oxygen species, into maternal circulation; these are able to trigger a broad intravascular inflammatory response, which is another essential step for the development of PE [247]. Like GDM, PE shares risk factors with metabolic syndrome including IR, subclinical inflammation and obesity [248] and women with a history of hypertensive pregnancy disorders present a 1.4 to 3-times higher risk of future cardiovascular diseases compared to women with normotensive pregnancies [249].

Chemerin

Despite its high expression in human placenta [74] and its well-known association with obesity, glucose metabolism and metabolic syndrome [64], data concerning the possible involvement of chemerin in physiological and pathological pregnancy is really poor. To the best of our knowledge, only one study in a small number of subjects has investigated chemerin in PE. Interestingly, maternal serum chemerin concentrations were significantly increased in preeclamptic women compared to healthy pregnant ones [250] (Figure 14). Furthermore, patients with severe PE had higher chemerin levels than those with mild PE, and circulating chemerin was independently correlated with markers of dyslipidaemia and PE severity, suggesting that chemerin regulation of glycolipid metabolism may contribute to the pathogenesis of this pathological condition [250] (Figure 14). Chemerin is also known as a pro-inflammatory adipokine, induced by TNF-alpha and enhancing macrophage adhesion [19], and as a potent angiogenic factor, inducing gelatinolytic activity of endothelial cells [64,154]. Hence, its role in PE might be more relevant and involve other aspects of its physiopathology, which deserve more in depth investigation.

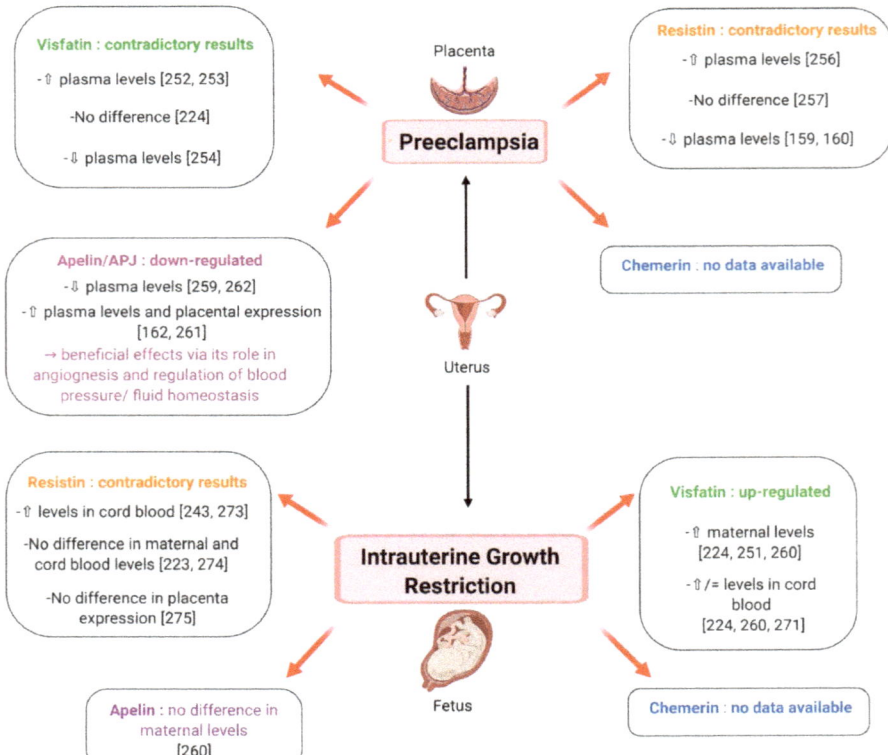

Figure 14. Putative involvement of plasma levels of chemerin, visfatin, resistin and apelin in preeclampsia and intrauterine growth restriction. ⇧ Increase/stimulation. ⇩ Decrease/inhibition.

Visfatin

The presence of visfatin transcript and protein has been detected in human foetal membranes and placenta [154] and pregnant women present higher circulating visfatin levels compared to non-pregnant subjects [234]. Notably, in normal pregnancies, median maternal plasma visfatin concentrations peak in the second trimester of gestation, between 19 and 26 weeks, and show a nadir between 27 and 34 weeks [234,251]. In women with PE, circulating visfatin levels have been reported to be increased [252,253] (Figure 14), similar [224] (Figure 14) or decreased [254] (Figure 14) compared to healthy pregnant women. Notably, Fasshauer et al. found that, after multivariate analysis, PE remained a significant predictor of circulating visfatin, independent of HOMA-IR and BMI [252]. Moreover, in the Mazaki-Tovi et al. study of patients with PE, there was no significant difference in maternal visfatin concentration between those with or without an SGA neonate, suggesting that the effect of FGR, which is known to increase visfatin levels (as described later), was overwhelmed by PE [224]. The authors proposed that in the presence of common risk factors for PE and SGA, high maternal visfatin concentrations could have beneficial metabolic effects, resulting in increased insulin-sensitivity and thus protecting mothers from PE [224]. Nevertheless, Hu et al. reported contrasting results, i.e., markedly decreased visfatin levels in preeclamptic women, irrespective of their BMI, and speculated an involvement of this adipokine in the exaggerated IR that characterises this pathological condition [254] (Figure 14). In light of these data and because visfatin is known to improve glucose tolerance, it has been suggested that the up-regulation of maternal visfatin concentration in IR-associated pregnancy complications may be part of a physiological feedback mechanism aimed at improving insulin signalling [223,251]. Furthermore, visfatin expression has recently been shown to be significantly related to TNF-alpha and IL-6 mRNA expression in placental tissues [223] and recombinant visfatin treatment of human foetal membranes causes a significant increase in inflammatory cytokines including IL-1β, TNF-alpha and IL-6 [154]. Thus, elevated visfatin levels observed in PE could additionally be associated with the pro-inflammatory state characteristic of this and other pregnancy complications.

Resistin

Resistin is expressed in human placenta, and mainly in trophoblastic cells [246]. Plasma resistin levels in pregnant women are significantly higher compared to those in non-pregnant controls and resistin gene expression, as well as its circulating concentrations, is more prominent as pregnancy advances [160]. As resistin gene expression is higher in the placenta than in adipose tissue, where it remains unchanged throughout pregnancy [160], it has been postulated that placental resistin may contribute to the physiological decrease in insulin-sensitivity occurring in the second half of human pregnancy [255]. Data about resistin levels in PE are discordant. Indeed, Haugen et al. reported higher resistin concentrations in women affected by PE compared to normal pregnant controls [256] Figure 14). However, such a difference was lost after controlling for IR and, as resistin placental gene expression was unchanged, it probably mostly depended on altered renal function in preeclamptic patients, which contributes to elevate resistin plasma concentrations [256]. In contrast to this report, Cortelazzi et al. and Chen et al. found that circulating resistin levels were lower in preeclamptic women than in the normotensive healthy pregnant ones, possibly due to reduced placental production because of the smaller size of the placenta [161,162] (Figure 14). Finally, Hendler et al. failed to find a difference in serum resistin concentrations between pregnant women with and without PE [257] (Figure 14). Hence, according to these data, resistin does not seem to be the main determinant of IR observed in PE [223]. However, as resistin is known to exert pro-inflammatory effects and stimulates IL-6 and TNF-alpha synthesis [258], it may be involved in the exaggerated maternal inflammatory response associated with PE pathogenesis.

Apelin

Because of its cardiovascular protective action and its role in the regulation of fluid homeostasis and insulin metabolism, the apelin/APJ system has been supposed to play a role in adaptation to pregnancy and regulation of foetal growth [259]. Additionally, embryonic expression studies in animals indicate that apelin is an important angiogenic factor required for normal blood vessel growth and endothelial cell proliferation [223]. Nevertheless, reports studying the expression and the function of this adipokine in human pregnancy are very few. Although apelin is known to be up-regulated in obesity and hyperinsulinaemia states in humans and mice [50], apelin fat mRNA expression seems to increase only in the early period in pregnant rats, suggesting that it may not be associated with physiological IR occurring in late pregnancy [223]. Furthermore, a recent study analysing maternal apelin concentrations in pregnant women failed to show any significant correlation between apelin and insulin levels [260]. In light of these data, apelin contribution to the regulation of maternal insulin sensitivity therefore seems limited. Nevertheless, several recent works have highlighted the important role of apelin in PE physiopathology. Indeed, although some authors showed higher maternal levels [261] (Figure 14) and increased placenta expression [164] (Figure 14) of apelin in preeclamptic pregnant women compared to healthy ones, most of the reports demonstrated a down-regulation of the apelin/APJ system in hypertensive pregnant disorders [259,262] (Figure 14). Notably, Yamaleyeva et al. found 30% lower content of apelin in the chorionic villi of preeclamptic patients compared to villi obtained from women with a normal gestation and proposed that lower apelin levels in the preeclamptic placenta might diminish its opposing modulation of vasoconstrictor mediators, which results in the increased blood pressure defining PE [259]. Indeed, the blood pressure-lowering action of apelin is well documented in several animal models and in patients with heart failure [263] and apelin is known to act on vascular smooth muscle cells, inducing either vasodilatation or vasoconstriction via different pathways [259]. Additionally, in the study of Yamaleyeva et al., apelin release from the chorionic villi was reduced by angiotensin II administration, suggesting a potential interaction between apelin and the renin-angiotensin system [259]. The beneficial effects of apelin in PE have also been suggested by a very recent report using a rat model in which PE symptoms were induced by reducing uterine perfusion pressure. In this model, apelin treatment significantly reversed the elevation in blood pressure and increased the total foetal weight, resulting in higher embryo survival rates [263]. Interestingly, these effects were obtained by improving the impaired eNOS/NO (endothelial nitric oxide synthase/nitric oxide) signalling pathway and preventing the activation of oxidative stress, which is one of the key features of PE pathogenesis [263].

Noteworthy, very recently, another component of the apelin-APJ system, named elabela has been postulated to be actively involved in PE development. Indeed, elabela is a new endogenous peptide ligand for the APJ receptor, which seems to play a crucial role in embryonic development [229]. Ho et al. demonstrated that deletion of the *elabela* gene in mice caused PE-like symptoms and that the administration of elabela to pregnant *elabela*-null mice prevented the increase in maternal blood pressure, proteinuria and FGR [264]. The authors thus proposed that the loss of *Elabela* might perturb early placental development, resulting in its inadequate perfusion. However, whether this effect is obtained via a paracrine role in angiogenesis or, indirectly, by inducing vasodilatation and regulating fluid balance, is currently unknown [264,265]. It needs to be underlined that these results have not been confirmed in humans, as no difference was found in placental transcript abundance or circulating levels of elabela in preeclamptic women compared to controls [266].

In conclusion, because of its involvement in angiogenesis and the regulation of blood pressure and fluid balance, the apelin/APJ system might play an important role in PE pathogenesis, encouraging further studies about its physiological relevance in pregnancy and its complications.

7.2.3. Intra-Uterine Growth Retardation

Foetal growth restriction (FGR) is defined by an estimated foetal weight less than the 10th percentile for the population at a given gestational age. It is a common complication of gestation, affecting up to 25% of pregnancies in low- to middle-income countries [267]. It derives from a placental failure to adequately supply oxygen and nutrients to the developing foetus, thus resulting in stunted foetal growth [268]. This phenomenon, named placental insufficiency, is idiopathic in up to 60% of cases and it is due to a physiological deficiency in uterine spiral arteries remodelling, resulting in restricted uteroplacental perfusion. In the foetus, hypoxia results in so-called brain-sparing, which is the preferential blood flow redistribution to vital organs like the brain, myocardium and adrenal glands, inducing a decrease in foetal weight and an altered foetal organ development that are associated with increased rates of neonatal mortality and morbidity [268]. Interestingly, in addition to placental insufficiency, FGR shares with PE several mechanisms of disease, including the anti-angiogenic state, the increased maternal intravascular inflammatory response [224] and the excessive maternal IR [269]. Furthermore, SGA neonates are more likely to develop metabolic complications, such as glucose metabolism disorders and adipose tissue dysfunction, later in life [270]. Several maternal adipokines are already known to link maternal nutrient status and adipose tissue metabolism to placental nutrient transport, thus contributing to foetal organ development and growth patterns in utero [222].

Chemerin

Although chemerin is actively involved in glucose and lipid metabolism [64] and its expression is elevated in the human placenta [74], its role in foetal growth has poorly been studied and, to the best of our knowledge, no report about chemerin involvement in FGR is currently available.

Visfatin

Given its insulin-mimetic action and as its expression in human placenta is limited to the villous capillary of the foetal endothelium, visfatin has been proposed to play a role in the transfer of glucose from the maternal to the foetal circulation [246]. The existence of a relationship between this adipokine and foetal growth has further been suggested by recent findings of elevated visfatin concentrations in cord blood [255]. Remarkably, all of the authors studying visfatin in the third trimester of pregnancies complicated by FGR reported higher maternal levels compared to control pregnant women with appropriate-for-gestational-age infants [224,251,260] (Figure 14). Visfatin has thus been proposed as a novel marker that is up-regulated in pregnant women with SGA neonates [251] (Figure 14). With regard to visfatin concentration in cord blood, however, data are more controversial. Indeed, while Ibanez et al. and Malamitsi-Puchner et al. found higher visfatin levels in SGA neonates compared to the appropriate-for-gestational-age ones [260,271] (Figure 14), Mazaki-Tovi et al. failed to highlight any difference between these two groups [224] (Figure 14). Similarly, the latter authors reported that visfatin concentration in foetal circulation was lower than in the maternal one and observed no significant correlation between the two [224] (Figure 14). This finding is in contrast with Malamitsi-Puchner et al., who showed that maternal and foetal visfatin concentrations were similar and significantly correlated each other [260] (Figure 14). Interestingly, Mazaki-Tovi et al. proposed that increased visfatin levels in SGA neonates might be linked to their different and/or altered visceral adiposity, which seems to contribute to the development of IR and impaired glucose metabolism in adulthood [224,272] (Figure 14).

Resistin

As resistin gene expression is higher in term placenta than in first trimester placental tissue and its levels in cord blood samples are elevated, resistin has been postulated to be involved in the control of foetal energy expenditure and deposition of adipose tissue [255]. Indeed, resistin is supposed to act as a feedback regulator of adipogenesis, exerting an inhibitory effect on adipose conversion [255]. Cord serum resistin levels have been found to be higher in growth-restricted pregnancies and lower in macrosomic foetuses when compared to normal ones [243,273] (Figure 14), further suggesting the existence of a negative correlation between maternal and cord blood resistin and birth weight. However, these results are not confirmed by other authors, who demonstrated no difference in resistin maternal [223] (Figure 14) and cord blood [274] (Figure 14) concentrations, as well as in placental resistin expression [275] (Figure 14) between FGR and normal pregnancies. Furthermore, in the study of Yeung et al., who analysed adipokines in newborn dried blood spots, resistin was inconsistently associated with birth size after accounting for the other measures [276]. In light of the currently available data, therefore, it is difficult to speculate on a specific role for resistin in foetal energy metabolism.

Apelin

Apelin and APJ have been identified at high levels in human placenta and, notably, in cytotrophoblasts, syncytiotrophoblasts and foetal endothelial cells, suggesting that apelin may have a paracrine action on human chorionic villi [164]. As apelin concentration is twice as high in umbilical cord blood than in maternal circulation [260] (Figure 14) and a positive correlation between maternal and foetal plasma apelin was observed in full-term normal pregnancies, a transplacental transfer of this adipokine with a potential impact on foetal growth has been suggested [259]. Notably, Mayeur et al. demonstrated that maternal intravenous apelin administration increased transplacental transport of glucose in a rodent model, either inducing the vasodilatation of placental vessels or, indirectly, modulating maternal blood pressure [167]. Interestingly, reducing the food intake of rat mothers significantly decreased their apelin levels, while a higher apelin expression was observed at the foeto-maternal interface, evoking a possible compensatory response of FGR foetuses to increase their glucose supply and improve their growth [167]. In light of these data, apelin seems to therefore have a beneficial role in foetal glucose homeostasis. However, despite such promising results in animals, to the best of our knowledge, only one study in humans has investigated this adipokine in pregnancies complicated by FGR and it did not find any difference in maternal apelin levels between FGR and normal pregnancies [260].

8. Adipokines and Male Reproductive Pathologies

In recent years, interest in the role of novel adipokines in male fertility has steadily grown. Indeed, a recent meta-analysis suggested that resistin and visfatin affect spermatogenesis [277] and a new study demonstrated that long treatment of human cultured Sertoli cells with chemerin, visfatin and resistin at high concentrations, which are often observed in obese men, significantly suppressed FSH receptor expression and up-regulated that of the cytochrome P450 CYP26A1, inducing a phenotype characteristic of the pre-pubertal state [278]. Thus, it has been postulated that these adipokines negatively affect Sertoli cell maturation, possibly contributing to testis dysfunction and fertility perturbations associated with obesity [278]. However, although the presence of chemerin and visfatin has been detected in the human testis, data concerning the pathogenic role of novel adipokines in male reproductive disorders are currently very poor.

With regard to chemerin, Thomas et al. reported that its concentration in seminal fluid was negatively correlated with spermatic motility and positively correlated with sperm concentration [139], while Bobjer et al. showed a negative correlation between plasma chemerin and LH, oestradiol and SHBG levels [279]. Furthermore, they found that, even after adjusting for BMI, serum chemerin concentration was lower in subfertile men compared to healthy controls, suggesting that, despite its positive association with BMI, this adipokine is independently linked to reproductive function [279]. Interestingly, vasectomised patients presented lower sperm chemerin levels than healthy men [139], evoking a local secretion of chemerin in the male genital tract, although chemerin levels in seminal fluid have repeatedly been found to be significantly lower than in blood plasma [135,139].

In light of the current knowledge, the expression of resistin in the testis has been detected only in rodents [20]. However, collectively, the studies carried out in men suggest a negative role of this adipokine in male fertility. Indeed, while some authors found no significant correlation between plasma resistin levels and sperm parameters [139], our laboratory recently showed that circulating resistin is negatively correlated with sperm vitality and normomorphic sperm percentage [135]. This finding agrees with the results obtained by Moretti et al., who highlighted a negative correlation between resistin levels in seminal fluid and sperm vitality and motility [280]. Very interestingly, they also demonstrated that seminal resistin was increased in patients presenting a leukocytospermia or a varicocele, two pathological conditions characterised by a local pro-inflammatory state, and positively correlated with levels of pro-inflammatory markers such as elastase, TNF-alpha and IL-6 [280]. Resistin could thus represent a marker of inflammation in the male genital tract and its increased levels in pathological situations like leukocytospermia might be related to alterations in sperm parameters [20].

Although visfatin has been demonstrated to be produced by human spermatozoa, notably the immature ones [137], and its levels are 100 times higher in seminal fluid than in blood plasma [139], no consistent data are available regarding its role in male reproductive disorders. In a very recent study carried out in obese and diabetic rats, plasma visfatin was negatively correlated with semen quality parameters, testosterone and LH levels and degenerative changes in the testis, suggesting that this adipokine may play a role in the physiopathology of male infertility associated with obesity and diabetes [281]. It must, however, be kept in mind that several authors failed to find any significant correlation between seminal and plasma visfatin and sperm parameters in humans [139].

As for visfatin, the literature for apelin is very poor and limited to animal studies. Notably, Sandal et al. demonstrated that the intracerebroventricular infusion of apelin-13 in male rats significantly suppressed LH release and decreased the number of Leydig cells, both resulting in a reduction in plasma testosterone levels [143]. However, at present, this possible role of apelin in the central regulation of male reproduction has not been confirmed, especially in humans.

9. Conclusions

Adipokines (chemerin, resistin, visfatin and apelin) and their cognate receptors (CMKLR1, GPR1, CCRL2 for chemerin and APJ for apelin) are expressed in peripheral tissues but also in the reproductive tract (from hypothalamus-pituitary, gonads) in both males and females of different species, including humans. Thus, these hormones could contribute to regulate the reproductive functions and consequently participate to explain some reproductive disorders. However, until now, most of the data come from in vitro experiments, and in vivo studies are limited. Sometimes, the in vitro data are contradictory, which can be explained by differences depending on the species but also by the use of different concentrations of tested adipokines and/or different experimental design. Transgenic mice where these adipokines or adipokine receptors are specifically deleted in the reproductive cells do not yet exist. Therefore, it is difficult to discriminate the effects of local adipokines production from systemic production. Moreover, most of these adipokines exist under various forms (ex-chemerin and apelin) and until now it has not been possible to detect all of these specific forms. Thus, the concentration in plasma as well as in the follicular fluid and seminal plasma of these various forms of adipokines as well as their effect in the reproductive tract remain to be investigated. For chemerin, some recombinant forms and specific enzyme-linked immunosorbent assays (ELISAs) have been developed in humans and mice but future studies are needed to further define the potential mechanistic role of these isoforms in reproduction. Interestingly, plasma and/or tissue expression of chemerin, resistin, visfatin and apelin might be associated with various female reproductive disorders including PCOS syndrome, gestational diabetes, preeclampsia, and uterine growth restriction. The involvement of these adipokines has been less studied in male reproductive pathologies. Finally, all of the data suggest that additional studies are necessary to better understand the role and molecular mechanism of adipokines in the control of fertility in order to potentially use them as prognostic markers and/or therapeutic targets in different reproductive disorders.

Author Contributions: The authors' responsibilities were as follows: A.E., A.B., M.R. and J.D. prepared the original draft, and wrote it. A.E., A.B., M.R., C.R., P.-H.D., P.F. and J.D. reviewed and edited the manuscript. J.D. got the funding and realized the project administration. J.D. had primary responsibility for the final content.

Funding: Agence de Biomedecine: 32000695. Region Centre Val de Loire Projet PREVADI: 32000820.

Acknowledgments: The authors thank to BIORENDER for the figures. This work was financially supported by Région Centre Val de Loire (PREVADI project number 32000820 and HAPOERTI project number 32000496) and Agence de Biomedecine (obesité et qualité des spermatozoïdes humains: importance des adipocytokines, project number: 32000822).

Conflicts of Interest: The authors declare no conflict of interest. The funders had no role in the design of the study; in the collection, analyses, or interpretation of data; in the writing of the manuscript, or in the decision to publish the results.

Abbreviations

ACE2	Angiotensin converting enzyme 2
ADSF	Adipocyte-specific secretory factor
Akt	Retroviral *oncogene also named Protein Kinase B*
AMPK	AMP-activated Protein Kinase
APJ	Tissue Inhibitors of MetalloProteinases
APLNR	Apelin receptor
BAT	Brown Adipose Tissue
BeWo	Placental cell line
BMI	Body Mass Index
CCRL2	C-C Motif Chemokine Receptor Like 2
ChemR23	Chemerin Receptor 23
CHO cells	Chinese hamster ovary cells
CL	Corpus Luteum
CMKLR1	Chemokine-Like Receptor 1
COV 434	Cellosaurus cell line 43 (immortalized ovarian cells)
CSF	CerebroSpinal Fluid
DCN	Decorin
DHT	Dihydrotestosterone
E2	Estradiol
ERK1/2	Extracellular signal-Regulated Kinases 1 & 2
EVTs	Extravillous *trophoblasts*
FSH	Follicle Stimulating Hormone
Gata4	GATA binding protein 4.
GnRH	Gonadotropin-Releasing Hormone
GPCR	G protein-coupled receptors
GPR1	G protein-coupled receptor 1
hCG	human Chorionic Gonadotropin
HCR	C-terminal receptor binding domain
HIV	Human Immunodeficiency Virus
HSD3B	3β-Hydroxysteroid dehydrogenase
HUVECs	Human umbilical vein endothelial cells
IGF-1	Insulin like Growth Factor 1
IGF-1-R	Insulin-like growth factor 1 receptor
IL17/22	Interleukin 17/22
Insl3	Insulin-like 3
IR	Insulin Resistance
KGN	Steroidogenic human granulosa-like tumor *cell* line
LH	Luteinizing Hormone
MAPK	Mitogen-Activated Protein Kinases
mTOR	mammalian Target Of Rapamycin Complex 1 or mechanistic target of rapamycin
NAD	Nicotinamide Adenine Dinucleotide
NadV	Nicotinamide phosphoribosyltransferase NadV
NAMPT	Nicotinamide phosphoribosyltransferase
NFkB	Transcription factor Nuclear Factor-kappa B
NK cells	Natural Killer cells
NMN	Nicotinamide MonoNucleotide
ORF	Open reading frame
P4	Progesterone
P450 CYP26A1	Cytochrome P450 CYP26A1
PBEF	Pre-B-cell colony-enhancing factor
PBMCS	Peripheral Blood Mononuclear Cells
PE	PreEclempsia

PGF2alpha	Prostaglandin F2alpha
PlGF	Placental growth factor
PKA	Protein Kinase A
PKC	Protein Kinase C
PPAR	Peroxisome Proliferator-Activated Receptor
PPAR gamma	Peroxisome proliferator-activated receptor gamma
PTEN	Phosphatase and TENsin homolog
PTX sensitive	Pertussis Toxin sensitive
RARRES2	Retinoic Acid Receptor Responder protein 2
Retn	Resistin
RhoA	Ras homolog gene family, member A
ROR1	Receptor tyrosine kinase-like orphan receptor 1
SF1	Steroidogenic Factor 1
SHBG	Sex Hormone-Binding Globulin
SIRT1	Member of the sirtuin family
SIV	Simian Immunodeficiency Virus
StAR	Steroid Acute Regulatory protein
STAT3	Signal transducer and activator of transcription 3
T2DM	Type 2 Diabetes Mellitus
TLR4	Toll Like Receptor 4
TNF alpha	Tumor Necrosis Factor alpha
VEGF	Vascular endothelial growth factor
VEGFR2	Vascular endothelial growth factor receptor 2
WAT	White Adipose Tissue
WT	Wild Type

References

1. Wade, G.N.; Schneider, J.E. Metabolic fuels and reproduction in female mammals. *Neurosci. Biobehav. Rev.* **1992**, *16*, 235–272. [CrossRef]
2. Schneider, J.E. Energy balance and reproduction. *Physiol. Behav.* **2004**, *81*, 289–317. [CrossRef] [PubMed]
3. Scheja, L.; Heeren, J. The endocrine function of adipose tissues in health and cardiometabolic disease. *Nat. Rev. Endocrinol.* **2019**, *15*, 507–524. [CrossRef] [PubMed]
4. Ntaios, G.; Gatselis, N.K.; Makaritsis, K.; Dalekos, G.N. Adipokines as mediators of endothelial function and atherosclerosis. *Atherosclerosis* **2013**, *227*, 216–221. [CrossRef] [PubMed]
5. Trujillo, M.E.; Scherer, P.E. Adipose tissue-derived factors: Impact on health and disease. *Endocr. Rev.* **2006**, *27*, 762–778. [CrossRef] [PubMed]
6. Pandit, R.; Beerens, S.; Adan, R.A.H. Role of leptin in energy expenditure: The hypothalamic perspective. *Am. J. Physiol. Regul. Integr. Comp. Physiol.* **2017**, *312*, R938–R947. [CrossRef]
7. Luo, L.; Liu, M. Adipose tissue in control of metabolism. *J. Endocrinol.* **2016**, *231*, R77–R99. [CrossRef] [PubMed]
8. Lee, B.; Shao, J. Adiponectin and energy homeostasis. *Rev. Endocr. Metab. Disord.* **2014**, *15*, 149–156. [CrossRef]
9. Messinis, I.E.; Milingos, S.D. Leptin in human reproduction. *Hum. Reprod. Update* **1999**, *5*, 52–63. [CrossRef]
10. Chehab, F.F. Leptin as a regulator of adipose mass and reproduction. *Trends Pharmacol. Sci.* **2000**, *21*, 309–314. [CrossRef]
11. Tena-Sempere, M.; Barreiro, M.L. Leptin in male reproduction: The testis paradigm. *Mol. Cell. Endocrinol.* **2002**, *188*, 9–13. [CrossRef]
12. Barbe, A.; Bongrani, A.; Mellouk, N.; Estienne, A.; Kurowska, P.; Grandhaye, J.; Elfassy, Y.; Levy, R.; Rak, A.; Froment, P.; et al. Mechanisms of Adiponectin Action in Fertility: An Overview from Gametogenesis to Gestation in Humans and Animal Models in Normal and Pathological Conditions. *Int. J. Mol. Sci.* **2019**, *20*, 1526. [CrossRef] [PubMed]
13. Kawwass, J.F.; Summer, R.; Kallen, C.B. Direct effects of leptin and adiponectin on peripheral reproductive tissues: A critical review. *Mol. Hum. Reprod.* **2015**, *21*, 617–632. [CrossRef] [PubMed]
14. Fang, H.; Judd, R.L. Adiponectin Regulation and Function. *Compr. Physiol.* **2018**, *8*, 1031–1063. [CrossRef] [PubMed]

15. Bertrand, C.; Valet, P.; Castan-Laurell, I. Apelin and energy metabolism. *Front. Physiol.* **2015**, *6*, 115. [CrossRef] [PubMed]
16. Rourke, J.L.; Muruganandan, S.; Dranse, H.J.; McMullen, N.M.; Sinal, C.J. Gpr1 is an active chemerin receptor influencing glucose homeostasis in obese mice. *J. Endocrinol.* **2014**, *222*, 201–215. [CrossRef] [PubMed]
17. Zhang, L.Q.; Van Haandel, L.; Xiong, M.; Huang, P.; Heruth, D.P.; Bi, C.; Gaedigk, R.; Jiang, X.; Li, D.-Y.; Wyckoff, G.; et al. Metabolic and molecular insights into an essential role of nicotinamide phosphoribosyltransferase. *Cell Death Dis.* **2017**, *8*, e2705. [CrossRef] [PubMed]
18. Meier, U.; Gressner, A.M. Endocrine regulation of energy metabolism: Review of pathobiochemical and clinical chemical aspects of leptin, ghrelin, adiponectin, and resistin. *Clin. Chem.* **2004**, *50*, 1511–1525. [CrossRef]
19. Tsatsanis, C.; Dermitzaki, E.; Avgoustinaki, P.; Malliaraki, N.; Mytaras, V.; Margioris, A.N. The impact of adipose tissue-derived factors on the hypothalamic-pituitary-gonadal (HPG) axis. *Hormones (Athens)* **2015**, *14*, 549–562. [CrossRef]
20. Elfassy, Y.; Bastard, J.P.; McAvoy, C.; Fellahi, S.; Dupont, J.; Levy, R. Adipokines in Semen: Physiopathology and Effects on Spermatozoas. *Int. J. Endocrinol.* **2018**, *2018*, 3906490. [CrossRef]
21. Reverchon, M.; Rame, C.; Bertoldo, M.; Dupont, J. Adipokines and the female reproductive tract. *Int. J. Endocrinol.* **2014**, *2014*, 232454. [CrossRef] [PubMed]
22. Campos, D.B.; Palin, M.F.; Bordignon, V.; Murphy, B.D. The 'beneficial' adipokines in reproduction and fertility. *Int. J. Obes. (Lond.)* **2008**, *32*, 223–231. [CrossRef] [PubMed]
23. Meder, W.; Wendland, M.; Busmann, A.; Kutzleb, C.; Spodsberg, N.; John, H.; Richter, R.; Schleuder, D.; Meyer, M.; Forssmann, W.G. Characterization of human circulating TIG2 as a ligand for the orphan receptor ChemR23. *FEBS Lett.* **2003**, *555*, 495–499. [CrossRef]
24. Wittamer, V.; Franssen, J.D.; Vulcano, M.; Mirjolet, J.F.; Le Poul, E.; Migeotte, I.; Brezillon, S.; Tyldesley, R.; Blanpain, C.; Detheux, M.; et al. Specific recruitment of antigen-presenting cells by chemerin, a novel processed ligand from human inflammatory fluids. *J. Exp. Med.* **2003**, *198*, 977–985. [CrossRef] [PubMed]
25. Zabel, B.A.; Allen, S.J.; Kulig, P.; Allen, J.A.; Cichy, J.; Handel, T.M.; Butcher, E.C. Chemerin activation by serine proteases of the coagulation, fibrinolytic, and inflammatory cascades. *J. Biol. Chem.* **2005**, *280*, 34661–34666. [CrossRef] [PubMed]
26. Mattern, A.; Zellmann, T.; Beck-Sickinger, A.G. Processing, signaling, and physiological function of chemerin. *IUBMB Life* **2014**, *66*, 19–26. [CrossRef]
27. Kennedy, A.J.; Davenport, A.P. International Union of Basic and Clinical Pharmacology CIII: Chemerin Receptors CMKLR1 (Chemerin1) and GPR1 (Chemerin2) Nomenclature, Pharmacology, and Function. *Pharmacol. Rev.* **2018**, *70*, 174–196. [CrossRef] [PubMed]
28. Rourke, J.L.; Dranse, H.J.; Sinal, C.J. Towards an integrative approach to understanding the role of chemerin in human health and disease. *Obes. Rev.* **2013**, *14*, 245–262. [CrossRef]
29. Samal, B.; Sun, Y.; Stearns, G.; Xie, C.; Suggs, S.; McNiece, I. Cloning and characterization of the cDNA encoding a novel human pre-B-cell colony-enhancing factor. *Mol. Cell. Biol.* **1994**, *14*, 1431–1437. [CrossRef]
30. Martin, P.R.; Shea, R.J.; Mulks, M.H. Identification of a plasmid-encoded gene from Haemophilus ducreyi which confers NAD independence. *J. Bacteriol.* **2001**, *183*, 1168–1174. [CrossRef]
31. Rongvaux, A.; Shea, R.J.; Mulks, M.H.; Gigot, D.; Urbain, J.; Leo, O.; Andris, F. Pre-B-cell colony-enhancing factor, whose expression is up-regulated in activated lymphocytes, is a nicotinamide phosphoribosyltransferase, a cytosolic enzyme involved in NAD biosynthesis. *Eur. J. Immunol.* **2002**, *32*, 3225–3234. [CrossRef]
32. Wang, T.; Zhang, X.; Bheda, P.; Revollo, J.R.; Imai, S.; Wolberger, C. Structure of Nampt/PBEF/visfatin, a mammalian NAD+ biosynthetic enzyme. *Nat. Struct. Mol. Biol.* **2006**, *13*, 661–662. [CrossRef] [PubMed]
33. Revollo, J.R.; Grimm, A.A.; Imai, S. The NAD biosynthesis pathway mediated by nicotinamide phosphoribosyltransferase regulates Sir2 activity in mammalian cells. *J. Biol. Chem.* **2004**, *279*, 50754–50763. [CrossRef] [PubMed]
34. Berndt, J.; Klöting, N.; Kralisch, S.; Kovacs, P.; Fasshauer, M.; Schön, M.R.; Stumvoll, M.; Blüher, M. Plasma visfatin concentrations and fat depot-specific mRNA expression in humans. *Diabetes* **2005**, *54*, 2911–2916. [CrossRef]
35. Revollo, J.R.; Grimm, A.A.; Imai, S. The regulation of nicotinamide adenine dinucleotide biosynthesis by Nampt/PBEF/visfatin in mammals. *Curr. Opin. Gastroenterol.* **2007**, *23*, 164–170. [CrossRef] [PubMed]

36. Yoon, M.J.; Yoshida, M.; Johnson, S.; Takikawa, A.; Usui, I.; Tobe, K.; Nakagawa, T.; Yoshino, J.; Imai, S. SIRT1-Mediated eNAMPT Secretion from Adipose Tissue Regulates Hypothalamic NAD+ and Function in Mice. *Cell Metab.* **2015**, *21*, 706–717. [CrossRef] [PubMed]
37. Audrito, V.; Manago, A.; Zamporlini, F.; Rulli, E.; Gaudino, F.; Madonna, G.; D'Atri, S.; Antonini Cappellini, G.C.; Ascierto, P.A.; Massi, D.; et al. Extracellular nicotinamide phosphoribosyltransferase (eNAMPT) is a novel marker for patients with BRAF-mutated metastatic melanoma. *Oncotarget* **2018**, *9*, 18997–19005. [CrossRef] [PubMed]
38. Sun, Y.; Zhu, S.; Wu, Z.; Huang, Y.; Liu, C.; Tang, S.; Wei, L. Elevated serum visfatin levels are associated with poor prognosis of hepatocellular carcinoma. *Oncotarget* **2017**, *8*, 23427–23435. [CrossRef]
39. Grolla, A.A.; Torretta, S.; Gnemmi, I.; Amoruso, A.; Orsomando, G.; Gatti, M.; Caldarelli, A.; Lim, D.; Penengo, L.; Brunelleschi, S.; et al. Nicotinamide phosphoribosyltransferase (NAMPT/PBEF/visfatin) is a tumoural cytokine released from melanoma. *Pigment Cell Melanoma Res.* **2015**, *28*, 718–729. [CrossRef]
40. Kim, K.H.; Lee, K.; Moon, Y.S.; Sul, H.S. A cysteine-rich adipose tissue-specific secretory factor inhibits adipocyte differentiation. *J. Biol. Chem.* **2001**, *276*, 11252–11256. [CrossRef] [PubMed]
41. Holcomb, I.N.; Kabakoff, R.C.; Chan, B.; Baker, T.W.; Gurney, A.; Henzel, W.; Nelson, C.; Lowman, H.B.; Wright, B.D.; Skelton, N.J.; et al. FIZZ1, a novel cysteine-rich secreted protein associated with pulmonary inflammation, defines a new gene family. *EMBO J.* **2000**, *19*, 4046–4055. [CrossRef] [PubMed]
42. Steppan, C.M.; Brown, E.J.; Wright, C.M.; Bhat, S.; Banerjee, R.R.; Dai, C.Y.; Enders, G.H.; Silberg, D.G.; Wen, X.; Wu, G.D.; et al. A family of tissue-specific resistin-like molecules. *Proc. Natl. Acad. Sci. USA* **2001**, *98*, 502–506. [CrossRef] [PubMed]
43. Wang, H.; Chu, W.S.; Hemphill, C.; Elbein, S.C. Human resistin gene: Molecular scanning and evaluation of association with insulin sensitivity and type 2 diabetes in Caucasians. *J. Clin. Endocrinol. Metab.* **2002**, *87*, 2520–2524. [CrossRef] [PubMed]
44. Banerjee, R.R.; Lazar, M.A. Dimerization of resistin and resistin-like molecules is determined by a single cysteine. *J. Biol. Chem.* **2001**, *276*, 25970–25973. [CrossRef] [PubMed]
45. Patel, S.D.; Rajala, M.W.; Rossetti, L.; Scherer, P.E.; Shapiro, L. Disulfide-dependent multimeric assembly of resistin family hormones. *Science* **2004**, *304*, 1154–1158. [CrossRef] [PubMed]
46. Codoner-Franch, P.; Alonso-Iglesias, E. Resistin: Insulin resistance to malignancy. *Clin. Chim. Acta* **2015**, *438*, 46–54. [CrossRef] [PubMed]
47. Panidis, D.; Koliakos, G.; Kourtis, A.; Farmakiotis, D.; Mouslech, T.; Rousso, D. Serum resistin levels in women with polycystic ovary syndrome. *Fertil. Steril.* **2004**, *81*, 361–366. [CrossRef]
48. Tatemoto, K.; Hosoya, M.; Habata, Y.; Fujii, R.; Kakegawa, T.; Zou, M.X.; Kawamata, Y.; Fukusumi, S.; Hinuma, S.; Kitada, C.; et al. Isolation and characterization of a novel endogenous peptide ligand for the human APJ receptor. *Biochem. Biophys. Res. Commun.* **1998**, *251*, 471–476. [CrossRef]
49. Medhurst, A.D.; Jennings, C.A.; Robbins, M.J.; Davis, R.P.; Ellis, C.; Winborn, K.Y.; Lawrie, K.W.; Hervieu, G.; Riley, G.; Bolaky, J.E.; et al. Pharmacological and immunohistochemical characterization of the APJ receptor and its endogenous ligand apelin. *J. Neurochem.* **2003**, *84*, 1162–1172. [CrossRef]
50. Boucher, J.; Masri, B.; Daviaud, D.; Gesta, S.; Guigne, C.; Mazzucotelli, A.; Castan-Laurell, I.; Tack, I.; Knibiehler, B.; Carpene, C.; et al. Apelin, a newly identified adipokine up-regulated by insulin and obesity. *Endocrinology* **2005**, *146*, 1764–1771. [CrossRef]
51. Huang, Z.; Luo, X.; Liu, M.; Chen, L. Function and regulation of apelin/APJ system in digestive physiology and pathology. *J. Cell. Physiol.* **2019**, *234*, 7796–7810. [CrossRef] [PubMed]
52. Roche, J.; Rame, C.; Reverchon, M.; Mellouk, N.; Cornuau, M.; Guerif, F.; Froment, P.; Dupont, J. Apelin (APLN) and Apelin Receptor (APLNR) in Human Ovary: Expression, Signaling, and Regulation of Steroidogenesis in Primary Human Luteinized Granulosa Cells. *Biol. Reprod.* **2016**, *95*, 104. [CrossRef] [PubMed]
53. Pitkin, S.L.; Maguire, J.J.; Bonner, T.I.; Davenport, A.P. International Union of Basic and Clinical Pharmacology. LXXIV. Apelin receptor nomenclature, distribution, pharmacology, and function. *Pharmacol. Rev.* **2010**, *62*, 331–342. [CrossRef] [PubMed]
54. Maguire, J.J.; Kleinz, M.J.; Pitkin, S.L.; Davenport, A.P. [Pyr1]apelin-13 identified as the predominant apelin isoform in the human heart: Vasoactive mechanisms and inotropic action in disease. *Hypertension* **2009**, *54*, 598–604. [CrossRef] [PubMed]

55. El Messari, S.; Iturrioz, X.; Fassot, C.; De Mota, N.; Roesch, D.; Llorens-Cortes, C. Functional dissociation of apelin receptor signaling and endocytosis: Implications for the effects of apelin on arterial blood pressure. *J. Neurochem.* **2004**, *90*, 1290–1301. [CrossRef]
56. Gantz, I.; Konda, Y.; Yang, Y.K.; Miller, D.E.; Dierick, H.A.; Yamada, T. Molecular cloning of a novel receptor (CMKLR1) with homology to the chemotactic factor receptors. *Cytogenet. Cell Genet.* **1996**, *74*, 286–290. [CrossRef] [PubMed]
57. Samson, M.; Edinger, A.L.; Stordeur, P.; Rucker, J.; Verhasselt, V.; Sharron, M.; Govaerts, C.; Mollereau, C.; Vassart, G.; Doms, R.W.; et al. ChemR23, a putative chemoattractant receptor, is expressed in monocyte-derived dendritic cells and macrophages and is a coreceptor for SIV and some primary HIV-1 strains. *Eur. J. Immunol.* **1998**, *28*, 1689–1700. [CrossRef]
58. Shimada, T.; Matsumoto, M.; Tatsumi, Y.; Kanamaru, A.; Akira, S. A novel lipopolysaccharide inducible C-C chemokine receptor related gene in murine macrophages. *FEBS Lett.* **1998**, *425*, 490–494. [CrossRef]
59. Fan, P.; Kyaw, H.; Su, K.; Zeng, Z.; Augustus, M.; Carter, K.C.; Li, Y. Cloning and characterization of a novel human chemokine receptor. *Biochem. Biophys. Res. Commun.* **1998**, *243*, 264–268. [CrossRef]
60. Marchese, A.; Cheng, R.; Lee, M.C.; Porter, C.A.; Heiber, M.; Goodman, M.; George, S.R.; O'Dowd, B.F. Mapping studies of two G protein-coupled receptor genes: An amino acid difference may confer a functional variation between a human and rodent receptor. *Biochem. Biophys. Res. Commun.* **1994**, *205*, 1952–1958. [CrossRef]
61. Barnea, G.; Strapps, W.; Herrada, G.; Berman, Y.; Ong, J.; Kloss, B.; Axel, R.; Lee, K.J. The genetic design of signaling cascades to record receptor activation. *Proc. Natl. Acad. Sci. USA* **2008**, *105*, 64–69. [CrossRef] [PubMed]
62. Zabel, B.A.; Nakae, S.; Zuniga, L.; Kim, J.Y.; Ohyama, T.; Alt, C.; Pan, J.; Suto, H.; Soler, D.; Allen, S.J.; et al. Mast cell-expressed orphan receptor CCRL2 binds chemerin and is required for optimal induction of IgE-mediated passive cutaneous anaphylaxis. *J. Exp. Med.* **2008**, *205*, 2207–2220. [CrossRef] [PubMed]
63. Arita, M.; Bianchini, F.; Aliberti, J.; Sher, A.; Chiang, N.; Hong, S.; Yang, R.; Petasis, N.A.; Serhan, C.N. Stereochemical assignment, antiinflammatory properties, and receptor for the omega-3 lipid mediator resolvin E1. *J. Exp. Med.* **2005**, *201*, 713–722. [CrossRef] [PubMed]
64. Bozaoglu, K.; Bolton, K.; McMillan, J.; Zimmet, P.; Jowett, J.; Collier, G.; Walder, K.; Segal, D. Chemerin is a novel adipokine associated with obesity and metabolic syndrome. *Endocrinology* **2007**, *148*, 4687–4694. [CrossRef] [PubMed]
65. Kaur, J.; Adya, R.; Tan, B.K.; Chen, J.; Randeva, H.S. Identification of chemerin receptor (ChemR23) in human endothelial cells: Chemerin-induced endothelial angiogenesis. *Biochem. Biophys. Res. Commun.* **2010**, *391*, 1762–1768. [CrossRef] [PubMed]
66. Herrera, B.S.; Ohira, T.; Gao, L.; Omori, K.; Yang, R.; Zhu, M.; Muscara, M.N.; Serhan, C.N.; Van Dyke, T.E.; Gyurko, R. An endogenous regulator of inflammation, resolvin E1, modulates osteoclast differentiation and bone resorption. *Br. J. Pharmacol.* **2008**, *155*, 1214–1223. [CrossRef] [PubMed]
67. Reverchon, M.; Cornuau, M.; Rame, C.; Guerif, F.; Royere, D.; Dupont, J. Chemerin inhibits IGF-1-induced progesterone and estradiol secretion in human granulosa cells. *Hum. Reprod.* **2012**, *27*, 1790–1800. [CrossRef]
68. Migeotte, I.; Franssen, J.D.; Goriely, S.; Willems, F.; Parmentier, M. Distribution and regulation of expression of the putative human chemokine receptor HCR in leukocyte populations. *Eur. J. Immunol.* **2002**, *32*, 494–501. [CrossRef]
69. Oostendorp, J.; Hylkema, M.N.; Luinge, M.; Geerlings, M.; Meurs, H.; Timens, W.; Zaagsma, J.; Postma, D.S.; Boddeke, H.W.; Biber, K. Localization and enhanced mRNA expression of the orphan chemokine receptor L-CCR in the lung in a murine model of ovalbumin-induced airway inflammation. *J. Histochem. Cytochem.* **2004**, *52*, 401–410. [CrossRef]
70. Shimizu, N.; Soda, Y.; Kanbe, K.; Liu, H.Y.; Jinno, A.; Kitamura, T.; Hoshino, H. An orphan G protein-coupled receptor, GPR1, acts as a coreceptor to allow replication of human immunodeficiency virus types 1 and 2 in brain-derived cells. *J. Virol.* **1999**, *73*, 5231–5239.
71. Peng, L.; Yu, Y.; Liu, J.; Li, S.; He, H.; Cheng, N.; Ye, R.D. The chemerin receptor CMKLR1 is a functional receptor for amyloid-beta peptide. *J. Alzheimer's Dis.* **2015**, *43*, 227–242. [CrossRef] [PubMed]
72. Yang, Y.L.; Ren, L.R.; Sun, L.F.; Huang, C.; Xiao, T.X.; Wang, B.B.; Chen, J.; Zabel, B.A.; Ren, P.; Zhang, J.V. The role of GPR1 signaling in mice corpus luteum. *J. Endocrinol.* **2016**, *230*, 55–65. [CrossRef] [PubMed]
73. Rourke, J.L.; Dranse, H.J.; Sinal, C.J. CMKLR1 and GPR1 mediate chemerin signaling through the RhoA/ROCK pathway. *Mol. Cell. Endocrinol.* **2015**, *417*, 36–51. [CrossRef] [PubMed]

74. Goralski, K.B.; McCarthy, T.C.; Hanniman, E.A.; Zabel, B.A.; Butcher, E.C.; Parlee, S.D.; Muruganandan, S.; Sinal, C.J. Chemerin, a novel adipokine that regulates adipogenesis and adipocyte metabolism. *J. Biol. Chem.* **2007**, *282*, 28175–28188. [CrossRef] [PubMed]
75. Li, J.J.; Yin, H.K.; Guan, D.X.; Zhao, J.S.; Feng, Y.X.; Deng, Y.Z.; Wang, X.; Li, N.; Wang, X.F.; Cheng, S.Q.; et al. Chemerin suppresses hepatocellular carcinoma metastasis through CMKLR1-PTEN-Akt axis. *Br. J. Cancer* **2018**, *118*, 1337–1348. [CrossRef] [PubMed]
76. Sell, H.; Laurencikiene, J.; Taube, A.; Eckardt, K.; Cramer, A.; Horrighs, A.; Arner, P.; Eckel, J. Chemerin is a novel adipocyte-derived factor inducing insulin resistance in primary human skeletal muscle cells. *Diabetes* **2009**, *58*, 2731–2740. [CrossRef] [PubMed]
77. Xie, H.; Tang, S.Y.; Luo, X.H.; Huang, J.; Cui, R.R.; Yuan, L.Q.; Zhou, H.D.; Wu, X.P.; Liao, E.Y. Insulin-like effects of visfatin on human osteoblasts. *Calcif. Tissue Int.* **2007**, *80*, 201–210. [CrossRef] [PubMed]
78. Adya, R.; Tan, B.K.; Chen, J.; Randeva, H.S. Nuclear factor-kappaB induction by visfatin in human vascular endothelial cells: Its role in MMP-2/9 production and activation. *Diabetes Care* **2008**, *31*, 758–760. [CrossRef] [PubMed]
79. Brown, J.E.; Onyango, D.J.; Ramanjaneya, M.; Conner, A.C.; Patel, S.T.; Dunmore, S.J.; Randeva, H.S. Visfatin regulates insulin secretion, insulin receptor signalling and mRNA expression of diabetes-related genes in mouse pancreatic beta-cells. *J. Mol. Endocrinol.* **2010**, *44*, 171–178. [CrossRef]
80. Jacques, C.; Holzenberger, M.; Mladenovic, Z.; Salvat, C.; Pecchi, E.; Berenbaum, F.; Gosset, M. Proinflammatory actions of visfatin/nicotinamide phosphoribosyltransferase (Nampt) involve regulation of insulin signaling pathway and Nampt enzymatic activity. *J. Biol. Chem.* **2012**, *287*, 15100–15108. [CrossRef]
81. Lee, S.; Lee, H.C.; Kwon, Y.W.; Lee, S.E.; Cho, Y.; Kim, J.; Lee, S.; Kim, J.Y.; Lee, J.; Yang, H.M.; et al. Adenylyl cyclase-associated protein 1 is a receptor for human resistin and mediates inflammatory actions of human monocytes. *Cell Metab.* **2014**, *19*, 484–497. [CrossRef] [PubMed]
82. Benomar, Y.; Gertler, A.; De Lacy, P.; Crepin, D.; Ould Hamouda, H.; Riffault, L.; Taouis, M. Central resistin overexposure induces insulin resistance through Toll-like receptor 4. *Diabetes* **2013**, *62*, 102–114. [CrossRef] [PubMed]
83. Daquinag, A.C.; Zhang, Y.; Amaya-Manzanares, F.; Simmons, P.J.; Kolonin, M.G. An isoform of decorin is a resistin receptor on the surface of adipose progenitor cells. *Cell Stem Cell* **2011**, *9*, 74–86. [CrossRef] [PubMed]
84. Sanchez-Solana, B.; Laborda, J.; Baladron, V. Mouse resistin modulates adipogenesis and glucose uptake in 3T3-L1 preadipocytes through the ROR1 receptor. *Mol. Endocrinol.* **2012**, *26*, 110–127. [CrossRef] [PubMed]
85. O'Dowd, B.F.; Heiber, M.; Chan, A.; Heng, H.H.; Tsui, L.C.; Kennedy, J.L.; Shi, X.; Petronis, A.; George, S.R.; Nguyen, T. A human gene that shows identity with the gene encoding the angiotensin receptor is located on chromosome 11. *Gene* **1993**, *136*, 355–360. [CrossRef]
86. O'Carroll, A.M.; Lolait, S.J.; Howell, G.M. Transcriptional regulation of the rat apelin receptor gene: Promoter cloning and identification of an Sp1 site necessary for promoter activity. *J. Mol. Endocrinol.* **2006**, *36*, 221–235. [CrossRef] [PubMed]
87. Masri, B.; Morin, N.; Pedebernade, L.; Knibiehler, B.; Audigier, Y. The apelin receptor is coupled to Gi1 or Gi2 protein and is differentially desensitized by apelin fragments. *J. Biol. Chem.* **2006**, *281*, 18317–18326. [CrossRef]
88. Helfer, G.; Ross, A.W.; Thomson, L.M.; Mayer, C.D.; Stoney, P.N.; McCaffery, P.J.; Morgan, P.J. A neuroendocrine role for chemerin in hypothalamic remodelling and photoperiodic control of energy balance. *Sci. Rep.* **2016**, *6*, 26830. [CrossRef]
89. Gonzalez-Alvarez, R.; Garza-Rodriguez Mde, L.; Delgado-Enciso, I.; Trevino-Alvarado, V.M.; Canales-Del-Castillo, R.; Martinez-De-Villarreal, L.E.; Lugo-Trampe, A.; Tejero, M.E.; Schlabritz-Loutsevitch, N.E.; Rocha-Pizana Mdel, R.; et al. Molecular evolution and expression profile of the chemerine encoding gene RARRES2 in baboon and chimpanzee. *Biol. Res.* **2015**, *48*, 31. [CrossRef]
90. Brunetti, L.; Orlando, G.; Ferrante, C.; Recinella, L.; Leone, S.; Chiavaroli, A.; Di Nisio, C.; Shohreh, R.; Manippa, F.; Ricciuti, A.; et al. Peripheral chemerin administration modulates hypothalamic control of feeding. *Peptides* **2014**, *51*, 115–121. [CrossRef]
91. Wilkinson, M.; Wilkinson, D.; Wiesner, G.; Morash, B.; Ur, E. Hypothalamic resistin immunoreactivity is reduced by obesity in the mouse: Co-localization with alpha-melanostimulating hormone. *Neuroendocrinology* **2005**, *81*, 19–30. [CrossRef] [PubMed]

92. Maillard, V.; Elis, S.; Desmarchais, A.; Hivelin, C.; Lardic, L.; Lomet, D.; Uzbekova, S.; Monget, P.; Dupont, J. Visfatin and resistin in gonadotroph cells: Expression, regulation of LH secretion and signalling pathways. *Reprod. Fertil. Dev.* **2017**, *29*, 2479–2495. [CrossRef] [PubMed]
93. Nogueiras, R.; Barreiro, M.L.; Caminos, J.E.; Gaytan, F.; Suominen, J.S.; Navarro, V.M.; Casanueva, F.F.; Aguilar, E.; Toppari, J.; Dieguez, C.; et al. Novel expression of resistin in rat testis: Functional role and regulation by nutritional status and hormonal factors. *J. Cell Sci.* **2004**, *117*, 3247–3257. [CrossRef] [PubMed]
94. Hallschmid, M.; Randeva, H.; Tan, B.K.; Kern, W.; Lehnert, H. Relationship between cerebrospinal fluid visfatin (PBEF/Nampt) levels and adiposity in humans. *Diabetes* **2009**, *58*, 637–640. [CrossRef] [PubMed]
95. Pope, G.R.; Roberts, E.M.; Lolait, S.J.; O'Carroll, A.M. Central and peripheral apelin receptor distribution in the mouse: Species differences with rat. *Peptides* **2012**, *33*, 139–148. [CrossRef] [PubMed]
96. Rozycka, M.; Kurowska, P.; Grzesiak, M.; Kotula-Balak, M.; Tworzydlo, W.; Rame, C.; Gregoraszczuk, E.; Dupont, J.; Rak, A. Apelin and apelin receptor at different stages of corpus luteum development and effect of apelin on progesterone secretion and 3beta-hydroxysteroid dehydrogenase (3beta-HSD) in pigs. *Anim. Reprod. Sci.* **2018**, *192*, 251–260. [CrossRef]
97. Roche, J.; Rame, C.; Reverchon, M.; Mellouk, N.; Rak, A.; Froment, P.; Dupont, J. Apelin (APLN) regulates progesterone secretion and oocyte maturation in bovine ovarian cells. *Reproduction* **2017**, *153*, 589–603. [CrossRef]
98. Martini, A.C.; Tissera, A.; Estofan, D.; Molina, R.I.; Mangeaud, A.; de Cuneo, M.F.; Ruiz, R.D. Overweight and seminal quality: A study of 794 patients. *Fertil. Steril.* **2010**, *94*, 1739–1743. [CrossRef]
99. Wang, Q.; Kim, J.Y.; Xue, K.; Liu, J.Y.; Leader, A.; Tsang, B.K. Chemerin, a novel regulator of follicular steroidogenesis and its potential involvement in polycystic ovarian syndrome. *Endocrinology* **2012**, *153*, 5600–5611. [CrossRef]
100. Wang, Q.; Leader, A.; Tsang, B.K. Inhibitory roles of prohibitin and chemerin in FSH-induced rat granulosa cell steroidogenesis. *Endocrinology* **2013**, *154*, 956–967. [CrossRef]
101. Reverchon, M.; Bertoldo, M.J.; Rame, C.; Froment, P.; Dupont, J. CHEMERIN (RARRES2) decreases in vitro granulosa cell steroidogenesis and blocks oocyte meiotic progression in bovine species. *Biol. Reprod.* **2014**, *90*, 102. [CrossRef] [PubMed]
102. Mellouk, N.; Rame, C.; Delaveau, J.; Rat, C.; Marchand, M.; Mercerand, F.; Travel, A.; Brionne, A.; Chartrin, P.; Ma, L.; et al. Food restriction but not fish oil increases fertility in hens: Role of RARRES2? *Reproduction* **2018**, *155*, 321–331. [CrossRef] [PubMed]
103. Diot, M.; Reverchon, M.; Rame, C.; Froment, P.; Brillard, J.P.; Briere, S.; Leveque, G.; Guillaume, D.; Dupont, J. Expression of adiponectin, chemerin and visfatin in plasma and different tissues during a laying season in turkeys. *Reprod. Biol. Endocrinol.* **2015**, *13*, 81. [CrossRef] [PubMed]
104. Maillard, V.; Froment, P.; Rame, C.; Uzbekova, S.; Elis, S.; Dupont, J. Expression and effect of resistin on bovine and rat granulosa cell steroidogenesis and proliferation. *Reproduction* **2011**, *141*, 467–479. [CrossRef] [PubMed]
105. Spicer, L.J.; Schreiber, N.B.; Lagaly, D.V.; Aad, P.Y.; Douthit, L.B.; Grado-Ahuir, J.A. Effect of resistin on granulosa and theca cell function in cattle. *Anim. Reprod. Sci.* **2011**, *124*, 19–27. [CrossRef] [PubMed]
106. Rak-Mardyla, A.; Durak, M.; Lucja Gregoraszczuk, E. Effects of resistin on porcine ovarian follicle steroidogenesis in prepubertal animals: An in vitro study. *Reprod. Biol. Endocrinol.* **2013**, *11*, 45. [CrossRef] [PubMed]
107. Singh, A.; Suragani, M.; Ehtesham, N.Z.; Krishna, A. Localization of resistin and its possible roles in the ovary of a vespertilionid bat, Scotophilus heathi. *Steroids* **2015**, *95*, 17–23. [CrossRef] [PubMed]
108. Singh, A.; Suragani, M.; Krishna, A. Effects of resistin on ovarian folliculogenesis and steroidogenesis in the vespertilionid bat, Scotophilus heathi. *Gen. Comp. Endocrinol.* **2014**, *208*, 73–84. [CrossRef]
109. Niles, L.P.; Lobb, D.K.; Kang, N.H.; Armstrong, K.J. Resistin expression in human granulosa cells. *Endocrine* **2012**, *42*, 742–745. [CrossRef] [PubMed]
110. Reverchon, M.; Cornuau, M.; Rame, C.; Guerif, F.; Royere, D.; Dupont, J. Resistin decreases insulin-like growth factor I-induced steroid production and insulin-like growth factor I receptor signaling in human granulosa cells. *Fertil. Steril.* **2013**, *100*, 247–255.e3. [CrossRef] [PubMed]
111. Chalvatzas, N.; Dafopoulos, K.; Kosmas, G.; Kallitsaris, A.; Pournaras, S.; Messinis, I.E. Effect of ovarian hormones on serum adiponectin and resistin concentrations. *Fertil. Steril.* **2009**, *91*, 1189–1194. [CrossRef] [PubMed]

112. Munir, I.; Yen, H.W.; Baruth, T.; Tarkowski, R.; Azziz, R.; Magoffin, D.A.; Jakimiuk, A.J. Resistin stimulation of 17alpha-hydroxylase activity in ovarian theca cells in vitro: Relevance to polycystic ovary syndrome. *J. Clin. Endocrinol. Metab.* **2005**, *90*, 4852–4857. [CrossRef] [PubMed]
113. Annie, L.; Gurusubramanian, G.; Roy, V.K. Estrogen and progesterone dependent expression of visfatin/NAMPT regulates proliferation and apoptosis in mice uterus during estrous cycle. *J. Steroid Biochem. Mol. Biol.* **2019**, *185*, 225–236. [CrossRef] [PubMed]
114. Messini, C.I.; Vasilaki, A.; Korona, E.; Anifandis, G.; Georgoulias, P.; Dafopoulos, K.; Garas, A.; Daponte, A.; Messinis, I.E. Effect of resistin on estradiol and progesterone secretion from human luteinized granulosa cells in culture. *Syst. Biol. Reprod. Med.* **2019**. [CrossRef] [PubMed]
115. Seow, K.M.; Juan, C.C.; Hsu, Y.P.; Ho, L.T.; Wang, Y.Y.; Hwang, J.L. Serum and follicular resistin levels in women with polycystic ovarian syndrome during IVF-stimulated cycles. *Hum. Reprod.* **2005**, *20*, 117–121. [CrossRef] [PubMed]
116. Varnagy, A.; Bodis, J.; Kovacs, G.L.; Sulyok, E.; Rauh, M.; Rascher, W. Metabolic hormones in follicular fluid in women undergoing in vitro fertilization. *J. Reprod. Med.* **2013**, *58*, 305–311. [PubMed]
117. Chen, D.; Fang, Q.; Chai, Y.; Wang, H.; Huang, H.; Dong, M. Serum resistin in gestational diabetes mellitus and early postpartum. *Clin. Endocrinol. (Oxf.)* **2007**, *67*, 208–211. [CrossRef]
118. Ons, E.; Gertler, A.; Buyse, J.; Lebihan-Duval, E.; Bordas, A.; Goddeeris, B.; Dridi, S. Visfatin gene expression in chickens is sex and tissue dependent. *Domest. Anim. Endocrinol.* **2010**, *38*, 63–74. [CrossRef]
119. Diot, M.; Reverchon, M.; Rame, C.; Baumard, Y.; Dupont, J. Expression and effect of NAMPT (visfatin) on progesterone secretion in hen granulosa cells. *Reproduction* **2015**, *150*, 53–63. [CrossRef]
120. Reverchon, M.; Rame, C.; Bunel, A.; Chen, W.; Froment, P.; Dupont, J. VISFATIN (NAMPT) Improves In Vitro IGF1-Induced Steroidogenesis and IGF1 Receptor Signaling Through SIRT1 in Bovine Granulosa Cells. *Biol. Reprod.* **2016**, *94*, 54. [CrossRef]
121. Choi, K.H.; Joo, B.S.; Sun, S.T.; Park, M.J.; Son, J.B.; Joo, J.K.; Lee, K.S. Administration of visfatin during superovulation improves developmental competency of oocytes and fertility potential in aged female mice. *Fertil. Steril.* **2012**, *97*, 1234–1241.e3. [CrossRef] [PubMed]
122. Shen, C.J.; Tsai, E.M.; Lee, J.N.; Chen, Y.L.; Lee, C.H.; Chan, T.F. The concentrations of visfatin in the follicular fluids of women undergoing controlled ovarian stimulation are correlated to the number of oocytes retrieved. *Fertil. Steril.* **2010**, *93*, 1844–1850. [CrossRef] [PubMed]
123. Plati, E.; Kouskouni, E.; Malamitsi-Puchner, A.; Boutsikou, M.; Kaparos, G.; Baka, S. Visfatin and leptin levels in women with polycystic ovaries undergoing ovarian stimulation. *Fertil. Steril.* **2010**, *94*, 1451–1456. [CrossRef] [PubMed]
124. Reverchon, M.; Cornuau, M.; Cloix, L.; Rame, C.; Guerif, F.; Royere, D.; Dupont, J. Visfatin is expressed in human granulosa cells: Regulation by metformin through AMPK/SIRT1 pathways and its role in steroidogenesis. *Mol. Hum. Reprod.* **2013**, *19*, 313–326. [CrossRef] [PubMed]
125. O'Carroll, A.M.; Selby, T.L.; Palkovits, M.; Lolait, S.J. Distribution of mRNA encoding B78/apj, the rat homologue of the human APJ receptor, and its endogenous ligand apelin in brain and peripheral tissues. *Biochim. Biophys. Acta* **2000**, *1492*, 72–80. [CrossRef]
126. Shirasuna, K.; Shimizu, T.; Sayama, K.; Asahi, T.; Sasaki, M.; Berisha, B.; Schams, D.; Miyamoto, A. Expression and localization of apelin and its receptor APJ in the bovine corpus luteum during the estrous cycle and prostaglandin F2alpha-induced luteolysis. *Reproduction* **2008**, *135*, 519–525. [CrossRef] [PubMed]
127. Rak, A.; Drwal, E.; Rame, C.; Knapczyk-Stwora, K.; Slomczynska, M.; Dupont, J.; Gregoraszczuk, E.L. Expression of apelin and apelin receptor (APJ) in porcine ovarian follicles and in vitro effect of apelin on steroidogenesis and proliferation through APJ activation and different signaling pathways. *Theriogenology* **2017**, *96*, 126–135. [CrossRef] [PubMed]
128. Altinkaya, S.O.; Nergiz, S.; Kucuk, M.; Yuksel, H. Apelin levels in relation with hormonal and metabolic profile in patients with polycystic ovary syndrome. *Eur. J. Obstet. Gynecol. Reprod. Biol.* **2014**, *176*, 168–172. [CrossRef]
129. Chang, C.Y.; Tsai, Y.C.; Lee, C.H.; Chan, T.F.; Wang, S.H.; Su, J.H. Lower serum apelin levels in women with polycystic ovary syndrome. *Fertil. Steril.* **2011**, *95*, 2520–2523.e2. [CrossRef]
130. Li, L.; Huang, C.; Zhang, X.; Wang, J.; Ma, P.; Liu, Y.; Xiao, T.; Zabel, B.A.; Zhang, J.V. Chemerin-derived peptide C-20 suppressed gonadal steroidogenesis. *Am. J. Reprod. Immunol.* **2014**, *71*, 265–277. [CrossRef]

131. Li, L.; Ma, P.; Huang, C.; Liu, Y.; Zhang, Y.; Gao, C.; Xiao, T.; Ren, P.G.; Zabel, B.A.; Zhang, J.V. Expression of chemerin and its receptors in rat testes and its action on testosterone secretion. *J. Endocrinol.* **2014**, *220*, 155–163. [CrossRef] [PubMed]
132. Chen, H.; Jin, S.; Guo, J.; Kombairaju, P.; Biswal, S.; Zirkin, B.R. Knockout of the transcription factor Nrf2: Effects on testosterone production by aging mouse Leydig cells. *Mol. Cell. Endocrinol.* **2015**, *409*, 113–120. [CrossRef] [PubMed]
133. Ivars, J.; Butruille, L.; Knauf, C.; Bouckenooghe, T.; Mayeur, S.; Vieau, D.; Valet, P.; Deruelle, P.; Lesage, J. Maternal hypertension induces tissue-specific modulations of the apelinergic system in the fetoplacental unit in rat. *Peptides* **2012**, *35*, 136–138. [CrossRef]
134. Zhao, H.; Yan, D.; Xiang, L.; Huang, C.; Li, J.; Yu, X.; Huang, B.; Wang, B.; Chen, J.; Xiao, T.; et al. Chemokine-like receptor 1 deficiency leads to lower bone mass in male mice. *Cell. Mol. Life Sci.* **2019**, *76*, 355–367. [CrossRef] [PubMed]
135. Bongrani, A.; Elfassy, Y.; Brun, J.S.; Rame, C.; Mellouk, N.; Fellahi, S.; Bastard, J.P.; Levy, R.; Vasseur, C.; Froment, P.; et al. Expression of adipokines in seminal fluid of men of normal weight. *Asian J. Androl.* **2019**. [CrossRef]
136. Jeremy, M.; Gurusubramanian, G.; Roy, V.K. Localization pattern of visfatin (NAMPT) in d-galactose induced aged rat testis. *Ann. Anat.* **2017**, *211*, 46–54. [CrossRef] [PubMed]
137. Riammer, S.; Garten, A.; Schaab, M.; Grunewald, S.; Kiess, W.; Kratzsch, J.; Paasch, U. Nicotinamide phosphoribosyltransferase production in human spermatozoa is influenced by maturation stage. *Andrology* **2016**, *4*, 1045–1053. [CrossRef]
138. Ocon-Grove, O.M.; Krzysik-Walker, S.M.; Maddineni, S.R.; Hendricks, G.L., 3rd; Ramachandran, R. NAMPT (visfatin) in the chicken testis: Influence of sexual maturation on cellular localization, plasma levels and gene and protein expression. *Reproduction* **2010**, *139*, 217–226. [CrossRef]
139. Thomas, S.; Kratzsch, D.; Schaab, M.; Scholz, M.; Grunewald, S.; Thiery, J.; Paasch, U.; Kratzsch, J. Seminal plasma adipokine levels are correlated with functional characteristics of spermatozoa. *Fertil. Steril.* **2013**, *99*, 1256–1263.e3. [CrossRef]
140. Hameed, W.; Yousaf, I.; Latif, R.; Aslam, M. Effect of visfatin on testicular steroidogenesis in purified Leydig cells. *J. Ayub Med. Coll. Abbottabad* **2012**, *24*, 62–64.
141. Roumaud, P.; Martin, L.J. Roles of leptin, adiponectin and resistin in the transcriptional regulation of steroidogenic genes contributing to decreased Leydig cells function in obesity. *Horm. Mol. Biol. Clin. Investig.* **2015**, *24*, 25–45. [CrossRef] [PubMed]
142. Bauer, S.; Bala, M.; Kopp, A.; Eisinger, K.; Schmid, A.; Schneider, S.; Neumeier, M.; Buechler, C. Adipocyte chemerin release is induced by insulin without being translated to higher levels in vivo. *Eur. J. Clin. Investig.* **2012**, *42*, 1213–1220. [CrossRef] [PubMed]
143. Sandal, S.; Tekin, S.; Seker, F.B.; Beytur, A.; Vardi, N.; Colak, C.; Tapan, T.; Yildiz, S.; Yilmaz, B. The effects of intracerebroventricular infusion of apelin-13 on reproductive function in male rats. *Neurosci. Lett.* **2015**, *602*, 133–138. [CrossRef] [PubMed]
144. Zaitseva, M.; Vollenhoven, B.J.; Rogers, P.A. Retinoids regulate genes involved in retinoic acid synthesis and transport in human myometrial and fibroid smooth muscle cells. *Hum. Reprod.* **2008**, *23*, 1076–1086. [CrossRef]
145. Carlino, C.; Trotta, E.; Stabile, H.; Morrone, S.; Bulla, R.; Soriani, A.; Iannitto, M.L.; Agostinis, C.; Mocci, C.; Minozzi, M.; et al. Chemerin regulates NK cell accumulation and endothelial cell morphogenesis in the decidua during early pregnancy. *J. Clin. Endocrinol. Metab.* **2012**, *97*, 3603–3612. [CrossRef]
146. Mumtaz, S.; AlSaif, S.; Wray, S.; Noble, K. Inhibitory effect of visfatin and leptin on human and rat myometrial contractility. *Life Sci.* **2015**, *125*, 57–62. [CrossRef] [PubMed]
147. Dall'Aglio, C.; Scocco, P.; Maranesi, M.; Petrucci, L.; Acuti, G.; De Felice, E.; Mercati, F. Immunohistochemical identification of resistin in the uterus of ewes subjected to different diets: Preliminary results. *Eur. J. Histochem.* **2019**, *63*, 3020. [CrossRef]
148. Kawamata, Y.; Habata, Y.; Fukusumi, S.; Hosoya, M.; Fujii, R.; Hinuma, S.; Nishizawa, N.; Kitada, C.; Onda, H.; Nishimura, O.; et al. Molecular properties of apelin: Tissue distribution and receptor binding. *Biochim. Biophys. Acta* **2001**, *1538*, 162–171. [CrossRef]
149. Hehir, M.P.; Morrison, J.J. The adipokine apelin and human uterine contractility. *Am. J. Obstet. Gynecol* **2012**, *206*, 359.e1–359.e5. [CrossRef]

150. Kacar, E.; Ercan, Z.; Serhatlioglu, I.; Sumer, A.; Kelestimur, H.; Kutlu, S. The effects of apelin on myometrium contractions in pregnant rats. *Cell. Mol. Biol. (Noisy-Le-Grand)* **2018**, *64*, 74–79. [CrossRef]
151. Kasher-Meron, M.; Mazaki-Tovi, S.; Barhod, E.; Hemi, R.; Haas, J.; Gat, I.; Zilberberg, E.; Yinon, Y.; Karasik, A.; Kanety, H. Chemerin concentrations in maternal and fetal compartments: Implications for metabolic adaptations to normal human pregnancy. *J. Perinat. Med.* **2014**, *42*, 371–378. [CrossRef] [PubMed]
152. Wang, L.; Yang, T.; Ding, Y.; Zhong, Y.; Yu, L.; Peng, M. Chemerin plays a protective role by regulating human umbilical vein endothelial cell-induced nitric oxide signaling in preeclampsia. *Endocrine* **2015**, *48*, 299–308. [CrossRef] [PubMed]
153. Huang, B.; Huang, C.; Zhao, H.; Zhu, W.; Wang, B.; Wang, H.; Chen, J.; Xiao, T.; Niu, J.; Zhang, J. Impact of GPR1 signaling on maternal high-fat feeding and placenta metabolism in mice. *Am. J. Physiol. Endocrinol. Metab.* **2019**, *316*, E987–E997. [CrossRef] [PubMed]
154. Ognjanovic, S.; Bryant-Greenwood, G.D. Pre-B-cell colony-enhancing factor, a novel cytokine of human fetal membranes. *Am. J. Obstet. Gynecol.* **2002**, *187*, 1051–1058. [CrossRef] [PubMed]
155. Ognjanovic, S.; Tashima, L.S.; Bryant-Greenwood, G.D. The effects of pre–B-cell colony–enhancing factor on the human fetal membranes by microarray analysis. *Am. J. Obstet. Gynecol.* **2003**, *189*, 1187–1195. [CrossRef]
156. Lappas, M. Visfatin regulates the terminal processes of human labour and delivery via activation of the nuclear factor-kappaB pathway. *Mol. Cell. Endocrinol.* **2012**, *348*, 128–134. [CrossRef] [PubMed]
157. Astern, J.M.; Collier, A.C.; Kendal-Wright, C.E. Pre-B cell colony enhancing factor (PBEF/NAMPT/Visfatin) and vascular endothelial growth factor (VEGF) cooperate to increase the permeability of the human placental amnion. *Placenta* **2013**, *34*, 42–49. [CrossRef]
158. Zhang, Y.; Huo, Y.; He, W.; Liu, S.; Li, H.; Li, L. Visfatin is regulated by interleukin6 and affected by the PPARgamma pathway in BeWo cells. *Mol. Med. Rep.* **2019**, *19*, 400–406. [CrossRef]
159. Caja, S.; Martinez, I.; Abelenda, M.; Puerta, M. Resistin expression and plasma concentration peak at different times during pregnancy in rats. *J. Endocrinol.* **2005**, *185*, 551–559. [CrossRef]
160. Yura, S.; Sagawa, N.; Itoh, H.; Kakui, K.; Nuamah, M.A.; Korita, D.; Takemura, M.; Fujii, S. Resistin is expressed in the human placenta. *J. Clin. Endocrinol. Metab.* **2003**, *88*, 1394–1397. [CrossRef]
161. Chen, D.; Dong, M.; Fang, Q.; He, J.; Wang, Z.; Yang, X. Alterations of serum resistin in normal pregnancy and pre-eclampsia. *Clin. Sci. (Lond.)* **2005**, *108*, 81–84. [CrossRef] [PubMed]
162. Cortelazzi, D.; Corbetta, S.; Ronzoni, S.; Pelle, F.; Marconi, A.; Cozzi, V.; Cetin, I.; Cortelazzi, R.; Beck-Peccoz, P.; Spada, A. Maternal and foetal resistin and adiponectin concentrations in normal and complicated pregnancies. *Clin. Endocrinol. (Oxf.)* **2007**, *66*, 447–453. [CrossRef] [PubMed]
163. Di Simone, N.; Di Nicuolo, F.; Marzioni, D.; Castellucci, M.; Sanguinetti, M.; D'Lppolito, S.; Caruso, A. Resistin modulates glucose uptake and glucose transporter-1 (GLUT-1) expression in trophoblast cells. *J. Cell. Mol. Med.* **2009**, *13*, 388–397. [CrossRef] [PubMed]
164. Cobellis, L.; De Falco, M.; Mastrogiacomo, A.; Giraldi, D.; Dattilo, D.; Scaffa, C.; Colacurci, N.; De Luca, A. Modulation of apelin and APJ receptor in normal and preeclampsia-complicated placentas. *Histol. Histopathol.* **2007**, *22*, 1–8. [CrossRef] [PubMed]
165. Van Mieghem, T.; van Bree, R.; Van Herck, E.; Pijnenborg, R.; Deprest, J.; Verhaeghe, J. Maternal apelin physiology during rat pregnancy: The role of the placenta. *Placenta* **2010**, *31*, 725–730. [CrossRef]
166. Lim, R.; Barker, G.; Riley, C.; Lappas, M. Apelin is decreased with human preterm and term labor and regulates prolabor mediators in human primary amnion cells. *Reprod. Sci.* **2013**, *20*, 957–967. [CrossRef] [PubMed]
167. Mayeur, S.; Wattez, J.S.; Lukaszewski, M.A.; Lecoutre, S.; Butruille, L.; Drougard, A.; Eberle, D.; Bastide, B.; Laborie, C.; Storme, L.; et al. Apelin Controls Fetal and Neonatal Glucose Homeostasis and Is Altered by Maternal Undernutrition. *Diabetes* **2016**, *65*, 554–560. [CrossRef]
168. Vaughan, O.R.; Powell, T.L.; Jansson, T. Apelin is a novel regulator of human trophoblast amino acid transport. *Am. J. Physiol. Endocrinol. Metab.* **2019**, *316*, E810–E816. [CrossRef]
169. Teede, H.; Deeks, A.; Moran, L. Polycystic ovary syndrome: A complex condition with psychological, reproductive and metabolic manifestations that impacts on health across the lifespan. *BMC Med.* **2010**, *8*, 41. [CrossRef]
170. Teede, H.J.; Misso, M.L.; Costello, M.F.; Dokras, A.; Laven, J.; Moran, L.; Piltonen, T.; Norman, R.J.; International, P.N. Recommendations from the international evidence-based guideline for the assessment and management of polycystic ovary syndrome. *Fertil. Steril.* **2018**, *110*, 364–379. [CrossRef]

171. Toulis, K.A.; Goulis, D.G.; Farmakiotis, D.; Georgopoulos, N.A.; Katsikis, I.; Tarlatzis, B.C.; Papadimas, I.; Panidis, D. Adiponectin levels in women with polycystic ovary syndrome: A systematic review and a meta-analysis. *Hum. Reprod. Update* **2009**, *15*, 297–307. [CrossRef] [PubMed]
172. Pasquali, R.; Gambineri, A.; Pagotto, U. The impact of obesity on reproduction in women with polycystic ovary syndrome. *BJOG* **2006**, *113*, 1148–1159. [CrossRef] [PubMed]
173. Barber, T.M.; McCarthy, M.I.; Wass, J.A.; Franks, S. Obesity and polycystic ovary syndrome. *Clin. Endocrinol. (Oxf.)* **2006**, *65*, 137–145. [CrossRef] [PubMed]
174. Benrick, A.; Chanclon, B.; Micallef, P.; Wu, Y.; Hadi, L.; Shelton, J.M.; Stener-Victorin, E.; Wernstedt Asterholm, I. Adiponectin protects against development of metabolic disturbances in a PCOS mouse model. *Proc. Natl. Acad. Sci. USA* **2017**, *114*, E7187–E7196. [CrossRef] [PubMed]
175. Dumesic, D.A.; Padmanabhan, V.; Abbott, D.H. Polycystic ovary syndrome and oocyte developmental competence. *Obstet. Gynecol. Surv.* **2008**, *63*, 39–48. [CrossRef] [PubMed]
176. Azziz, R.; Carmina, E.; Dewailly, D.; Diamanti-Kandarakis, E.; Escobar-Morreale, H.F.; Futterweit, W.; Janssen, O.E.; Legro, R.S.; Norman, R.J.; Taylor, A.E.; et al. Positions statement: Criteria for defining polycystic ovary syndrome as a predominantly hyperandrogenic syndrome: An Androgen Excess Society guideline. *J. Clin. Endocrinol. Metab.* **2006**, *91*, 4237–4245. [CrossRef]
177. Tan, B.K.; Chen, J.; Farhatullah, S.; Adya, R.; Kaur, J.; Heutling, D.; Lewandowski, K.C.; O'Hare, J.P.; Lehnert, H.; Randeva, H.S. Insulin and metformin regulate circulating and adipose tissue chemerin. *Diabetes* **2009**, *58*, 1971–1977. [CrossRef]
178. Ernst, M.C.; Sinal, C.J. Chemerin: At the crossroads of inflammation and obesity. *Trends Endocrinol. Metab.* **2010**, *21*, 660–667. [CrossRef]
179. Kort, D.H.; Kostolias, A.; Sullivan, C.; Lobo, R.A. Chemerin as a marker of body fat and insulin resistance in women with polycystic ovary syndrome. *Gynecol. Endocrinol.* **2015**, *31*, 152–155. [CrossRef]
180. Guvenc, Y.; Var, A.; Goker, A.; Kuscu, N.K. Assessment of serum chemerin, vaspin and omentin-1 levels in patients with polycystic ovary syndrome. *J. Int. Med. Res.* **2016**, *44*, 796–805. [CrossRef]
181. Huang, R.; Yue, J.; Sun, Y.; Zheng, J.; Tao, T.; Li, S.; Liu, W. Increased serum chemerin concentrations in patients with polycystic ovary syndrome: Relationship between insulin resistance and ovarian volume. *Clin. Chim. Acta* **2015**, *450*, 366–369. [CrossRef] [PubMed]
182. Guzel, E.C.; Celik, C.; Abali, R.; Kucukyalcin, V.; Celik, E.; Guzel, M.; Yilmaz, M. Omentin and chemerin and their association with obesity in women with polycystic ovary syndrome. *Gynecol. Endocrinol.* **2014**, *30*, 419–422. [CrossRef] [PubMed]
183. Martinez-Garcia, M.A.; Montes-Nieto, R.; Fernandez-Duran, E.; Insenser, M.; Luque-Ramirez, M.; Escobar-Morreale, H.F. Evidence for masculinization of adipokine gene expression in visceral and subcutaneous adipose tissue of obese women with polycystic ovary syndrome (PCOS). *J. Clin. Endocrinol. Metab.* **2013**, *98*, E388–E396. [CrossRef] [PubMed]
184. Wang, Y.; Huang, R.; Li, X.; Zhu, Q.; Liao, Y.; Tao, T.; Kang, X.; Liu, W.; Li, S.; Sun, Y. High concentration of chemerin caused by ovarian hyperandrogenism may lead to poor IVF outcome in polycystic ovary syndrome: A pilot study. *Gynecol. Endocrinol.* **2019**. [CrossRef] [PubMed]
185. Tang, M.; Huang, C.; Wang, Y.F.; Ren, P.G.; Chen, L.; Xiao, T.X.; Wang, B.B.; Pan, Y.F.; Tsang, B.K.; Zabel, B.A.; et al. CMKLR1 deficiency maintains ovarian steroid production in mice treated chronically with dihydrotestosterone. *Sci. Rep.* **2016**, *6*, 21328. [CrossRef] [PubMed]
186. Lima, P.D.A.; Nivet, A.L.; Wang, Q.; Chen, Y.A.; Leader, A.; Cheung, A.; Tzeng, C.R.; Tsang, B.K. Polycystic ovary syndrome: Possible involvement of androgen-induced, chemerin-mediated ovarian recruitment of monocytes/macrophages. *Biol. Reprod.* **2018**, *99*, 838–852. [CrossRef] [PubMed]
187. Kim, J.Y.; Xue, K.; Cao, M.; Wang, Q.; Liu, J.Y.; Leader, A.; Han, J.Y.; Tsang, B.K. Chemerin suppresses ovarian follicular development and its potential involvement in follicular arrest in rats treated chronically with dihydrotestosterone. *Endocrinology* **2013**, *154*, 2912–2923. [CrossRef] [PubMed]
188. Chen, M.P.; Chung, F.M.; Chang, D.M.; Tsai, J.C.; Huang, H.F.; Shin, S.J.; Lee, Y.J. Elevated plasma level of visfatin/pre-B cell colony-enhancing factor in patients with type 2 diabetes mellitus. *J. Clin. Endocrinol. Metab.* **2006**, *91*, 295–299. [CrossRef]
189. Pagano, C.; Soardo, G.; Pilon, C.; Milocco, C.; Basan, L.; Milan, G.; Donnini, D.; Faggian, D.; Mussap, M.; Plebani, M.; et al. Increased serum resistin in nonalcoholic fatty liver disease is related to liver disease severity and not to insulin resistance. *J. Clin. Endocrinol. Metab.* **2006**, *91*, 1081–1086. [CrossRef]

190. Farshchian, F.; Ramezani Tehrani, F.; Amirrasouli, H.; Rahimi Pour, H.; Hedayati, M.; Kazerouni, F.; Soltani, A. Visfatin and resistin serum levels in normal-weight and obese women with polycystic ovary syndrome. *Int. J. Endocrinol. Metab.* **2014**, *12*, e15503. [CrossRef]
191. Chang, Y.H.; Chang, D.M.; Lin, K.C.; Shin, S.J.; Lee, Y.J. Visfatin in overweight/obesity, type 2 diabetes mellitus, insulin resistance, metabolic syndrome and cardiovascular diseases: A meta-analysis and systemic review. *Diabetes Metab. Res. Rev.* **2011**, *27*, 515–527. [CrossRef] [PubMed]
192. Ozkaya, M.; Cakal, E.; Ustun, Y.; Engin-Ustun, Y. Effect of metformin on serum visfatin levels in patients with polycystic ovary syndrome. *Fertil. Steril.* **2010**, *93*, 880–884. [CrossRef] [PubMed]
193. Kim, J.J.; Choi, Y.M.; Hong, M.A.; Kim, M.J.; Chae, S.J.; Kim, S.M.; Hwang, K.R.; Yoon, S.H.; Ku, S.Y.; Suh, C.S.; et al. Serum visfatin levels in non-obese women with polycystic ovary syndrome and matched controls. *Obstet. Gynecol. Sci.* **2018**, *61*, 253–260. [CrossRef] [PubMed]
194. Gumus, U.; Guzel, A.I.; Topcu, H.O.; Timur, H.; Yilmaz, N.; Danisman, N. Plasma Visfatin Levels in Adolescents with Polycystic Ovary Syndrome: A Prospective Case-Control Study. *J. Pediatr. Adolesc. Gynecol.* **2015**, *28*, 249–253. [CrossRef] [PubMed]
195. Sun, Y.; Wu, Z.; Wei, L.; Liu, C.; Zhu, S.; Tang, S. High-visfatin levels in women with polycystic ovary syndrome: Evidence from a meta-analysis. *Gynecol. Endocrinol.* **2015**, *31*, 808–814. [CrossRef] [PubMed]
196. Cekmez, F.; Cekmez, Y.; Pirgon, O.; Canpolat, F.E.; Aydinoz, S.; Metin Ipcioglu, O.; Karademir, F. Evaluation of new adipocytokines and insulin resistance in adolescents with polycystic ovary syndrome. *Eur. Cytokine Netw.* **2011**, *22*, 32–37. [CrossRef] [PubMed]
197. Chan, T.F.; Chen, Y.L.; Chen, H.H.; Lee, C.H.; Jong, S.B.; Tsai, E.M. Increased plasma visfatin concentrations in women with polycystic ovary syndrome. *Fertil. Steril.* **2007**, *88*, 401–405. [CrossRef] [PubMed]
198. Gen, R.; Akbay, E.; Muslu, N.; Sezer, K.; Cayan, F. Plasma visfatin level in lean women with PCOS: Relation to proinflammatory markers and insulin resistance. *Gynecol. Endocrinol.* **2009**, *25*, 241–245. [CrossRef]
199. Kowalska, I.; Straczkowski, M.; Nikolajuk, A.; Adamska, A.; Karczewska-Kupczewska, M.; Otziomek, E.; Wolczynski, S.; Gorska, M. Serum visfatin in relation to insulin resistance and markers of hyperandrogenism in lean and obese women with polycystic ovary syndrome. *Hum. Reprod.* **2007**, *22*, 1824–1829. [CrossRef]
200. Panidis, D.; Farmakiotis, D.; Rousso, D.; Katsikis, I.; Delkos, D.; Piouka, A.; Gerou, S.; Diamanti-Kandarakis, E. Plasma visfatin levels in normal weight women with polycystic ovary syndrome. *Eur. J. Intern. Med.* **2008**, *19*, 406–412. [CrossRef]
201. Tan, B.K.; Chen, J.; Digby, J.E.; Keay, S.D.; Kennedy, C.R.; Randeva, H.S. Increased visfatin messenger ribonucleic acid and protein levels in adipose tissue and adipocytes in women with polycystic ovary syndrome: Parallel increase in plasma visfatin. *J. Clin. Endocrinol. Metab.* **2006**, *91*, 5022–5028. [CrossRef] [PubMed]
202. Tsouma, I.; Kouskouni, E.; Demeridou, S.; Boutsikou, M.; Hassiakos, D.; Chasiakou, A.; Hassiakou, S.; Baka, S. Correlation of visfatin levels and lipoprotein lipid profiles in women with polycystic ovary syndrome undergoing ovarian stimulation. *Gynecol. Endocrinol.* **2014**, *30*, 516–519. [CrossRef] [PubMed]
203. Ek, I.; Arner, P.; Ryden, M.; Holm, C.; Thorne, A.; Hoffstedt, J.; Wahrenberg, H. A unique defect in the regulation of visceral fat cell lipolysis in the polycystic ovary syndrome as an early link to insulin resistance. *Diabetes* **2002**, *51*, 484–492. [CrossRef] [PubMed]
204. Hug, C.; Lodish, H.F. Medicine. Visfatin: A new adipokine. *Science* **2005**, *307*, 366–367. [CrossRef] [PubMed]
205. Moschen, A.R.; Kaser, A.; Enrich, B.; Mosheimer, B.; Theurl, M.; Niederegger, H.; Tilg, H. Visfatin, an adipocytokine with proinflammatory and immunomodulating properties. *J. Immunol.* **2007**, *178*, 1748–1758. [CrossRef] [PubMed]
206. Majuri, A.; Santaniemi, M.; Rautio, K.; Kunnari, A.; Vartiainen, J.; Ruokonen, A.; Kesaniemi, Y.A.; Tapanainen, J.S.; Ukkola, O.; Morin-Papunen, L. Rosiglitazone treatment increases plasma levels of adiponectin and decreases levels of resistin in overweight women with PCOS: A randomized placebo-controlled study. *Eur. J. Endocrinol.* **2007**, *156*, 263–269. [CrossRef] [PubMed]
207. Schwartz, D.R.; Lazar, M.A. Human resistin: Found in translation from mouse to man. *Trends Endocrinol. Metab.* **2011**, *22*, 259–265. [CrossRef] [PubMed]
208. Gul, O.O.; Cander, S.; Gul, B.; Acikgoz, E.; Sarandol, E.; Ersoy, C. Evaluation of insulin resistance and plasma levels for visfatin and resistin in obese and non-obese patients with polycystic ovary syndrome. *Eur. Cytokine Netw.* **2015**, *26*, 73–78. [CrossRef] [PubMed]

209. Yilmaz, M.; Bukan, N.; Demirci, H.; Ozturk, C.; Kan, E.; Ayvaz, G.; Arslan, M. Serum resistin and adiponectin levels in women with polycystic ovary syndrome. *Gynecol. Endocrinol.* **2009**, *25*, 246–252. [CrossRef]
210. Zhang, J.; Zhou, L.; Tang, L.; Xu, L. The plasma level and gene expression of resistin in polycystic ovary syndrome. *Gynecol. Endocrinol.* **2011**, *27*, 982–987. [CrossRef]
211. Urbanek, M.; Du, Y.; Silander, K.; Collins, F.S.; Steppan, C.M.; Strauss, J.F., 3rd; Dunaif, A.; Spielman, R.S.; Legro, R.S. Variation in resistin gene promoter not associated with polycystic ovary syndrome. *Diabetes* **2003**, *52*, 214–217. [CrossRef] [PubMed]
212. Baldani, D.P.; Skrgatic, L.; Kasum, M.; Zlopasa, G.; Kralik Oguic, S.; Herman, M. Altered leptin, adiponectin, resistin and ghrelin secretion may represent an intrinsic polycystic ovary syndrome abnormality. *Gynecol. Endocrinol.* **2019**, *35*, 401–405. [CrossRef] [PubMed]
213. Mahde, A.; Shaker, M.; Al-Mashhadani, Z. Study of Omentin1 and Other Adipokines and Hormones in PCOS Patients. *Oman Med. J.* **2009**, *24*, 108–118. [CrossRef] [PubMed]
214. Seow, K.M.; Juan, C.C.; Wu, L.Y.; Hsu, Y.P.; Yang, W.M.; Tsai, Y.L.; Hwang, J.L.; Ho, L.T. Serum and adipocyte resistin in polycystic ovary syndrome with insulin resistance. *Hum. Reprod.* **2004**, *19*, 48–53. [CrossRef] [PubMed]
215. Seow, K.M.; Juan, C.C.; Ho, L.T.; Hsu, Y.P.; Lin, Y.H.; Huang, L.W.; Hwang, J.L. Adipocyte resistin mRNA levels are down-regulated by laparoscopic ovarian electrocautery in both obese and lean women with polycystic ovary syndrome. *Hum. Reprod.* **2007**, *22*, 1100–1106. [CrossRef] [PubMed]
216. Olszanecka-Glinianowicz, M.; Madej, P.; Nylec, M.; Owczarek, A.; Szanecki, W.; Skalba, P.; Chudek, J. Circulating apelin level in relation to nutritional status in polycystic ovary syndrome and its association with metabolic and hormonal disturbances. *Clin. Endocrinol. (Oxf.)* **2013**, *79*, 238–242. [CrossRef]
217. Choi, Y.S.; Yang, H.I.; Cho, S.; Jung, J.A.; Jeon, Y.E.; Kim, H.Y.; Seo, S.K.; Lee, B.S. Serum asymmetric dimethylarginine, apelin, and tumor necrosis factor-alpha levels in non-obese women with polycystic ovary syndrome. *Steroids* **2012**, *77*, 1352–1358. [CrossRef] [PubMed]
218. Goren, K.; Sagsoz, N.; Noyan, V.; Yucel, A.; Caglayan, O.; Bostanci, M.S. Plasma apelin levels in patients with polycystic ovary syndrome. *J. Turk. Ger. Gynecol. Assoc.* **2012**, *13*, 27–31. [CrossRef]
219. Benk Silfeler, D.; Gokce, C.; Keskin Kurt, R.; Yilmaz Atilgan, N.; Ozturk, O.H.; Turhan, E.; Baloglu, A. Does polycystic ovary syndrome itself have additional effect on apelin levels? *Obstet. Gynecol. Int.* **2014**, *2014*, 536896. [CrossRef]
220. Franks, S.; Stark, J.; Hardy, K. Follicle dynamics and anovulation in polycystic ovary syndrome. *Hum. Reprod. Update* **2008**, *14*, 367–378. [CrossRef]
221. Taheri, S.; Murphy, K.; Cohen, M.; Sujkovic, E.; Kennedy, A.; Dhillo, W.; Dakin, C.; Sajedi, A.; Ghatei, M.; Bloom, S. The effects of centrally administered apelin-13 on food intake, water intake and pituitary hormone release in rats. *Biochem. Biophys. Res. Commun.* **2002**, *291*, 1208–1212. [CrossRef] [PubMed]
222. Howell, K.R.; Powell, T.L. Effects of maternal obesity on placental function and fetal development. *Reproduction* **2017**, *153*, R97–R108. [CrossRef] [PubMed]
223. Briana, D.D.; Malamitsi-Puchner, A. Reviews: Adipocytokines in normal and complicated pregnancies. *Reprod. Sci.* **2009**, *16*, 921–937. [CrossRef] [PubMed]
224. Mazaki-Tovi, S.; Romero, R.; Kim, S.K.; Vaisbuch, E.; Kusanovic, J.P.; Erez, O.; Chaiworapongsa, T.; Gotsch, F.; Mittal, P.; Nhan-Chang, C.L.; et al. Could alterations in maternal plasma visfatin concentration participate in the phenotype definition of preeclampsia and SGA? *J. Matern. Fetal Neonatal. Med.* **2010**, *23*, 857–868. [CrossRef] [PubMed]
225. Plows, J.F.; Stanley, J.L.; Baker, P.N.; Reynolds, C.M.; Vickers, M.H. The Pathophysiology of Gestational Diabetes Mellitus. *Int. J. Mol. Sci.* **2018**, *19*, 3342. [CrossRef] [PubMed]
226. Parsons, J.A.; Brelje, T.C.; Sorenson, R.L. Adaptation of islets of Langerhans to pregnancy: Increased islet cell proliferation and insulin secretion correlates with the onset of placental lactogen secretion. *Endocrinology* **1992**, *130*, 1459–1466. [CrossRef] [PubMed]
227. Retnakaran, R.; Ye, C.; Connelly, P.W.; Hanley, A.J.; Sermer, M.; Zinman, B. Impact of Changes Over Time in Adipokines and Inflammatory Proteins on Changes in Insulin Sensitivity, Beta-Cell Function, and Glycemia in Women with Previous Gestational Dysglycemia. *Diabetes Care* **2017**, *40*, e101–e102. [CrossRef] [PubMed]
228. Hare, K.J.; Bonde, L.; Svare, J.A.; Randeva, H.S.; Asmar, M.; Larsen, S.; Vilsboll, T.; Knop, F.K. Decreased plasma chemerin levels in women with gestational diabetes mellitus. *Diabet. Med.* **2014**, *31*, 936–940. [CrossRef]
229. Zhou, Z.; Chen, H.; Ju, H.; Sun, M. Circulating chemerin levels and gestational diabetes mellitus: A systematic review and meta-analysis. *Lipids Health Dis.* **2018**, *17*, 169. [CrossRef]

230. Fasshauer, M.; Bluher, M.; Stumvoll, M. Adipokines in gestational diabetes. *Lancet Diabetes Endocrinol.* **2014**, *2*, 488–499. [CrossRef]
231. Van Poppel, M.N.; Zeck, W.; Ulrich, D.; Schest, E.C.; Hirschmugl, B.; Lang, U.; Wadsack, C.; Desoye, G. Cord blood chemerin: Differential effects of gestational diabetes mellitus and maternal obesity. *Clin. Endocrinol. (Oxf.)* **2014**, *80*, 65–72. [CrossRef] [PubMed]
232. Krzyzanowska, K.; Krugluger, W.; Mittermayer, F.; Rahman, R.; Haider, D.; Shnawa, N.; Schernthaner, G. Increased visfatin concentrations in women with gestational diabetes mellitus. *Clin. Sci. (Lond.)* **2006**, *110*, 605–609. [CrossRef] [PubMed]
233. Lewandowski, K.C.; Stojanovic, N.; Press, M.; Tuck, S.M.; Szosland, K.; Bienkiewicz, M.; Vatish, M.; Lewinski, A.; Prelevic, G.M.; Randeva, H.S. Elevated serum levels of visfatin in gestational diabetes: A comparative study across various degrees of glucose tolerance. *Diabetologia* **2007**, *50*, 1033–1037. [CrossRef] [PubMed]
234. Mazaki-Tovi, S.; Romero, R.; Kusanovic, J.P.; Vaisbuch, E.; Erez, O.; Than, N.G.; Chaiworapongsa, T.; Nhan-Chang, C.L.; Pacora, P.; Gotsch, F.; et al. Maternal visfatin concentration in normal pregnancy. *J. Perinat. Med.* **2009**, *37*, 206–217. [CrossRef] [PubMed]
235. Ferreira, A.F.; Rezende, J.C.; Vaikousi, E.; Akolekar, R.; Nicolaides, K.H. Maternal serum visfatin at 11–13 weeks of gestation in gestational diabetes mellitus. *Clin. Chem.* **2011**, *57*, 609–613. [CrossRef] [PubMed]
236. Haider, D.G.; Handisurya, A.; Storka, A.; Vojtassakova, E.; Luger, A.; Pacini, G.; Tura, A.; Wolzt, M.; Kautzky-Willer, A. Visfatin response to glucose is reduced in women with gestational diabetes mellitus. *Diabetes Care* **2007**, *30*, 1889–1891. [CrossRef]
237. Akturk, M.; Altinova, A.E.; Mert, I.; Buyukkagnici, U.; Sargin, A.; Arslan, M.; Danisman, N. Visfatin concentration is decreased in women with gestational diabetes mellitus in the third trimester. *J. Endocrinol. Investig.* **2008**, *31*, 610–613. [CrossRef]
238. Kuzmicki, M.; Telejko, B.; Szamatowicz, J.; Zonenberg, A.; Nikolajuk, A.; Kretowski, A.; Gorska, M. High resistin and interleukin-6 levels are associated with gestational diabetes mellitus. *Gynecol. Endocrinol.* **2009**, *25*, 258–263. [CrossRef]
239. Megia, A.; Vendrell, J.; Gutierrez, C.; Sabate, M.; Broch, M.; Fernandez-Real, J.M.; Simon, I. Insulin sensitivity and resistin levels in gestational diabetes mellitus and after parturition. *Eur. J. Endocrinol.* **2008**, *158*, 173–178. [CrossRef]
240. Abell, S.K.; De Courten, B.; Boyle, J.A.; Teede, H.J. Inflammatory and Other Biomarkers: Role in Pathophysiology and Prediction of Gestational Diabetes Mellitus. *Int. J. Mol. Sci.* **2015**, *16*, 13442–13473. [CrossRef]
241. Lowe, L.P.; Metzger, B.E.; Lowe, W.L., Jr.; Dyer, A.R.; McDade, T.W.; McIntyre, H.D.; HAPO Study Cooperative Research Group. Inflammatory mediators and glucose in pregnancy: Results from a subset of the Hyperglycemia and Adverse Pregnancy Outcome (HAPO) Study. *J. Clin. Endocrinol. Metab.* **2010**, *95*, 5427–5434. [CrossRef] [PubMed]
242. Lobo, T.F.; Torloni, M.R.; Gueuvoghlanian-Silva, B.Y.; Mattar, R.; Daher, S. Resistin concentration and gestational diabetes: A systematic review of the literature. *J. Reprod. Immunol.* **2013**, *97*, 120–127. [CrossRef] [PubMed]
243. Lappas, M.; Yee, K.; Permezel, M.; Rice, G.E. Release and regulation of leptin, resistin and adiponectin from human placenta, fetal membranes, and maternal adipose tissue and skeletal muscle from normal and gestational diabetes mellitus-complicated pregnancies. *J. Endocrinol.* **2005**, *186*, 457–465. [CrossRef] [PubMed]
244. Telejko, B.; Kuzmicki, M.; Wawrusiewicz-Kurylonek, N.; Szamatowicz, J.; Nikolajuk, A.; Zonenberg, A.; Zwierz-Gugala, D.; Jelski, W.; Laudanski, P.; Wilczynski, J.; et al. Plasma apelin levels and apelin/APJ mRNA expression in patients with gestational diabetes mellitus. *Diabetes Res. Clin. Pr.* **2010**, *87*, 176–183. [CrossRef] [PubMed]
245. Abalos, E.; Cuesta, C.; Grosso, A.L.; Chou, D.; Say, L. Global and regional estimates of preeclampsia and eclampsia: A systematic review. *Eur. J. Obstet. Gynecol. Reprod. Biol.* **2013**, *170*, 1–7. [CrossRef] [PubMed]
246. Miehle, K.; Stepan, H.; Fasshauer, M. Leptin, adiponectin and other adipokines in gestational diabetes mellitus and pre-eclampsia. *Clin. Endocrinol. (Oxf.)* **2012**, *76*, 2–11. [CrossRef] [PubMed]
247. Mayrink, J.; Costa, M.L.; Cecatti, J.G. Preeclampsia in 2018: Revisiting Concepts, Physiopathology, and Prediction. *Sci. World J.* **2018**, *2018*, 6268276. [CrossRef]

248. Sibai, B.; Dekker, G.; Kupferminc, M. Pre-eclampsia. *Lancet* **2005**, *365*, 785–799. [CrossRef]
249. Mannisto, T.; Mendola, P.; Vaarasmaki, M.; Jarvelin, M.R.; Hartikainen, A.L.; Pouta, A.; Suvanto, E. Elevated blood pressure in pregnancy and subsequent chronic disease risk. *Circulation* **2013**, *127*, 681–690. [CrossRef]
250. Duan, D.M.; Niu, J.M.; Lei, Q.; Lin, X.H.; Chen, X. Serum levels of the adipokine chemerin in preeclampsia. *J. Perinat. Med.* **2011**, *40*, 121–127. [CrossRef]
251. Fasshauer, M.; Bluher, M.; Stumvoll, M.; Tonessen, P.; Faber, R.; Stepan, H. Differential regulation of visfatin and adiponectin in pregnancies with normal and abnormal placental function. *Clin. Endocrinol. (Oxf.)* **2007**, *66*, 434–439. [CrossRef] [PubMed]
252. Fasshauer, M.; Waldeyer, T.; Seeger, J.; Schrey, S.; Ebert, T.; Kratzsch, J.; Lossner, U.; Bluher, M.; Stumvoll, M.; Faber, R.; et al. Serum levels of the adipokine visfatin are increased in pre-eclampsia. *Clin. Endocrinol. (Oxf.)* **2008**, *69*, 69–73. [CrossRef] [PubMed]
253. Adali, E.; Yildizhan, R.; Kolusari, A.; Kurdoglu, M.; Bugdayci, G.; Sahin, H.G.; Kamaci, M. Increased visfatin and leptin in pregnancies complicated by pre-eclampsia. *J. Matern. Fetal Neonatal Med.* **2009**, *22*, 873–879. [CrossRef] [PubMed]
254. Hu, W.; Wang, Z.; Wang, H.; Huang, H.; Dong, M. Serum visfatin levels in late pregnancy and pre-eclampsia. *Acta Obstet. Gynecol. Scand.* **2008**, *87*, 413–418. [CrossRef] [PubMed]
255. Sartori, C.; Lazzeroni, P.; Merli, S.; Patianna, V.D.; Viaroli, F.; Cirillo, F.; Amarri, S.; Street, M.E. From Placenta to Polycystic Ovarian Syndrome: The Role of Adipokines. *Mediat. Inflamm.* **2016**, *2016*, 4981916. [CrossRef] [PubMed]
256. Haugen, F.; Ranheim, T.; Harsem, N.K.; Lips, E.; Staff, A.C.; Drevon, C.A. Increased plasma levels of adipokines in preeclampsia: Relationship to placenta and adipose tissue gene expression. *Am. J. Physiol. Endocrinol. Metab.* **2006**, *290*, E326–E333. [CrossRef] [PubMed]
257. Hendler, I.; Blackwell, S.C.; Mehta, S.H.; Whitty, J.E.; Russell, E.; Sorokin, Y.; Cotton, D.B. The levels of leptin, adiponectin, and resistin in normal weight, overweight, and obese pregnant women with and without preeclampsia. *Am. J. Obstet. Gynecol.* **2005**, *193*, 979–983. [CrossRef]
258. Bokarewa, M.; Nagaev, I.; Dahlberg, L.; Smith, U.; Tarkowski, A. Resistin, an adipokine with potent proinflammatory properties. *J. Immunol.* **2005**, *174*, 5789–5795. [CrossRef]
259. Yamaleyeva, L.M.; Chappell, M.C.; Brosnihan, K.B.; Anton, L.; Caudell, D.L.; Shi, S.; McGee, C.; Pirro, N.; Gallagher, P.E.; Taylor, R.N.; et al. Downregulation of apelin in the human placental chorionic villi from preeclamptic pregnancies. *Am. J. Physiol. Endocrinol. Metab.* **2015**, *309*, E852–E860. [CrossRef]
260. Malamitsi-Puchner, A.; Briana, D.D.; Boutsikou, M.; Kouskouni, E.; Hassiakos, D.; Gourgiotis, D. Perinatal circulating visfatin levels in intrauterine growth restriction. *Pediatrics* **2007**, *119*, e1314–e1318. [CrossRef]
261. Kucur, M.; Tuten, A.; Oncul, M.; Acikgoz, A.S.; Yuksel, M.A.; Imamoglu, M.; Balci Ekmekci, O.; Yilmaz, N.; Madazli, R. Maternal serum apelin and YKL-40 levels in early and late-onset pre-eclampsia. *Hypertens. Pregnancy* **2014**, *33*, 467–475. [CrossRef] [PubMed]
262. Bortoff, K.D.; Qiu, C.; Runyon, S.; Williams, M.A.; Maitra, R. Decreased maternal plasma apelin concentrations in preeclampsia. *Hypertens. Pregnancy* **2012**, *31*, 398–404. [CrossRef] [PubMed]
263. Wang, C.; Liu, X.; Kong, D.; Qin, X.; Li, Y.; Teng, X.; Huang, X. Apelin as a novel drug for treating preeclampsia. *Exp. Ther. Med.* **2017**, *14*, 5917–5923. [CrossRef] [PubMed]
264. Ho, L.; van Dijk, M.; Chye, S.T.J.; Messerschmidt, D.M.; Chng, S.C.; Ong, S.; Yi, L.K.; Boussata, S.; Goh, G.H.; Afink, G.B.; et al. ELABELA deficiency promotes preeclampsia and cardiovascular malformations in mice. *Science* **2017**, *357*, 707–713. [CrossRef] [PubMed]
265. Zhou, Q.; Zhang, K.; Guo, Y.; Chen, L.; Li, L. Elabela-APJ axis contributes to embryonic development and prevents pre-eclampsia in pregnancy. *Acta Biochim. Biophys. Sin. (Shanghai)* **2018**, *50*, 319–321. [CrossRef]
266. Pritchard, N.; Kaitu'u-Lino, T.J.; Gong, S.; Dopierala, J.; Smith, G.C.S.; Charnock-Jones, D.S.; Tong, S. ELABELA/APELA Levels Are Not Decreased in the Maternal Circulation or Placenta among Women with Preeclampsia. *Am. J. Pathol.* **2018**, *188*, 1749–1753. [CrossRef] [PubMed]
267. Miller, S.L.; Huppi, P.S.; Mallard, C. The consequences of fetal growth restriction on brain structure and neurodevelopmental outcome. *J. Physiol.* **2016**, *594*, 807–823. [CrossRef]
268. Malhotra, A.; Allison, B.J.; Castillo-Melendez, M.; Jenkin, G.; Polglase, G.R.; Miller, S.L. Neonatal Morbidities of Fetal Growth Restriction: Pathophysiology and Impact. *Front. Endocrinol. (Lausanne)* **2019**, *10*, 55. [CrossRef]
269. Brodsky, D.; Christou, H. Current concepts in intrauterine growth restriction. *J. Intensiv. Care Med.* **2004**, *19*, 307–319. [CrossRef]

270. Goto, E. Blood adiponectin concentration at birth in small for gestational age neonates: A meta-analysis. *Diabetes Metab. Syndr. Clin. Res. Rev.* **2019**, *13*, 183–188. [CrossRef]
271. Ibanez, L.; Sebastiani, G.; Lopez-Bermejo, A.; Diaz, M.; Gomez-Roig, M.D.; de Zegher, F. Gender specificity of body adiposity and circulating adiponectin, visfatin, insulin, and insulin growth factor-I at term birth: Relation to prenatal growth. *J. Clin. Endocrinol. Metab.* **2008**, *93*, 2774–2778. [CrossRef] [PubMed]
272. Rotteveel, J.; van Weissenbruch, M.M.; Twisk, J.W.; Delemarre-Van de Waal, H.A. Infant and childhood growth patterns, insulin sensitivity, and blood pressure in prematurely born young adults. *Pediatrics* **2008**, *122*, 313–321. [CrossRef] [PubMed]
273. Wang, J.; Shang, L.X.; Dong, X.; Wang, X.; Wu, N.; Wang, S.H.; Zhang, F.; Xu, L.M.; Xiao, Y. Relationship of adiponectin and resistin levels in umbilical serum, maternal serum and placenta with neonatal birth weight. *Aust. N. Z. J. Obstet. Gynaecol.* **2010**, *50*, 432–438. [CrossRef] [PubMed]
274. Martos-Moreno, G.A.; Barrios, V.; Saenz de Pipaon, M.; Pozo, J.; Dorronsoro, I.; Martinez-Biarge, M.; Quero, J.; Argente, J. Influence of prematurity and growth restriction on the adipokine profile, IGF1, and ghrelin levels in cord blood: Relationship with glucose metabolism. *Eur. J. Endocrinol.* **2009**, *161*, 381–389. [CrossRef] [PubMed]
275. Struwe, E.; Berzl, G.M.; Schild, R.L.; Dotsch, J. Gene expression of placental hormones regulating energy balance in small for gestational age neonates. *Eur. J. Obstet. Gynecol. Reprod. Biol.* **2009**, *142*, 38–42. [CrossRef] [PubMed]
276. Yeung, E.H.; McLain, A.C.; Anderson, N.; Lawrence, D.; Boghossian, N.S.; Druschel, C.; Bell, E. Newborn Adipokines and Birth Outcomes. *Paediatr. Perinat. Epidemiol.* **2015**, *29*, 317–325. [CrossRef] [PubMed]
277. Syriou, V.; Papanikolaou, D.; Kozyraki, A.; Goulis, D.G. Cytokines and male infertility. *Eur. Cytokine Netw.* **2018**, *29*, 73–82. [CrossRef] [PubMed]
278. Wagner, I.V.; Yango, P.; Svechnikov, K.; Tran, N.D.; Soder, O. Adipocytokines may delay pubertal maturation of human Sertoli cells. *Reprod. Fertil. Dev.* **2019**. [CrossRef]
279. Bobjer, J.; Katrinaki, M.; Dermitzaki, E.; Margioris, A.N.; Giwercman, A.; Tsatsanis, C. Serum chemerin levels are negatively associated with male fertility and reproductive hormones. *Hum. Reprod.* **2018**, *33*, 2168–2174. [CrossRef] [PubMed]
280. Moretti, E.; Collodel, G.; Mazzi, L.; Campagna, M.; Iacoponi, F.; Figura, N. Resistin, interleukin-6, tumor necrosis factor-alpha, and human semen parameters in the presence of leukocytospermia, smoking habit, and varicocele. *Fertil. Steril.* **2014**, *102*, 354–360. [CrossRef]
281. Abdel-Fadeil, M.R.; Abd Allah, E.S.H.; Iraqy, H.M.; Elgamal, D.A.; Abdel-Ghani, M.A. Experimental obesity and diabetes reduce male fertility: Potential involvement of hypothalamic Kiss-1, pituitary nitric oxide, serum vaspin and visfatin. *Pathophysiology* **2019**. [CrossRef] [PubMed]

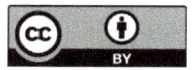

© 2019 by the authors. Licensee MDPI, Basel, Switzerland. This article is an open access article distributed under the terms and conditions of the Creative Commons Attribution (CC BY) license (http://creativecommons.org/licenses/by/4.0/).

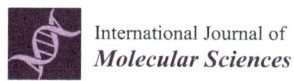

Article

Expression of Chemerin and Its Receptors in the Porcine Hypothalamus and Plasma Chemerin Levels during the Oestrous Cycle and Early Pregnancy

Nina Smolinska, Marta Kiezun, Kamil Dobrzyn, Edyta Rytelewska, Katarzyna Kisielewska, Marlena Gudelska, Ewa Zaobidna, Krystyna Bogus-Nowakowska, Joanna Wyrebek, Kinga Bors, Grzegorz Kopij, Barbara Kaminska and Tadeusz Kaminski *

Department of Animal Anatomy and Physiology, Faculty of Biology and Biotechnology, University of Warmia and Mazury in Olsztyn, Oczapowskiego 1A, 10-719 Olsztyn-Kortowo, Poland;
nina.smolinska@uwm.edu.pl (N.S.); marta.kiezun@uwm.edu.pl (M.K.); kamil.dobrzyn@uwm.edu.pl (K.D.);
edyta.rytelewska@uwm.edu.pl (E.R.); katarzyna.kisielewska@uwm.edu.pl (K.K.);
marlena.gudelska@uwm.edu.pl (M.G.); ewa.zaobidna@uwm.edu.pl (E.Z.); boguska@uwm.edu.pl (K.B.-N.);
joanna.wyrebek@uwm.edu.pl (J.W.); kinga.bors@uwm.edu.pl (K.B.); grzegorzkopij@gmail.com (G.K.);
barbara.kaminska@uwm.edu.pl (B.K.)
* Correspondence: tkam@uwm.edu.pl

Received: 22 July 2019; Accepted: 6 August 2019; Published: 9 August 2019

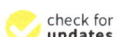

Abstract: Chemerin (CHEM) may act as an important link integrating energy homeostasis and reproductive functions of females, and its actions are mediated by three receptors: chemokine-like receptor 1 (CMKLR1), G protein-coupled receptor 1 (GPR1), and C-C motif chemokine receptor-like 2 (CCRL2). The aim of the current study was to compare the expression of CHEM and its receptor (CHEM system) mRNAs (quantitative real-time PCR) and proteins (Western blotting and fluorescent immunohistochemistry) in the selected areas of the porcine hypothalamus responsible for gonadotropin-releasing hormone production and secretion: the mediobasal hypothalamus, preoptic area and stalk median eminence during the oestrous cycle and early pregnancy. Moreover, plasma CHEM concentrations were determined using ELISA. The expression of CHEM system has been demonstrated in the porcine hypothalamus throughout the luteal phase and follicular phase of the oestrous cycle, and during early pregnancy from days 10 to 28. Plasma CHEM levels and concentrations of transcripts and proteins of CHEM system components in the hypothalamus fluctuated throughout pregnancy and the oestrous cycle. Our study was the first experiment to demonstrate the presence of CHEM system mRNAs and proteins in the porcine hypothalamus and the correlations between the expression levels and physiological hormonal milieu related to the oestrous cycle and early pregnancy.

Keywords: chemerin; chemerin receptors; hypothalamus; oestrous cycle; early pregnancy; pig

1. Introduction

Chemerin (CHEM), encoded by the gene retinoic acid receptor responder 2 (*RARRES2*) or tazarotene-induced gene 2 (*TIG2*), is a chemotactic factor for immune cells engaged in the processes of innate and acquired immunity [1]. CHEM is also an adipokine protein produced and secreted by the adipose tissue, which is considered to be involved in the major metabolic and inflammatory processes [2,3]. In mammalian cells, CHEM is initially synthesised as a 163 amino acid (aa) pre-prochemerin. The N-terminal truncation of 20 aa signal peptide results in the release of 143 residue prochemerin into the blood. Several isoforms of CHEM have been reported that are dependent on the proteolytic cleavage at its C-terminus by various serine and cysteine proteases. Thus, this process serves as a key regulatory mechanism to determine the local and systemic concentrations of active CHEM which exerts local biological actions [4]. In the plasma from healthy humans, inert CHEM precursor is the dominant isoform. However, the different CHEM isoforms in human blood (CHEM-A155, -S157 and -K158), cerebrospinal fluid (CHEM-K158), hemofiltrate (CHEM-F154) and synovial fluid (CHEM-K158) have also been reported, thus indicating that complex prochemerin processing occurs in vivo [5].

CHEM binds with three G-protein coupled receptors: chemokine-like receptor 1 (CMKLR1), in humans also termed as chemerin receptor 23 (ChemR23), G protein-coupled receptor 1 (GPR1), and C-C motif chemokine receptor-like 2 (CCRL2). Of these, CMKLR1 has been the best investigated, and it uses ERK1/2 and Akt kinases for signal transduction. GPR1 is structurally similar to CMKLR1 but its biological function has not been fully investigated. Nevertheless, GPR1 probably has different functions from CMKLR1, because of its presence in different tissues. CCRL2 is clearly different from the two other receptors. It is unable to transduce signals, but binds the N-terminal region of CHEM, exposing the C-terminal region of the hormone molecule to CMKLR1 receptors on the adjacent cells. Therefore, its role is limited to presenting the adipokine to the neighbouring cells with CMKLR1 receptors. The various CHEM isoforms are implied to regulate a biochemical cascade by competition binding to the corresponding receptors. Of these, CHEM-S157 and CHEM-F156 demonstrate the highest affinity to CMKLR1, while other isoforms such as prochemerin, CHEM-K158, or CHEM-F154 bind to the receptor with lower affinity (for review see [6]).

Of all four components of the CHEM system (the hormone and its three receptors), most studies have been focused on CHEM alone and CMKLR1. The adipokine mRNA expression was found mainly in the mouse liver, white adipose tissue and placenta, with lower levels also in the ovaries [2], and in the human liver and pancreas [7]. The expression of the *RARRES2* gene was also found in the ovaries of women [8] and rodents [2,9], and in the hypothalamus of mice and rats [10,11]. CMKLR1 gene expression in mice was detected mainly in the white adipose tissue, with lower levels found in the lungs, heart and placenta [2]. In humans, the highest expression of this receptor was identified in the lymph nodes and spleen [8]. The expression of CMKLR1 was identified in the ovaries of women [8] and rats [9], and in the hypothalamus of rats [11,12]. GPR1 is predominantly expressed in the central nervous system of humans [13] although the expression was also found in the mouse adipose tissue, human skin [14] and granulosa cells [8]. The third CHEM receptor, CCRL2, was also found in the hypothalamus of rats [11]. Most of the research focused on the expression of the CHEM system has been carried out on humans and rodents and data related to farm animals, including pigs, are still missing.

There is a close relationship between nutritional status and reproductive success in animals. The metabolic processes and reproductive system functions are controlled by a number of hormones. It can be assumed that in addition to hormones affecting only the selected metabolic processes or reproductive organs or structures, there are also other hormones creating a link controlling both the metabolic status and reproductive system functions. Based on sparse literature data, a hypothesis can be put forward that CHEM is one such hormone. CHEM is likely to have pleiotropic properties. It influences, for example, food intake, energy homeostasis, adipose tissue function, obesity-related parameters (BMI, blood pressure, cholesterol level), and modulates insulin sensitivity [6,15]. Reduced feed intake, body mass and adiposity, and higher glucose tolerance was found in mice with a disrupted *CMKLR1* gene as compared to the control animals [16]. Moreover, the adipokine is closely related to the female reproductive process. It was described as an important regulator of ovarian steroidogenesis and follicular development [8,9,17,18]. High circulating CHEM levels appear to be associated with pregnancy disorders such as polycystic ovary syndrome (PCOS) [19], pre-eclampsia [20] and endometriosis [21]. It has been also reported that CHEM production in the uterus is up-regulated during decidualization, and that CHEM could play a crucial role in vascular remodelling during early pregnancy of women [22].

In the existing body of research, there are no studies investigating the expression of the CHEM system in the hypothalamic structures responsible for the synthesis of gonadotropin-releasing hormone (GnRH) and the possible impact of hormonal status of the animals connected with the phase of the oestrous cycle and early pregnancy on CHEM and its receptors expression. For this reason, the aim of the present study was to investigate the expression of CHEM system genes and proteins in the specialised hypothalamic structures (mediobasal hypothalamus—MBH, preoptic area—POA, stalk median eminence—SME) involved in the synthesis and secretion of GnRH (the key hypothalamic factor controlling the pituitary gland and, indirectly, ovaries), and serum CHEM levels during the oestrous cycle and early pregnancy, associated with the implantation of embryos.

2. Results

2.1. The Distribution of CHEM, CMKLR1, GPR1 and CCRL2 in the Porcine Hypothalamus

The immunofluorescence staining has shown the presence of CHEM and its 3 receptors—CMKLR1, GPR1 and CCRL2—in some regions of the pig hypothalamus both during the oestrous cycle (days 10 to 12; Figures 1 and 2) as well as during early gestation (days 15 to 16 of pregnancy; Figures 3 and 4). CHEM-immunoreactive (CHEM-IR) (Figure 1G,H and Figure 3G,H), GPR1-immunoreactive (GPR1-IR) (Figure 1C,D and Figure 3C,D) and CCRL2-immunoreactive (CCRL2-IR) (Figure 1E,F and Figure 3E,F) neurons were the most abundant in the paraventricular nucleus, which is the part of MBH, both during early gestation and during the oestrous cycle. However, CMKLR1-immunoreactive (CMKLR1-IR) cells in this brain region displayed slightly weaker immunoreactivity (Figure 1A,B and Figure 3A,B). Other hypothalamic regions which showed immunoreactivity of CHEM and its receptors were the preoptic region (Figures 2 and 4) and the anterior hypothalamic area. POA exhibited high immunoreactivity of CHEM (Figure 2G,H and Figure 4G,H), GPR1 (Figure 2C,D and Figure 4C,D), CCRL2 (Figure 2E,F and Figure 4E,F) and CMKLR1 (Figure 2A,B and Figure 4A,B). In the anterior hypothalamic area, only single CHEM-IR and CMKLR1-IR cells were identified. Additionally, in the diagonal band of Broca, a part of POA, GPR1 showed very high immunoreactivity (Figure 4C), whereas CHEM-IR and CMKLR1-IR cells were observed sporadically.

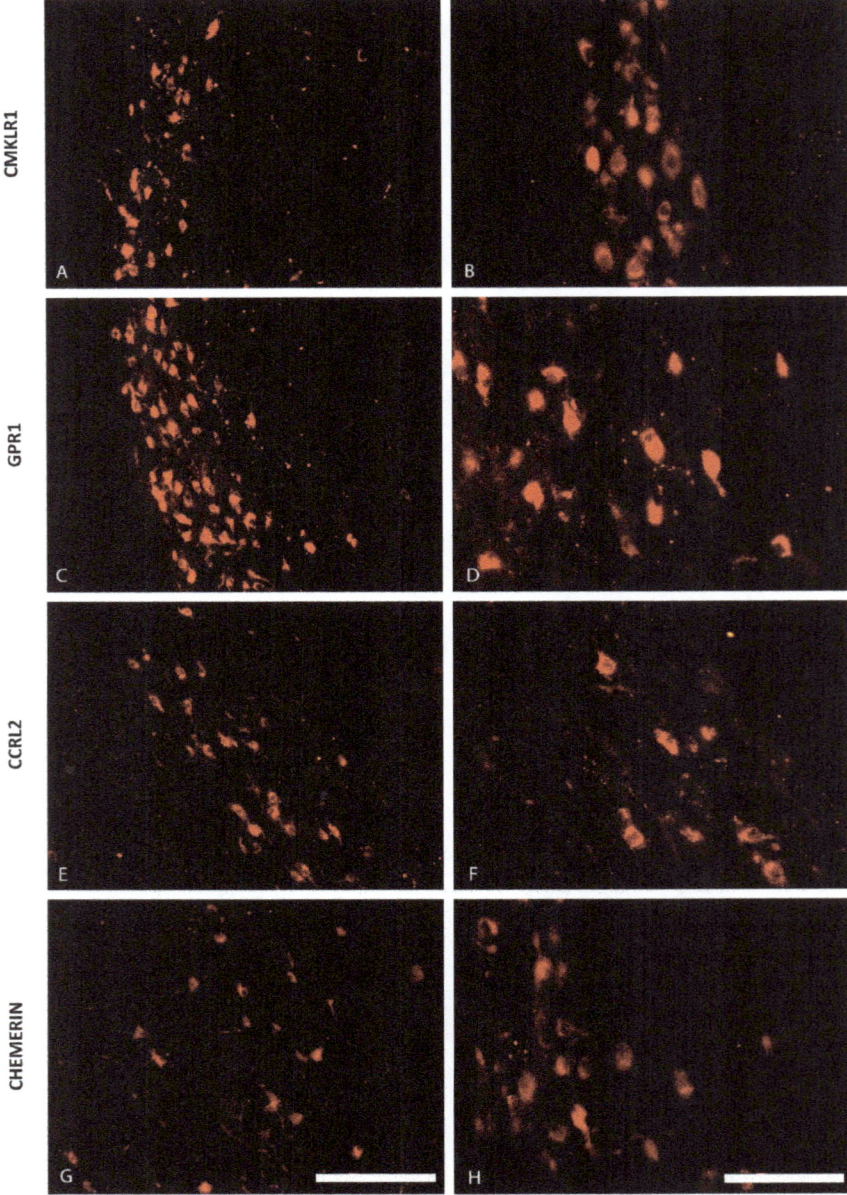

Figure 1. The distribution of the chemerin system in the porcine mediobasal hypothalamus (MBH) during the oestrous cycle. Immunoreactivity of chemokine-like receptor 1 (CMKLR1; **A** and **B**), G protein-coupled receptor 1 (GPR1; **C** and **D**), C-C motif chemokine receptor-like 2 (CCRL2; **E** and **F**) and chemerin (**G** and **H**) during the oestrous cycle (days 10 to 12) in the hypothalamus of the pig at the level of the paraventricular nucleus. Scale bar: 200 μm, applies to A, C, E, G; scale bar: 100 μm, applies to B, D, F, H.

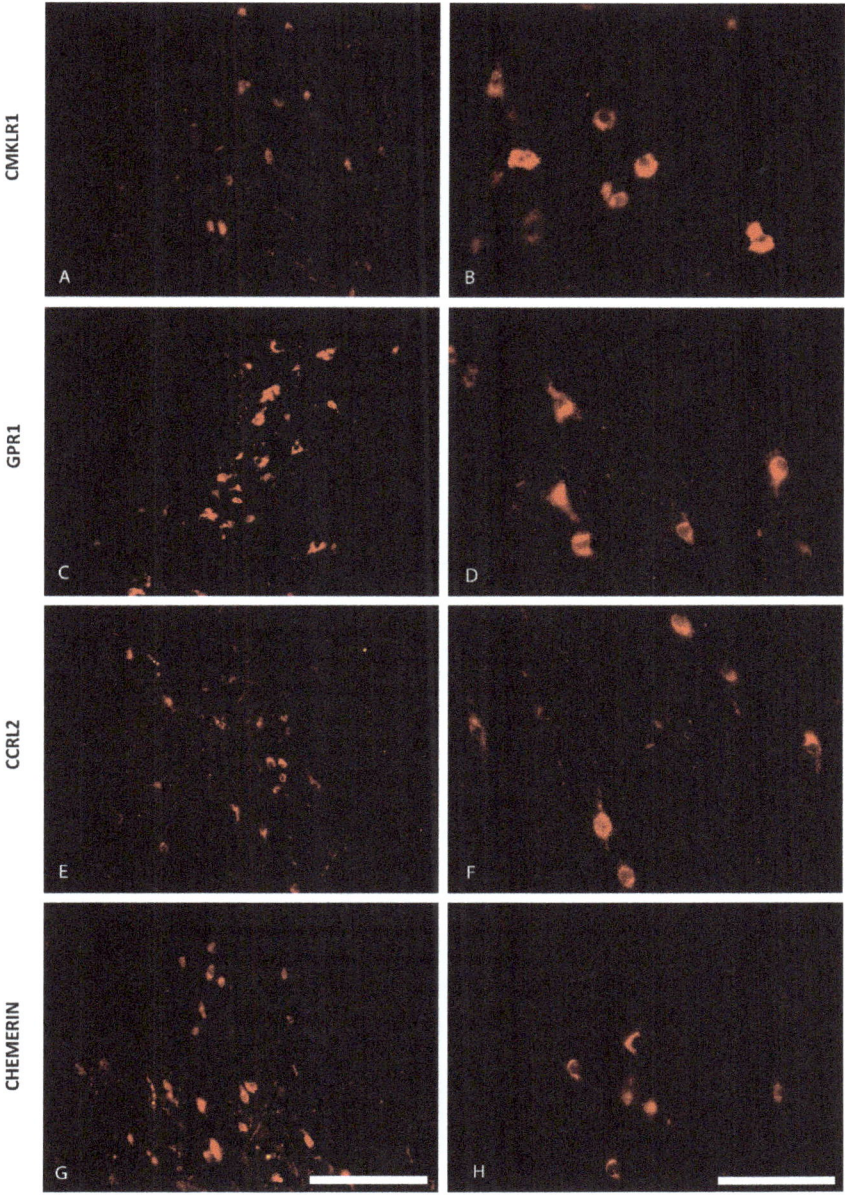

Figure 2. The distribution of the chemerin system in the porcine preoptic area (POA) during the oestrous cycle. Immunoreactivity of chemokine-like receptor 1 (CMKLR1; **A** and **B**), G protein-coupled receptor 1 (GPR1; **C** and **D**), C-C motif chemokine receptor-like 2 (CCRL2; **E** and **F**) and chemerin (**G** and **H**) during the oestrous cycle (days 10 to 12) in the hypothalamus of the pig at the level of the preoptic area. Scale bar: 200 μm, applies to A, C, E, G; scale bar: 100 μm, applies to B, D, F, H.

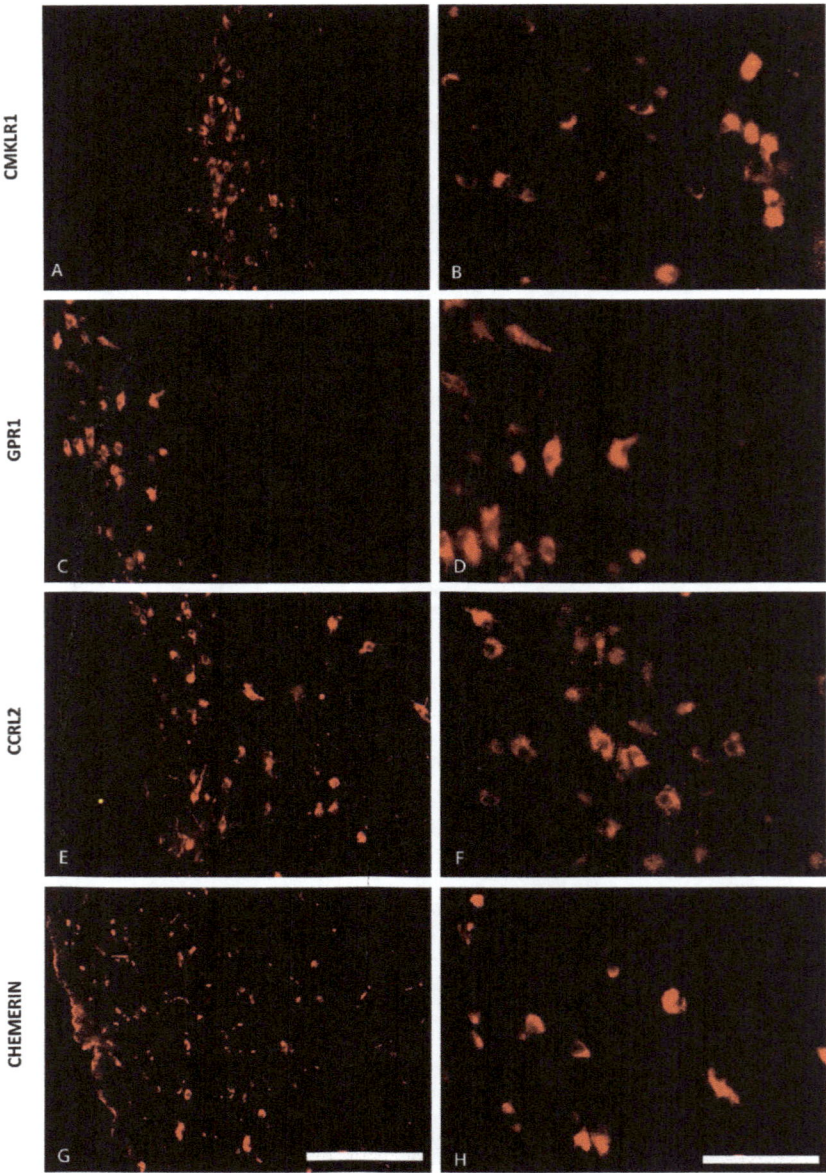

Figure 3. The distribution of the chemerin system in the porcine mediobasal hypothalamus (MBH) during early pregnancy. Immunoreactivity of chemokine-like receptor 1 (CMKLR1; **A** and **B**), G protein-coupled receptor 1 (GPR1; **C** and **D**), C-C motif chemokine receptor-like 2 (CCRL2; **E** and **F**) and chemerin (**G** and **H**) during early pregnancy (days 15 to 16) in the hypothalamus of the pig at the level of the paraventricular nucleus. Scale bar: 200 µm, applies to A, C, E, G; scale bar: 100 µm, applies to B, D, F, H.

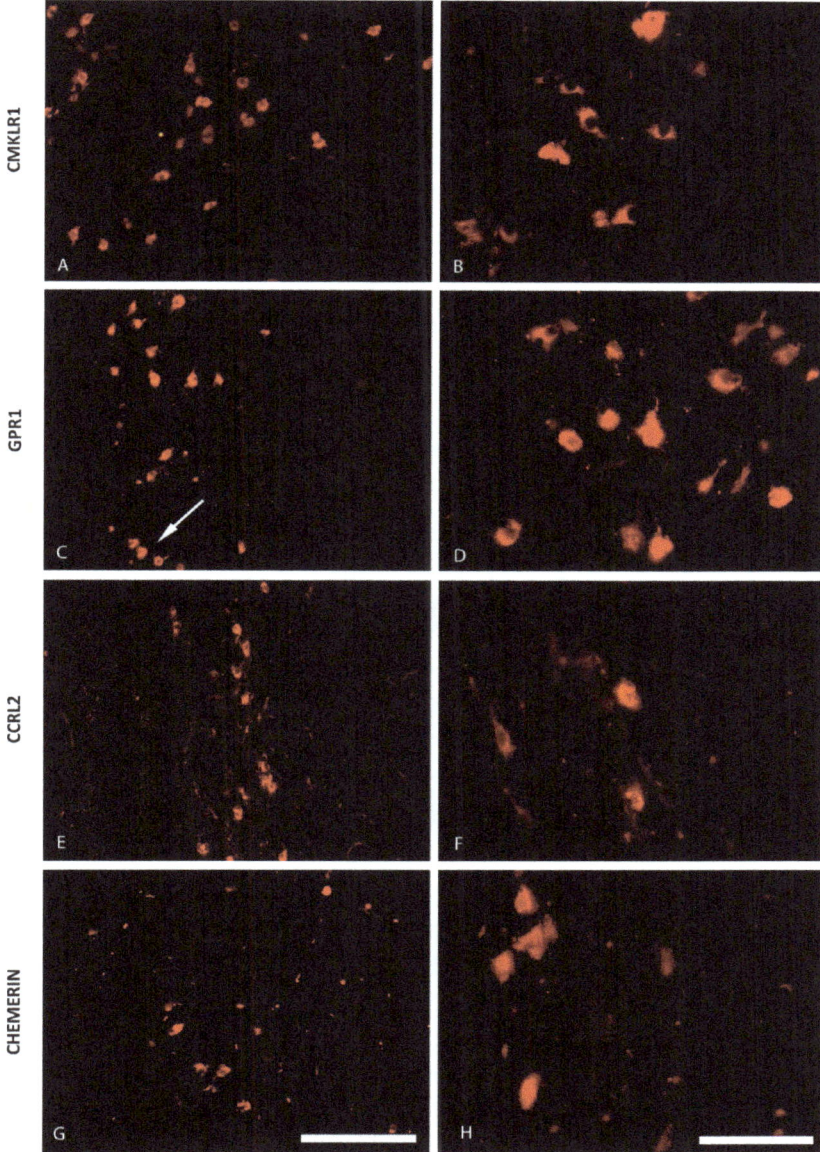

Figure 4. The distribution of the chemerin system in the porcine preoptic area (POA) during early pregnancy. Immunoreactivity of chemokine-like receptor 1 (CMKLR1; **A** and **B**), G protein-coupled receptor 1 (GPR1; **C** and **D**), C-C motif chemokine receptor-like 2 (CCRL2; **E** and **F**) and chemerin (**G** and **H**) during early pregnancy (days 15 to 16) in the hypothalamus of the pig at the level of the preoptic area. The white arrow indicates the diagonal band of Broca. Scale bar: 200 µm, applies to A, C, E, G; scale bar: 100 µm, applies to B, D, F, H.

2.2. CHEM System Gene and Protein Expression in MBH during the Oestrous Cycle

During the oestrous cycle, the concentrations of *CMKLR1* mRNA were significantly higher on days 17 to 19 when compared to days 2 to 3, whereas protein contents of this receptor were higher on days 10 to 12 of the cycle than in other studied periods of the cycle (Figure 5A,B; $p < 0.05$). *GPR1* gene expression during the cycle was the highest on days 2 to 3 in relation to days 14 to 16 and 17 to 19. The protein contents of GPR1 were the highest on days 17 to 19 when compared to other studied periods of the cycle ($p < 0.05$; Figure 5C,D). Higher *CCRL2* mRNA expression was noted on days 2 to 3 and 14 to 16, whereas protein contents of this receptor were greater on days 10 to 12 in comparison to days 2 to 3 and 14 to 16 ($p < 0.05$; Figure 5E,F). The highest expression of *RARRES2* was observed on days 2 to 3 and 10 to 12 when compared to days 17 to 19 of the cycle ($p < 0.05$; Figure 5G).

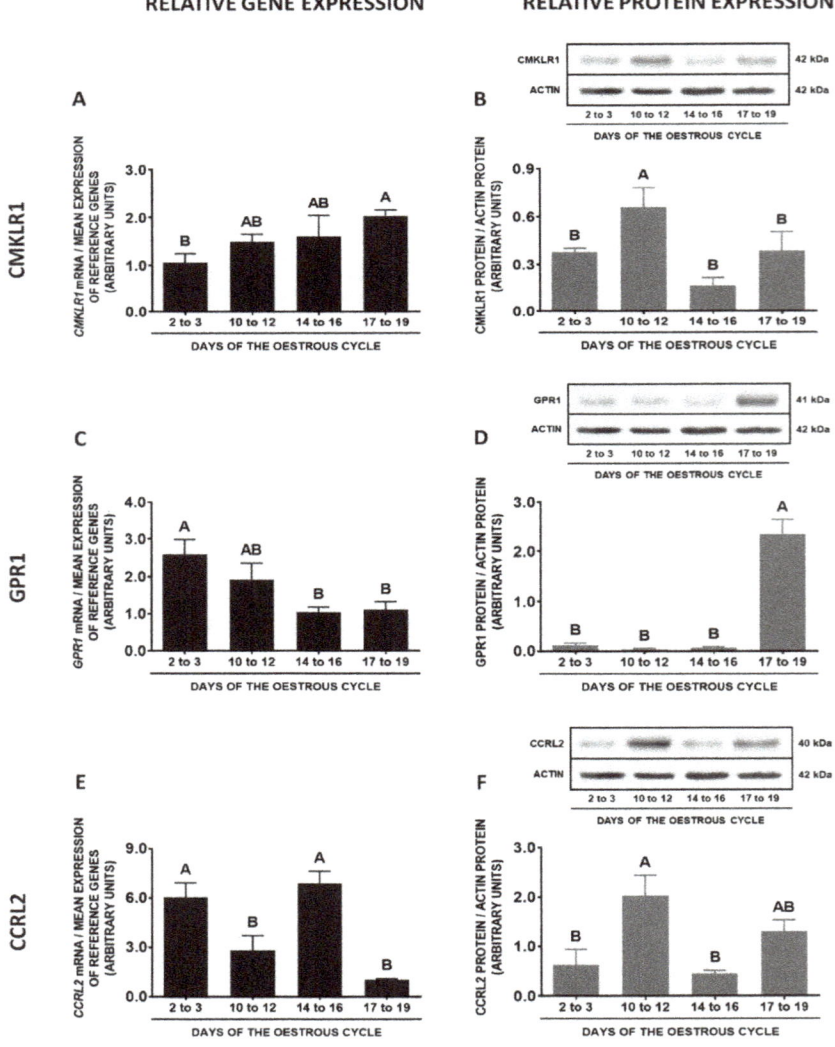

Figure 5. *Cont.*

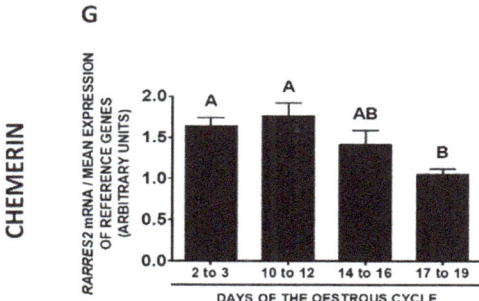

Figure 5. Chemerin system expression in the porcine mediobasal hypothalamus (MBH) during the oestrous cycle. Gene and protein expression of chemokine-like receptor 1 (CMKLR1; **A** and **B**), G protein-coupled receptor 1 (GPR1; **C** and **D**) and C-C motif chemokine receptor-like 2 (CCRL2; **E** and **F**), as well as chemerin (*RARRES2*) mRNA content (**G**) in the porcine MBH on days: 2 to 3, 10 to 12, 14 to 16 and 17 to 19 of the oestrous cycle. Gene expression was determined by qPCR. Protein expression was determined by Western blotting; upper panels: representative immunoblots; lower panels: densitometric analysis of CMKLR1/GPR1/CCRL2 proteins relative to actin protein. Representative actin blots are identical for all chemerin receptors though proteins have been analysed on different gels. Results are presented as means ± SEM ($n = 5$). Bars with different superscripts differ (one-way ANOVA at $p < 0.05$ followed by Tuckey *post-hoc* test at $p < 0.05$).

2.3. CHEM System Gene and Protein Expression in MBH during Pregnancy

During pregnancy, the highest *CMKLR* gene expression was observed on days 15 to 16, lower on days 12 to 13, and the lowest on days 10 to 11 and 27 to 28. CMKLR1 protein contents in MBH were greater on days 27 to 28 when compared to days 10 to 11 and 12 to 13 of gestation ($p < 0.05$; Figure 6A,B). The lowest *GPR1* gene expression was noted on days 10 to 11 in relation to other studied stages of pregnancy. Similarly, the lowest protein contents were observed on days 10 to 11, higher on days 15 to 16, and the highest on days 27 to 28 of pregnancy ($p < 0.05$; Figure 6C,D). The expression of *CCRL2* gene was higher on days 15 to 16 related to other studied periods of gestation, whereas protein contents were elevated on days 12 to 13 and 15 to 16 in comparison to days 10 to 11 ($p < 0.05$; Figure 6E,F). The highest expression of *RARRES2* gene was observed on days 12 to 13, lower on days 10 to 11, and the lowest on days 15 to 16 and 27 to 28 of pregnancy ($p < 0.05$; Figure 6G).

2.4. CHEM System Gene and Protein Expression in MBH—Pregnancy vs. Oestrous Cycle

Comparing the studied stages of early pregnancy and days 10 to 12 of the oestrous cycle, significantly higher expression of *CMKLR1* gene in MBH was observed on days 15 to 16 and 12 to 13 of gestation in relation to days 10 to 12 of the oestrous cycle. The protein concentrations of this receptor were lower on days 12 to 13 of gestation, compared to days 10 to 12 of the cycle ($p < 0.05$; Figure 7A,B). The expression of the *GPR1* gene was enhanced on days 12 to 13, 15 to 16 and 27 to 28 of pregnancy when compared to days 10 to 12 of the cycle. Significantly higher GPR1 protein contents were observed on days 27 to 28 and 15 to 16 of gestation in relation to days 10 to 12 of the oestrous cycle ($p < 0.05$; Figure 7C,D). The expression of the *CCRL2* gene was elevated on days 15 to 16 of pregnancy compared to the cycle. The protein contents of this receptor were higher on days 10 to 12 of the cycle compared to the studied stages of pregnancy ($p < 0.05$; Figure 7E,F). Higher levels of *RARRES2* mRNA contents were observed on days 10 to 12 of the cycle than during the studied stages of gestation ($p < 0.05$; Figure 7G).

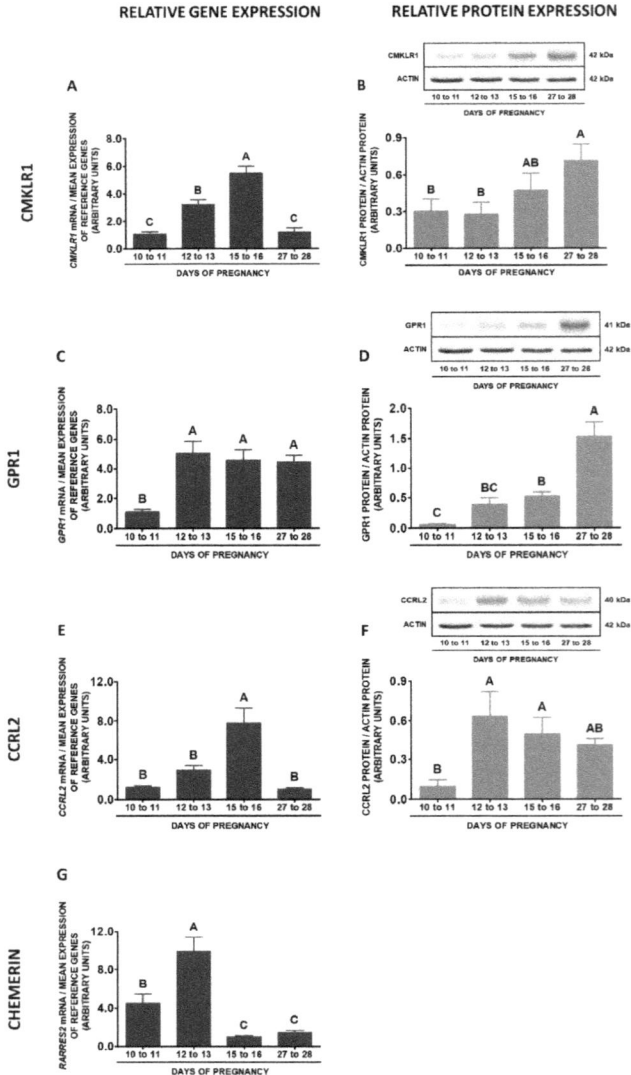

Figure 6. Chemerin system expression in the porcine mediobasal hypothalamus (MBH) during early pregnancy. Gene and protein expression of chemokine-like receptor 1 (CMKLR1; **A** and **B**), G protein-coupled receptor 1 (GPR1; **C** and **D**) and C-C motif chemokine receptor-like 2 (CCRL2; **E** and **F**), as well as chemerin (*RARRES2*) mRNA content (**G**) in the porcine MBH on days: 10 to 11, 12 to 13, 15 to 16 and 27 to 28 of pregnancy. Gene expression was determined by qPCR. Protein expression was determined by Western blotting; upper panels: representative immunoblots; lower panels: densitometric analysis of CMKLR1/GPR1/CCRL2 proteins relative to actin protein. Representative actin blots are identical for all chemerin receptors though proteins have been analysed on different gels. Results are presented as means ± SEM ($n = 5$). Bars with different superscripts differ (one-way ANOVA at $p < 0.05$ followed by Tuckey *post-hoc* test at $p < 0.05$).

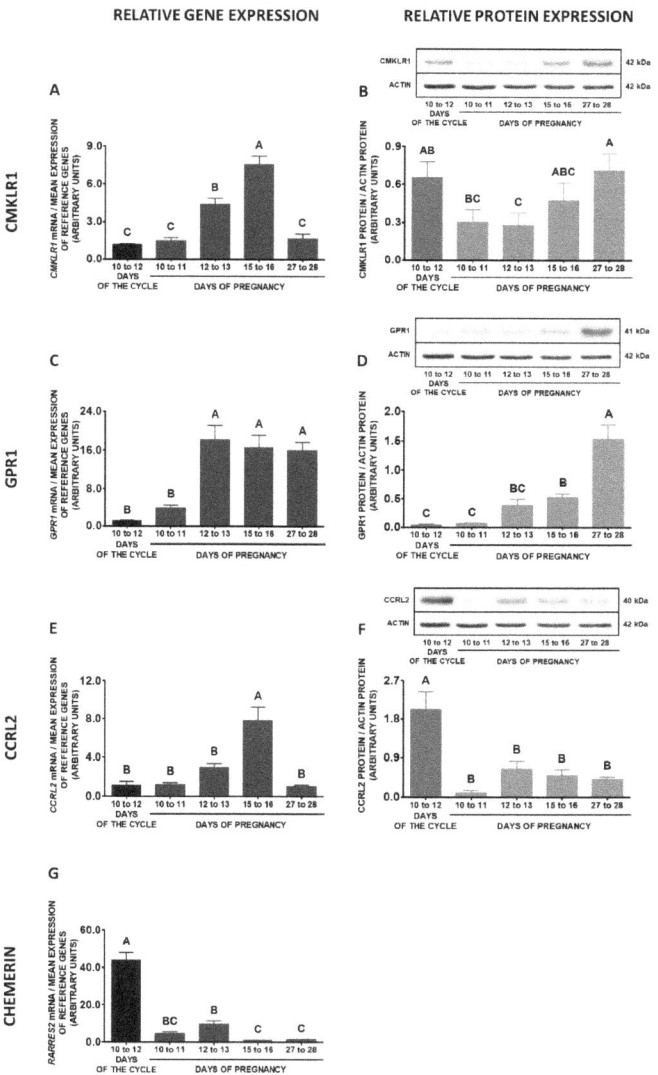

Figure 7. Chemerin system expression in the porcine mediobasal hypothalamus (MBH)—pregnancy vs. oestrous cycle. Gene and protein expression of chemokine-like receptor 1 (CMKLR1; **A** and **B**), G protein-coupled receptor 1 (GPR1; **C** and **D**) and C-C motif chemokine receptor-like 2 (CCRL2; **E** and **F**), as well as chemerin (*RARRES2*) mRNA content (**G**) in the porcine MBH on days: 10 to 11, 12 to 13, 15 to 16 and 27 to 28 of pregnancy, and on days 10 to 12 of the oestrous cycle. Gene expression was determined by qPCR. Protein expression was determined by Western blotting; upper panels: representative immunoblots; lower panels: densitometric analysis of CMKLR1/GPR1/CCRL2 proteins relative to actin protein. Representative actin blots are identical for all chemerin receptors though proteins have been analysed on different gels. Results are presented as means ± SEM ($n = 5$). Bars with different superscripts differ (one-way ANOVA at $p < 0.05$ followed by Tuckey *post-hoc* test at $p < 0.05$).

2.5. CHEM System Gene and Protein Expression in POA during the Oestrous Cycle

In the porcine POA, the highest *CMKLR1* gene expression was observed on days 17 to 19 of the cycle when compared to days 2 to 3 and 10 to 12, whereas the lowest on days 10 to 12 of the cycle in relation to days 14 to 16 and 17 to 19. The highest protein contents of this receptor were noted on days 10 to 12 compared to other phases of the cycle ($p < 0.05$; Figure 8A,B). Although the differences in *GPR1* gene expression between the studied phases of the oestrous cycle were negligible, the higher protein concentrations were observed on days 14 to 16 compared to days 2 to 3 and 17 to 19 of the cycle ($p < 0.05$; Figure 8C,D). The expression of the *CCRL2* gene was higher on days 17 to 19 than on days 14 to 16 of the oestrous cycle. The protein concentrations of CCRL2 were higher on days 10 to 12 compared to other phases of the cycle ($p < 0.05$; Figure 8E,F). In POA, higher *RARRES2* gene expression was noted on days 2 to 3 of the cycle than in the other studied phases of pregnancy ($p < 0.05$; Figure 8G).

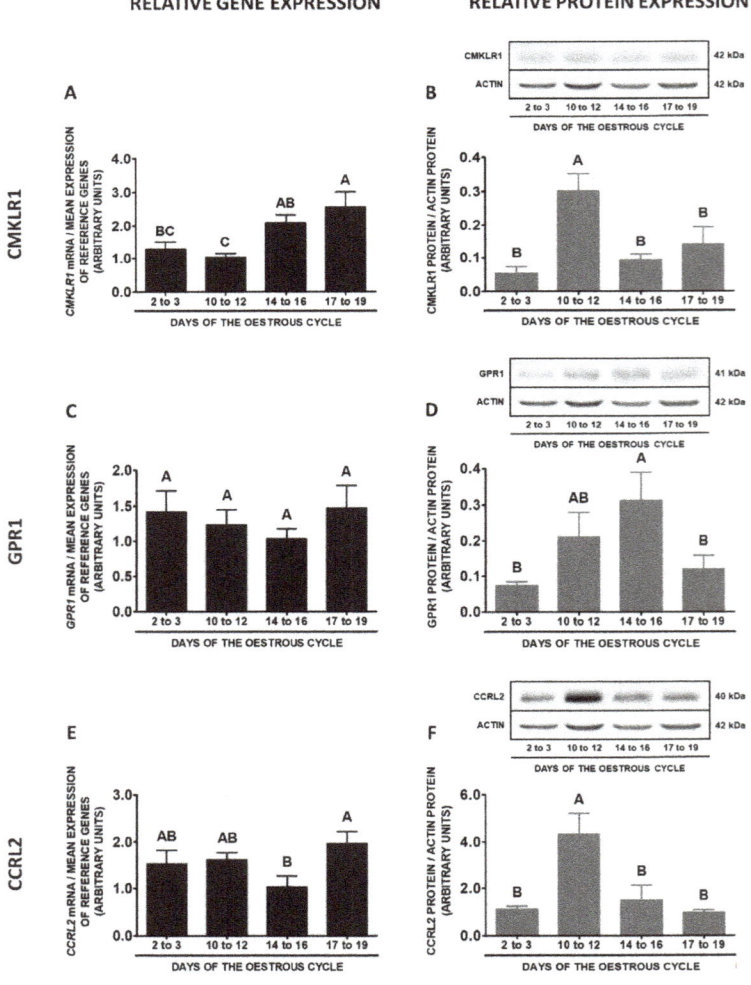

Figure 8. *Cont.*

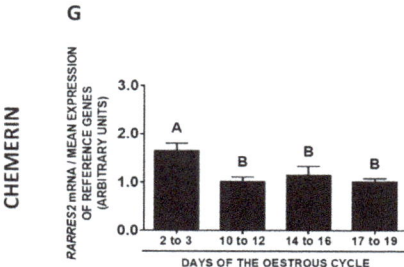

Figure 8. Chemerin system expression in the porcine preoptic area (POA) during the oestrous cycle. Gene and protein expression of chemokine-like receptor 1 (CMKLR1; **A** and **B**), G protein-coupled receptor 1 (GPR1; **C** and **D**) and C-C motif chemokine receptor-like 2 (CCRL2; **E** and **F**), as well as chemerin (*RARRES2*) mRNA content (**G**) in the porcine POA on days: 2 to 3, 10 to 12, 14 to 16 and 17 to 19 of the oestrous cycle. Gene expression was determined by qPCR. Protein expression was determined by Western blotting; upper panels: representative immunoblots; lower panels: densitometric analysis of CMKLR1/GPR1/CCRL2 proteins relative to actin protein. Representative actin blots are identical for all chemerin receptors though proteins have been analysed on different gels. Results are presented as means ± SEM ($n = 5$). Bars with different superscripts differ (one-way ANOVA at $p < 0.05$ followed by Tuckey *post-hoc* test at $p < 0.05$).

2.6. CHEM System Gene and Protein Expression in POA during Pregnancy

During early pregnancy in POA, the highest *CMKLR1* gene expression was observed on days 10 to 11, lower on days 27 to 28, and the lowest on days 15 to 16 when compared to days 10 to 11 and 27 to 28 of gestation. Protein contents of this receptor were higher on days 27 to 28 related to days 10 to 11 of pregnancy ($p < 0.05$; Figure 9A,B). The contents of the *GPR1* mRNA were the highest on days 27 to 28 compared to other stages of pregnancy, whereas the lowest on days 15 to 16 in relation to days 10 to 11 and 27 to 28 of gestation. Similarly, the highest protein concentrations of GPR1 were noted on days 27 to 28, lower on days 12 to 13 and the lowest on days 10 to 11 and 15 to 16 of pregnancy ($p < 0.05$; Figure 9C,D). The expression of the *CCRL2* gene in this tissue was the highest on days 27 to 28, lower on days 10 to 11, whereas the lowest on days 12 to 13 and 15 to 16 of gestation. The protein concentrations of this receptor were higher on days 27 to 28 than on days 10 to 11 of pregnancy ($p < 0.05$; Figure 9E,F). The expression of the *RARRES2* gene was much more pronounced on days 27 to 28 than in other studied stages of pregnancy ($p < 0.05$; Figure 9G).

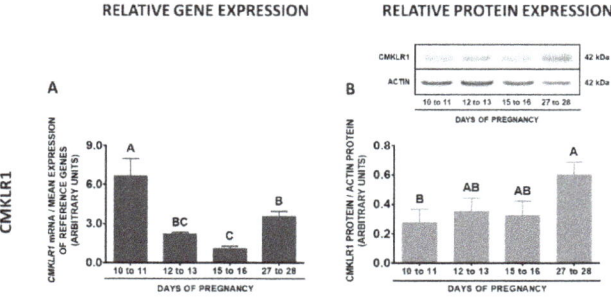

Figure 9. *Cont.*

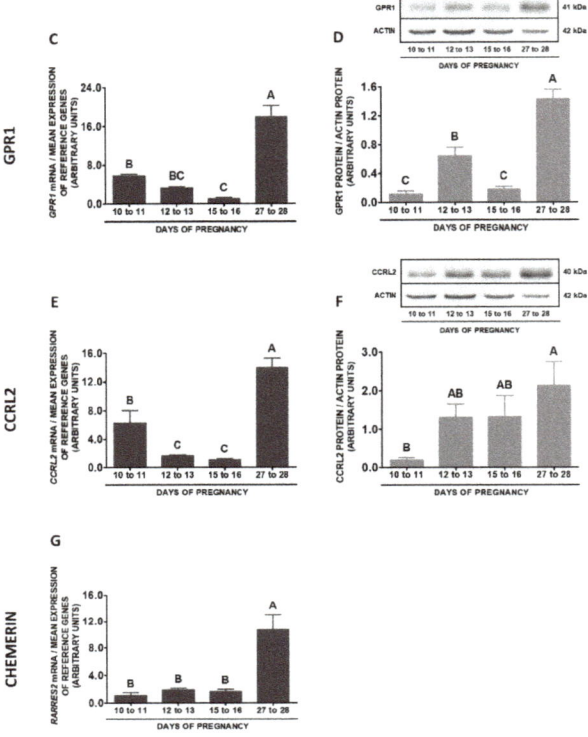

Figure 9. Chemerin system expression in the porcine preoptic area (POA) during early pregnancy. Gene and protein expression of chemokine-like receptor 1 (CMKLR1; **A** and **B**), G protein-coupled receptor 1 (GPR1; **C** and **D**) and C-C motif chemokine receptor-like 2 (CCRL2; **E** and **F**), as well as chemerin (*RARRES2*) mRNA content (**G**) in the porcine POA on days: 10 to 11, 12 to 13, 15 to 16 and 27 to 28 of pregnancy. Gene expression was determined by qPCR. Protein expression was determined by Western blotting; upper panels: representative immunoblots; lower panels: densitometric analysis of CMKLR1/GPR1/CCRL2 proteins relative to actin protein. Representative actin blots are identical for all chemerin receptors though proteins have been analysed on different gels. Results are presented as means ± SEM (*n* = 5). Bars with different superscripts differ (one-way ANOVA at $p < 0.05$ followed by Tuckey *post-hoc* test at $p < 0.05$).

2.7. CHEM System Gene and Protein Expression in POA—Pregnancy vs. Oestrous Cycle

Comparing the studied stages of pregnancy and days 10 to 12 of the oestrous cycle, higher *CMKLR1* gene expression was noted on days 10 to 11 of pregnancy, whereas lower on days 15 to 16 in relation to days 10 to 12 of the cycle. Protein concentrations of this receptor were higher on days 27 to 28 of pregnancy compared to days 10 to 12 of the cycle ($p < 0.05$; Figure 10A,B). The expression of *GPR1* gene during the mid-luteal phase was lower than on days 27 to 28 and 10 to 11 of pregnancy. Protein contents of this receptor on days 10 to 12 of the cycle were lower than on days 27 to 28 of pregnancy and days 12 to 13 of pregnancy ($p < 0.05$; Figure 10C,D). Higher contents of *CCRL2* mRNA were observed on days 27 to 28 of and 10 to 11 of gestation in relation to days 10 to 12 of the cycle. The highest protein concentrations of this receptor were noted on days 10 to 12 of the cycle in comparison to the studied stages of gestation ($p < 0.05$; Figure 10E,F). An elevated expression of the *RARRES2* gene was observed on days 10 to 12 of the cycle in relation to days 10 to 11, 12 to 13 and 15 to 16 of gestation ($p < 0.05$; Figure 10G).

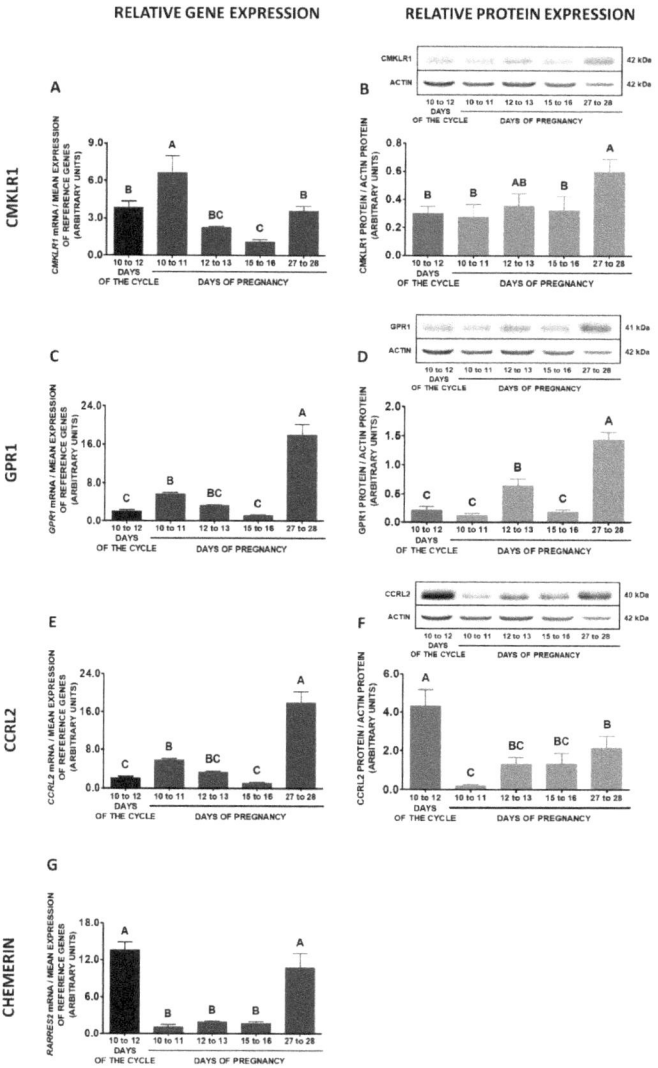

Figure 10. Chemerin system expression in the porcine preoptic area (POA)—pregnancy vs. oestrous cycle. Gene and protein expression of chemokine-like receptor 1 (CMKLR1; **A** and **B**), G protein-coupled receptor 1 (GPR1; **C** and **D**) and C-C motif chemokine receptor-like 2 (CCRL2; **E** and **F**), as well as chemerin (*RARRES2*) mRNA content (**G**) in the porcine POA on days: 10 to 11, 12 to 13, 15 to 16 and 27 to 28 of pregnancy, and on days 10 to 12 of the oestrous cycle. Gene expression was determined by qPCR. Protein expression was determined by Western blotting; upper panels: representative immunoblots; lower panels: densitometric analysis of CMKLR1/GPR1/CCRL2 proteins relative to actin protein. Representative actin blots are identical for all chemerin receptors though proteins have been analysed on different gels. Results are presented as means ± SEM ($n = 5$). Bars with different superscripts differ (one-way ANOVA at $p < 0.05$ followed by Tuckey *post-hoc* test at $p < 0.05$).

2.8. CHEM System Gene and Protein Expression in SME during the Oestrous Cycle

During the oestrous cycle, the expression of the *CMKLR1* gene in SME was significantly decreased on days 2 to 3 in relation to other phases of the cycle. However, the protein concentrations of this receptor were increased only on days 10 to 12 compared to other phases of the cycle ($p < 0.05$; Figure 11A,B). The highest *GPR1* mRNA contents were noted on days 17 to 19 compared to days 2 to 3 and 14 to 16, whereas the lowest on days 2 to 3 in relation to days 10 to 12 and 17 to 19 of the cycle. The differences in this receptor protein concentrations during the oestrous cycle were negligible ($p < 0.05$; Figure 11C,D). The expression of the *CCRL2* gene was the highest on days 10 to 12, lower on days 17 to 19, whereas the lowest on days 2 to 3 and 14 to 16 of the cycle. An elevated contents of CCRL2 protein were observed on days 14 to 16 and 17 to 19 in relation to days 2 to 3 and 10 to 12 of the cycle ($p < 0.05$; Figure 11E,F). The expression of *RARRES2* gene was enhanced on days 17 to 19 when compared to other studied stages of the cycle ($p < 0.05$; Figure 11G).

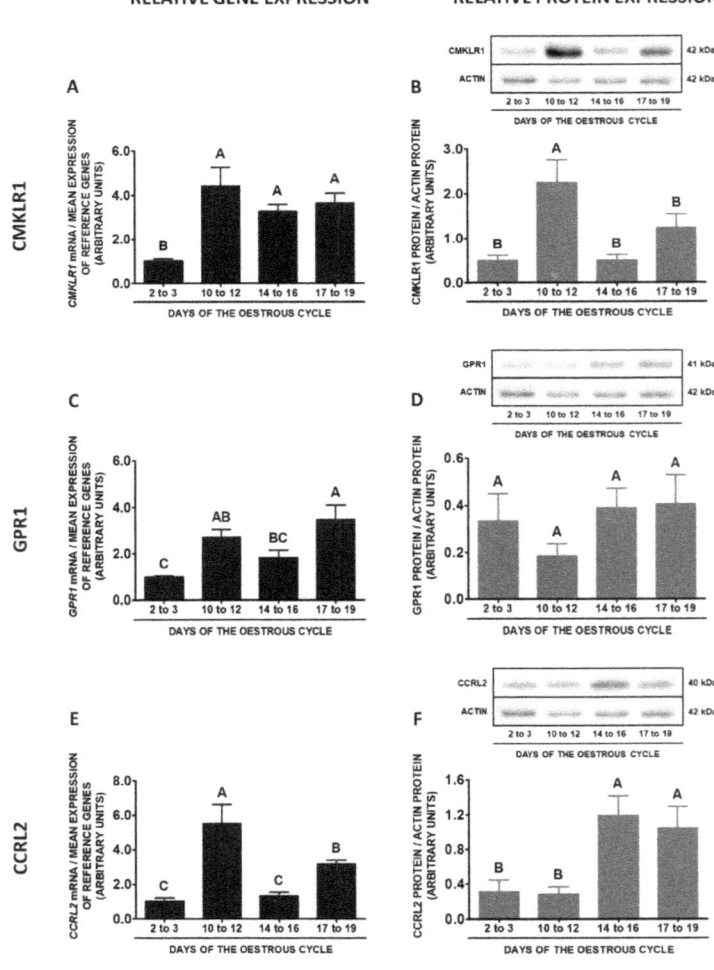

Figure 11. *Cont.*

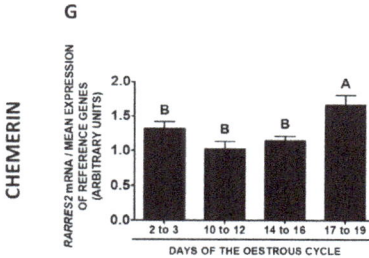

Figure 11. Chemerin system expression in the porcine stalk median eminence (SME) during the oestrous cycle. Gene and protein expression of chemokine-like receptor 1 (CMKLR1; **A** and **B**), G protein-coupled receptor 1 (GPR1; **C** and **D**) and C-C motif chemokine receptor-like 2 (CCRL2; **E** and **F**), as well as chemerin (*RARRES2*) mRNA content (**G**) in the porcine SME on days: 2 to 3, 10 to 12, 14 to 16 and 17 to 19 of the oestrous cycle. Gene expression was determined by qPCR. Protein expression was determined by Western blotting; upper panels: representative immunoblots; lower panels: densitometric analysis of CMKLR1/GPR1/CCRL2 proteins relative to actin protein. Representative actin blots are identical for all chemerin receptors though proteins have been analysed on different gels. Results are presented as means ± SEM ($n = 5$). Bars with different superscripts differ (one-way ANOVA at $p < 0.05$ followed by Tuckey *post-hoc* test at $p < 0.05$).

2.9. CHEM System Gene and Protein Expression in SME during Pregnancy

During pregnancy, an elevated levels of *CMKLR1* mRNA were observed on days 27 to 28 comparing to other stages of early pregnancy. Protein concentrations of this receptor were the highest on days 12 to 13 in relation to days 10 to 11 and 27 to 28, and the lowest on days 10 to 11 compared to days 12 to 13 and 15 to 16 of pregnancy ($p < 0.05$; Figure 12A,B). The expression of the *GPR1* gene was the highest on days 27 to 28 of pregnancy, lower on days 15 to 16, whereas the lowest on days 10 to 11 and 12 to 13 of gestation. The concentrations of GPR1 protein were elevated on days 12 to 13 and 27 to 28 of pregnancy in relation to the remaining stages of pregnancy ($p < 0.05$; Figure 12C,D). The highest *CCRL2* gene expression was noted on days 27 to 28, whereas the lowest on days 10 to 11 when compared to days 15 to 16 and 27 to 28 of pregnancy. The protein contents of this receptor were the highest on days 27 to 28 in relation to days 10 to 11 and 15 to 16, whereas the lowest on days 10 to 11 compared to days 12 to 13 and 27 to 28 of pregnancy ($p < 0.05$; Figure 12E,F). The highest expression of the *RARRES2* gene was observed on days 27 to 28 of gestation, whereas the lowest on days 12 to 13 in relation to days 15 to 16 and 27 to 28 of pregnancy ($p < 0.05$; Figure 12G).

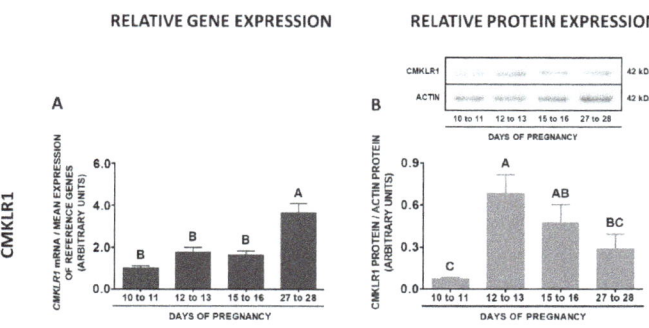

Figure 12. *Cont.*

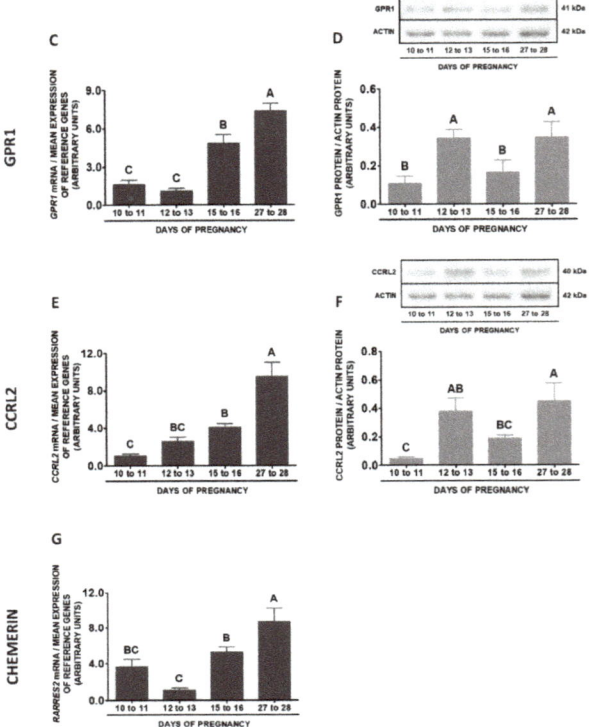

Figure 12. Chemerin system expression in the porcine stalk median eminence (SME) during early pregnancy. Gene and protein expression of chemokine-like receptor 1 (CMKLR1; **A** and **B**), G protein-coupled receptor 1 (GPR1; **C** and **D**) and C-C motif chemokine receptor-like 2 (CCRL2; **E** and **F**), as well as chemerin (*RARRES2*) mRNA content (**G**) in the porcine SME on days: 10 to 11, 12 to 13, 15 to 16 and 27 to 28 of pregnancy. Gene expression was determined by qPCR. Protein expression was determined by Western blotting; upper panels: representative immunoblots; lower panels: densitometric analysis of CMKLR1/GPR1/CCRL2 proteins relative to actin protein. Representative actin blots are identical for all chemerin receptors though proteins have been analysed on different gels. Results are presented as means ± SEM ($n = 5$). Bars with different superscripts differ (one-way ANOVA at $p < 0.05$ followed by Tuckey *post-hoc* test at $p < 0.05$).

2.10. CHEM System Gene and Protein Expression in SME—Pregnancy vs. Oestrous Cycle

Comparing the studied stages of pregnancy and days 10 to 12 of the oestrous cycle, significantly lower *CMKLR1* gene expression was noted on days 10 to 12 of the oestrous cycle in relation to days 12 to 13, 15 to 16 and 27 to 28 of gestation. Protein concentrations of this receptor were significantly higher on days 10 to 12 of the cycle compared to the studied stages of pregnancy ($p < 0.05$; Figure 13A,B). The expression of the *GPR1* gene during the mid-luteal phase of the cycle was lower than on days 15 to 16 and 27 to 28 of gestation. Protein contents of this receptor on days 10 to 12 of the oestrous cycle did not differ from the studied stages of gestation ($p < 0.05$; Figure 13C,D). The gene expression of *CCRL2* was lower on days 10 to 12 of the cycle compared to days 15 to 16 and 27 to 28 of pregnancy. Protein contents of this receptor on days 10 to 12 of the oestrous cycle did not differ from the studied stages of gestation ($p < 0.05$; Figure 13E,F). The gene expression of *RARRES2* on days 10 to 12 of the cycle was higher than on days 12 to 13 of pregnancy, whereas lower than on days 27 to 28 of gestation ($p < 0.05$; Figure 13G).

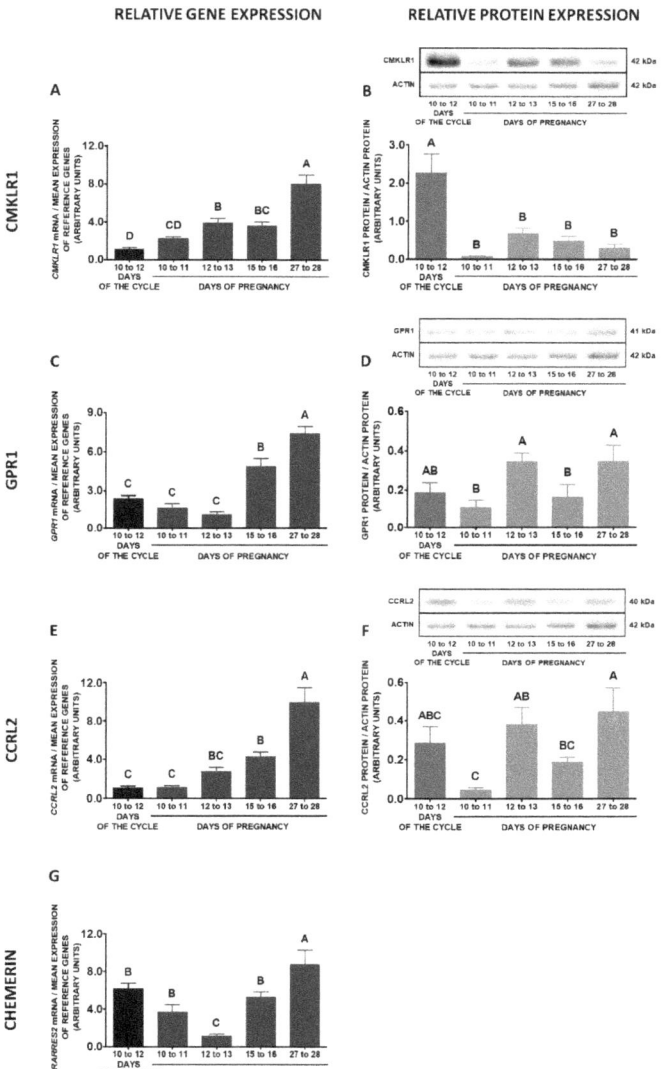

Figure 13. Chemerin system expression in the porcine stalk median eminence (SME)—pregnancy vs. oestrous cycle. Gene and protein expression of chemokine-like receptor 1 (CMKLR1; **A** and **B**), G protein-coupled receptor 1 (GPR1; **C** and **D**) and C-C motif chemokine receptor-like 2 (CCRL2; **E** and **F**), as well as chemerin (*RARRES2*) mRNA content (**G**) in the porcine SME on days: 10 to 11, 12 to 13, 15 to 16 and 27 to 28 of pregnancy, and on days 10 to 12 of the oestrous cycle. Gene expression was determined by qPCR. Protein expression was determined by Western blotting; upper panels: representative immunoblots; lower panels: densitometric analysis of CMKLR1/GPR1/CCRL2 proteins relative to actin protein. Representative actin blots are identical for all chemerin receptors though proteins have been analysed on different gels. Results are presented as means ± SEM ($n = 5$). Bars with different superscripts differ (one-way ANOVA at $p < 0.05$ followed by Tuckey *post-hoc* test at $p < 0.05$).

2.11. CHEM Concentrations in the Blood Plasma

During the oestrous cycle, the highest concentrations of CHEM in the blood plasma were observed on days 2 to 3 ($p < 0.05$; Figure 14A). During early pregnancy, significantly higher CHEM contents in the plasma were noted on days 15 to 16 comparing to days 10 to 11 and 27 to 28 ($p < 0.05$; Figure 14B). Comparing the studied stages of early pregnancy and days 10 to 12 of the cycle, significantly higher concentrations of CHEM in the blood plasma were observed on days 15 to 16 of gestation in relation to the cycle ($p < 0.05$; Figure 14C).

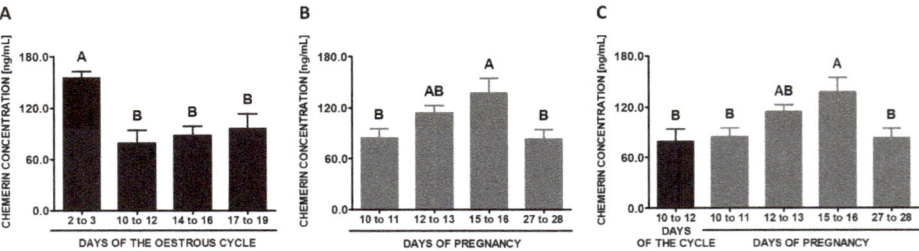

Figure 14. Chemerin concentrations in the porcine blood plasma. Concentrations of chemerin in the porcine blood plasma was determined during the oestrous cycle on days: 2 to 3, 10 to 12, 14 to 16 and 17 to 19 (**A**), during early pregnancy on days: 10 to 11, 12 to 13, 15 to 16 and 27 to 28 (**B**) and compared between early pregnancy and days 10 to 12 of the oestrous cycle (**C**). The hormone content in blood plasma was evaluated using ELISA. Results are presented as means ± SEM ($n = 5$). Bars with different superscripts differ (one-way ANOVA at $p < 0.05$ followed by Tuckey *post-hoc* test at $p < 0.05$).

3. Discussion

The present study was the first experiment to report the expression of CHEM and its receptors genes and proteins in the porcine hypothalamic structures, MBH, POA and SME, responsible for GnRH production and secretion, during the oestrous cycle and early pregnancy. In our immunohistochemical analyses, CHEM and its receptors were localised in the porcine paraventricular nucleus, which is the part of mediobasal hypothalamus and in the preoptic region during the oestrous cycle and early pregnancy. In the diagonal band of Broca, a part of preoptic region, very high immunoreactivity of GPR1 was observed. To date, the *RARRES2* gene was expressed in the hypothalamus of mice and rats [10,11]. In the brain of mice, *RARRES2* mRNA expression was restricted to the dorsal ventricular wall of the anterior, medial and posterior hypothalamus [10]. In turn, in the brain of rats, *RARRES2* mRNA was present in the tanycytes and ependymal cells layer lining the ventral third ventricle and SME of the hypothalamus, and *CMKLR1* transcript was found in the prefrontal cortex, hippocampus, cerebellum, ependymal cell layer and SME [11,12]. The transcripts of *RARRES2* were also present in the hypothalamus of baboons and chimpanzees [23]. GPR1 is expressed abundantly in the human brain, such as hippocampus, glioblastoma cells, brain-derived fibroblast-like cells lines and microglia [13]. In the ependymal cell layer and SME of rats, the gene expression of third CHEM receptor, *CCRL2* is also localised [11]. After CHEM injection, the expression of the cytoskeletal protein vimentin, a marker for estimating hypothalamic plasticity, was increased in the ependymal cell region of rats. It has been suggested that CHEM plays an important role in the structural remodelling of the hypothalamus [11]. The above and our studies indicate that the hypothalamus is capable of synthesising the discussed adipokine. The local production of CHEM and the presence of specific receptors suggest that the hormone exerts a direct effect on the hypothalamus with possible autocrine and/or paracrine action of CHEM in the brain.

CHEM is also delivered to the central nervous system (CNS) with the blood. It was found in the cerebrospinal fluid (CSF) of humans and the CHEM-158K protein is the dominant CHEM isoform. The total levels of cleaved and noncleaved CHEM were significantly lower in the CSF samples from patients with a variety of CNS diseases than in the plasma. In turn, in normal human plasma, the prochemerin form (CHEM-163S) dominated, whereas CHEM-158K represented only a small percentage of the total CHEM, and CHEM-157S was barely detectable. Thus, under normal conditions, the majority of circulating CHEM exists in the relatively inactive prochemerin form and requires proteolytic processing to bioactive CHEM isoforms. Only about 18% of CHEM is cleaved in normal plasma, whereas in CSF samples the fraction ranges about 50%. It has been implied that considerable proteolysis of CHEM is taking place in this extravascular compartment. Moreover, the differences between the total amount of CHEM as well as the extent of its cleavage that was found in the CSF supported the hypothesis of local CHEM synthesis and processing [24].

In the human blood, relatively high levels of CHEM (100–200 ng/mL) have been detected [25]. Plasma CHEM levels are correlated with BMI, body mass and adipose tissue mass. A statistically significant correlation has also been found between the adipokine level, and age and sex. Higher CHEM levels were found in women and older subjects than in men and younger subjects [3]. Our present studies indicate the higher levels of porcine plasma CHEM during the early-luteal phase (oestradiol (E_2) and progesterone (P_4) plasma concentrations are at moderate levels) than during the mid- and late-luteal phases (P_4 levels are high in the porcine blood) and follicular phase (E_2 levels are high in the porcine blood) of the oestrous cycle. The above results suggest that sex hormones, particularly gonadal steroids, may affect the synthesis of CHEM. Such a correlation has been documented for androgens increasing the levels of CHEM in women [19,26] and female rats [17]. A stimulatory effect of insulin on the synthesis of CHEM and its plasma levels was also demonstrated [19]. The levels of CHEM also change throughout pregnancy and between pregnancy and the oestrous cycle. In the present study, during the beginning of implantation, porcine plasma CHEM contents were enhanced compared to the period of embryos migration within the uterus, end of implantation and mid-luteal phase of the oestrous cycle. In the blood of pregnant women, CHEM levels were significantly higher than in the non-pregnant ones [27]. Moreover, plasma levels of CHEM were significantly elevated during late gestation when compared to the early gestation of humans [27], but the reverse correlation was found in rats [28]. This may indicate species–specific differences in the activity of CHEM.

To our knowledge, this is the first study that compares CHEM system genes expression and proteins concentrations in the hypothalamus within the oestrous cycle and early pregnancy and between these physiological periods. Our obtained results indicate that CHEM expression levels were determined by the stage of the oestrous cycle and early pregnancy and these results confirmed the hypothesis that steroid hormones may regulate the synthesis of CHEM. The expression of CMKLR1 and CCLR2 proteins in most hypothalamic structures increased during the mid-luteal phase of the oestrous cycle, which seems to suggest the up-regulating effect of P_4. In POA, the expression of GPR1 protein was also stimulated during the luteal phase of the cycle. However, GPR1 protein contents in MBH were enhanced during the follicular phase, when plasma levels of oestrogens are very high. In addition, the concentrations of CHEM receptors proteins in the porcine hypothalamic structures generally increase with the advancement of pregnancy from days 10 to days 28. In our previous study, in the porcine peripheral blood plasma from days 10 to days 28 of pregnancy, a statistically significant decrease in the mean of P_4 levels was observed [29]. These results may suggest an inverse pattern between the expression of CHEM receptors and the levels of P_4 during pregnancy. The role of steroids in the regulation of CHEM system was also investigated in humans and the results are also unclear. The findings of an inverse association of E_2 and CHEM levels have been observed in a clinical study comprising both lean and overweight men and women [30], but no significant effects of steroids on CHEM protein production in the control human subcutaneous adipose tissue explants were reported [19]. It cannot be ruled out that other hormones regulating the oestrous cycle, such as the pituitary luteinizing hormone (LH), may be involved in the regulation of CHEM expression. Men with elevated LH levels had lower CHEM contents in relation to those with the normal range of LH [31]. Further studies would be recommended to identify the exact mechanisms of the relationship between the contents of CHEM and steroid/other hormones. Moreover, in our study, we have also observed the higher GPR1 and lower CCRL2 protein concentrations in the porcine MBH and POA during the early pregnancy versus the oestrous cycle. These findings supported the idea that CHEM/GPR1/CCRL2 could be the one of the regulators of pregnancy at the hypothalamic level. However, the possible roles of CHEM in the maintenance of pregnancy should be investigated in further studies.

Some lines of evidence suggest that CHEM regulates hypothalamic hormones secretion connected with feeding behaviour. A direct stimulating effect of CHEM on hypothalamic agouti-related peptide and pro-opiomelanocortin gene expression was observed in rats after injecting a single dose of CHEM (8 µg/kg) in the arcuate nucleus [32]. These results are in good agreement with reports indicating that the administration of the major dosage of CHEM (16 g/kg) increased mRNA contents of both cocaine and amphetamine-regulated transcript (CART) and neuropeptide Y [15]. The above results confirmed the role of CHEM in the regulation of hypothalamic modulators. However, there is a lack of data on the role of CHEM on the reproductive functions at the brain level, in the hypothalamus and pituitary through the regulation of GnRH, LH and follicle-stimulating hormone production. Several studies have reported the direct role of CHEM on the gonads. The expression of the *RARRES2* gene was found in the ovaries of women [8], rodents [2,9] and cows [33]. Mammalian ovaries are also sensitive to CHEM: CMKLR1 expression was identified in the ovaries of women [8] and rats [9], while CMKLR1, GPR1 and CCLR2 expression was noticed in the ovaries of cows [33]. A clear effect of CHEM on ovarian steroidogenesis was demonstrated and reflected by the inhibition of FSH-induced secretion of P_4 and E_2 by granulosa cells in rats [9,18], cows [33] and the insulin-like growth factor 1-induced secretion of both steroids in granulosa cells in women [8]. The presence of the CHEM system in hypothalamic structures responsible for GnRH synthesis and secretion observed in our study implies that the discussed hormone regulates GnRH generation. Therefore, it cannot be excluded that the adipokine can affect the gonads indirectly via effects on the central hypothalamic–pituitary–gonadal axis, i.e., by affecting the GnRH hypothalamic neurons and/or the gonadotrophs of the pituitary; however, this hypothesis needs to be verified.

4. Materials and Methods

4.1. Experimental Animals and Tissue Collection

Experimental animals were mature gilts (Large White × Polish Landrace), about 7–8 months old, weighing 120–130 kg, descended from private breeding. All individuals were given access to water and forage ad libitum. Forty animals were assigned to one of eight experimental groups ($n = 5$ in each group) as follows: days 2 to 3 (early luteal phase, the presence of corpora hemorrhagica), 10 to 12 (mid-luteal phase, the phase when the corpus luteum activity is high and similar to that noted during pregnancy), 14 to 16 (late luteal phase, the period of luteolysis) and 17 to 19 (follicular phase) of the oestrous cycle, and 10 to 11 (migration of the embryos within the uterus), 12 to 13 (maternal recognition of pregnancy), 15 to 16 (beginning of implantation) and 27 to 28 (end of implantation) of pregnancy. Cyclic gilts were monitored daily for an oestrous behaviour in the presence of a boar. The day of the onset of the second oestrous was designated as day 0 of the oestrous cycle. The phase of the oestrous cycle was also confirmed based on ovaries morphology [34]. In the case of pregnant pigs, the insemination was performed on days 1 to 2 of the oestrous cycle. Pregnancy was confirmed by the presence and morphology of conceptuses. On days 10 to 11 and 12 to 13 of pregnancy, conceptuses were obtained by the flushing of uterine horns with 20 mL of sterile phosphate-buffered saline (PBS), whereas on days 15 to 16 and 27 to 28 of pregnancy, by dissection from the endometrium. Within a few minutes after slaughter, blood samples were collected and the hypothalamus was dissected. Blood samples were placed into heparinised tubes, centrifuged (2500× g, 15 min, 4 °C) and the obtained plasma was stored at −80 °C. Each hypothalamic block was divided into: MBH, POA and SME as described by Sesti and Britt [35]. The mediobasal hypothalamus was defined as a block of tissue bound rostrally by the optic chiasma, caudally by mammillary body, laterally by the hypothalamic sulci and dorsally by a cut 5 mm deep. POA was limited rostrally approximately 5 mm anterior to the optic chiasma and caudally by the rostral border of MBH. The stalk median eminence was easily detached from the MBH and was cut away at its junction with the pituitary gland. Preoptic areas and MBH from days 15 to 16 of pregnancy and 10 to 12 of the cycle were divided in two parts, from which one half intended for immunofluorescent staining was placed in 4% buffered paraformaldehyde (pH = 7.4, 4 °C), whereas other halves, along with all the rest of the POAs, MBHs and SMEs were frozen in liquid nitrogen and stored at −80 °C until RNA and protein isolation.

Tissue samples were taken from animals intended for commercial slaughter and meat processing. All studies were conducted in accordance with ethical standards of the Animal Ethics Committee at the University of Warmia and Mazury in Olsztyn. The animals used in the study were reared and transported under conditions specified in the "Act on the protection of animals used for scientific or educational purposes" (Poland, 2015).

4.2. Fluorescent Immunohistochemistry of the Porcine Hypothalamus

The tissue blocks were fixed by immersion for 24 h in 4% buffered paraformaldehyde (pH = 7.4; 4 °C). Following fixation, the brains were washed in 0.1 M PBS and then cryoprotected for 3–5 days in graded solutions (19% and 30%) of sucrose (Sigma Aldrich, St. Louis, MO, USA) at 4 °C until they sank. The tissue blocks comprised of the hypothalamus and adjoining structures were frozen and cut into 18 µm thick cryostat coronal sections and stored at −80 °C. Frozen sections were processed for double-labelling immunofluorescence by means of primary antisera raised in different species. The sections were air-dried for 30 min, washed 3 times in cold PBS and incubated for 1 h with blocking buffer (0.1 M PBS, 10% normal donkey serum, 0.01% bovine serum albumin, 1% Tween, 0.05% thimerosal, 0.01% NaN3). Then sections were incubated overnight at room temperature with a solution of rabbit polyclonal antibodies against CMKLR1 (0.5 µg/uL, ab230442, Abcam, Cambridge, UK), or GPR1 (1.25 µg/uL, ab188977, Abcam, Cambridge, UK), or CCRL2 (0.67 µg/uL, ab85224, Abcam, Cambridge, UK), or CHEM (0.5 µg/uL, ab203040, Abcam, Cambridge, UK). In order to show the binding sites of the antisera with antigens, the sections were incubated with the Alexa Fluor 555 donkey anti-rabbit antibodies (0.5 µg/uL, A-31572, Molecular Probes, Eugene, OR, USA). After staining, scraps were washed in PBS and mounted with carbonate-buffered glycerol (pH 8.6) and cover slipped. All steps of the staining procedures were conducted in humid chambers at room temperature. Standard controls, i.e., the omission and replacement of primary antisera by non-immune sera were applied to test antibody and method specificity. The lack of any immunoreactions indicated specificity. The sections were analysed with an Olympus BX51 microscope equipped with a CC-12 digital camera (Soft Imaging System GMBH, Münster, Germany). Images were acquired with Cell-F software (Olympus GmbH, Hamburg, Germany).

4.3. Quantitative Real-Time PCR

Total RNA from MBH, POA and SME samples was isolated using the peqGold TriFast isolation system (Peqlabs, Erlangen, Germany). RNA quantity and quality were determined spectrometrically (Infinite M200 Pro, Tecan, Männedorf, Switzerland). First strand cDNA was synthesised using the Omniscript RT Kit (Qiagen, Hilden, Germany) in a total volume of 20 µL with 1 µg of RNA, 0.5 µg oligo(dT)15 (Roche, Basel, Switzerland) at 37 °C for 1 h and was terminated by the incubation at 93 °C for 5 min. Specific primer pairs used to amplify parts of *RARRES2, CMKLR1, GPR1, CCRL2,* ubiquitin C (*UBC*) and 18S ribosomal RNA (*18sRNA*) genes are detailed in Table 1. Specific primers for *RARRES2, CMKLR1, GPR1* and *CCRL2* were designed with the Primer Express 3.0 software (Life Technologies, Camarillo, CA, USA) and their specificities were confirmed by comparison of their sequences with the sequences of corresponding genes deposited in a GenBank database. Due to the calculation of the statistical significance of the match, the Basic Local Alignment Search Tool (BLAST) was used. Quantitative real-time PCR (qPCR) analysis was carried out using PCR System 7300 (Applied Biosystems Inc., Foster, CA, USA), as described previously by Smolinska et. al. [36]. Briefly, the qPCR reaction included 10 ng of cDNA, the appropriate forward and reverse primers at the concentrations detailed in Table 1, 12.5 µL Power SYBR Green PCR Master Mix (Applied Biosystems Inc., Foster, CA, USA), and RNase-free water in a final volume of 25 µL. The constitutively expressed genes, *UBC* and *18sRNA*, were used as an internal control to verify the qPCR. To ensure that UBC and 18sRNA were suitable reference genes for this study, we revealed that their expression was stable between the tested tissues and during the oestrous cycle and early pregnancy. Real-time conditions were as follows: Initial denaturation and enzyme activation at 95 °C for 10 min, followed by 40 cycles of denaturation at 95 °C for 15 s, annealing at 60 °C for 1 min and elongation at 70 °C for 1 min. Negative controls were performed by substitution of cDNA with water. All samples were in duplicate. The specificity of amplification was tested at the end of the qPCR by melting curve analysis. Levels of gene expression were calculated using the ΔΔCt method and normalised using the geometrical means of reference gene expression levels: *UBC* and *18sRNA*. The Ct values for all non-template controls were under the detection threshold.

Table 1. Characteristics of primers used in the study.

Gene	Primers Sequences	Accession Number	Amplicon Length, bp	Primer, nM	Reference
RARRES2	F: 5′-TGGAGGAGTTCCACAAGCAC-3′ R: 5′-GCTTTCTTCCAGTCCCTCTTC-3′	EU660865	154	500 500	[The present study]
CCRL2	F: 5′-GAGCAGCAGCTACTTACTTCC-3′ R: 5′-CTGCCCACTGACCGAGTTC-3′	NM_001001617.1	196	200 200	[The present study]
CMKLR1	F: 5′-GGACTACCACTGGGTGTTCG-3′ R: 5′-GCCATGTAAGCCAGTCGGA-3′	EU660866	174	200 200	[The present study]
GPR1	F: 5′-ACCGACTTGGAGGAGAAAGC-3′ R: 5′-ATTGAGGAACCAGAGCGTGG-3′	FJ234899.1	159	200 200	[The present study]
UBC	F: 5′-GGAGGAATCTACTGGGGCGG-3′ R: 5′-CAGAAGAAACGCAGGCAAACT-3′	XM_003483411.3	103	400 400	[37]
18sRNA	F: 5′-TCCAATGGATCCTCGCGGAA-3′ R: 5′-GGCTACCACATCCAAGGAAG-3′	AY265350.1	149	400 400	[38]

RARRES2: chemerin; *CCRL2*: C-C motif chemokine receptor like 2; *CMLKR1*: chemokine-like receptor 1; *GPR1*: G protein-coupled receptor 1; *UBC*: Ubiquitin C; *18sRNA*: 18S ribosomal RNA; F: forward; R: reverse.

4.4. Western Blotting

Tissue preparation and lysis, as well as Western blotting analysis was performed essentially as described by Smolinska et al. [39] with a few modifications. Briefly, equal amounts of porcine MBH, POA and SME protein lysates (30 µg of total proteins) were resolved by SDS-PAGE (12.5% gel) for separating CMKLR1, GPR1, CCRL2 and actin, and then transferred to PVDF membranes and blocked for 1 h at room temperature in Tris-buffered saline Tween-20 (TBST) containing 5% skimmed milk powder. After blocking, PVDF membranes were incubated overnight with rabbit polyclonal CMKLR1 (1 µg/uL, ab230442, Abcam, Cambridge, UK), CCRL2 (3.33 µg/uL, ab85224, Abcam, Cambridge, UK), actin (6.58 µg/uL, A2066, Sigma-Aldrich, St. Louis, MO, USA) antibodies or mouse polyclonal GPR1 (2.0 µg/uL, ab169331, Abcam, UK) in TBST. Actin immunoblots were used as an internal control for equal loading and to quantify porcine CMKLR1, GPR1 and CCRL2 proteins. In order to examine immunoreactive bands, PVDF membranes were incubated with goat anti-rabbit antibodies for CMKLR1, CCRL2 and actin (0.25 µg/uL, sc-2054, Santa Cruz, Santa Cruz, CA, USA) or goat anti-mouse antibodies for GPR1 (0.5 µg/uL, 115-035-003, Jackson ImmunoResearch Laboratories Inc., West Grove, PA, USA) conjugated with horse radish peroxidase (HRP) diluted in TBST containing 5% skimmed milk. PVDF membranes were incubated with Immobilon Western Chemiluminescent HRP Substrate (Merck Millipore, Burlington, MA, USA) and visualised using G: Box EF Gel Documentation System (Syngene, Cambridge, UK) with GeneSnap software. The same protocol was performed in relation to the adipose tissue used as the positive controls. The quality of the experiment was confirmed using reference protein, actin, the expression of which did not vary across the oestrous cycle and pregnancy or between the studied tissues. The results of Western blotting analyses were quantified by densitometric scanning of immunoblots with Image Studio™ Lite version

5.2 software (LI-COR, Lincoln, NE, USA). Data were expressed as the ratio of CHEM receptors proteins relative to actin proteins in arbitrary optical density units.

4.5. Enzyme-Linked Immune-Sorbent Assay (ELISA) of CHEM

The concentrations of CHEM protein in plasma were determined using a commercial ELISA kit (FineTest, Wuhan Fine Biotech Co., Ltd., Wuhan, China) according to the manufacturer's protocol. The range of standard curve was 0.156–10 ng/mL. The sensitivity of the assay was defined as the least protein concentration that could be differentiated from zero samples, which was <0.1 ng/mL. According to the manufacturer, no significant cross-reactivity or interference between CHEM and homologous proteins assayed has been observed. Species cross-reactivity has not been specifically determined. Absorbance values were measured at 450 nm using an Infinite M200 Pro reader with Tecan i-control software (Tecan, Männedorf, Switzerland). The data were linearised by plotting the log of CHEM concentrations versus the log of the optical density and the best fit line was determined by regression analysis. Intra-assay coefficient of variation of the ELISA assay for CHEM was 3.89%.

4.6. Statistical Analysis

Data are presented as means ± S.E.M. from five different observations. Differences between groups were analysed by one-way ANOVA followed by Tukey's honest significant difference *post-hoc* test. Statistical analyses were performed using Statistica Software (StatSoft Inc., Tulsa, OH, USA). Values for $p < 0.05$ were considered statistically significant.

5. Conclusions

The presented data indicated, for the first time, the presence of CHEM and its receptors in the hypothalamic structures responsible for GnRH production and secretion, which suggest that the adipokine exerts autocrine/paracrine effects on GnRH synthesis and/or secretion. Moreover, the observed changes in CHEM system expression levels may be dependent on the influence of ovarian steroids and other hormones controlling reproductive processes. Our present findings expand our knowledge of the potential role of CHEM as a key neuromodulator of reproductive functions.

Author Contributions: Conceptualization: N.S., T.K.; methodology, N.S., M.K., K.D., M.G., K.K., E.R, and K.B.-N.; formal analysis, N.S., M.K., M.G., and E.Z.; investigation, N.S., M.K. and K.D.; resources, K.B., J.W. and G.K.; data curation, M.K., E.Z, and B.K.; writing—original draft preparation, N.S.; writing—review and editing, N.S., M.K., T.K., B.K. and K.D.; supervision, N.S., T.K.; project administration, N.S., T.K.; funding acquisition, N.S., T.K.

Funding: This research was supported by the National Science Centre (Project no.: 2015/17/B/NZ9/03595). The publication was written as a result of the author's internship in Department of Physiology, Center for Research in Molecular Medicine and Chronic Diseases (CiMUS), University of Santiago de Compostela, Spain, co-financed by the European Union under the European Social Fund (Operational Program Knowledge Education Development), carried out in the project Development Program at the University of Warmia and Mazury in Olsztyn (POWR.03.05. 00-00-Z310/17).

Conflicts of Interest: The authors declare no conflict of interest.

References

1. Ernst, M.C.; Sinal, C.J. Chemerin: At the crossroads of inflammation and obesity. *Trends Endocrinol. Metab.* **2010**, *21*, 660–667. [CrossRef] [PubMed]
2. Goralski, K.B.; McCarthy, T.C.; Hanniman, E.A.; Zabel, B.A.; Butcher, E.C.; Parlee, S.D.; Muruganandan, S.; Sinal, C.J. Chemerin, a novel adipokine that regulates adipogenesis and adipocyte metabolism. *J. Biol. Chem.* **2007**, *282*, 28175–28188. [CrossRef] [PubMed]
3. Bozaoglu, K.; Bolton, K.; McMillan, J.; Zimmet, P.; Jowett, J.; Collier, G.; Walder, K.; Segal, D. Chemerin is a novel adipokine associated with obesity and metabolic syndrome. *Endocrinology* **2007**, *148*, 4687–4694. [CrossRef] [PubMed]
4. Du, X.Y.; Leungl, L.L. Proteolytic regulatory mechanism of chemerin bioactivity. *Acta Biochim. Biophys. Sin.* **2009**, *41*, 973–979. [CrossRef] [PubMed]

5. Rourke, J.L.; Dranse, H.J.; Sinal, C.J. Towards an integrative approach to understanding the role of chemerin in human health and disease. *Obes. Rev.* **2013**, *14*, 245–262. [CrossRef] [PubMed]
6. Mattern, A.; Zellmann, T.; Beck-Sickinger, A.G. Processing, signaling, and physiological function of chemerin. *IUBMB Life* **2014**, *66*, 19–26. [CrossRef] [PubMed]
7. Chamberland, J.P.; Berman, R.L.; Aronis, K.N.; Mantzoros, C.S. Chemerin is expressed mainly in pancreas and liver, is regulated by energy deprivation, and lacks day/night variation in humans. *Eur. J. Endocrinol.* **2013**, *169*, 453–462. [CrossRef] [PubMed]
8. Reverchon, M.; Cornuau, M.; Rame, C.; Guerif, F.; Royere, D.; Dupont, J. Chemerin inhibits IGF-1-induced progesterone and estradiol secretion in human granulosa cells. *Hum. Reprod.* **2012**, *27*, 1790–1800. [CrossRef] [PubMed]
9. Wang, Q.; Kim, J.Y.; Xue, K.; Liu, J.-Y.; Leader, A.; Tsang, B.K. Chemerin, a novel regulator of follicular steroidogenesis and its potential involvement in polycystic ovarian syndrome. *Endocrinology* **2012**, *153*, 5600–5611. [CrossRef]
10. Miranda-Angulo, A.L.; Byerly, M.S.; Mesa, J.; Wang, H.; Blackshaw, S. Rax regulates hypothalamic tanycyte differentiation and barrier function in mice. *J. Comp. Neurol.* **2014**, *522*, 876–899. [CrossRef]
11. Helfer, G.; Ross, A.W.; Thomson, L.M.; Mayer, C.D.; Stoney, P.N.; McCaffery, P.J.; Morgan, P.J. A neuroendocrine role for chemerin in hypothalamic remodelling and photoperiodic control of energy balance. *Sci. Rep.* **2016**, *6*, 26830. [CrossRef] [PubMed]
12. Guo, X.; Fu, Y.; Xu, Y.; Weng, S.; Liu, D.; Cui, D.; Yu, S.; Liu, X.; Jiang, K.; Dong, Y. Chronic mild restraint stress rats decreased CMKLR1 expression in distinct brain region. *Neurosci. Lett.* **2012**, *524*, 25–29. [CrossRef] [PubMed]
13. Shimizu, N.; Soda, Y.; Kanbe, K.; Liu, H.-Y.; Jinno, A.; Kitamura, T.; Hoshino, H. An orphan G protein-coupled receptor, GPR1, acts as a coreceptor to allow replication of human immunodeficiency virus types 1 and 2 in brain-derived cells. *J. Virol.* **1999**, *73*, 5231–5239.
14. Banas, M.; Zegar, A.; Kwitniewski, M.; Zabieglo, K.; Marczynska, J.; Kapinska-Mrowiecka, M.; LaJevic, M.; Zabel, B.A.; Cichy, J. The expression and regulation of chemerin in the epidermis. *PLoS One* **2015**, *10*, e0117830. [CrossRef]
15. Brunetti, L.; Orlando, G.; Ferrante, C.; Recinella, L.; Leone, S.; Chiavaroli, A.; Nisio, C.D.; Shohreh, R.; Manippa, F.; Ricciuti, A.; et al. Peripheral chemerin administration modulates hypothalamic control of feeding. *Peptides* **2014**, *51*, 115–121. [CrossRef]
16. Ernst, M.C.; Haidl, I.D.; Zuniga, L.A.; Dranse, H.J.; Rourke, J.L.; Zabel, B.A.; Butcher, E.C.; Sinal, C.J. Disruption of the chemokine-like receptor 1 (CMKLR1) gene is associated with reduced adiposity and glucose intolerance. *Endocrinology* **2012**, *153*, 672–682. [CrossRef] [PubMed]
17. Kim, J.Y.; Xue, K.; Cao, M.; Wang, Q.; Liu, J.-Y.; Leader, A.; Han, J.Y.; Tsang, B.K. Chemerin suppresses ovarian follicular development and its potential involvement in follicular arrest in rats treated chronically with dihydrotestosterone. *Endocrinology* **2013**, *154*, 2912–2923. [CrossRef]
18. Wang, Q.; Leader, A.; Tsang, B.K. Inhibitory roles of prohibitin and chemerin in FSH-induced rat granulosa cell steroidogenesis. *Endocrinology* **2013**, *154*, 956–967. [CrossRef]
19. Tan, B.K.; Chen, J.; Farhatullah, S.; Adya, R.; Kaur, J.; Heutling, D.; Lewandowski, K.C.; O'Hare, J.P.; Lehnert, H.; Randeva, H.S. Insulin and metformin regulate circulating and adipose tissue chemerin. *Diabetes* **2009**, *58*, 1971–1977. [CrossRef]
20. Duan, D.M.; Niu, J.M.; Lei, Q.; Lin, X.H.; Chen, X. Serum levels of the adipokine chemerin in preeclampsia. *J. Perinat. Med.* **2011**, *40*, 121–127. [CrossRef]
21. Jin, C.H.; Yi, K.W.; Ha, Y.R.; Shin, J.H.; Park, H.T.; Kim, T.; Hur, J.Y. Chemerin expression in the peritoneal fluid, serum, and ovarian endometrioma of women with endometriosis. *Am. J. Reprod. Immunol.* **2015**, *74*, 379–386. [CrossRef] [PubMed]
22. Carlino, C.; Trotta, E.; Stabile, H.; Morrone, S.; Bulla, R.; Soriani, A.; Iannitto, M.L.; Agostinis, C.; Mocci, C.; Minozzi, M.; et al. Chemerin regulates NK cell accumulation and endothelial cell morphogenesis in the decidua during early pregnancy. *J. Clin. Endocrinol. Metab.* **2012**, *97*, 3603–3612. [CrossRef] [PubMed]
23. Gonzalez-Alvarez, R.; Garza-Rodriguez Mde, L.; Delgado-Enciso, I.; Trevino-Alvarado, V.M.; Canales-Del-Castillo, R.; Martinez-De-Villarreal, L.E.; Lugo-Trampe, A.; Tejero, M.E.; Schlabritz-Loutsevitch, N.E.; Rocha-Pizana Mdel, R.; et al. Molecular evolution and expression profile of the chemerine encoding gene RARRES2 in baboon and chimpanzee. *Biol. Res.* **2015**, *48*, 31. [CrossRef] [PubMed]

24. Zhao, L.; Yamaguchi, Y.; Sharif, S.; Du, X.Y.; Song, J.J.; Lee, D.M.; Recht, L.D.; Robinson, W.H.; Morser, J.; Leung, L.L. Chemerin158K protein is the dominant chemerin isoform in synovial and cerebrospinal fluids but not in plasma. *J. Biol. Chem.* **2011**, *286*, 39520–39527. [CrossRef] [PubMed]
25. Bozaoglu, K.; Curran, J.E.; Stocker, C.J.; Zaibi, M.S.; Segal, D.; Konstantopoulus, N.; Morrison, N.; Carless, M.; Dyer, T.D.; Cole, S.A.; et al. Chemerin, a novel adipokine in the regulation of angiogenesis. *J. Clin Endocrinol Metab.* **2010**, *95*, 2476–2485. [CrossRef] [PubMed]
26. Martinez-Garcia, M.A.; Montes-Nieto, R.; Fernandez-Duran, E.; Insenser, M.; Luque-Ramirez, M.; Escobar-Morreale, H.F. Evidence for masculinization of adipokine gene expression in visceral and subcutaneous adipose tissue of obese women with polycystic ovary syndrome (PCOS). *J. Clin. Endocrinol. Metab.* **2013**, *98*, E388–E396. [CrossRef] [PubMed]
27. Garces, M.F.; Sanchez, E.; Ruiz-Parra, A.I.; Rubio-Romero, J.A.; Angel-Muller, A.; Suarez, M.A.; Bohorquez, L.F.; Bravo, S.B.; Nogueiras, R.; Dieguez, C.; et al. Serum chemerin levels during normal human pregnancy. *Peptides* **2013**, *42*, 138–143. [CrossRef]
28. Garces, M.F.; Sanchez, E.; Acosta, B.J.; Angel, E.; Ruiz, A.I.; Rubio-Romero, J.A.; Dieguez, C.; Nogueiras, R.; Caminos, J.E. Expression and regulation of chemerin during rat pregnancy. *Placenta* **2012**, *33*, 373–378. [CrossRef]
29. Dobrzyn, K.; Smolinska, N.; Szeszko, K.; Kiezun, M.; Maleszka, A.; Rytelewska, E.; Kaminski, T. Effect of progesterone on adiponectin system in the porcine uterus during early pregnancy. *J. Anim. Sci.* **2017**, *95*, 338–352. [CrossRef]
30. Luque-Ramírez, M.; Martínez-García, M.Á.; Montes-Nieto, R.; Fernández-Durán, E.; Insenser, M.; Alpañés, M.; Escobar-Morreale, H.F. Sexual dimorphism in adipose tissue function as evidenced by circulating adipokine concentrations in the fasting state and after an oral glucose challenge. *Hum. Reprod.* **2013**, *28*, 1908–1918. [CrossRef]
31. Bobjer, J.; Katrinaki, M.; Dermitzaki, E.; Margioris, A.N.; Giwercman, A.; Tsatsanis, C. Serum chemerin levels are negatively associated with male fertility and reproductive hormones. *Hum. Reprod.* **2018**, *33*, 2168–2174. [CrossRef] [PubMed]
32. Brunetti, L.; Nisio, C.D.; Recinella, L.; Chiavaroli, A.; Leone, S.; Ferrante, C.; Orlando, G.; Vacca, M. Effects of vaspin, chemerin and omentin-1 on feeding behavior and hypothalamic peptidegene expression in the rat. *Peptides* **2011**, *32*, 1866–1871. [CrossRef] [PubMed]
33. Reverchon, M.; Bertoldo, M.J.; Rame, C.; Froment, P.; Dupont, J. Chemerin (RARRES2) decreases in vitro granulosa cell steroidogenesis and blocks oocyte meiotic progression in bovine species. *Biol. Reprod.* **2014**, *90*, 1–15. [CrossRef] [PubMed]
34. Akins, E.L.; Morrissette, M.C. Gross ovarian changes during estrous cycle of swine. *Am. J. Vet. Res.* **1968**, *29*, 1953–1957. [PubMed]
35. Sesti, L.A.; Britt, J.H. Relationship of secretion of GnRH in vitro to changes in pituitary concentrations of LH and FSH and serum concentrations of LH during lactation in sows. *J. Reprod. Fertil.* **1993**, *98*, 393–400. [CrossRef] [PubMed]
36. Smolinska, N.; Dobrzyn, K.; Kiezun, M.; Szeszko, K.; Maleszka, A.; Kaminski, T. Effect of adiponectin on the steroidogenic acute regulatory protein, P450 side chain cleavage enzyme and 3β-hydroxysteroid dehydrogenase genes expression, progesterone and androstenedione production by the porcine uterus during early pregnancy. *J. Physiol. Pharmacol.* **2016**, *67*, 443–456. [PubMed]
37. Martyniak, M.; Zglejc, K.; Franczak, A.; Kotwica, G. Expression of 3-hydroxysteroid dehydrogenase and P450 aromatase in porcine oviduct during the estrous cycle. *J. Anim. Feed Sci.* **2016**, *25*, 235–243. [CrossRef]
38. Martyniak, M.; Franczak, A.; Kotwica, G. Interleukin-1β system in the oviducts of pigs during the oestrous cycle and early pregnancy. *Theriogenology* **2017**, *96*, 31–41. [CrossRef]
39. Smolinska, N.; Kaminski, T.; Siawrys, G.; Przala, J. Long form of leptin receptor gene and protein expression in the porcine ovary during the estrous cycle and early pregnancy. *Reprod. Biol.* **2007**, *7*, 17–39.

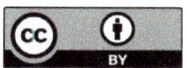

© 2019 by the authors. Licensee MDPI, Basel, Switzerland. This article is an open access article distributed under the terms and conditions of the Creative Commons Attribution (CC BY) license (http://creativecommons.org/licenses/by/4.0/).

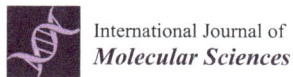

Article

Ovarian Expression of Adipokines in Polycystic Ovary Syndrome: A Role for Chemerin, Omentin, and Apelin in Follicular Growth Arrest and Ovulatory Dysfunction?

Alice Bongrani [1,2,3,4], Namya Mellouk [1,2,3,4], Christelle Rame [1,2,3,4], Marion Cornuau [5], Fabrice Guérif [1,2,3,4,5], Pascal Froment [1,2,3,4] and Joëlle Dupont [1,2,3,4,*]

1. Institut National de la Recherche Agronomique Unité Mixte de Recherche Physiology Department, Physiologie de la Reproduction et des Comportements, F-37380 Nouzilly, France
2. Centre National de la Recherche Scientifique, Life Science Department Physiologie de la Reproduction et des Comportements, F-37380 Nouzilly, France
3. Université François Rabelais de Tours, F-37041 Tours, France
4. Institut Français du Cheval et de l'équitation F-37380 Nouzilly, France
5. Service de Médecine et Biologie de la Reproduction, CHRU Bretonneau, 2, boulevard Tonnellé, F-37044 Tours, France
* Correspondence: Joelle.dupont@inra.fr; Tel.: +33-2-4742-7789; Fax: +33-2-4742-7743

Received: 12 July 2019; Accepted: 31 July 2019; Published: 2 August 2019

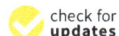

Abstract: Adipokines are a potential link between reproduction and energy metabolism and could partly explain some infertilities related to some pathophysiology, such as polycystic ovary syndrome (PCOS). However, adipokines were predominantly assessed in blood samples, while very little is known concerning their variations in follicular fluid (FF) and ovarian granulosa cells (GCs) of PCOS women. Thus, the objectives of our study were to investigate adiponectin, chemerin, resistin, visfatin, omentin, and apelin ovarian expression in PCOS women in comparison with controls and women with only a polycystic ovary morphology. In total, 78 women undergoing an in vitro fertilization procedure were divided into three groups: 23 PCOS women, 28 women presenting only ≥12 follicles per ovary (ECHO group), and 27 control women. Each group almost equally included normal weight and obese women. Follicular fluid (FF) concentration and granulosa cells (GCs) mRNA expression of adipokines and their receptors were assessed by ELISA and RT-qPCR, respectively. Omentin levels in FF and GC were higher in PCOS than in ECHO and control women, while apelin expression was increased in both PCOS and ECHO groups. FF chemerin concentration was predominant in normal-weight PCOS women compared to BMI (Body Mass Index)-matched ECHO and control women, while GC mRNA levels were higher in the obese PCOS group than in the ECHO one. Compared to PCOS, ECHO women had increased FF adiponectin concentrations and lower plasma AMH levels. The FF concentration of all adipokines was higher in obese subjects except for adiponectin, predominant in normal-weight women. In conclusion, women with PCOS expressed higher GC chemerin and omentin, whereas the ECHO group presented higher levels of FF adiponectin and apelin and lower plasma AMH and LH concentrations. Chemerin, omentin, and apelin expression was differently regulated in women with PCOS, suggesting their possible role in follicular growth arrest and ovulatory dysfunction characterizing PCOS pathogenesis.

Keywords: adipokines; PCOS; polycystic ovary morphology; follicular fluid; human granulosa cells

1. Introduction

Polycystic ovary syndrome (PCOS) is a very common endocrinopathy affecting 6% to 13% of women of reproductive age and is one of the leading causes of female poor fertility [1]. It was initially described as the association of anovulation and clinical and/or biological hyperandrogenism (1990 National Institutes of Health-Sponsored conference). In 2003, the Rotterdam Consensus Conference introduced polycystic ovaries on ultrasound (corresponding to a follicle number per ovary ≥12 and/or an ovarian volume ≥10 mL) as a supplementary, not mandatory, diagnostic criterion [2]. Thus, PCOS diagnosis currently requires the presence of at least two of these three criteria: Oligo/anovulation, hyperandrogenism, and polycystic ovaries morphology (PCOM) [3]. Despite its typical association with insulin resistance (IR), abdominal obesity [4], and an increased risk of developing type 2 diabetes [5], the causal relationship between reproductive and metabolic features in PCOS has not yet been fully elucidated. Adverse effects of obesity on fertility have largely been discussed and investigated [6,7]. Notably, in PCOS, it has been suggested that an original adipose tissue dysfunction, possibly due to in utero androgen hyperexposition and leading to excessive visceral fat depots, may play a key role in determining both IR and altered androgen metabolism [8].

It is well known that white adipose tissue can act as a metabolically active tissue able to synthetize and secrete many endocrine compounds called adipokines [9,10]. The involvement of these molecules in human fertility has been earning growing interest in the last years. Leptin implication in the interaction between energy metabolism and the reproductive system is nowadays widely admitted [11,12]. More recently, it has been demonstrated that several other adipokines may play a role in female reproductive function, and notably in ovarian physiology [13]. Indeed, in vitro investigations demonstrated that adiponectin receptors AdipoR1 and AdipoR2 [14], chemerin and its receptor chemerin chemokine-Like Receptor 1 (CMKLR1) [15], resistin [16], visfatin [17], omentin [18], apelin, and its receptor APJ (Apelin Receptor) [19] are expressed at both mRNA and protein levels in human granulosa cells (GCs). Moreover, some of these adipokines have been in vitro demonstrated to be implicated in human ovarian follicle function [20] and modulation of steroidogenesis [14–17,19,21]. Plasma levels of adiponectin [4], chemerin [22,23], resistin [24,25], visfatin [26,27], omentin [28,29], and apelin [19] seem to vary in women with PCOS, but the literature is poor, and results are often discordant [19,30–34]. Further, adipokines were predominantly assessed in blood samples, while very little is known concerning their variations in follicular fluid (FF) and GCs of women with PCOS [19,35–37].

The aim of our study was to investigate the concentration in FF and the mRNA expression in GC of adiponectin, chemerin, resistin, visfatin, omentin, and apelin and some of their receptors in PCOS women. Further, to improve the understanding of PCOS etiology that is still under debate, and to identify adipokines potentially involved in its physiopathology, we chose to compare PCOS subjects to a cohort of women presenting only PCOM on ultrasound, without any other characteristic feature of PCOS. This condition, which we named "ECHO", has in addition significant clinical interest, since it is well known that a high number of ovarian follicles is a major risk factor of ovarian hyperstimulation syndrome during a medically assisted reproduction (MAR) procedure [38].

2. Results

2.1. Anthropometric, Clinical, and Hormonal Data

Anthropometric, clinical, and hormonal data as well as IVF procedure outcomes are detailed in Table 1 and Figure 1. As expected, BMI was higher in obese groups and cycles were longer in PCOS compared to ECHO and control women. ECHO and PCOS groups were characterized by a greater follicle count compared to controls; a significant, not predictable difference was also found between normal-weight and obese women. Plasma AMH and LH levels were higher in PCOS women compared to controls. Interestingly, as regards AMH, we observed a highly statistically significant difference also between PCOS and ECHO groups. Concerning IVF procedure outcomes, oocytes and embryos numbers were greater in ECHO and PCOS women. No difference in plasma FSH and oestradiol levels was observed between the groups. No woman of the ECHO and control groups and only 6 out of 23 women with PCOS presented a clinical and/or biological hyperandrogenism. Plasma testosterone concentrations determined with the same kit for each group are reported in Table 1.

Table 1. Study population's ($n = 78$) clinical parameters, hormonal data, and in vitro fertilization procedure outcomes.

Parameter	Age (y)	BMI (kg/m^2)	Cycle Duration (d)	FSH (UI/L)	Estradiol (ng/L)	Testosterone (µg/L)
NW Controls ($n = 12$)	31.08 ± 3.82	21.77 ± 2.07	28.46 ± 2.15	6.78 ± 3.19	43.33 ± 14.29	0.33 ± 0.20 ($n = 5$)
NW ECHO ($n = 13$)	31.69 ± 5.88	20.84 ± 1.86	30.25 ± 2.54	6.40 ± 2.15	42.85 ± 16.01	0.28 ± 0.15 ($n = 6$)
NW PCOS ($n = 13$)	29.54 ± 3.36	20.68 ± 1.96	98.54 ± 67.77 *	5.86 ± 1.66	41.55 ± 14.85	0.88 ± 0.93 ($n = 6$)
Obese Controls ($n = 15$)	33.80 ± 4.62	33.13 ± 2.29	28.97 ± 2.21	6.71 ± 3.49	43.23 ± 17.24	0.41 ± 0.19 ($n = 5$)
Obese ECHO ($n = 15$)	32.73 ± 4.50	31.53 ± 3.33	29.89 ± 1.30	5.68 ± 1.09	35.23 ± 13.43	0.43 ± 0.08 ($n = 5$)
Obese PCOS ($n = 10$)	30.10 ± 3.25	33.38 ± 2.12	76.11 ± 61.79 #	4.86 ± 1.64	34.13 ± 6.99	0.49 ± 0.24 ($n = 7$)
Condition Effect	$p = 0.07$	$p = 0.14$	$p < 0.0001$	$p = 0.13$	$p = 0.38$	-
BMI Effect	$p = 0.15$	$p < 0.0001$	$p = 0.37$	$p = 0.28$	$p = 0.13$	-
Interaction	$p = 0.65$	$p = 0.32$	$p = 0.46$	$p = 0.78$	$p = 0.57$	-

Note: BMI = Body Mass Index; FSH = Follicle-Stimulating Hormone; NW = Normal-Weight; * indicated significant difference ($p < 0.001$) between Normal-Weight PCOS women and Normal-Weight ECHO/Control women; # indicated significant difference ($p < 0.001$) between Obese PCOS and Obese ECHO/Control women. The values are expressed as mean ± standard deviation.

2.2. FF Adiponectin and AdipoR1 Expression in GC Varied Mainly According to BMI

Adiponectin concentration in FF was clearly significantly higher in normal-weight women then in obese ones (Figure 2A). According to pathological status, we observed a significant difference only within the normal-weight group, with greater levels of adiponectin in ECHO as compared to PCOS women (Figure 2A). Likewise, AdipoR1 was predominantly expressed in GCs of normal-weight women (Figure 2B). However, differences in pathological condition were limited to the obese group, with ECHO and PCOS women showing greater AdipoR1 expression compared to controls (Figure 2B). Both adiponectin concentration in FF and AdipoR1 expression in GCs were negatively correlated with BMI (r = −0.748 and r = −0.288, respectively, Table 2). FF adiponectin was also negatively correlated with plasma E2 (r = −0.30, Table 2), while a positive correlation was observed between AdipoR1 expression and follicles (r = 0.554, $p < 0.001$), oocytes (r = 0.286, $p < 0.05$), and embryos number (r = 0.309, $p < 0.05$). No significant correlation was found between adiponectin concentration in FF and AdipoR1 expression.

Table 2. Correlations between follicular fluid concentration of adipokines and clinical parameters, hormonal data, and in vitro fertilization procedure outcomes ($n = 62$).

Parameter	Adiponectin	Chemerin	Resistin	Visfatin	Omentin	Apelin
BMI (kg/m^2)	r = −0.748 ***	r = 0.725 ***	r = 0.799 ***	r = 0.275 *	r = 0.446 ***	r = 0.441 ***
Cycle duration (d)	NS	NS	NS	NS	r = 0.421 ***	NS
Follicles Count (n)	NS	NS	NS	r = −0.352 **	NS	r = 0.480 **
AMH (ng/mL)	NS	NS	NS	r = −0.284 *	NS	NS
Estradiol (ng/L)	r = −0.300 *	NS	NS	NS	NS	r = −0.284 *
Oocytes Retrieved (n)	NS	NS	NS	r = −0.37 **	NS	r = 0.300 *
Embryos (n)	NS	NS	NS	r = −0.262 *	NS	r = 0.268 *

Note: BMI = Body Mass Index; AMH = Anti-Müllerian Hormone. NS = Not Statistically Significant; * $p < 0.05$; ** $p < 0.01$; *** $p < 0.001$.

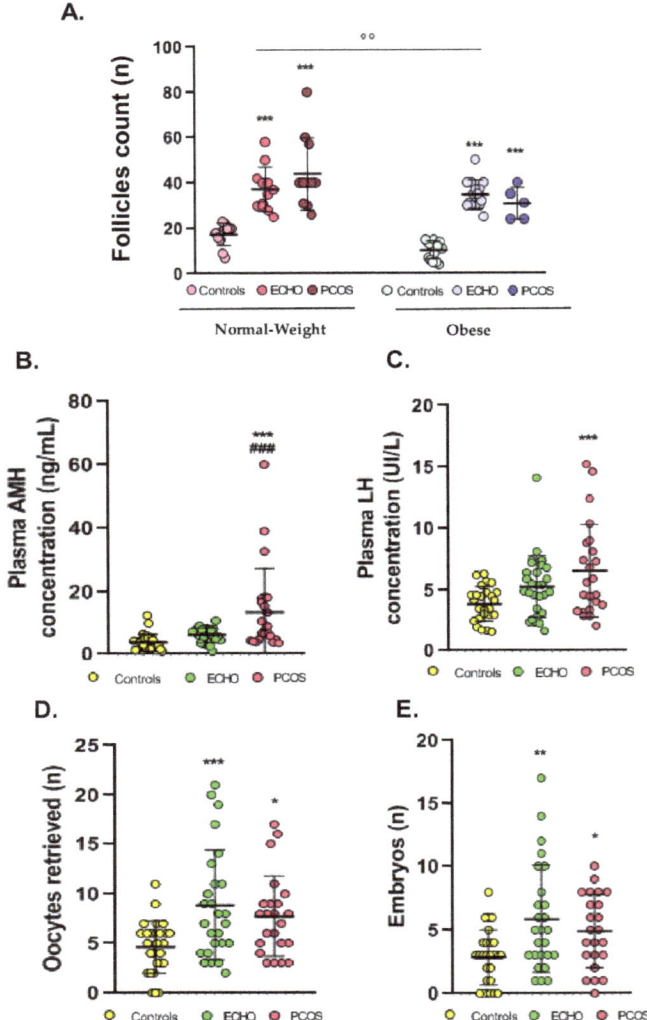

Figure 1. Clinical parameters, hormonal data, and in vitro fertilization procedure outcomes in patients of different studied groups. (**A**) Follicle counts assessed by transvaginal ultrasound, (**B**) plasma AMH concentration, (**C**) plasma LH concentration, (**D**) number of oocytes withdrawn during transvaginal retrieval, and (**E**) number of embryos obtained after in vitro fertilization. For A panel, see Table 1 for the data number per group. For the **B**, **C**, **D**, and **E** panels, the data were pooled in three groups ($n = 27$, $n = 28$, $n = 23$ for controls, ECHO, and PCOS groups, respectively) according to the pathological condition, as the BMI effect was not significant and no interaction between the BMI and pathological condition effect was found. The values are expressed as mean ± standard errors of means. °° indicates significant difference ($p < 0.01$) between normal-weight and obese subjects; * indicates significant difference vs. controls (* $p < 0.05$, ** $p < 0.01$, *** $p < 0.001$); ### indicates significant difference ($p < 0.001$) vs. ECHO women.

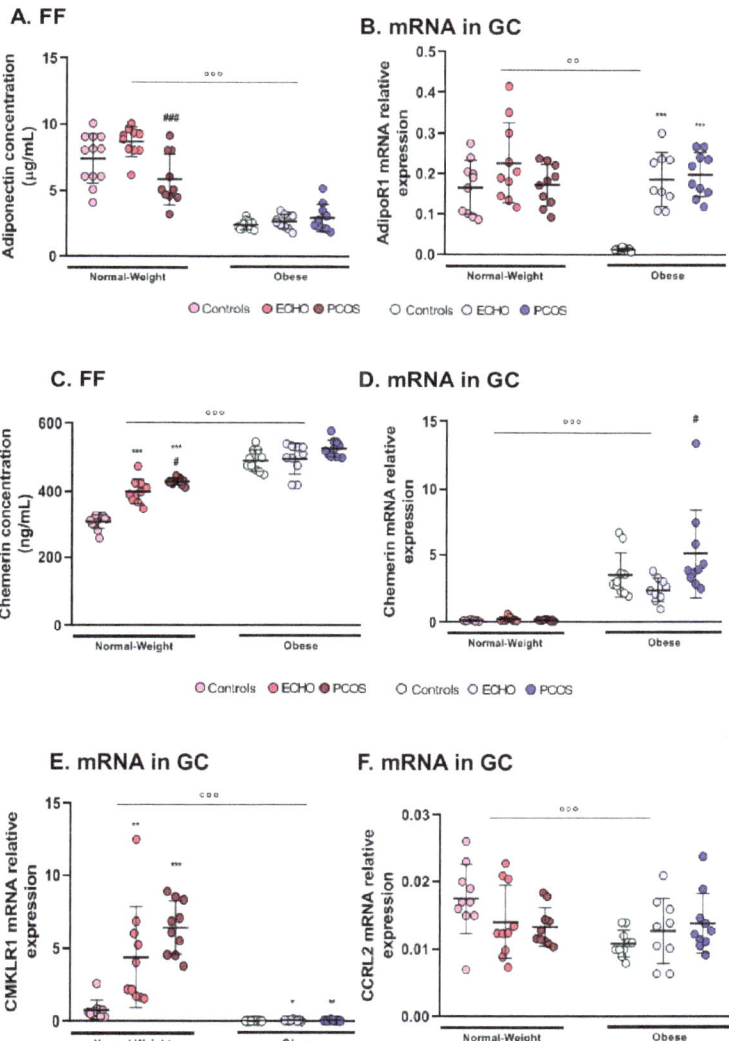

Figure 2. Follicular fluid adiponectin and chemerin concentration and mRNA expression of AdipoR1(Adiponectin receptor 1), CMKLR1, and CCRL2 in granulosa cells of obese and normal-weight PCOS, ECHO, and control groups. (**A**) Follicular fluid (FF) adiponectin concentration assessed by ELISA and (**B**) AdipoR1 mRNA levels in granulosa cells (GCs) quantified by RT-PCR within the six different groups; (**C, D**) chemerin levels in FF and GC; (**E, F**) mRNA levels of CMKLR1 and CCLR2 in GC. The values are expressed as mean ± standard errors of means (n = 12 for normal-weight controls, n = 13 for normal-weight ECHO, n = 13 for normal-weight PCOS, n = 15 for obese controls, n = 15 for obese ECHO, and n = 10 for obese PCOS). ° indicates significant difference between normal-weight and obese subjects (°° $p < 0.01$, °°° $p < 0.001$); * indicates significant difference vs. controls (*** $p < 0.001$); # indicates significant difference vs. ECHO women (# $p < 0.05$, # # # $p < 0.001$).

2.3. Chemerin (FF and GC mRNA Expression) Was Higher in Obese Subjects and in Women with PCOS

Chemerin expression both in FF and GC was greater in obese women than in normal-weight women (Figure 2C,D). Concerning pathological status, chemerin concentration in FF was clearly predominant in women with PCOS, but a statistically significant difference was found only in the normal-weight group (Figure 2C). Otherwise, chemerin expression in GC varied only within the obese group, with significantly higher levels in PCOS compared to ECHO women (Figure 2D). Interestingly, chemerin follicular concentration positively correlated with chemerin mRNA levels in GC ($r = 0.64$, $p < 0.001$) and both strongly positively correlated with BMI ($r = 0.725$ and $r = 0.694$, respectively, Table 2).

2.4. CMKLR1 and CCRL2 mRNA Expression in GC was Markedly Reduced in Obese Women

Contrary to chemerin, mRNA levels of its receptor, CMKLR1, were almost undetectable in obese women (Figure 2E). However, in line with what was seen for chemerin, in the normal-weight group, CMKLR1 expression was predominant in women with PCOS, even if the difference with the ECHO group failed to reach statistical significance (Figure 2E). C-C Chemokine Receptor-Like 2 (CCRL2) expression varied only according to BMI, with higher mRNA levels in GCs of normal-weight women compared to the obese ones (Figure 2F). No significant modification was observed according to pathological status. G Protein-Coupled Receptor 1 (GPR1) expression did not change in any condition (data not shown). A positive correlation was observed between CMKLR1 expression and follicle count ($r = 0.520$, $p < 0.001$), cycle duration ($r = 0.337$, $p = 0.01$), plasma AMH ($r = 0.353$, $p < 0.01$), plasma LH ($r = 0.306$, $p < 0.05$), and plasma E2 concentrations ($r = 0.091$, $p < 0.05$). Remarkably, CMKLR1 mRNA levels were negatively correlated with BMI ($r = -0.622$, $p < .001$). Indeed, chemerin expression both in FF and GC was negatively correlated with the mRNA levels of all its receptors, although statistical significance was found only between FF chemerin and CCRL2 ($r = 0.342$, $p < 0.05$) and between chemerin mRNA levels in GC and CMKLR1 ($r = -0.46$, $p < 0.001$).

2.5. FF Resistin Was Higher in Obese Women

Resistin concentration in FF was markedly higher in obese women than in the normal-weight ones (Figure 3A) and, interestingly, it was positively correlated with BMI ($r = 0.799$, Table 2). In the normal-weight group, the highest resistin levels were observed in ECHO and PCOS women (Figure 3A). Resistin mRNA levels in GCs did not vary according to either BMI or pathological condition. Unlike chemerin, FF resistin did not significantly correlate with resistin expression in GCs.

2.6. Visfatin Modifications Were Restrained to Its Concentration in FF

As for resistin, visfatin expression varied only in FF and mainly according to BMI, with higher levels in obese subjects compared to the normal-weight ones (Figure 3B). However, follicular concentration of visfatin was lower in ECHO and PCOS women compared to controls, especially in the obese group (Figure 3B). FF visfatin was positively correlated with BMI ($r = 0.275$, Table 2) and negatively correlated with plasma AMH concentration ($r = -0.284$) and follicles ($r = -0.352$), oocytes ($r = -0.37$), and embryo number ($r = -0.262$) (Table 2). No significant modification nor correlation was found for visfatin mRNA levels in GCs.

2.7. Omentin Expression (FF and GC mRNA) Was Markedly Predominant in Women with PCOS

Omentin concentration was significantly higher in the FF of obese women (Figure 3C). Remarkably, independently from BMI, omentin levels were markedly more elevated in PCOS than in ECHO and control women (Figure 3C). Interestingly, obese ECHO women showed lower omentin follicular concentrations than controls (Figure 3C). The same significant results were found concerning omentin expression in GCs (Figure 3D). Further, omentin concentration in FF was strongly positively correlated with omentin mRNA levels in GCs ($r = 0.824$, $p < 0.001$) and both positively correlated with BMI ($r = 0.446$ for follicular omentin, Table 2, and $r = 0.464$ for GC omentin mRNA levels, $p < 0.001$).

A positive correlation was also observed between follicular omentin concentration and cycle duration (r = 0.421, Table 2).

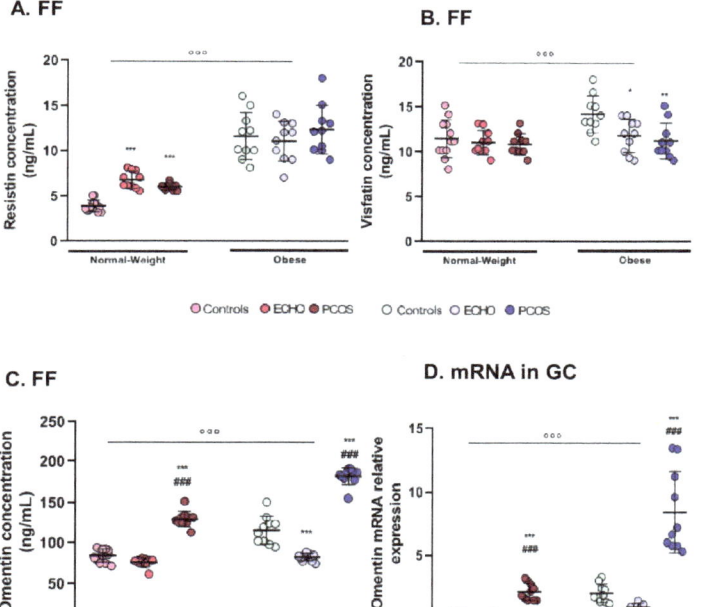

Figure 3. Follicular fluid resistin, visfatin, and omentin concentration and mRNA expression of omentin in granulosa cells of obese and normal-weight PCOS, ECHO, and control groups. (A) Follicular fluid (FF) resistin, (B) visfatin, and (C) omentin concentrations assessed by ELISA; (D) mRNA omentin levels in granulosa cells (GCs) quantified by RT-PCR within the six different groups. The values are expressed as mean ± standard errors of means ($n = 12$ for normal-weight controls, $n = 13$ for normal-weight ECHO, $n = 13$ for normal-weight PCOS, $n = 15$ for obese controls, $n = 15$ for obese ECHO, and $n = 10$ for obese PCOS). °°° indicates significant difference ($p < 0.001$) between normal-weight and obese subjects; * indicates significant difference vs. controls (* $p < 0.05$, ** $p < 0.01$, *** $p < 0.001$); ### indicates significant difference ($p < 0.001$) vs. ECHO women.

2.8. Apelin and Its Receptor APJ Were Mostly Expressed in Obese Subjects and in ECHO/PCOS Women

Both apelin FF levels and apelin expression in GCs were significantly higher in obese than in normal-weight women (Figure 4A and B) and positively correlated with BMI (r = 0.441, Table 2, and r = 0.554, $p < 0.001$, respectively). According to pathological status, apelin was mostly expressed in ECHO and PCOS women in both the normal-weight and obese groups (Figure 4A and 4B). Interestingly, limited to FF concentration, apelin was significantly lower in normal-weight PCOS than in ECHO women (Figure 4A). A positive correlation was found between follicle count and both apelin levels in FF (r = 0.480, Table 2) and apelin expression in GC (r = 0.301, $p < 0.05$). Follicular apelin also positively correlated with oocytes and embryo numbers (r = 0.30 and r = 0.268, respectively, Table 2) and negatively correlated with plasma E2 concentration (r = −0.284, Table 2). Apelin mRNA levels in GCs were correlated with cycle duration (positive correlation, r = 0.289, $p < 0.05$) and plasma FSH (negative correlation, r = −0.298, $p < 0.05$). Concerning APJ, we found the same significant results, with a predominant expression of this receptor in the obese group and women with PCOS (Figure 4C). Further, like apelin, mRNA levels of APJ positively correlated with BMI (r = 0.510, $p < 0.001$) and cycle duration (r = 0.402, $p < 0.01$) and negatively correlated with plasma FSH concentration (r = −0.282, $p < 0.05$). Notably, APJ expression was strongly positively correlated with apelin expression in GCs (r = 0.866, Figure 4G) and apelin concentration in FF (r = 0.749, Figure 4E right panel), which in turn were strongly positively correlated to each other (r = 0.821, Figure 4D).

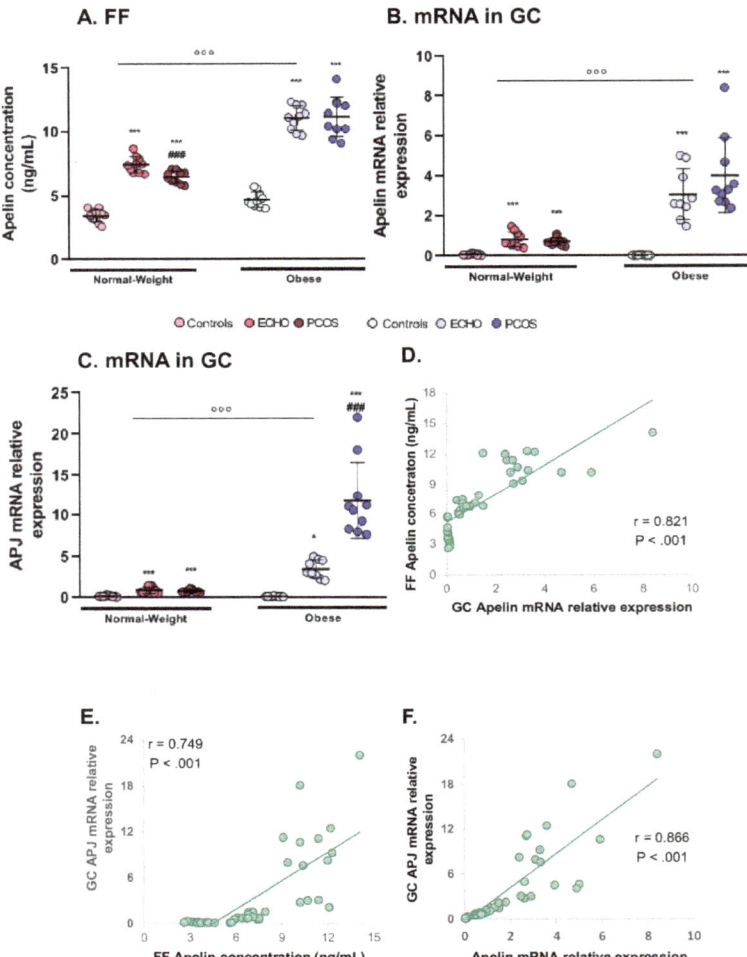

Figure 4. Follicular fluid apelin concentration, mRNA expression of apelin and its receptor, APJ, in GCs of obese and normal-weight PCOS, ECHO, and controls groups and correlations of apelin FF levels and apelin or APJ mRNA expression in GCs. (**A**) Follicular fluid (FF) apelin concentration assessed by ELISA; (**B**) apelin and (**C**) APJ mRNA levels in granulosa cells (GC) quantified by RT-PCR within the six different groups; (**D**) correlation between FF concentration and GC expression of apelin; correlations between APJ mRNA levels in GCs; and (**E**) apelin FF concentration and (**F**) apelin mRNA levels in GCs. The values are expressed as mean ± standard errors of means ($n = 12$ for normal-weight controls, $n = 13$ for normal-weight ECHO, $n = 13$ for normal-weight PCOS, $n = 15$ for obese controls, $n = 15$ for obese ECHO, and $n = 10$ for obese PCOS). °°° indicates significant difference ($p < 0.001$) between normal-weight and obese subjects; *** indicates significant difference ($p < 0.001$) vs. controls; ### indicates significant difference ($p < 0.001$) vs. ECHO women.

3. Discussion

Our study aimed to improve the understanding of PCOS etiology, and to identify adipokines potentially involved in its physiopathology. Thus, we analyzed the adipokines' profile at the ovarian level (FF and GC) in normal-weight and obese women with PCOS diagnosis in comparison with women presenting only a PCOM, a condition that we named "ECHO". This condition, as discussed above, has per se a significant clinical interest and, to the best of our knowledge, there are no data available about adipokines expression in the FF and GCs of these women. We evaluated adiponectin, chemerin, resistin, visfatin, omentin, and apelin concentrations in FF samples, as well as the expression of the same adipokines and some of their receptors in GCs. The results are discussed below for each single adipokine.

3.1. Adiponectin

Adiponectin is one of the better known and most abundant circulating adipokines. It is mainly produced by white adipocytes and secreted into plasma circulation as three oligomeric complexes, whose medium and high molecular weight isoforms represent 90% of circulating protein. It acts mainly through two G protein-coupled receptors, AdipoR1, which is ubiquitously expressed, and AdipoR2, which is mainly located in white adipose tissue and liver [30]. Its involvement in energy metabolism as an insulin-sensitizing, anti-inflammatory, and anti-atherogenic molecule is largely admitted [30] and obesity and insulin-resistant states have been associated with reduced plasma adiponectin concentrations [4]. In agreement with literature data, we found that adiponectin concentration in FF and AdipoR1 mRNA expression in GCs were markedly higher in normal-weight women then in the obese ones and both negatively correlated with BMI. Interestingly, we also observed that within the normal-weight group, FF adiponectin levels were significantly lower in PCOS compared to ECHO women. Consistent with our findings, despite some conflicting results [30], PCOS women have been reported to present lower adiponectin concentrations in serum [4,39] and FF [35,40], as well as a decreased expression of AdipoR1 and AdipoR2 in adipose tissue [5]. Although adiponectin dysregulation may be one of the possible mechanisms responsible for impairment of insulin-sensitivity in women with PCOS, the reduction of adiponectin levels in serum seems to be independent of IR severity [41]. Thus, adiponectin might play a role in the pathogenesis of other characteristic features of PCOS. In particular, several authors evoked a possible role of this adipokine in folliculogenesis [35,40]. Notably, Campos et al. reported that adiponectin acts directly and indirectly, through the interaction with LH and insulin, on GCs by inducing the expression of genes associated with periovulatory maturation of ovarian follicles [42]. It is therefore noteworthy that in our study, AdipoR1 expression in GCs was positively correlated with follicles, oocytes, and embryo count. On the other hand, contrary to what is reported in the literature [40], we did not find any significant difference in AdipoR2 expression. In addition, mRNA AdipoR1 levels varied only in the obese group, being greater in PCOS and ECHO women compared to controls. The meaning of our findings is currently unknown and deserves to be further elucidated. Although adiponectin involvement in PCOS pathogenesis is supported by several evidences, including genomic analyses [30], it is possible that the limited data we obtained are due to the fact that we only investigated GCs. In our study, we did not find any correlation between FF adiponectin concentration and AdipoR1/AdipoR2 expression in GCs. Hence, since adiponectin levels are twice higher in FF than in plasma [14], theca cells might represent the key actor in the metabolism of adiponectin as the main cell responsible for its production in FF and then the most likely target of its effects.

3.2. Resistin

Resistin is a small cysteine-rich protein mainly expressed by macrophages [43] and within adipose tissue, it is predominantly released by omental non-adipocyte resident inflammatory cells [44]. Its relevance and physiological role in humans are currently unclear. Notably, Panidis et al. showed that circulating resistin was higher in overweight women with PCOS but did not differ between PCOS and control women with a normal BMI, although the first were more insulin resistant [45]. Further, after stepwise multiple regression analysis, serum resistin levels were not associated with any parameter independent of BMI, suggesting that they correlated with IR as a consequence of obesity itself, rather than as an independent causative factor [45]. In accordance with these data, in our study, we found that resistin concentration in FF was significantly higher in obese women compared to the normal-weight ones and positively correlated with BMI. As regards PCOS women, some authors noted higher plasma resistin concentrations in overweight/obese patients compared to the normal-weight ones, independently from PCOS diagnosis [45]. However, others showed no difference in serum resistin levels between obese and non-obese PCOS women [25] and most of the studies failed to find a significant correlation between circulating resistin and BMI [37,46]. Interestingly, within the normal-weight group of patients, we observed higher resistin levels in the FF of ECHO and PCOS women compared to controls. Other studies, however, showed no difference in FF resistin concentration between PCOS and healthy normal-weight women [37]. Indeed, the association of resistin with PCOS is largely debated. Resistin mRNA and protein have been detected in granulosa, theca, cumulus cells, and oocytes from human ovarian follicles [16]. In human granulosa cells, recombinant resistin has been reported to decrease IGF-1-induced progesterone and estradiol secretion [16], which was associated with a reduction in P450scc and P450 aromatase levels [16], indicating a role for resistin in the regulation of ovarian steroidogenesis. However, data concerning serum resistin levels in women affected by PCOS are inconsistent. While some authors pointed out significantly higher resistin concentrations in the plasma of women with PCOS [24,25], no difference between PCOS and healthy women was reported by several others [37,45]. Interestingly, resistin mRNA levels in adipocytes were twice higher in women with PCOS compared to controls and significantly decreased after laparoscopic ovarian electrocautery [47,48], suggesting that although systemic resistin does not seem to be actively involved in PCOS pathogenesis, it may act as a local determining factor for this syndrome [45,48]. However, it is noteworthy that in agreement with previous literature data [37], in our study, FF resistin levels did not correlate with any reproductive outcome, making it unlikely that resistin plays a role in oocytes' maturation and development. Unlike other adipokines, we observed that resistin mRNA levels in GCs did not vary either according to BMI or pathological condition and did not correlate with FF concentration. Resistin levels in FF have been repeatedly found to be lower than in plasma [16,37]. It is therefore unlikely that human GCs, while expressing resistin protein [16], secrete it into FF or circulation. Furthermore, according to our findings and considering that follicular resistin seems to derive primarily from blood plasma, the regulation of resistin expression appears to be different at the systemic and ovarian level.

3.3. Visfatin

Visfatin, previously described as a growth factor for early B-cells called pre-B cell colony enhancing factor (PEBF) [49], was later characterized by Fukuhara et al. as a peptide predominantly expressed in and secreted from visceral adipose tissue in both humans and mice [50]. Although visfatin has been proposed as a potential link between visceral obesity and increased metabolic risk [51], data concerning the relationship between this adipokine, obesity, and IR are widely discordant. In our study, visfatin concentration in FF was significantly higher in the obese group than in the normal-weight one and positively correlated with BMI. Despite some conflicting results [52], a recent meta-analysis revealed that plasma visfatin is significantly increased in subjects presenting overweight/obesity, IR, metabolic syndrome, and cardiovascular diseases [53]. A positive association between circulating visfatin and BMI has been reported by several authors [26,27,34,51] but not confirmed by others [52]. On the contrary, the role of visfatin in the regulation of female reproductive functions is supported by several evidences. Indeed, it is expressed in human myometrium, placenta, and human fetal membranes, where it seems to be involved in placentation [17]. In the ovary, its presence has been demonstrated in human follicles, notably in oocytes, cumulus, and GCs and less abundantly in theca cells [17,53].

In human GCs, it has been reported to enhance IGF-1-induced progesterone and estradiol secretion, thus showing a positive effect on steroidogenesis [17]. In our study, we observed significantly lower levels of visfatin in the FF of obese ECHO and PCOS women compared to obese healthy controls, a result not in line with literature data. Indeed, in previous studies, FF visfatin was shown to be similar [54] or higher [36] in women with PCOS when compared to BMI-matched normally ovulatory women. Similarly, as regards circulating visfatin, although two studies failed to highlight a significant difference between PCOS and healthy women [34], most of the authors found significantly higher levels in women with PCOS [26,27,36,54,55]. The decrease in visfatin concentration observed in the FF of the PCOS and ECHO women of our study, which is characterized by a high antral follicle count deriving from follicular growth arrest, suggests a positive effect of visfatin on female reproductive function, and notably folliculogenesis. Indeed, Shen et al. found a significant positive correlation between visfatin concentration in FF and the number of retrieved oocytes [53] and the administration of visfatin during ovulation induction in aged female mice improved the developmental competency of oocytes [56]. However, it needs to be underlined that in our study, follicular visfatin was negatively correlated with follicle, oocyte, and embryo numbers, as well as with plasma AMH concentration. As for resistin, visfatin mRNA levels in GCs did not vary either according to BMI or pathological condition and did not correlate with FF concentration. Visfatin levels in FF have been shown to be similar [53] or lower [54] compared to those in plasma and no correlation was found between visfatin concentrations in plasma and FF [53]. In light of our results, the possibility of an ovarian origin for this adipokine, although previously evoked [53], seems thus unlikely.

3.4. Apelin

Apelin is a bioactive peptide originally identified in bovine stomach extract as the endogenous ligand of the orphan G protein-coupled receptor, APJ [57]. Its expression has been detected in several organs, like the stomach, brain, lung, uterus, and ovary, as well as in the endothelium of small arteries [57], indicating that the apelin/APJ system may play a pivotal role in multiple physiological functions. In particular, apelin seems to be involved in the regulation of food intake, energy metabolism, cardiovascular system, angiogenesis, and neuroendocrine functions [57]. In our study, we found that apelin concentration in FF as well as apelin and APJ mRNA expression in GCs were significantly higher in obese than in normal-weight women and positively correlated with BMI. These results already reported by Roche et al. [19] are consistent also with literature data about circulating apelin levels [58]. As the existence of a correlation between serum apelin levels and IR in PCOS is still a matter of debate [59], apelin, rather than as a marker of insulin sensitivity, may play a role in other characteristic features of PCOS, such as ovulatory dysfunction. Indeed, apelin and APJ expression has been detected in human ovarian follicles, GCs, theca cells, and oocytes and in vitro studies suggest a potential role of apelin in the control of several aspects of ovarian function [19]. Indeed, apelin enhances progesterone and estradiol secretion in human and porcine GC cultures [19,60], it improves rat, bovine, and porcine GC proliferation, and it seems to be involved in the regulation of the bovine corpus luteum luteolysis process [61] and oocyte maturation [62]. In our study, we demonstrated that both apelin concentration in FF and apelin/APJ mRNA expression in GCs positively correlated with antral follicle count and were significantly higher in PCOS and ECHO groups, both characterized by the accumulation of small antral follicles resulting from the failed selection of a dominant follicle. Thus, according to these observations, apelin may play a key role in follicular growth arrest at the origin of PCOM. In support of this hypothesis, apelin has been suggested to be implicated in bovine follicular atresia [63] and in different animal species; both protein and mRNA levels of apelin and APJ have been reported to change during follicular growth, with the highest expression in large follicles [60,63]. Folliculogenesis disruption in PCOS is thought to be due to an increased responsiveness to FSH in terms of oestradiol and progesterone production and to a premature responsiveness to LH in small follicles [64]. Consequently, in PCOS anovulatory women, plasma estradiol levels are slightly higher and FSH levels are lower than in the normal early follicular phase [64]. While keeping in mind that correlations may be merely spurious, without causative significance, very interestingly, we found that apelin mRNA levels in GCs were negatively correlated with plasma FSH levels and positively correlated with cycle duration, strongly supporting that apelin could also participate in hormonal disturbances at the origin of PCOS pathogenesis. Indeed, this adipokine has been identified in the arcuate supraoptic and paraventricular hypothalamic nuclei [62], it has been demonstrated to suppress LH secretion in rats [65], and a negative correlation between plasma apelin and LH levels has repeatedly been shown in humans [66,67]. In our study, FF concentration and GC mRNA expression of apelin was strongly positively correlated with each other and with APJ expression. Further, even if plasma apelin levels largely depend on the dosage method, FF apelin concentration seems to be higher than the plasma one [59]. Thus, follicular apelin may partly derive by GC production and act in a paracrine and/or autocrine manner on GCs themselves.

3.5. Omentin

Omentin, also known as intelectin-1, is a novel adipokine identified from the cDNA library of omental adipose tissue by Yang et al. and predominantly produced by visceral fat depots [68]. Despite some discordant results [29], serum omentin levels have been shown to be inversely related to obesity [69,70] and to increase after weight loss [71]. Contrarily to what was reported in plasma, in our study, we found that FF concentration and GC mRNA expression of omentin were significantly higher in obese women compared to the normal-weight ones and positively correlated with BMI. We also demonstrated that omentin expression in both FF and GCs was significantly higher in women with PCOS compared to controls and ECHO women. These results, already shown by Cloix et al. [18], once again disagree with literature data concerning plasma omentin levels. Indeed, most of the studies investigating omentin expression in PCOS women found lower plasma omentin concentrations [28,29,69,70], as well as decreased omentin mRNA and protein levels in adipose tissue [72]. Several factors have been evoked to explain such results. First, it has been repeatedly reported that serum omentin levels are inversely related with HOMA-IR/fasting insulin [29,69,70,72] and an in vitro study supported the role of hyperinsulinemia in lessening omentin expression in adipose tissue [72]. Hormonal disturbances, and notably hyperandrogenism, have been suggested as another key factor contributing to a decrease of omentin synthesis in PCOS women [29,70]. Indeed, as for some other adipokines, plasma omentin levels are higher in women than in men [73] and negatively correlate with androgens' levels [29,70]. At last, omentin may also be regulated by inflammation, as its expression is altered in inflammatory states [28] and PCOS is actually considered as a proinflammatory condition [74]. According to these observations, the higher omentin expression that we found in FF and GCs in PCOS women suggests that omentin production at the ovarian level is independent from insulin action and differently regulated in these patients. Furthermore, in our study, FF concentration and GC expression of omentin positively correlated with each other, strongly supporting the hypothesis that follicular omentin is at least partially produced by GCs. Interestingly, Cloix et al. showed that in PCOS women, but not in controls, omentin concentration is doubled in FF compared to in plasma [18]. Whether omentin is implicated in PCOS pathogenesis is, however, still to be demonstrated. In humans, omentin is expressed in reproductive tissues, including the placenta and ovary [70], and it has been shown to enhance, through induction of visfatin expression, GC IGF-1-induced steroidogenesis and IGF-1R signaling [18]. Thus, it has been suggested that omentin and visfatin, modulating insulin sensitivity in GC, could affect ovarian function. Indeed, insulin and IGF-1 act synergistically with FSH to increase GC estrogens' synthesis and with LH to enhance theca cells' androgen production [18]. Interestingly, circulating omentin has already been shown to be positively correlated with serum estradiol and negatively correlated with the LH/FSH ratio [29]. Mahde et al. also found higher serum omentin levels in PCOS women with irregular cycles compared to those with regular ones [69], data that agree with our finding of a positive correlation between follicular omentin and cycle duration, further confirming the possible role of this adipokine in ovulatory dysfunction characteristics of PCOS.

3.6. Chemerin

Chemerin, also known as Retinoic Acid Receptor Responder protein 2 (RARRES2), is a small chemotactic protein originally identified as the natural ligand of the G-protein coupled receptor CMKLR1 [75]. Initially known as a proinflammatory cytokine involved in adaptive and innate immunity [76], in 2007, it was discovered as a novel adipokine associated with obesity and metabolic syndrome [77] and shown to promote adipogenesis and adipocyte metabolism [78]. In addition to CMKLR1, two other receptors, GPR1 and CCRL2, were reported to bind chemerin with high affinity, but at present data concerning their functional relevance are poor [75]. In our study, chemerin expression in both FF and GCs was greater in obese women than in the normal-weight ones and strongly positively correlated with BMI. This is consistent with Bozaoglu et al.'s data, showing that chemerin and CMKLR1 were highly expressed in mature adipocytes and upregulated in the adipose tissue of obese animals [77]. Circulating chemerin levels have also been reported to be higher in obese subjects compared to those with a normal BMI and significantly correlated with metabolic syndrome parameters, such as BMI, triglycerides, and fasting serum insulin [23]. Nevertheless, BMI alone does not seem to be a predictive factor for circulating chemerin [31]. Indeed, the existence of a correlation between this adipokine and PCOS has repeatedly been evoked [79]. Our findings showed that both chemerin FF concentration and chemerin and CMKLR1 mRNA levels in GCs were predominant in women with PCOS. The same results have recently been found by Wang et al. in a cohort of non-obese women [21]. Further, serum and ovarian chemerin levels have been shown to be elevated in a dihydrotestosterone (DHT)-induced rat PCOS model [21] and, despite few discordant data [31], the literature widely reports higher chemerin levels in the plasma and adipose tissue of PCOS women [22]. Chemerin has been demonstrated to act as an important negative regulator of ovarian steroidogenesis [80], inhibiting IGF-1-induced secretion of progesterone and estradiol in human GCs [15] and suppressing FSH-induced expression of aromatase and P450scc in cultured rat preantral follicles and GCs [21,81]. Furthermore, in DHT-treated rats, elevated chemerin levels and down-regulated aromatase expression were positively related to increased GC apoptosis [80], suggesting that chemerin may be involved in the antral follicular growth arrest associated to the hyperandrogenic proinflammatory state characterizing PCOS [82]. While keeping in mind that correlations may be merely spurious, without causative significance, it is noteworthy that in our study CMKLR1 expression in GCs was significantly positively correlated with follicle count, cycle duration, and plasma AMH, LH, and estradiol levels. As for apelin and omentin, we found that the follicular concentration of chemerin strongly positively correlated with its mRNA levels in GCs, suggesting that follicular chemerin may be partly produced in the ovary. Indeed, chemerin and CMKLR1 expression has been demonstrated in human and mouse placenta [78], in human, mouse, and rat ovary [21], and more recently in human granulosa and theca cells [15]. In support of this hypothesis, the concentration of this adipokine has been shown to be higher in FF than in plasma [15] and the rise of follicular chemerin in PCOS women has been demonstrated to be independent of changes in its plasma concentration and adiposity, strongly indicating that chemerin is independently regulated at the ovarian level [82]. Interestingly, in our study, CMKLR1 and chemerin expression seemed to be inversely regulated as regards adiposity. Indeed, contrarily to chemerin, CMKLR1 mRNA levels were higher in GCs of normal-weight women and negatively correlated with BMI. Further, chemerin and CMKLR1 levels in GCs negatively correlated with each other, suggesting the possibility of a negative feedback between chemerin and its receptor. Such a regulatory mechanism has already been proposed by Bozaoglu et al. in adipose tissue, but finally, chemerin's role in the regulation of CMKLR1 expression in adipocytes seems quite limited [77]. As an alternative, these findings could be due to a resistance mechanism to chemerin action at the ovarian level. Indeed, as hyperinsulinemia in the IR states, the high chemerin levels found in obese women could be a compensatory response to the lack of CMKLR1 in GCs. This is, however, a pure hypothesis, since no data is at the moment available about whether and how this chemerin resistance may occur.

3.7. ECHO Condition

In our study, we chose to compare women with PCOS and controls to a third group of women presenting at least 12 small antral follicles per ovary without any other criterion necessary for PCOS diagnosis, i.e., hyperandrogenism and/or oligo-anovulation. Besides allowing us to better understand adipokines' role in PCOS physiopathology, the "ECHO condition" has relevant clinical interest. Indeed, despite some discordant results [83], it has repeatedly been reported to be associated with hyperandrogenism and IR [84,85]. PCOM is also encountered in about 30% of young asymptomatic women [85], but its actual meaning in this condition is currently unknown [86]. There is little evidence to suggest that its sole presence has any significant risk to subsequent health, except for circumstances in which women with PCOM require a gonadotropin treatment, such as during an IVF procedure [86]. Indeed, due to polycystic ovaries' extreme sensitivity to FSH, an antral follicle count greater than 24 is considered a major risk factor of ovarian hyperstimulation syndrome and nowadays is routinely recommended for the pre-treatment identification of patients at risk [38]. Interestingly, we found that FF concentration and GC mRNA expression of omentin, chemerin, and APJ (for the last two, these observations were limited to the obese group) were significantly lower in ECHO compared to PCOS women, suggesting that these molecules could play a physiopathological role in other main features of PCOS, such as anovulatory infertility. On the contrary, the ECHO group was characterized by higher FF adiponectin levels, possibly reflecting a lower IR compared to the PCOS group or, more intriguingly, a beneficial effect of adiponectin on follicular maturation and subsequent ovulation. Surprisingly, we also observed that, despite no difference in terms of follicle numbers between the two groups, ECHO women presented lower plasma AMH levels than women with PCOS. It has been demonstrated that AMH plays a key role in protecting growing follicles from premature maturation, directly by inhibiting the recruitment of primordial follicles and indirectly by opposing the effects of FSH. For this reason, it is considered an endocrine marker of the number of small antral follicles [87]. Indeed, plasma AMH concentration was reported to be two to three-fold higher in women with PCOS than in normal ovulatory women [88] and in vitro studies demonstrated that GCs of normo-ovulatory and anovulatory PCOS women produce, respectively, 4-fold and 75-fold higher AMH levels compared to controls [89]. Serum AMH levels are therefore considered to reflect the severity of PCOS [90] and notably, the ovulatory disturbances characteristic of this disease [87]. In addition, Homburg et al. reported that AMH levels can be used to differentiate women with PCOS from women with PCOM alone and controls [91], further strengthening our results. As for AMH, plasma LH levels in the ECHO group were intermediate between controls and women with PCOS. Women with PCOM had already been reported to present a hormonal profile, as well as a per-follicle AMH production, intermediate between normal and PCOS women, suggesting that isolated PCOM might represent a PCOS-like phenotype characterized by a mild GC dysfunction, not yet sufficient to affect the ovulatory process [86]. Our findings also agree with literature data showing a tight positive correlation between LH and AMH [86] and support the role of AMH in hormonal alterations at the origin of the ovulatory dysfunction observed in women with PCOS [92].

3.8. Limitations and Perspectives

Although this study provided meaningful information, it has some limitations. Firstly, it was a retrospective and observational study and, as such, it did not permit determination of whether the modifications in adipokines' concentration were at the origin of the development of polycystic ovaries in PCOS, or rather a consequence or a compensatory response. Secondly, we studied only women requiring IVF and hence under controlled ovarian stimulation, a condition that surely modifies the normal functions of the female reproductive system. Thus, our results might not be generalized to all PCOS and ECHO women. Finally, data about the IR state were not available for most of the women included in the study. This could have given us more information about patients' hormonal profile and, mostly, helped us to better understand and interpret adipokines' modifications. Our current understanding of the role of chemerin, omentin, and apelin in PCOS is far from complete and deserves further studies. Notably, it would be of importance to elucidate the molecular mechanisms involved in their effects on GCs and, above all, to study their expression and action on theca cells, which play a key role in the hyperandrogenism characterizing PCOS women.

4. Materials and Methods

4.1. Ethics Approval

Study was conducted according to principles set in the Declaration of Helsinki. Informed consent was signed by each participant and study protocol was approved by the Institutional Review Board (Authorization protocol 2016_075, 1 January 2016) Ethic Committee of University Hospital of Tours, France).

4.2. Study Population

Biological samples and clinical data of a total of 78 women undergoing an in vitro fertilization (IVF) procedure between 2011 and 2017 at the referral center for reproductive medicine of University Hospital of Tours were analyzed.

Three groups of patients were created: 23 women suffering from PCOS (PCOS group), 28 women presenting ≥12 follicles per ovary on transvaginal ultrasound without other criteria necessary for diagnosis of PCOS (ECHO group), and 27 women affected by another cause of infertility requiring a MAR procedure (control group). Each group almost equally included normal weight (BMI 18–25 kg/m^2) and obese (BMI > 30 kg/m^2) women. A total of 6 groups was then analyzed. Diagnosis of PCOS followed 2003 Rotterdam Consensus Conference Criteria [2]. All women with PCOS presented an oligo/anovulation and follicle count ≥12 per ovary. Clinical and/or biological hyperandrogenism was reported for 6 out of 23 of them. Signs of clinical hyperandrogenism included acne, alopecia, and hirsutism as evaluated by a physician experienced in the field. No woman included in the ECHO and control groups had clinical and/or biological hyperandrogenism and all were characterized by normal ovulatory cycles. They underwent an IVF procedure because of male infertility, tubal sterility, ovarian insufficiency, endometriosis, or a combination of male and female causes. The antral follicle number was assessed in the early follicular phase by transvaginal ultrasound scans of the ovaries performed by experienced sonographers. Blood samples for hormonal evaluations were collected between day 3 and day 5 of the menstrual cycle before the IVF stimulation protocol. Plasma levels of testosterone, oestradiol (E2), luteinizing hormone (LH), and follicle-stimulating hormone (FSH) were measured using an Immulite® 2500 immunoassay analyzer (Siemens, Munich, Germany). However, none of the control and ECHO women included in our study showed clinical and biological hyperandrogenism. Plasma anti-Mullerian hormone (AMH) was determined by Eurofin Biomnis (Lyon, France).

4.3. Collection of FF Samples and Isolation of GCs

GCs were obtained from preovulatory follicles during oocyte retrieval preceding IVF. The controlled ovarian stimulation protocol and IVF procedures employed have already been reported [93]. After isolation of cumulus-oocyte complexes, FF was recovered and centrifuged (400× g, 10 min) to separate cell remnants. The supernatant was stored at −80 °C for later analyses. GCs were isolated from erythrocytes with 20 min of centrifugation at 400× g on two layers of discontinuous Percoll gradient (40%, 60% in Ham's F-12 medium; GIBCO-BRL/Life Technologies, Lyon, France). The 40% fraction was collected and treated with hemolytic medium (NH4Cl 10 mM in Tris HCL, pH 7.5; Sigma Aldrich, Saint Quentin-Fallavier, France) to remove the remaining erythrocytes. Following centrifugation, the pellet was washed with fresh medium (Ham's F-12) and stored at −80 °C for later use.

4.4. Adipokines Concentration in FF

Adiponectin, chemerin, resistin, visfatin, omentin, and apelin concentrations were measured by ELISA in FF samples. ELISA R&D Bio-Techne Ltd. kits (Abingdon, United Kingdom, intra-assay coefficients of variations <6% and inter-assay coefficients of variations ≤8%) were used for all adipokines.

4.5. RNA Extraction and Real-Time Quantitative PCR (qPCR)

Total RNA from GCs was extracted with TRIzol reagent according to the manufacturer's procedure (Sigma Aldrich, Saint Quentin-Fallavier, France). The concentration and the purity of isolated RNA were determined with a NanoDrop spectrophotometer (Peqlab Biotechnologie GmbH, Erlangen, Germany). The integrity of RNA was checked on 1.25% agarose-formaldehyde gels. The cDNA was generated by reverse transcription (RT) of total RNA (1 µg) and real-time quantitative PCR was performed as reported previously [18]. Briefly, total RNA (1 µg) was denatured and reverse transcribed in a 20 µL reaction mixture containing 50 mM Tris-HCL (pH 8.3), 75 mM KCL, 3 mM $MgCl_2$, 200 mM of each deoxynucleotide triphosphate, 50 pmol of oligo(dT), 15.5 IU of ribonuclease inhibitor, and 15 IU of Moloney Murine Leukaemia Virus (M-MLV) reverse transcriptase. The mixture was incubated for 1 h at 37 °C. Targeted cDNAs were quantified by real-time PCR using SYBR Green Supermix (Bio-Rad, Marnes la Coquette, France) and 250 nM of specific primers (as mentioned below) in a total volume of 20 µL in a MyiQ Cycle device (Bio-Rad). Samples were tested in duplicate on the same plate and PCR amplification with water instead of cDNA was done systemically as a negative control. After incubation for 2 min at 50 °C and a denaturation step of 10 min at 95 °C, samples were subjected to 40 cycles (30 s at 95 °C, 30 s at 60 °C, 30 s at 72 °C), followed by the acquisition of the melting curve. The levels of mRNA expression were standardized to the geometric mean of three reference genes (GAPDH, beta-actin, and PPIA), which has been reported as an accurate normalization procedure [94]. The relative amounts of gene transcripts (R) were calculated according to the equation: $R = (E_{gene}^{-Ct\ gene})/$ (geometric mean $(E_{GAPDH}^{-Ct\ GAPDH}; E_{BETA\ ACTIN}^{-Ct\ BETA\ ACTIN}; E_{PPIA}^{-Ct\ PPIA}))$, where E is the primer efficiency and Ct is the cycle threshold.

The primers' efficiency (E) was performed from serial dilutions of a pool of obtained cDNA and ranged from 1.8 to 2. The specific primer pairs used were: Adiponectin: Fw (forward) 5'-GAAAGGAGATCCAGGTCTTATTG-3' and Rev (reverse) 5'-TCAGCAAAACCACTATGATGG-3'; AdipoR1: Fw 5'-TTCTTCCTCATGGCTGTGATGT-3' and Rev 5'-AAGAAGCGCTCAGG-AATTCG-3'; AdipoR2: Fw 5'-CCACCACCTTGCTTCATCTA-3' and Rev 5'-GATACTGAGGGGTGGCAAAC-3'; visfatin or NAMPT: Fw 5'-CAGCAGAACACAGTACCATA-3' and Rev 5'-CTCTAAGATAAGGTGGCAGC-3'; omentin: Fw 5'-GGATTTGTTCAGTTCAGGGTATTTAA-3' and Rev 5'-GCCTCTGGAAAGTATCCTCCT-3'; resistin Fw: 5'-GGACAGGAGCTAATACCCAGAAC-3' and Rev 5'-GGAAAAGGAGGGGAAATGAA-3'; apelin: Fw 5'-CTCTGGCTCTCCTTGACCG-3' and Rev 5'-GGCCCATTCCTTGACCCTC-3'; apelin receptor (APJ): Fw 5'-CTATCCTGTTTTCTGAGTGTGAGG-3' and Rev 5'-CTAAGGGCTGGAGCACTAATTATC-3'; chemerin (rarres2): Fw 5'-CCCAATGGGAGGAAACG-3' and Rev 5'-CCAGGGAAGTAGAAGCTGTG-3'; CMKLR1: Fw 5'-CCCAATCCATATCACCTATGCC-3' and Rev 5'-GTCCCGAAAACCCAGTGGTA-3'; CCRL2: Fw 5'-CACATAACTAGGAAGTGGCAGAAC-3' and Rev 5'-AGCGTAGGCTCTGACCAAAT-3'; GPR1:Fw 5'-CTGTCATTTGGTTCACAGGA-3' and Rev 5'-AACAACCTGAGGTCCACATC-3'; GADPH: Fw 5'-TGCACCACCAACTGCTTAGC-3' and Rev 5'GGCATGGACTGTGGTCATGAG-3'; PPIA: Fw 5'-CTGAGCACTGGAGAGAAAGG-3' and Rev 5'-AGGAATGATCTGGTGGTTAAG-3'; beta Actin; Fw 5'-CTTCTACAATGAGCTGCGTGTG-3' and Rev 5'- GTGAGGATCTTCATGAGGTAGTCAGTC-3'. PCR products were analyzed on an agarose gel (1.5%) stained with ethidium bromide and the cDNA fragment of interest was confirmed after sequencing by Genewiz (Leipzig, Germany).

4.6. Statistical Analyses

Values are reported as mean ± standard deviation (SD). Statistical analyses included two-way ANOVA, followed by Bonferroni post-hoc tests. For each parameter, we examined the effect of BMI and pathological condition, and the interaction between these two parameters. In case of a not-significant BMI effect and no interaction, the data for subsequent analysis were pooled in three groups according to pathological status (controls, PCOS, and ECHO). In all other cases, normal-weight and obese groups were investigated separately. Correlations were analyzed by simple regression analysis and the correlation-Z-test. Neither adjustment for age nor any other factor was made. StatView software (version version 9.3, Distributors: SAS Institute Inc., SAS Campus Drive, Cary NC 27513, USA) was used, with $p < 0.05$ as a threshold statistically significant level.

5. Conclusions

In conclusion, we showed in a cohort of women affected by infertility that chemerin and omentin expression in FF and GCs is electively increased in the PCOS group, while ECHO women are characterized by high levels of adiponectin, apelin, and APJ, as well as lower plasma AMH and LH levels. We also demonstrated that the regulation at the ovarian level of these adipokines differs from the systemic one, suggesting that follicular chemerin, omentin, and apelin may be at least partly produced by GCs and act in an autocrine and/or paracrine manner on ovarian follicles' cells, modulating their functions and, in particular, steroid production. FF concentration of all adipokines varied according to BMI, with resistin, visfatin, chemerin, omentin, and apelin levels higher in obese subjects in contrast with a predominant adiponectin expression in normal-weight women. Our findings thus provide novel insights into the role of chemerin, omentin, and apelin in follicular growth arrest and ovulatory dysfunction characterizing PCOS pathogenesis.

Author Contributions: The authors' responsibilities were as follows: J.D. and A.B. were involved in the conceptualization and the methodology of the research; N.M., C.R., M.C., F.G., P.F. and J.D. conducted the investigation; formal analysis. M.C. and F.G. recruited the patients and collected all biological data about these patients. A.B. and J.D. analyzed the data; A.B. prepared the original draft and wrote it. A.B., N.M., C.R., M.C., F.G., P.F. and J.D. reviewed and edited the manuscript; J.D. got the funding and realized the project administration. J.D. had primary responsibility for the final content.

Acknowledgments: We thank all the in vitro fertilization team and Anthony Estienne for the layout of the figures. This work was financially supported by Région Centre Val de Loire (PREVADI project number 32000820 and HAPOERTI project number 32000496) and Agence de Biomedecine.

Conflicts of Interest: The authors declare no conflict of interest. The funders had no role in the design of the study; in the collection, analyses, or interpretation of data; in the writing of the manuscript, or in the decision to publish the results.

References

1. Teede, H.; Deeks, A.; Moran, L. Polycystic ovary syndrome: A complex condition with psychological, reproductive and metabolic manifestations that impacts on health across the lifespan. *BMC Med.* **2010**, *8*, 41. [CrossRef] [PubMed]
2. Rotterdam ESHRE/ASRM-Sponsored PCOS Consensus Workshop Group. Revised 2003 consensus on diagnostic criteria and long-term health risks related to polycystic ovary syndrome. *Fertil. Steril.* **2004**, *81*, 19–25. [CrossRef] [PubMed]
3. Teede, H.J.; Misso, M.L.; Costello, M.F.; Dokras, A.; Laven, J.; Moran, L.; Piltonen, T.; Norman, R.J.; International, P.N. Recommendations from the international evidence-based guideline for the assessment and management of polycystic ovary syndrome. *Fertil. Steril.* **2018**, *110*, 364–379. [CrossRef] [PubMed]
4. Toulis, K.A.; Goulis, D.G.; Farmakiotis, D.; Georgopoulos, N.A.; Katsikis, I.; Tarlatzis, B.C.; Papadimas, I.; Panidis, D. Adiponectin levels in women with polycystic ovary syndrome: A systematic review and a meta-analysis. *Hum. Reprod. Update* **2009**, *15*, 297–307. [CrossRef] [PubMed]

5. Benrick, A.; Chanclon, B.; Micallef, P.; Wu, Y.; Hadi, L.; Shelton, J.M.; Stener-Victorin, E.; Wernstedt Asterholm, I. Adiponectin protects against development of metabolic disturbances in a PCOS mouse model. *Proc. Natl. Acad. Sci. USA* **2017**, *114*, E7187–E7196. [CrossRef] [PubMed]
6. Pasquali, R.; Pelusi, C.; Genghini, S.; Cacciari, M.; Gambineri, A. Obesity and reproductive disorders in women. *Hum. Reprod. Update* **2003**, *9*, 359–372. [CrossRef]
7. Norman, J.E. The adverse effects of obesity on reproduction. *Reproduction* **2010**, *140*, 343–345. [CrossRef] [PubMed]
8. Pasquali, R.; Gambineri, A.; Pagotto, U. The impact of obesity on reproduction in women with polycystic ovary syndrome. *BJOG* **2006**, *113*, 1148–1159. [CrossRef] [PubMed]
9. Bluher, M. Adipose tissue dysfunction in obesity. *Exp. Clin. Endocrinol. Diabetes* **2009**, *117*, 241–250. [CrossRef]
10. Ohashi, K.; Shibata, R.; Murohara, T.; Ouchi, N. Role of anti-inflammatory adipokines in obesity-related diseases. *Trends. Endocrinol. Metab.* **2014**, *25*, 348–355. [CrossRef]
11. Vazquez, M.J.; Romero-Ruiz, A.; Tena-Sempere, M. Roles of leptin in reproduction, pregnancy and polycystic ovary syndrome: Consensus knowledge and recent developments. *Metabolism* **2015**, *64*, 79–91. [CrossRef] [PubMed]
12. Landry, D.; Cloutier, F.; Martin, L.J. Implications of leptin in neuroendocrine regulation of male reproduction. *Reprod. Biol.* **2013**, *13*, 1–14. [CrossRef] [PubMed]
13. Dupont, J.; Pollet-Villard, X.; Reverchon, M.; Mellouk, N.; Levy, R. Adipokines in human reproduction. *Horm. Mol. Biol. Clin. Investig.* **2015**, *24*, 11–24. [CrossRef] [PubMed]
14. Chabrolle, C.; Tosca, L.; Rame, C.; Lecomte, P.; Royere, D.; Dupont, J. Adiponectin increases insulin-like growth factor I-induced progesterone and estradiol secretion in human granulosa cells. *Fertil. Steril.* **2009**, *92*, 1988–1996. [CrossRef] [PubMed]
15. Reverchon, M.; Cornuau, M.; Rame, C.; Guerif, F.; Royere, D.; Dupont, J. Chemerin inhibits IGF-1-induced progesterone and estradiol secretion in human granulosa cells. *Hum. Reprod.* **2012**, *27*, 1790–1800. [CrossRef] [PubMed]
16. Reverchon, M.; Cornuau, M.; Rame, C.; Guerif, F.; Royere, D.; Dupont, J. Resistin decreases insulin-like growth factor I-induced steroid production and insulin-like growth factor I receptor signaling in human granulosa cells. *Fertil. Steril.* **2013**, *100*, 247–255. [CrossRef] [PubMed]
17. Reverchon, M.; Cornuau, M.; Cloix, L.; Rame, C.; Guerif, F.; Royere, D.; Dupont, J. Visfatin is expressed in human granulosa cells: Regulation by metformin through AMPK/SIRT1 pathways and its role in steroidogenesis. *Mol. Hum. Reprod.* **2013**, *19*, 313–326. [CrossRef] [PubMed]
18. Cloix, L.; Reverchon, M.; Cornuau, M.; Froment, P.; Rame, C.; Costa, C.; Froment, G.; Lecomte, P.; Chen, W.; Royere, D.; et al. Expression and regulation of INTELECTIN1 in human granulosa-lutein cells: Role in IGF-1-induced steroidogenesis through NAMPT. *Biol. Reprod.* **2014**, *91*, 50. [CrossRef]
19. Roche, J.; Rame, C.; Reverchon, M.; Mellouk, N.; Cornuau, M.; Guerif, F.; Froment, P.; Dupont, J. Apelin (APLN) and Apelin Receptor (APLNR) in Human Ovary: Expression, Signaling, and Regulation of Steroidogenesis in Primary Human Luteinized Granulosa Cells. *Biol. Reprod.* **2016**, *95*, 104. [CrossRef]
20. Tang, M.; Huang, C.; Wang, Y.F.; Ren, P.G.; Chen, L.; Xiao, T.X.; Wang, B.B.; Pan, Y.F.; Tsang, B.K.; Zabel, B.A.; et al. CMKLR1 deficiency maintains ovarian steroid production in mice treated chronically with dihydrotestosterone. *Sci. Rep.* **2016**, *6*, 21328. [CrossRef]
21. Wang, Q.; Kim, J.Y.; Xue, K.; Liu, J.Y.; Leader, A.; Tsang, B.K. Chemerin, a novel regulator of follicular steroidogenesis and its potential involvement in polycystic ovarian syndrome. *Endocrinology* **2012**, *153*, 5600–5611. [CrossRef]
22. Tan, B.K.; Chen, J.; Farhatullah, S.; Adya, R.; Kaur, J.; Heutling, D.; Lewandowski, K.C.; O'Hare, J.P.; Lehnert, H.; Randeva, H.S. Insulin and metformin regulate circulating and adipose tissue chemerin. *Diabetes* **2009**, *58*, 1971–1977. [CrossRef]
23. Bozaoglu, K.; Segal, D.; Shields, K.A.; Cummings, N.; Curran, J.E.; Comuzzie, A.G.; Mahaney, M.C.; Rainwater, D.L.; VandeBerg, J.L.; MacCluer, J.W.; et al. Chemerin is associated with metabolic syndrome phenotypes in a Mexican-American population. *J. Clin. Endocrinol. Metab.* **2009**, *94*, 3085–3088. [CrossRef]
24. Munir, I.; Yen, H.W.; Baruth, T.; Tarkowski, R.; Azziz, R.; Magoffin, D.A.; Jakimiuk, A.J. Resistin stimulation of 17alpha-hydroxylase activity in ovarian theca cells in vitro: Relevance to polycystic ovary syndrome. *J. Clin. Endocrinol. Metab.* **2005**, *90*, 4852–4857. [CrossRef]

25. Baldani, D.P.; Skrgatic, L.; Kasum, M.; Zlopasa, G.; Kralik Oguic, S.; Herman, M. Altered leptin, adiponectin, resistin and ghrelin secretion may represent an intrinsic polycystic ovary syndrome abnormality. *Gynecol. Endocrinol.* **2019**, *35*, 401–405. [CrossRef]
26. Chan, T.F.; Chen, Y.L.; Chen, H.H.; Lee, C.H.; Jong, S.B.; Tsai, E.M. Increased plasma visfatin concentrations in women with polycystic ovary syndrome. *Fertil. Steril.* **2007**, *88*, 401–405. [CrossRef]
27. Panidis, D.; Farmakiotis, D.; Rousso, D.; Katsikis, I.; Delkos, D.; Piouka, A.; Gerou, S.; Diamanti-Kandarakis, E. Plasma visfatin levels in normal weight women with polycystic ovary syndrome. *Eur. J. Intern. Med.* **2008**, *19*, 406–412. [CrossRef]
28. Tan, B.K.; Adya, R.; Farhatullah, S.; Chen, J.; Lehnert, H.; Randeva, H.S. Metformin treatment may increase omentin-1 levels in women with polycystic ovary syndrome. *Diabetes* **2010**, *59*, 3023–3031. [CrossRef]
29. Orlik, B.; Madej, P.; Owczarek, A.; Skalba, P.; Chudek, J.; Olszanecka-Glinianowicz, M. Plasma omentin and adiponectin levels as markers of adipose tissue dysfunction in normal weight and obese women with polycystic ovary syndrome. *Clin. Endocrinol. (Oxf)* **2014**, *81*, 529–535. [CrossRef]
30. Barbe, A.; Bongrani, A.; Mellouk, N.; Estienne, A.; Kurowska, P.; Grandhaye, J.; Elfassy, Y.; Levy, R.; Rak, A.; Froment, P.; et al. Mechanisms of Adiponectin Action in Fertility: An Overview from Gametogenesis to Gestation in Humans and Animal Models in Normal and Pathological Conditions. *Int. J. Mol. Sci.* **2019**, *20*. [CrossRef]
31. Guvenc, Y.; Var, A.; Goker, A.; Kuscu, N.K. Assessment of serum chemerin, vaspin and omentin-1 levels in patients with polycystic ovary syndrome. *J. Int. Med. Res.* **2016**, *44*, 796–805. [CrossRef]
32. Farshchian, F.; Ramezani Tehrani, F.; Amirrasouli, H.; Rahimi Pour, H.; Hedayati, M.; Kazerouni, F.; Soltani, A. Visfatin and resistin serum levels in normal-weight and obese women with polycystic ovary syndrome. *Int. J. Endocrinol. Metab.* **2014**, *12*, e15503. [CrossRef]
33. Akbarzadeh, S.; Ghasemi, S.; Kalantarhormozi, M.; Nabipour, I.; Abbasi, F.; Aminfar, A.; Jaffari, S.M.; Motamed, N.; Movahed, A.; Mirzaei, M.; et al. Relationship among plasma adipokines, insulin and androgens level as well as biochemical glycemic and lipidemic markers with incidence of PCOS in women with normal BMI. *Gynecol. Endocrinol.* **2012**, *28*, 521–524. [CrossRef]
34. Kim, J.J.; Choi, Y.M.; Hong, M.A.; Kim, M.J.; Chae, S.J.; Kim, S.M.; Hwang, K.R.; Yoon, S.H.; Ku, S.Y.; Suh, C.S.; et al. Serum visfatin levels in non-obese women with polycystic ovary syndrome and matched controls. *Obstet. Gynecol. Sci.* **2018**, *61*, 253–260. [CrossRef]
35. Tao, T.; Xu, B.; Liu, W. Ovarian HMW adiponectin is associated with folliculogenesis in women with polycystic ovary syndrome. *Reprod. Biol. Endocrinol.* **2013**, *11*, 99. [CrossRef]
36. Tsouma, I.; Kouskouni, E.; Demeridou, S.; Boutsikou, M.; Hassiakos, D.; Chasiakou, A.; Hassiakou, S.; Baka, S. Correlation of visfatin levels and lipoprotein lipid profiles in women with polycystic ovary syndrome undergoing ovarian stimulation. *Gynecol. Endocrinol.* **2014**, *30*, 516–519. [CrossRef]
37. Seow, K.M.; Juan, C.C.; Hsu, Y.P.; Ho, L.T.; Wang, Y.Y.; Hwang, J.L. Serum and follicular resistin levels in women with polycystic ovarian syndrome during IVF-stimulated cycles. *Hum. Reprod.* **2005**, *20*, 117–121. [CrossRef]
38. Practice Committee of the American Society for Reproductive Medicine. Prevention and treatment of moderate and severe ovarian hyperstimulation syndrome: A guideline. *Fertil. Steril.* **2016**, *106*, 1634–1647. [CrossRef]
39. Li, S.; Huang, X.; Zhong, H.; Peng, Q.; Chen, S.; Xie, Y.; Qin, X.; Qin, A. Low circulating adiponectin levels in women with polycystic ovary syndrome: An updated meta-analysis. *Tumour. Biol.* **2014**, *35*, 3961–3973. [CrossRef]
40. Artimani, T.; Saidijam, M.; Aflatoonian, R.; Ashrafi, M.; Amiri, I.; Yavangi, M.; SoleimaniAsl, S.; Shabab, N.; Karimi, J.; Mehdizadeh, M. Downregulation of adiponectin system in granulosa cells and low levels of HMW adiponectin in PCOS. *J. Assist. Reprod. Genet.* **2016**, *33*, 101–110. [CrossRef]
41. O'Connor, A.; Phelan, N.; Tun, T.K.; Boran, G.; Gibney, J.; Roche, H.M. High-molecular-weight adiponectin is selectively reduced in women with polycystic ovary syndrome independent of body mass index and severity of insulin resistance. *J. Clin. Endocrinol. Metab.* **2010**, *95*, 1378–1385. [CrossRef]
42. Campos, D.B.; Palin, M.F.; Bordignon, V.; Murphy, B.D. The 'beneficial' adipokines in reproduction and fertility. *Intj. Obes. (Lond.)* **2008**, *32*, 223–231. [CrossRef]

43. Patel, L.; Buckels, A.C.; Kinghorn, I.J.; Murdock, P.R.; Holbrook, J.D.; Plumpton, C.; Macphee, C.H.; Smith, S.A. Resistin is expressed in human macrophages and directly regulated by PPAR gamma activators. *Biochem. Biophys. Res. Commun.* **2003**, *300*, 472–476. [CrossRef]
44. Fain, J.N.; Cheema, P.S.; Bahouth, S.W.; Lloyd Hiler, M. Resistin release by human adipose tissue explants in primary culture. *Biochem. Biophys. Res. Commun.* **2003**, *300*, 674–678. [CrossRef]
45. Panidis, D.; Koliakos, G.; Kourtis, A.; Farmakiotis, D.; Mouslech, T.; Rousso, D. Serum resistin levels in women with polycystic ovary syndrome. *Fertil. Steril.* **2004**, *81*, 361–366. [CrossRef]
46. Lee, J.H.; Chan, J.L.; Yiannakouris, N.; Kontogianni, M.; Estrada, E.; Seip, R.; Orlova, C.; Mantzoros, C.S. Circulating resistin levels are not associated with obesity or insulin resistance in humans and are not regulated by fasting or leptin administration: Cross-sectional and interventional studies in normal, insulin-resistant, and diabetic subjects. *J. Clin. Endocrinol. Metab.* **2003**, *88*, 4848–4856. [CrossRef]
47. Seow, K.M.; Juan, C.C.; Hsu, Y.P.; Hwang, J.L.; Huang, L.W.; Ho, L.T. Amelioration of insulin resistance in women with PCOS via reduced insulin receptor substrate-1 Ser312 phosphorylation following laparoscopic ovarian electrocautery. *Hum. Reprod.* **2007**, *22*, 1003–1010. [CrossRef]
48. Seow, K.M.; Juan, C.C.; Wu, L.Y.; Hsu, Y.P.; Yang, W.M.; Tsai, Y.L.; Hwang, J.L.; Ho, L.T. Serum and adipocyte resistin in polycystic ovary syndrome with insulin resistance. *Hum. Reprod.* **2004**, *19*, 48–53. [CrossRef]
49. Samal, B.; Sun, Y.; Stearns, G.; Xie, C.; Suggs, S.; McNiece, I. Cloning and characterization of the cDNA encoding a novel human pre-B-cell colony-enhancing factor. *Mol. Cell. Biol.* **1994**, *14*, 1431–1437. [CrossRef]
50. Fukuhara, A.; Matsuda, M.; Nishizawa, M.; Segawa, K.; Tanaka, M.; Kishimoto, K.; Matsuki, Y.; Murakami, M.; Ichisaka, T.; Murakami, H.; et al. Visfatin: A protein secreted by visceral fat that mimics the effects of insulin. *Science* **2005**, *307*, 426–430. [CrossRef]
51. Berndt, J.; Kloting, N.; Kralisch, S.; Kovacs, P.; Fasshauer, M.; Schon, M.R.; Stumvoll, M.; Bluher, M. Plasma visfatin concentrations and fat depot-specific mRNA expression in humans. *Diabetes* **2005**, *54*, 2911–2916. [CrossRef]
52. Chen, M.P.; Chung, F.M.; Chang, D.M.; Tsai, J.C.; Huang, H.F.; Shin, S.J.; Lee, Y.J. Elevated plasma level of visfatin/pre-B cell colony-enhancing factor in patients with type 2 diabetes mellitus. *J. Clin. Endocrinol. Metab.* **2006**, *91*, 295–299. [CrossRef]
53. Shen, C.J.; Tsai, E.M.; Lee, J.N.; Chen, Y.L.; Lee, C.H.; Chan, T.F. The concentrations of visfatin in the follicular fluids of women undergoing controlled ovarian stimulation are correlated to the number of oocytes retrieved. *Fertil. Steril.* **2010**, *93*, 1844–1850. [CrossRef]
54. Plati, E.; Kouskouni, E.; Malamitsi-Puchner, A.; Boutsikou, M.; Kaparos, G.; Baka, S. Visfatin and leptin levels in women with polycystic ovaries undergoing ovarian stimulation. *Fertil. Steril.* **2010**, *94*, 1451–1456. [CrossRef]
55. Tan, B.K.; Chen, J.; Digby, J.E.; Keay, S.D.; Kennedy, C.R.; Randeva, H.S. Increased visfatin messenger ribonucleic acid and protein levels in adipose tissue and adipocytes in women with polycystic ovary syndrome: Parallel increase in plasma visfatin. *J. Clin. Endocrinol. Metab.* **2006**, *91*, 5022–5028. [CrossRef]
56. Choi, K.H.; Joo, B.S.; Sun, S.T.; Park, M.J.; Son, J.B.; Joo, J.K.; Lee, K.S. Administration of visfatin during superovulation improves developmental competency of oocytes and fertility potential in aged female mice. *Fertil. Steril.* **2012**, *97*, 1234–1241. [CrossRef]
57. Tatemoto, K.; Hosoya, M.; Habata, Y.; Fujii, R.; Kakegawa, T.; Zou, M.X.; Kawamata, Y.; Fukusumi, S.; Hinuma, S.; Kitada, C.; et al. Isolation and characterization of a novel endogenous peptide ligand for the human APJ receptor. *Biochem. Biophys. Res. Commun.* **1998**, *251*, 471–476. [CrossRef]
58. Boucher, J.; Masri, B.; Daviaud, D.; Gesta, S.; Guigne, C.; Mazzucotelli, A.; Castan-Laurell, I.; Tack, I.; Knibiehler, B.; Carpene, C.; et al. Apelin, a newly identified adipokine up-regulated by insulin and obesity. *Endocrinology* **2005**, *146*, 1764–1771. [CrossRef]
59. Chang, Y.H.; Chang, D.M.; Lin, K.C.; Shin, S.J.; Lee, Y.J. Visfatin in overweight/obesity, type 2 diabetes mellitus, insulin resistance, metabolic syndrome and cardiovascular diseases: A meta-analysis and systemic review. *Diabetes Metab. Res. Rev.* **2011**, *27*, 515–527. [CrossRef]
60. Rak, A.; Drwal, E.; Rame, C.; Knapczyk-Stwora, K.; Slomczynska, M.; Dupont, J.; Gregoraszczuk, E.L. Expression of apelin and apelin receptor (APJ) in porcine ovarian follicles and in vitro effect of apelin on steroidogenesis and proliferation through APJ activation and different signaling pathways. *Theriogenology* **2017**, *96*, 126–135. [CrossRef]

61. Shirasuna, K.; Shimizu, T.; Sayama, K.; Asahi, T.; Sasaki, M.; Berisha, B.; Schams, D.; Miyamoto, A. Expression and localization of apelin and its receptor APJ in the bovine corpus luteum during the estrous cycle and prostaglandin F2alpha-induced luteolysis. *Reproduction* **2008**, *135*, 519–525. [CrossRef]
62. Roche, J.; Rame, C.; Reverchon, M.; Mellouk, N.; Rak, A.; Froment, P.; Dupont, J. Apelin (APLN) regulates progesterone secretion and oocyte maturation in bovine ovarian cells. *Reproduction* **2017**, *153*, 589–603. [CrossRef]
63. Shimizu, T.; Kosaka, N.; Murayama, C.; Tetsuka, M.; Miyamoto, A. Apelin and APJ receptor expression in granulosa and theca cells during different stages of follicular development in the bovine ovary: Involvement of apoptosis and hormonal regulation. *Anim. Reprod. Sci.* **2009**, *116*, 28–37. [CrossRef]
64. Franks, S.; Stark, J.; Hardy, K. Follicle dynamics and anovulation in polycystic ovary syndrome. *Hum. Reprod. Update* **2008**, *14*, 367–378. [CrossRef]
65. Taheri, S.; Murphy, K.; Cohen, M.; Sujkovic, E.; Kennedy, A.; Dhillo, W.; Dakin, C.; Sajedi, A.; Ghatei, M.; Bloom, S. The effects of centrally administered apelin-13 on food intake, water intake and pituitary hormone release in rats. *Biochem. Biophys. Res. Commun.* **2002**, *291*, 1208–1212. [CrossRef]
66. Altinkaya, S.O.; Nergiz, S.; Kucuk, M.; Yuksel, H. Apelin levels in relation with hormonal and metabolic profile in patients with polycystic ovary syndrome. *Eur.J. Obstet. Gynecol. Reprod. Biol.* **2014**, *176*, 168–172. [CrossRef]
67. Olszanecka-Glinianowicz, M.; Madej, P.; Nylec, M.; Owczarek, A.; Szanecki, W.; Skalba, P.; Chudek, J. Circulating apelin level in relation to nutritional status in polycystic ovary syndrome and its association with metabolic and hormonal disturbances. *Clin. Endocrinol. (Oxf)* **2013**, *79*, 238–242. [CrossRef]
68. Yang, R.Z.; Lee, M.J.; Hu, H.; Pray, J.; Wu, H.B.; Hansen, B.C.; Shuldiner, A.R.; Fried, S.K.; McLenithan, J.C.; Gong, D.W. Identification of omentin as a novel depot-specific adipokine in human adipose tissue: Possible role in modulating insulin action. *Am. J. Physiol. Endocrinol. Metab.* **2006**, *290*, E1253–E1261. [CrossRef]
69. Mahde, A.; Shaker, M.; Al-Mashhadani, Z. Study of Omentin1 and Other Adipokines and Hormones in PCOS Patients. *Oman. Med. J.* **2009**, *24*, 108–118. [CrossRef]
70. Choi, J.H.; Rhee, E.J.; Kim, K.H.; Woo, H.Y.; Lee, W.Y.; Sung, K.C. Plasma omentin-1 levels are reduced in non-obese women with normal glucose tolerance and polycystic ovary syndrome. *Eur. J. Endocrinol.* **2011**, *165*, 789–796. [CrossRef]
71. Moreno-Navarrete, J.M.; Catalan, V.; Ortega, F.; Gomez-Ambrosi, J.; Ricart, W.; Fruhbeck, G.; Fernandez-Real, J.M. Circulating omentin concentration increases after weight loss. *Nutr. Metab. (Lond)* **2010**, *7*, 27. [CrossRef]
72. Tan, B.K.; Pua, S.; Syed, F.; Lewandowski, K.C.; O'Hare, J.P.; Randeva, H.S. Decreased plasma omentin-1 levels in Type 1 diabetes mellitus. *Diabet. Med.* **2008**, *25*, 1254–1255. [CrossRef]
73. de Souza Batista, C.M.; Yang, R.Z.; Lee, M.J.; Glynn, N.M.; Yu, D.Z.; Pray, J.; Ndubuizu, K.; Patil, S.; Schwartz, A.; Kligman, M.; et al. Omentin plasma levels and gene expression are decreased in obesity. *Diabetes* **2007**, *56*, 1655–1661. [CrossRef]
74. Spritzer, P.M.; Lecke, S.B.; Satler, F.; Morsch, D.M. Adipose tissue dysfunction, adipokines, and low-grade chronic inflammation in polycystic ovary syndrome. *Reproduction* **2015**, *149*, R219–R227. [CrossRef]
75. De Henau, O.; Degroot, G.N.; Imbault, V.; Robert, V.; De Poorter, C.; McHeik, S.; Gales, C.; Parmentier, M.; Springael, J.Y. Signaling Properties of Chemerin Receptors CMKLR1, GPR1 and CCRL2. *PLoS ONE* **2016**, *11*, e0164179. [CrossRef]
76. Wittamer, V.; Franssen, J.D.; Vulcano, M.; Mirjolet, J.F.; Le Poul, E.; Migeotte, I.; Brezillon, S.; Tyldesley, R.; Blanpain, C.; Detheux, M.; et al. Specific recruitment of antigen-presenting cells by chemerin, a novel processed ligand from human inflammatory fluids. *J. Exp. Med.* **2003**, *198*, 977–985. [CrossRef]
77. Bozaoglu, K.; Bolton, K.; McMillan, J.; Zimmet, P.; Jowett, J.; Collier, G.; Walder, K.; Segal, D. Chemerin is a novel adipokine associated with obesity and metabolic syndrome. *Endocrinology* **2007**, *148*, 4687–4694. [CrossRef]
78. Goralski, K.B.; McCarthy, T.C.; Hanniman, E.A.; Zabel, B.A.; Butcher, E.C.; Parlee, S.D.; Muruganandan, S.; Sinal, C.J. Chemerin, a novel adipokine that regulates adipogenesis and adipocyte metabolism. *J. Biol. Chem.* **2007**, *282*, 28175–28188. [CrossRef]
79. Kort, D.H.; Kostolias, A.; Sullivan, C.; Lobo, R.A. Chemerin as a marker of body fat and insulin resistance in women with polycystic ovary syndrome. *Gynecol. Endocrinol.* **2015**, *31*, 152–155. [CrossRef]

80. Tsatsanis, C.; Dermitzaki, E.; Avgoustinaki, P.; Malliaraki, N.; Mytaras, V.; Margioris, A.N. The impact of adipose tissue-derived factors on the hypothalamic-pituitary-gonadal (HPG) axis. *Horm. (Athens)* **2015**, *14*, 549–562. [CrossRef]
81. Kim, J.Y.; Xue, K.; Cao, M.; Wang, Q.; Liu, J.Y.; Leader, A.; Han, J.Y.; Tsang, B.K. Chemerin suppresses ovarian follicular development and its potential involvement in follicular arrest in rats treated chronically with dihydrotestosterone. *Endocrinology* **2013**, *154*, 2912–2923. [CrossRef]
82. Lima, P.D.A.; Nivet, A.L.; Wang, Q.; Chen, Y.A.; Leader, A.; Cheung, A.; Tzeng, C.R.; Tsang, B.K. Polycystic ovary syndrome: Possible involvement of androgen-induced, chemerin-mediated ovarian recruitment of monocytes/macrophages. *Biol. Reprod.* **2018**, *99*, 838–852. [CrossRef]
83. Dunaif, A. Insulin resistance and the polycystic ovary syndrome: Mechanism and implications for pathogenesis. *Endocr. Rev.* **1997**, *18*, 774–800. [CrossRef]
84. Panidis, D.; Tziomalos, K.; Misichronis, G.; Papadakis, E.; Betsas, G.; Katsikis, I.; Macut, D. Insulin resistance and endocrine characteristics of the different phenotypes of polycystic ovary syndrome: A prospective study. *Hum. Reprod.* **2012**, *27*, 541–549. [CrossRef]
85. Dewailly, D.; Pigny, P.; Soudan, B.; Catteau-Jonard, S.; Decanter, C.; Poncelet, E.; Duhamel, A. Reconciling the definitions of polycystic ovary syndrome: The ovarian follicle number and serum anti-Mullerian hormone concentrations aggregate with the markers of hyperandrogenism. *J. Clin. Endocrinol. Metab.* **2010**, *95*, 4399–4405. [CrossRef]
86. Dewailly, D.; Lujan, M.E.; Carmina, E.; Cedars, M.I.; Laven, J.; Norman, R.J.; Escobar-Morreale, H.F. Definition and significance of polycystic ovarian morphology: A task force report from the Androgen Excess and Polycystic Ovary Syndrome Society. *Hum. Reprod. Update* **2014**, *20*, 334–352. [CrossRef]
87. Pigny, P.; Merlen, E.; Robert, Y.; Cortet-Rudelli, C.; Decanter, C.; Jonard, S.; Dewailly, D. Elevated serum level of anti-mullerian hormone in patients with polycystic ovary syndrome: Relationship to the ovarian follicle excess and to the follicular arrest. *J. Clin. Endocrinol. Metab.* **2003**, *88*, 5957–5962. [CrossRef]
88. Teede, H.; Misso, M.; Tassone, E.C.; Dewailly, D.; Ng, E.H.; Azziz, R.; Norman, R.J.; Andersen, M.; Franks, S.; Hoeger, K.; et al. Anti-Mullerian Hormone in PCOS: A Review Informing International Guidelines. *Trends Endocrinol. Metab.* **2019**, *30*, 467–478. [CrossRef]
89. Victoria, M.; Labrosse, J.; Krief, F.; Cedrin-Durnerin, I.; Comtet, M.; Grynberg, M. Anti Mullerian Hormone: More than a biomarker of female reproductive function. *J. Gynecol. Obstet. Hum. Reprod.* **2019**, *48*, 19–24. [CrossRef]
90. Pierre, A.; Peigne, M.; Grynberg, M.; Arouche, N.; Taieb, J.; Hesters, L.; Gonzales, J.; Picard, J.Y.; Dewailly, D.; Fanchin, R.; et al. Loss of LH-induced down-regulation of anti-Mullerian hormone receptor expression may contribute to anovulation in women with polycystic ovary syndrome. *Hum. Reprod.* **2013**, *28*, 762–769. [CrossRef]
91. Homburg, R.; Crawford, G. The role of AMH in anovulation associated with PCOS: A hypothesis. *Hum. Reprod.* **2014**, *29*, 1117–1121. [CrossRef]
92. Cimino, I.; Casoni, F.; Liu, X.; Messina, A.; Parkash, J.; Jamin, S.P.; Catteau-Jonard, S.; Collier, F.; Baroncini, M.; Dewailly, D.; et al. Novel role for anti-Mullerian hormone in the regulation of GnRH neuron excitability and hormone secretion. *Nat. Commun.* **2016**, *7*, 10055. [CrossRef]
93. Guerif, F.; Bidault, R.; Gasnier, O.; Couet, M.L.; Gervereau, O.; Lansac, J.; Royere, D. Efficacy of blastocyst transfer after implantation failure. *Reprod. Biomed. Online* **2004**, *9*, 630–636. [CrossRef]
94. Vandesompele, J.; De Preter, K.; Pattyn, F.; Poppe, B.; Van Roy, N.; De Paepe, A.; Speleman, F. Accurate normalization of real-time quantitative RT-PCR data by geometric averaging of multiple internal control genes. *Genome Biol.* **2002**, *3*, RESEARCH0034. [CrossRef]

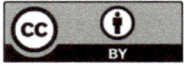

© 2019 by the authors. Licensee MDPI, Basel, Switzerland. This article is an open access article distributed under the terms and conditions of the Creative Commons Attribution (CC BY) license (http://creativecommons.org/licenses/by/4.0/).

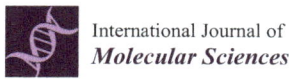

Review

The Adipokine Network in Rheumatic Joint Diseases

Mar Carrión [1], Klaus W. Frommer [2], Selene Pérez-García [1], Ulf Müller-Ladner [2], Rosa P. Gomariz [1] and Elena Neumann [2,*]

[1] Department of Cellular Biology, Faculty of Biology, Complutense University, 28040 Madrid, Spain
[2] Department of Rheumatology and Clinical Immunology, Justus-Liebig-University Giessen, Campus Kerckhoff, 61231 Bad Nauheim, Germany
* Correspondence: e.neumann@kerckhoff-klinik.de; Tel.: +49-6032-996-2801

Received: 31 July 2019; Accepted: 19 August 2019; Published: 22 August 2019

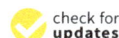

Abstract: Rheumatic diseases encompass a diverse group of chronic disorders that commonly affect musculoskeletal structures. Osteoarthritis (OA) and rheumatoid arthritis (RA) are the two most common, leading to considerable functional limitations and irreversible disability when patients are unsuccessfully treated. Although the specific causes of many rheumatic conditions remain unknown, it is generally accepted that immune mechanisms and/or uncontrolled inflammatory responses are involved in their etiology and symptomatology. In this regard, the bidirectional communication between neuroendocrine and immune system has been demonstrated to provide a homeostatic network that is involved in several pathological conditions. Adipokines represent a wide variety of bioactive, immune and inflammatory mediators mainly released by adipocytes that act as signal molecules in the neuroendocrine-immune interactions. Adipokines can also be synthesized by synoviocytes, osteoclasts, osteoblasts, chondrocytes and inflammatory cells in the joint microenvironment, showing potent modulatory properties on different effector cells in OA and RA pathogenesis. Effects of adiponectin, leptin, resistin and visfatin on local and systemic inflammation are broadly described. However, more recently, other adipokines, such as progranulin, chemerin, lipocalin-2, vaspin, omentin-1 and nesfatin, have been recognized to display immunomodulatory actions in rheumatic diseases. This review highlights the latest relevant findings on the role of the adipokine network in the pathophysiology of OA and RA.

Keywords: adipokine; rheumatic diseases; inflammation; osteoarthritis; rheumatoid arthritis

---

1. Introduction

According to the World Health Organization "Musculoskeletal disorders comprise more than 150 diagnoses that affect the locomotor system—that is, muscles, bones, joints and associated tissues such as tendons and ligaments—and are the second largest contributor to disability worldwide [1]. Musculoskeletal conditions generally comprise disorders that affect joints such as osteoarthritis (OA) and rheumatoid arthritis (RA). Although both diseases have an inflammatory component, the underlying pathological mechanisms are different.

OA is the most common joint disease affecting 18% of the population above 60 years of age although young individuals, especially juvenile athletes, can also suffer from this disorder [2]. It has been demonstrated that it is triggered mainly by biomechanical stress and joint overload, although obesity and metabolic disease are also considered key risk factors for its development [3–5]. Cartilage, subchondral bone, and synovium are the main tissues involved in OA pathogenesis. In recent years, the important contribution of pro-inflammatory mediators such as cytokines, reactive oxygen species (ROS), nitric oxide, and matrix degrading enzymes have been reported [6].

RA is a severe autoimmune disorder, characterized by chronic inflammation of diarthrodial joints, leading to cartilage and bone destruction. RA affects 1% of the population worldwide and is related to loss of physical function, quality of life and high prevalence of comorbid conditions [7]. RA develops in genetically susceptible individuals, under the influence of environmental factors, as well as with the involvement of epigenetic mechanisms. It is a heterogeneous disorder with diverse pathogenic mechanisms and variable clinical forms [8,9].

Unraveling the mechanisms that underlie both immune regulation and resolution of inflammation is crucial for the design of new strategies to treat these two highly prevalent rheumatic disorders. One of the approaches to understand these mechanisms is the study of the neuro-endocrine-immune systems balance, which is crucial for the maintenance of homeostasis and the effective adaptation to stressors [10,11]. This intricate communication and their regulatory mechanisms rely in the presence of common mediators such as neurotransmitters, cytokines, hormones and their receptors. In this sense, on the one hand, dysregulation in immune-endocrine integrated circuitries have been involved in the development of chronic metabolic diseases, comprising obesity, diabetes, and metabolic syndrome [12]. On the other hand, RA has been defined as an example of a disease resulting from abnormal interactions between these systems [13]. Reversal of abnormal cellular phenotypes in this disease has also been shown: As an example, synovial fibroblasts (SF) from RA patients (RASF) could be reprogrammed from a cartilage-degrading phenotype towards a regulatory type by hormones/neurotransmitters [14].

Interestingly, adipose tissue has been shown to be not only involved in the energetic homeostasis but also to act as an endocrine organ by secreting a diverse array of factors referred as adipocytokines. Products of adipose tissue include adipokines, cytokines, chemokines and complement factors [15]. Adipokines are bioactive proteins, which have emerged as modulators of inflammatory and immune response, exerting key roles in rheumatic diseases, both at local and systemic level. Adipose tissue is not the only source of adipokines. Immune cells, chondrocytes as well as synoviocytes also synthesize these mediators. In musculoskeletal disorders, autocrine, paracrine and endocrine pathways acting on target cells and tissues such as bone, cartilage and synovial membrane have been described [16]. Higher levels of adipokines in both serum and synovial fluid from RA patients compared with healthy controls have been reported [17,18]. Moreover, an inflammatory profile in the infrapatellar fat pad (IPFP) of OA patients has been described [19]. Overall, increasing evidence postulates that adipokines play an important role in both immune-mediated rheumatic disease and in degenerative disorders such as OA. In the next sections, we will disclose the most recent data about the role played by these mediators in these two rheumatic diseases.

2. Pathophysiology of Osteoarthritis and Rheumatoid Arthritis

2.1. Osteoarthritis

OA is a chronic rheumatic disease, considered one of the leading causes of substantial physical and psychological disability worldwide. OA is a complex multifactorial disorder [20,21], where mechanical, genetic, biological, biochemical and metabolic factors are involved. It is characterized by cell stress and extracellular matrix (ECM) degradation, resulting in an imbalance in joint tissue metabolism [22–24]. Although cartilage degradation is the main event in the pathology, OA affects the whole joint, including the remodeling of adjacent subchondral bone, osteophyte formation and synovial inflammation, which might culminate in pain, loss of joint function, and disability in advanced stages [21,24–31].

OA cartilage is characterized by an increase of ECM remodeling, cartilage calcification and angiogenesis [32,33]. Chondrocytes have receptors for responding to mechanical stress and inflammatory mediators, many of which are also receptors for ECM components, including cartilage-degradation products [31,34–36]. Activated chondrocytes acquire a hypertrophic phenotype, proliferating and increasing the release of inflammatory cytokines and chemokines, stress-induced intracellular signals, ROS, and matrix-degrading enzymes, including aggrecanases and matrix metalloproteinases (MMPs). In addition, ECM protein production is decreased. Depletion of aggrecan and degradation of type II collagen are the main events in cartilage destruction when the process becomes irreversible [37–40].

Changes in subchondral bone are related to cartilage remodeling, thus playing an important role in OA progression by the release of catabolic mediators that promote an abnormal metabolism in chondrocytes [30,41]. Production of inflammatory and degradative mediators by joint cells also induces the synovial inflammation. Synovitis is characterized by synovial hyperplasia, with SF and synovial macrophage proliferation, as well as immune cell infiltration. These cells release inflammatory mediators including interleukin-1β (IL-1β) and tumor necrosis factor-α (TNF-α), among other cytokines and chemokines which aggravate inflammation [31,42,43]. In addition, SF produce matrix-degrading enzymes, also contributing to cartilage ECM degradation [28,29,44].

2.2. Rheumatoid Arthritis

RA is a severe and chronic systemic inflammatory autoimmune disease with unknown etiology that mainly affects peripheral joints symmetrically, leading to progressive articular damage and joint dysfunction. One of the hallmarks of RA is the persistent inflammatory infiltration of the synovial sublining layer that contributes to generate a microenvironment in which stromal cells display a hyper-activated phenotype, releasing several pro-inflammatory and tissue damaging mediators to the joint space [45,46]. Although many of the underlying causes of RA are still unclear, systemic and local immune dysregulation is considered to orchestrate its pathogenesis. In fact, this disease is characterized by the production of autoantibodies such as anti-citrullinated protein antibody (ACPA) and rheumatoid factor (RF), as well as by increased levels of e.g., TNF-α, IL-1β and IL-6 which are recognised as central pro-inflammatory cytokines involved in chronic synovitis, osteoclast formation and subsequent erosive joint damage. In this context, SF and synovial macrophages are recognized to play a key role in driving RA pathology [8,47,48].

RASF characteristically exhibit an autonomous pathogenic phenotype that includes the capability for hyperproliferation and migration, thus contributing to synovial hyperplasia and spreading RA to unaffected joints [8,47,49]. Likewise, resident and monocyte-derived RA synovial macrophages display a pro-inflammatory profile that has been linked to the pathological activity of RASF, and the number of these cells in the synovium of affected joints has been shown to correlate with disease activity and joint erosion [50–52]. Furthermore, it is generally accepted that endothelial cells under synovial inflammatory conditions also contribute to chronic synovitis via angiogenesis and recruitment of immune cells in RA [53].

3. Adiponectin

Adiponectin has previously been described as an anti-inflammatory adipokine mainly produced and secreted by adipocytes [54]. The highly complex adiponectin molecules exist in different isoforms, the globular form, the trimer (low molecular weight, LMW), the hexamer (middle molecular weight, MMW) and the multimeric (high molecular weight, HMW) adiponectin. LMW, MMW and HMW represent the main circulating forms of adiponectin while the monomer only seems to occur as an intermediate in adipocytes [55].

Two receptors are mainly responsible for adiponectin signaling and the adiponectin isoforms differ in their affinity to the respective receptors [56]. Other receptors such as T cadherin [57–60] and PAQR3 [61] have also been discussed. Mainly anti-inflammatory effects at the systemic level have been described for adiponectin in atherosclerosis but also for example in metabolic syndrome, type 2 diabetes mellitus [56,62]. In contrast, adiponectin seems to have opposing effects on effector cells of arthritis. Adiponectin was one of the first adipokines to be evaluated in the pathophysiology of arthritis. Numerous studies found that cultured RASF respond to adiponectin by an increase of pro-inflammatory factors including prostaglandin E2, IL-6, IL-8, MMPs-1, -13 [56,62]. However, a stronger pro-inflammatory effect of the HMW isoforms has been described in contrast to LMW adiponectin in these cells [56,62]. For some cell types, even opposing effects have been described for specific adiponectin isoforms. For example, IL-6 secretion was induced by HMW adiponectin in human monocytes (but had no such effect on lipopolysaccharide (LPS)-activated monocytes), while LMW adiponectin reduced IL-6 and increased IL-10 secretion in LPS-activated monocytes [63]. Other cell types including chondrocytes, endothelial cells and lymphocytes showed a mainly pro-inflammatory response to adiponectin [56,62]. Bone cells are affected as well by adiponectin in both OA and RA [15].

3.1. Adiponectin in OA

A recent meta-analysis showed that the systemic adiponectin concentration is higher in OA patients compared to healthy controls [64] and a cross-sectional study described that serum adiponectin and leptin were significantly and negatively associated with bone mineral density in OA of the knee in contrast to resistin [65]. Furthermore, serum adiponectin levels were found to be significantly lower in OA patients with metabolic syndrome when compared to OA without metabolic syndrome [66] independent of the body mass index (BMI) [67]. In the context of OA, adiponectin was associated with pain while resistin and visfatin were mainly associated with disability [68]. Interestingly, adiponectin serum levels were shown to be negatively associated with serum MMP-13 in OA-related knee structural abnormalities [69]. The synovial tissue and IPFP of OA patients with metabolic syndrome secreted less adiponectin compared to those OA patients with metabolic syndrome, whereas leptin was increased in OA patients with metabolic syndrome. Adipokine secretion by tissue reflected the systemic adipokine levels observed in these patients [66]. In another study, evaluation of perisynovial and infrapatellar adipose tissue depots revealed differences that were influenced by the BMI of the patient. Compared to adipocytes in the IPFP and synovium of lean OA patients, obese patients showed significantly larger adipocytes with increased synovial fibrosis, macrophage infiltration and toll-like receptor (TLR) 4 gene expression in those patients while adiponectin expression in the synovium was lower in obese patients compared to lean patients [70].

3.2. Adiponectin in RA

Systemic adiponectin levels have been described to be increased in chronic-inflammatory RA and to be associated with disease activity and radiographic disease progression [56,62]. However, the correlation with disease activity has been shown in some studies but not by others [62], a discrepancy which still needs to be elucidated. Besides serum levels, synovial fluid concentrations of adiponectin are increased in RA [17,71]. In RA patients, subcutaneous abdominal adipose tissue has been found to secrete more adiponectin compared to subcutaneous abdominal adiposetissue from OA patients, and the amount of adiponectin secreted from this tissue positively correlated with the 28-joint disease activity score (DAS28) and disease duration [72].

Interestingly, RA patients with higher baseline adiponectin showed a more pronounced improvement in inflammatory parameters after anti-TNF-α treatment [73]. Along this line, anti-IL-6 treatment significantly increased adiponectin and reduced chemerin levels in RA patients independently of the disease treatment response [74].

In another recent study, adiponectin indirectly affected T follicular helper cells (Tfh), which did not directly respond to adiponectin, by activating these cells via adiponectin stimulation of RASF, mainly through IL-6. Liu et al. confirm that intraarticular injection of adiponectin increased synovial inflammation with an increased frequency of Tfh in adiponectin-treated collagen-induced arthritis (CIA) mice [75]. Targeting specific adiponectin isoforms using therapeutic antibodies specifically against MMW/HMW adiponectin reduced the IL-6 and IL-8 induction in osteoblasts induced by those isoforms [76]. In addition, Lee et al. showed that antibodies against MMW/HMW as well as against MMW alone significantly ameliorated CIA in mice and that hence both these adiponectin isoforms may contribute to progression of arthritis.

In another recent study, Qian and colleagues suggested a potential cardiovascular protective role of IL-6 inhibition. Adiponectin and osteopontin (OPN) levels were increased and associated with each other in RA serum [77], and RASF stimulation with adiponectin led to a dose-dependent increase in OPN, which in turn caused increased monocyte (RAW264.7) migration. This increased migration could be inhibited by blocking OPN. In vivo, OPN silencing reduced the amount of tartrate-resistant acid phosphatase positive osteoclasts and bone erosion in collagen-induced arthritis (CIA) mice. Therefore, enhanced bone erosion in RA is suggested to be mediated by the induction of OPN in SF, thus increasing the differentiation and recruitment of osteoclast precursors [77].

4. Leptin

Discovered in 1994 by Jeffrey Friedman et al. [78], leptin is the main adipokine secreted by adipocytes, with a positive correlation with white adipose tissue mass [79,80]. It is a 16kDa non-glycosylated protein encoded by the *LEP* (*ob*) gene, involved in appetite and obesity regulation by the induction of anorexigenic factors and suppression of orexigenic neuropeptides. Leptin is also implicated in basal metabolism, insulin secretion, bone mass, and reproduction among other functions [78,80,81]. In addition to food intake- and eating-related hormones, leptin synthesis is regulated by energy status, sex hormones and inflammatory mediators [82]. Leptin is mainly secreted by adipose tissue but it is able to act peripherally and centrally, in the hypothalamus, by its release to circulation [83]. Its biological effects are mediated by binding to the long form of leptin receptor (LEPR), which belongs to the class I cytokine receptor superfamily [84].

Leptin is considered a pro-inflammatory adipokine involved in the "low-grade inflammatory state" described in overweight and obese people [85]. In the immune system, leptin modulates both innate and adaptive immunity: it activates proliferation and phagocytosis of monocytes and macrophages, regulates cytotoxicity of natural killer (NK) cells, modulates neutrophils chemotaxis, induces proliferation and inhibits memory T CD4 cells, suppresses type 2 T helper (Th2) phenotype in favour of Th1, and modulates T regulatory (Treg) activity [80,86]. Most immune cells express LEPR at their surface, which has also been described for chondrocytes, SF and osteoblasts [87,88]. In addition, pro-inflammatory cytokines induce leptin synthesis in acute infection and sepsis [89]. Involvement of leptin has been described in several physiological and pathophysiological conditions, including vascular function, reproduction, immunity, and inflammation, as well as in rheumatic diseases [80,90–94].

4.1. Leptin in OA

Increased leptin levels in serum and synovial fluid from OA patients have been described to be involved in the physiopathology [95–99] and to be associated with pain and disease severity [99,100]. Single nucleotide polymorphisms (SNP) in the leptin gene and its receptor are linked to OA development [101,102]. Moreover, DNA methylation in OA chondrocytes correlates with leptin expression [103], which associates with the BMI [96]. Fan et al. reported different genes associated with the leptin-induced OA phenotype in rats by microarray analysis, including genes related to MMPs, inflammatory factors, growth factors, apoptosis, and osteogenesis [104].

In OA chondrocytes, leptin increased the production of the pro-inflammatory cytokine IL-1β, as well as matrix-degrading enzymes, including MMP-1, -3, -9, and -13 [80,96,103], suggesting a role in the inflammatory and degradative process that takes place during OA. Accordingly, leptin also increased MMP-2, MMP-9, a disintegrin and metalloproteinase with thrombospondin motifs (ADAMTS)-4 and ADAMTS-5, while it decreased fibroblast growth factor (FGF) and proteoglycan synthesis in rats cartilage [105]. Moreover, leptin induced activation of type 2 nitric oxide synthase (NOS2) in human and mouse chondrocytes, with the involvement of JAK2, PI3K, MEK1 and p38 MAPK signaling [106,107]. By contrast, Dumond et al. showed an anabolic effect of leptin in rat chondrocytes [108]. Leptin also induced changes in chondrogenic progenitor cells causing senescence by the inhibition of their migratory and chondrogenic potential, and the induction of their osteogenic transformation [109].

A role of leptin in OA subchondral bone has also been described, showing an increased expression which is related to high levels of alkaline phosphatase, osteocalcin, collagen type I and transforming growth factor β (TGF-β) [110]. Finally, in relation to the inflammatory process, an increase of IL-6, IL-8 and chemokine ligand 3 (CCL3) by leptin has been described in CD4$^+$T cells from OA patients [111]. In addition, Griffin et al. showed that leptin-impaired mice did not develop knee OA inflammation [112].

4.2. Leptin in RA

In RA, higher leptin serum levels are related to disease course and activity [113–116]. In addition to the activity, leptin in serum and synovial fluid has also been linked to disease duration and joint erosion [117].

Several authors have reported the involvement of leptin in joint inflammation by the modulation of different inflammatory mediators. Correlation of leptin and IL-17 has been reported in plasma from RA patients [118]. In addition, leptin induced IL-6 and IL-8 expression in SF from RA and OA patients, where JAK2/STAT3, NF κB, and AP-1 signaling pathways were involved [119,120]. Leptin also increased expression of the vascular cell adhesion molecule (VCAM)-1 in human and murine chondrocytes, and is involved in leukocyte extravasation during RA and OA inflammatory processes. JAK2, PI3K and MAPK intracellular signaling was shown to play a role in this context [87]. Moreover, induction of MAPK signaling by leptin has also been described in RASF [120].

Correlation of leptin with RA pathology has been shown in animal models. Busso et al. reported less severe arthritis in leptin-deficient mice, accompanied with a reduction in IL-1β and TNF-α levels [121]. In addition, leptin injection in CIA mice increased Th17 response, exacerbating RA severity and increasing synovial hyperplasia and joint damage [122]. Serum leptin concentrations also correlated with body fat percentage in RA patients, working as an obesity marker [123]. Cardiovascular risk is another factor associated to obesity and RA pathology. Accordingly, Batun et al. reported an association between leptin and IL-6 concentrations with cardiovascular risk in these patients [124].

5. Resistin

Resistin is a dimeric cysteine-rich protein that circulates as a 108-amino acid homodimer in human blood [125]. In humans, this adipokine is mainly produced by macrophages whereas in mice it is primarily secreted by adipocytes [126]. In line with this, human resistin has been primarily associated with inflammatory responses by promoting immune cell recruitment [127–129], whereas in mice it has been mostly linked to the development of type 2 diabetes and obesity-mediated insulin resistance [130,131]. However, conflicting results have been published regarding the modulatory role of resistin on inflammatory responses, and whether this adipokine induces anti- or pro-inflammatory effects on cells may depend on both the tissue and organ context and the disease studied [125]. Nevertheless, it is accepted that resistin is generally involved in inflammation and insulin resistance, and subsequently in the development of different pathologies such as coronary artery disease, atherosclerosis, type 2 diabetes, psoriasis and colorectal cancer [132–136]. In this sense, resistin has also emerged as an adipokine implicated in the pathogenesis of OA and RA given its immunomodulatory effects and the ability to enhance the activated phenotype of the effector cells involved in these rheumatic diseases [98,129].

5.1. Resistin in OA

Numerous clinical studies have revealed that serum, plasma and synovial fluid resistin levels are increased in OA patients compared with healthy subjects [98,137], suggesting that this adipokine may act as a linker between the inflammatory process and the altered metabolism of joint tissues in the pathogenesis of OA [138].

Resistin levels in the synovial fluid of OA joints have been found to exhibit a positive association with symptomatic and radiographic severity as well as with articular cartilage damage. Moreover, such levels of resistin have been reported to correlate with resistin released from cultured OA cartilage [139–141]. Likewise, presence of inflammatory and catabolic factors in synovial fluid, including IL-6, MMP-1, MMP-3 and collagen type II C-telopeptide fragments, also exhibited a positive correlation with synovial fluid resistin levels [141,142]. Furthermore, these adipokine levels have been linked with pain and disability in OA patients with join effusion [143], although no association with knee cartilage volume has been found [97,144].

Interestingly, in vitro studies have shown that resistin-stimulated human articular chondrocytes display an upregulated expression of several pro-inflammatory mediators, including TNF-α, IL-6 and IL-12 [145], and different cartilage catabolic enzymes and mediators, such as MMP1, MMP3, ADAMTS-4 and inducible cyclooxygenase (COX)-2, as well as a decreased production of some components of cartilage ECM such as type II collagen and the proteoglycan aggrecan [146–148]. This ability of resistin to promote catabolic over anabolic activity in OA chondrocytes has been confirmed in a recent study, which further found that resistin modulates the expression of several microRNAs (miRNA) involved in the pathogenesis of OA [149]. Accordingly, resistin stimulation of meniscal tissue explants from OA patients resulted in a significant increase of sulfated glycosaminoglycan depletion [150] similar to the dose-dependent loss of proteoglycan in murine cartilage [148]. Furthermore, resistin has also has been found to induce the expression of monocyte chemoattractant protein-1 (MCP-1) by SF from OA patients and to subsequently promote the monocyte migration and infiltration in synovium [151].

However, some inconsistent results have been published regarding the involvement of resistin circulating levels in the pathophysiology of OA. On the one hand, serum levels of resistin have demonstrated a positive correlation with bone marrow lesions and cartilage degradation, also showing an association with different scoring systems for measuring severity, progression and pain in OA [141,152]. Likewise, plasma resistin levels in OA were shown to be associated with progression of radiographic knee [153]. On the other hand, other authors have not found any significant relationship between serum resistin and OA radiographic severity, bone mineral density, pain or cartilage damage [65,97,98,142,154]. Nevertheless, such serum levels exhibited a weak but positive association with histological signs of synovial inflammation in OA patients [98]. Therefore, while the potential pathogenic role of serum/plasma resistin levels needs to be further investigated, there is evidence of the involvement of synovial fluid resistin in OA pathogenic mechanisms by promoting pro-inflammatory responses and cartilage catabolic activity.

5.2. Resistin in RA

Resistin is present in blood plasma or serum, synovial fluid, and synovial tissue of RA patients. Synovial stromal cells, including SF, and infiltrating immune cells, such as macrophages and B cells, express resistin in joints affected by RA [155,156]. Higher resistin levels in synovial sublining layers and also in synovial fluid from RA patients compared with OA have been described [17,155,157]. Regarding the potential pathological impact of synovial resistin levels in RA, it has been shown that increased levels correlate with RA disease activity, joint damage [71], and inflammation intensity defined by the intra-articular leukocytes count and IL-6 levels [128]. Conversely, in another study, synovial fluid resistin did not show any significant relationship with inflammation degree based on C-reactive protein (CRP) levels [155].

Besides, the available data concerning the circulating resistin levels in RA patients have also generated conflicting conclusions. Although most studies describe no differences between serum or plasma resistin levels in RA patients and controls [71,113,128,156,158], other authors have reported higher resistin serum levels in RA when compared with healthy controls or with OA patients [155,159]. There is evidence that resistin serum levels in RA patients are positively correlated with inflammatory markers, such as erythrocyte sedimentation rate (ESR) and CRP levels, as well as with the degree of disease activity measured by DAS28 [113,155,160]. Another study also demonstrated a positive correlation between circulating levels of this adipokine and TNF-α levels in blood from RA patients [161], whereas no relationship with TNF-α, CRP levels, leukocytes counts, or with other pro-inflammatory cytokines such as IL6, IL8, or MCP-1 was found by other authors [128,155].

Despite these controversial results regarding correlations between resistin levels in circulating blood or in the joint with parameters of disease activity, there is a general agreement that this adipokine is involved in the pathogenesis of RA. In fact, the intra-articular injection of recombinant resistin in healthy mice induced leukocyte infiltration and hyperplasia of the synovia, leading to a joint inflammation similar to human arthritis [128]. Furthermore, in vitro stimulation of human synovial fluid leukocytes and peripheral blood mononuclear cells (PBMC) with resistin induced the secretion of IL-6, IL-1 and TNF-α by an NF κB-dependent pathway, providing a positive feedback circuit in PBMC by stimulating also its own production [128]. Likewise, stimulatory effect of this adipokine on IL-12 and TNF-α release by both murine and human macrophages was demonstrated to be mediated by the NF κB pathway [127]. More recently, the ability of resistin to increase the production of pro-inflammatory chemokines by SF has been shown [162]. Moreover, resistin has been considered as a key factor triggering angiogenesis in RA affected joints through the upregulation of vascular endothelial growth factor (VEGF) expression in endothelial progenitor cells and causing the homing of these cells to the synovium [163].

The potential involvement of resistin in the RA inflammatory cascade is also sustained by the rapid reduction of its serum levels observed in patients after anti-TNF-α therapy, showing a close association with the inflammation marker CRP [164,165]. Accordingly, a downregulation of resistin gene expression in CD4 Th lymphocytes and CD14 monocytes in RA patients responding to TNF-α inhibitor therapy has recently been demonstrated, showing an increased expression in patients who failed to respond to the therapy [166]. In addition, recent studies in a Chinese population have demonstrated the association of SNP in the resistin gene with RA susceptibility as well as with its clinicopathological characteristics [167,168].

6. Visfatin

Visfatin is also called pre-B-cell colony-enhancing factor (PBEF) for its ability to promote B cell precursor differentiation (in synergy with IL-7) or nicotinamide phosphoribosyl-transferase (Nampt) due to its enzymatic activity. However, whether altered systemic or local visfatin levels are associated with changes in the nicotinamide adenine dinucleotide content due to the Nampt activity of visfatin is not well studied. It is produced by adipose tissue but also other tissues such as the liver, bone marrow, and muscle tissue. Visfatin can be induced by inflammatory factors such as TNF-α, IL-1β, IL-6, LPS and chemokines as well as itself [15,56,62].

Hypoxia as found in inflamed joints may also play a role since hypoxia-inducible factor 2alpha (HIF-2α) directly induced visfatin in chondrocytes [169]. In turn, visfatin is able to induce a pro-inflammatory response in a large number of different cell types [115]. In contrast to adiponectin, visfatin is primarily pro-inflammatory. These pro-inflammatory responses have also been described in the effector cells of joints affected by arthritis, for example in SF, lymphocytes, monocytes, chondrocytes or bone cells [15,170]. However, although visfatin is increased in both OA and RA, compared to healthy controls, the levels differ between these two diseases. Likewise, the potential to respond to visfatin is similar in OA- and RA-derived cells but the responses, although pro-inflammatory in both cases, differ in strength between RA and OA [11,29].

Visfatin is also associated with insulin-like effects: It regulates insulin secretion, insulin receptor phosphorylation and insulin-related intracellular signaling [171,172] but the work by Fukuhara et al. (2007) that originally reported visfatin to interact with the insulin receptor was retracted. Therefore, as of now, visfatin does not have a known receptor and several studies showed that its effects are at least in part due to its Nampt activity [173].

Another mechanism includes its influence on insulin-like growth factor-1 (IGF-1) function. Amongst others, IGF-1 is involved in cartilage synthesis and repair by stimulating proteoglycan and collagen type II synthesis. Visfatin has been shown to inhibit these IGF-1 functions, independently of IGF-1 receptor activation [174]. Altered levels of miRNAs may be another means how visfatin mediates its effects as a range of miRNAs were either increased (miR-155, -34a, -181a) or decreased (miR-140, -146a) in OA chondrocytes by visfatin [149].

6.1. Visfatin in OA

Systemic visfatin levels are increased in OA patients compared to healthy controls [175,176] but serum levels are lower compared to chronic-inflammatory diseases such as RA. However, OASF respond to visfatin even at low concentrations with increased secretion of pro-inflammatory factors such as IL-8, MCP-1 and other chemokines [170]. Visfatin also induced IL-6 and TNF-α in SF from OA patients, which was mediated by the repression of the miRNA miR-199a-5p via different signaling pathways including ERK, p38, and JNK [177].

A cell culture study on OA suggests a catabolic effect of visfatin because treatment of human chondrocytes with IL-1β resulted in an increased synthesis of the matrix-degrading enzymes MMP-3, MMP-13, ADAMTS-4 and ADAMTS-5 and a decreased synthesis of the extracellular matrix component aggrecan [178]. In line with these effects, visfatin significantly reduced viability, induced apoptosis as well as MMP-1 and MMP-13 secretion in OA chondrocytes [149].

6.2. Visfatin in RA

In RA patients, systemic visfatin levels have been shown to be increased in comparison to OA patients and healthy donors and a positive correlation between visfatin and RA disease activity and inflammatory parameters such as CRP has been described [56,62,115]. According to a recent study, visfatin expression is associated with reduced atherosclerotic risk in RA patients [179].

Animal models have also shown a potential role of visfatin in RA. In a murine CIA model, visfatin-deficient mice displayed reduced bone destruction, inflammation and disease progression [180]. In this study from Li and coworkers, visfatin has been shown to be required for osteoclastogenesis. In another study, use of the selective inhibitor APO866, which inhibits the Nampt activity of visfatin, reduced the severity of arthritis in a CIA mouse model and the production of pro-inflammatory cytokines in the affected mouse joints [173].

7. Other Adipokines in OA and RA

7.1. Progranulin

Human progranulin (PGRN, also known as granulin/epithelin precursor) is a glycoprotein of approximately 75–80 kDa which is composed of seven granulin/epithelin repeats (granulins) that can undergo enzymatic proteolysis into small homologous subunits. Both full-length protein and its constituent granulin peptides are biologically active although often with anti- and pro-inflammatory actions, respectively [181]. PGRN was originally described as an autocrine growth factor that stimulates chondrocyte differentiation and proliferation [182], as well as endochondral ossification [183,184]. Moreover, PGRN has also been identified as an adipokine with anti-inflammatory properties mainly mediated by its competitive binding to TNF-α receptors (TNFR1 and TNFR2), which disturbs TNF-α-induced responses [80,185].

Multiple studies have reported significantly increased PGRN levels in cartilage, synovial fluid, as well as in serum from OA and RA patients compared with healthy donors, with higher levels in RA [186–188]. Regarding the potential pathogenic role of PGRN, a correlation between circulating PGRN levels and disease activity has been shown in RA patients [189]. In this sense, a recent study in Hispanic RA patients found a correlation between changes in serum PGRN levels and RA progression scores over time, although serum concentrations of PGRN did not predict the clinical response to TNF-α-antagonist therapy [190]. The presence of antibodies against PGRN (PGRN-abs) has been detected in sera from patients with different rheumatic diseases, including RA, showing neutralizing effects on PGRN plasma levels [191]. More recently, it has been proved that PGRN-abs positive RA patients exhibit higher disease activity compared to negative patients, and that a pattern of increased rates of PGRN-abs is observed in the serum of RA patients with poorer outcome [192].

PGRN is secreted by a broad spectrum of cells, including adipocytes, macrophages and chondrocytes [193], and an increased expression of this adipokine has been found during chondrocytes differentiation in vitro, in the IPFP from OA patients [186], as well as in cells infiltrating the sublining layer of RA synovium [187]. Hence, the increased expression of PGRN at local sites of inflammation is suggested to be linked to its ability to initiate immune activation by recruiting fibroblasts, macrophages and neutrophils at the site of inflammation [194]. However, on the other hand, it is now generally accepted that PGRN is also an important mediator in the maintenance of cartilage integrity. This adipokine is able to inhibit the ADAMTS-7/-12 mediated degradation of cartilage oligomeric matrix protein by interfering with direct interactions between these catabolic enzymes and their substrate, as well as by inhibiting the TNF-α-induced expression of both ADAMTS in human chondrocytes [195]. Furthermore, treatment with PGRN has been demonstrated to inhibit proteoglycan loss and the expression of catabolic inflammatory biomarkers induced by TNF-α in cultured human cartilage [196]. In fact, PGRN has been described to trigger anabolic pathways in human cartilage and primary chondrocytes by binding to TNFR2, and to inhibit the IL-1β and LPS induced catabolic metabolism in chondrocytes by blocking TNFR1 [193,197]. In addition, a negative modulation of Wnt/catenin signaling by PGRN has been shown, with the consequent reduction of osteophyte formation and cartilage degeneration [198,199]. PGRN has also demonstrated a protective effect on osteoblast differentiation under an inflammatory milieu by blocking the inhibitory effects of TNF-α on this process [200]. Despite its chondro- and osteoprotective potential, increased PGRN levels as observed in both OA and RA patients are obviously not sufficient to compensate for the catabolic effect of other mediators [181].

Interestingly, an association between serum PGRN levels, functional impairment and disease activity has been found in RA patients [189], in which the balance between PGRN and TNF-α also showed a direct correlation with disease progression [186]. In this regard, different animal models of both OA and RA have demonstrated that loss of PGRN expression results in hyper-susceptibility to develop more severe disease phenotypes [185,196]. Along this line, a recent study has showed that the miR-29b-3p promotes disease development and chondrocyte apoptosis in an OA rat model by modulating PGRN expression [201]. Accordingly, administration of recombinant PGRN or the PGRN-derived atsttrin in OA and RA animal models protected against the development of such rheumatic disorders by, at least in part, inhibiting the TNF-α/TNFR signaling in vivo [183,185,196,202–204]. Moreover, atsttrin-transduced mesenchymal stem cells have demonstrated to inhibit cartilage degeneration in an OA murine model after intra-articular injection, and to reduce the TNF-α induced expression of pro-inflammatory molecules by human primary chondrocytes [197].

Other studies in animal arthritis models have shown that PGRN also exerts its immunosuppressive effect by promoting the differentiation, proliferation and recruitment of Treg cells under inflammatory conditions, as well as by inducing IL-10 production [185,205,206]. In this regard, more recently, a study described higher levels of PGRN and human B regulatory cells in RA patients, but without finding a correlation between them [189].

7.2. Chemerin

Chemerin is expressed as a 163 amino acid residues-long adipokine that becomes activated after hydrolization by cysteine or serine proteases [207]. The precursor is composed of a hydrophobic signal peptide sequence, a cystatin fold-containing domain, and a labile C terminus. Removal of the signal sequence results in a 143-amino acid secreted preform (prochemerin or chem163S) with low biological activity. Different cleaved isoforms of chemerin have been described depending on the location. Cleavage of the last four amino acids from chem163S rise to chem158K, and removal of the C-terminal lysine from chem158K, results in chem157S, the most active chemerin form. In addition, chem156F, a chemerin C-terminal peptide, is functionally active in vitro [208,209]. Anti-inflammatory properties have been described by mouse chem156S, homologous to human chem157S, on macrophage [210] and in a LPS-induced acute lung injury model [211]. Chemerin plays an important role in the development of coronary atherosclerosis, metabolic syndrome and other diseases [212]. It is also involved in innate and adaptative immunity working as a chemoattractant for NK cells, macrophages and dendritic cells [213,214].

In relation to rheumatic diseases, chondrocytes and SF from RA and OA patients express both chemerin and its receptor chemokine-like receptor 1 (CMKLR1) [208,215,216]. In addition, Zhao et al. described the presence of chem156F in synovial fluid samples from patients with OA and RA [208]. Chemerin induced expression of inflammatory and degradative mediators in these cells, including IL-6, CCL2, and MMP-3 in RASF, CCL2, and TLR4 in SF from RA and OA patients, and IL-1β in chondrocytes. In addition, chemerin stimulated SF motility and leukocyte migration to the joint [209,216–218].

Cleaved isoforms of chemerin have been described in synovial fluid samples from RA and OA patients [208]. Ma et al. reported higher levels of chemerin in the synovial fluid and synovial membrane of knee OA patients compared to controls. Chemerin levels also correlated with serum levels of CRP and OA severity [219,220]. Similar results were obtained in patients with OA of the temporomandibular joint, with higher levels this adipokine in synovial fluid and correlation with OA severity and pain [221]. A recent study in a rat OA model showed that chemerin aggravated the disease by inducing activation of Akt/ERK signaling, and by increasing the expression of MMP-1, MMP-3, and MMP-13 in IL-1β activated chondrocytes as well as by decreasing their proliferative capability [222].

In RA, chemerin plasma levels correlated with disease activity and BMI, which is a risk factor in the pathology, arising as a biomarker of meta-inflammation [223]. In addition, the IL-6 inhibitor tocilizumab has an anti-inflammatory and antithrombotic/fibrinolytic role and is able to decrease serum chemerin levels in RA patients [74].

7.3. Lipocalin-2

LCN2 is an adipokine produced in joint tissues in response to both mechanical loading and inflammatory mediators [218,224,225]. Specifically, LCN2 expression in chondrocytes is induced by IL-1β, LPS, dexamethasone, adipokines (leptin and adiponectin) [218,226,227] and by osteoblast conditioned medium [228], establishing also a feedback regulatory loop with the catabolic factor nitric oxide [229]. In osteoblasts, the inflammatory molecules TNF-α and IL-17 [230] can induce an upregulated expression of this adipokine, which is able to shift the balance between pro- and anti-osteoclastogenic factors toward a more catabolic metabolism [227,231]. In this sense, a recent study confirmed the catabolic effects of LCN2 in osteoblasts and chondrocytes from OA osteochondral junctions, also showing that osteoblasts induced its expression in a paracrine manner [228].

Although there are data pointing to the involvement of LCN2 in the joint pathophysiology of OA and RA, further studies are needed to elucidate its role in human development of such rheumatic diseases. LCN2 concentration was found to be elevated in synovial fluid of patients with OA and RA, with higher levels in RA [224,225,232]. In OA patients, elevated LCN2 levels in synovial fluid and cartilage have been linked to cartilage matrix destruction given its ability to reduce chondrocyte proliferation and to form a covalent complex with MMP-9 that blocks its auto-degradation [224,225,227]. However, studies in mice have shown that LCN2 overexpression in mouse cartilage is not enough to induce OA pathogenesis, and that its absence has no consequences in the induction of cartilage destruction in *Lcn2*-knockout mice [233]. Regarding RA patients, serum levels of this adipokine have been reported to be an indicator for structural damage in early-stage RA, but not for monitoring disease activity [234]. Likewise, induced LCN2 expression in neutrophils by the granulocyte macrophage colony-stimulating factor has been linked with synovial cell proliferation and inflammatory cell infiltration in RA synovium [225]. Of note, glucocorticoids (normally used to treat OA and RA) have been described to induce the expression of LCN2 by mouse chondrocytes in synergy with IL-1, suggesting that this adipokine may mediate some of the degradative effects on cartilage described after prolonged treatment with such drugs [235].

7.4. Vaspin

The adipokine vaspin belongs to a serine protease inhibitor family known to be associated with insulin resistance as well as metabolic syndrome [236]. Also, a link between vaspin and artherosclerosis and cardiovascular disease has been suggested [237]. Vaspin is expressed in several tissues including subcutaneous adipose tissue, skin, stomach and skeletal muscle [238]. In OA patients undergoing joint surgery, it was detected in cartilage, synovium and osteophytes [239]. In the same study, it was found that vaspin serum levels exceeded synovial fluid levels in paired samples.

Studies investigating potential inflammation-related effects of this adipokine are not always in agreement, which may be due to differences between the studied diseases including RA, OA, PsA, juvenile idiopathic arthritis and ankylosing spondylitis. For example, vaspin has been shown to be involved in skeletal muscle inflammation [238] and its serum levels were associated with inflammation in RA [165,240] and with the development of clinically manifest RA after follow up (in contrast to other adipokines) [241]. In an animal study, Transgenic mice overexpressing vaspin showed specific changes in metabolism- and inflammation-related markers: Glucose tolerance was improved, the mice were resistant to high-fat diet induced obesity and had lower systemic IL-6 levels [242]. Cellular effects for this adipokine have also been observed, mainly in the context of metabolism. For example, vaspin has been described to modulate adipocyte differentiation and glucose homeostasis [243]. In the context of human coronary atheromatous plaques, the pro-inflammatory phenotype of human macrophages was suppressed by vaspin [244].

Systemically, serum levels of vaspin were found to be higher in psoriatic arthritis (PsA) patients compared to healthy controls [245], whereas levels were lower in OA patients compared to healthy controls [239]. In synovial fluid, vaspin levels were significantly higher in RA compared to OA patients with a tendency to correlate with DAS28 in the RA group [246]. However, an association of serum vaspin with the inflammation markers CRP or ESR could not be identified in this study. Interestingly, inhibiting inflammation in RA patients by short-term treatment with high-dose glucocorticoids increased vaspin levels [165], suggesting an association with inflammation albeit probably not in a causal manner. On the other hand, in juvenile idiopathic arthritis, vaspin level did not differ significantly compared to healthy controls [247] and there was no association between disease activity and vaspin serum levels [248]. Interestingly, in patients with ankylosing spondylitis low vaspin levels were related to endothelial dysfunction [249].

However, vaspin also affected bone cells and chondrocytes *in vitro*: Human osteoblasts were protected from apoptosis [250] and osteoclastogenesis was inhibited in the pre-osteoblast cell line MC3T3-E1 [251], the murine macrophage cell line RAW264.7 and bone marrow-derived cells. Furthermore, in the RAW264.7 cells, vaspin reduced the RANKL-induced expression of cathepsin K and MMP-9 [252]. Vaspin was also able to inhibit the IL-1β [253] as well as the leptin [254] induced production of catabolic and pro-inflammatory mediators in murine or rat chondrocytes, respectively. These are potential pathomechanisms by which vaspin might contribute to certain arthritic diseases.

7.5. Omentin-1

Omentin was discovered as a secretory glycoprotein binding to galactofuranosyl residues on microorganisms as well as a lactoferrin-binding protein. Its role in omental adipose tissue, hence its name, was described in patients with Crohn's disease. But omentin is also highly abundant in plasma of healthy donors [255]. Most studies point towards omentin as an anti-inflammatory molecule. For example, this adipokine showed anti-inflammatory and anti-atherogenic properties in obese individuals [256] and a negative association with inflammatory bowel disease and metabolic syndrome has been described [255,257,258].

As far as rheumatic diseases are concerned, the role of omentin is rather inconclusive. In serum, omentin was found to be higher in juvenile idiopathic arthritis (JIA) [247] and PsA [248] patients compared to healthy controls. Furthermore, serum levels were higher in JIA patients with active synovitis in comparison to those without active joints [247]. On the other hand, in synovial fluid, omentin levels were found to be lower in chronic-inflammatory RA compared to OA [246]. For RA, an association of omentin with the inflammation marker CRP at baseline has been reported [241]. The level of omentin-1 in synovial fluid of OA patients negatively correlated with self-reported pain and physical disability (as measured by the WOMAC score) in OA patients [259], intended to reflect symptomatic severity in OA. This is in line with the observed inverse correlation between synovial fluid omentin-1 and radiographic severity as assessed by the Kellgren-Lawrence grading [260].

In synovial tissue, omentin was expressed in the synovial lining layer as well as perivascularly; however, no difference was detectable between RA and OA tissues [261]. In RA, omentin concentrations were inversely associated with MMP-3 levels and influenced by different factors such as disease activity but showed no association with endothelial activation and atherosclerosis in this study [262].

The knowledge regarding specific effects of omentin on different cell types in synovial tissue and systemic inflammation is very limited. For example, the response of RA and OA SF towards omentin was very low [67], suggesting that other effector cells may respond to omentin. Interestingly, Calvet et al. observed a non-significant trend between adiponectin and omentin levels was observed when other adipokines were included in the multivariate linear statistical model using the partial correlation coefficient (PCC) for interpretation [143].

7.6. Nesfatin

Nesfatin-1 (nesfastin) is an N-terminal 82-amino-acid peptide nucleobindin-2-derived adipokine, involved in satiety induction and energy homeostasis. Nesfatin was first described as an anorexigenic molecule secreted by the hypothalamus [263] but it is also secreted by subcutaneous adipose tissue, gastric mucosa, pancreatic cells, and testes [264].

Higher nesfatin levels have been detected in serum from OA patients compared to controls [265,266]. Moreover, nesfatin serum and synovial fluid concentrations have been associated with radiographic severity in OA [266], where its levels also correlated with CRP and IL-18 in serum and synovial fluid, respectively. In addition, nesfatin has been detected in human and murine chondrocytes, inducing pro-inflammatory mediators such as COX-2, IL-8, IL-6, and CCL3 in chondrocytes from OA patients [95]. In contrast, recent studies also described this adipokine as an anti-inflammatory molecule [264,267] able to reduce cardiovascular risk [268,269].

In relation to RA, a study demonstrated a positive association between nesfastin and rheumatoid factor in RA patients. In addition, nesfatin concentration correlated with MMP-2, and reduced atherosclerosis in these patients [179].

Akour et al. also described nesfatin activation by the endocrine growth factor FGF21 [270], which has been described as a new adipokine related to BMI in RA patients [271]. Association between FGF21 and rheumatic diseases would be of interest as FGF21 ameliorates CIA by regulating oxidative stress and inflammatory response [272,273]. In addition, FGF21, also inhibits macrophage-mediated inflammation [274] and down-regulates Th17-IL17 axis in CIA mice [275]. In relation to OA, FGF21 concentration in serum and synovial fluid is associated with radiographic knee bone loss [276].

8. Concluding Remarks

Common consequences of two of the most prevalent rheumatic diseases, OA and RA, are severe long-term pain and loss of locomotor function, with the subsequent negative impact on health care burden and social system. In order to reduce such socio-economic costs it is necessary to progress in the diagnosis, treatment and in the identification of disease severity biomarkers which requires a more detailed understanding of the diverse factors involved in the initiation and progression of these joint diseases. While the complex etiology of OA and RA are still unclear, and despite the differences between the pathophysiology underlying these joint degenerative diseases, it is now generally accepted that they share similar inflammatory pathways that contribute to synovitis and the loss of balance between cartilage and subchondral bone, leading to the progressive destruction of affected joints [6,8,31,45].

This review summarized the more relevant clinical and experimental lines of evidence for the connection between classic and novel adipokines and the cellular and molecular pathogenic characteristics of two of the most common rheumatic diseases, OA and RA. However, given the pleiotropic action of these molecules and their immunomodulatory effects at both local and systemic levels, the study of their role in the pathogenesis and progression of rheumatic diseases is very complex and has generated conflicting results. In this sense, both pro- and anti-inflammatory effects have been associated with the same adipokine, evidencing that their biological actions depend on the inflammatory context and the disease conditions (Figure 1). Moreover, the correlation between the levels of a particular adipokine in the synovial fluid and the activity/progression of a rheumatic disease may disappear when circulating levels are considered. In fact, when it has been studied whether there is an relationship between synovial and serum levels of adipokines with the development of arthritis in autoantibody-positive individuals at risk of RA, only a significant association between serum levels of vaspin and the disease development was found [241], thus evidencing the complexity of assessing their potential as diagnostic biomarkers.

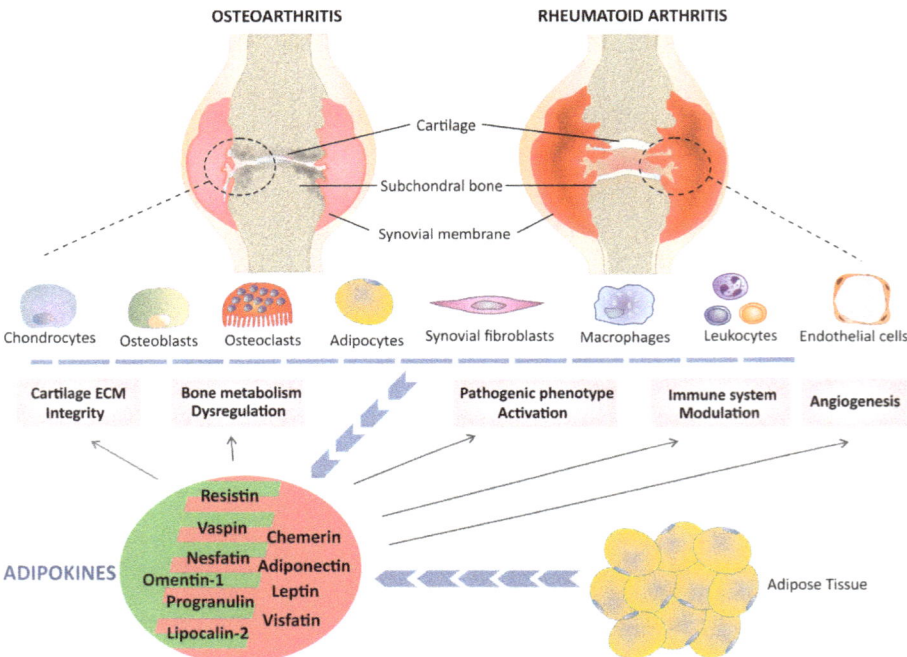

Figure 1. Graphical schematic representation of the role of classic and novel adipokines in two rheumatic diseases: osteoarthritis (OA) and rheumatoid arthritis (RA). A variety of adipokines produced by adipose tissue (blue line of arrows) as well as by chondrocytes, osteoclasts, osteoblasts, synoviocytes and inflammatory cells (blue dashed line and blue line formed by arrows), contribute to multiple pathological mechanisms (solid arrows) involved in the development of OA and RA. Although there are differences between the pathogenesis of OA and RA, common mechanisms have also been identified that affect cartilage extracellular matrix (ECM) integrity, dysregulation of bone metabolism, the pathogenic phenotype of synovial fibroblasts and macrophages, modulation of the immune system and synovial angiogenesis. Depending on the context, both pro- and anti-inflammatory effects have been associated with some adipokines, such as visfatin and resistin. Adipokines with a dominant pro-inflammatory role in arthritis are shown with a light red background, whereas those in which an anti-inflammatory action predominates are shown with a green background.

All in all, it is worthy to note that the contribution of adipokines to the pathogenesis of rheumatic diseases should be understood as cross-talking networks that coordinate with other molecular mediators to orchestrate the activity of effector cells involved in OA and RA. In this regard, activated resident cells in joints affected by these rheumatic diseases are probably the main contributors to the increased levels of adipokines detected in synovium, consequently suggesting that antagonizing local specific adipokines may be a viable option for the development of new therapeutic strategies. However, further research is needed to determine the exact contribution of the adipokine network to rheumatic disorders, which would also help to identify which adipokine could be considered a potential diagnostic and/or prognostic biomarker for OA and RA.

Author Contributions: Conceptualization, M.C., R.P.G. and E.N.; writing—original draft preparation, M.C., K.W.F., S.P.-G., U.M.-L., R.P.G., and E.N.; writing—review and editing, M.C., K.W.F., S.P.-G., U.M.-L., R.P.G., and E.N.; figures M.C. All authors contributed by proof-reading the manuscript and approving the final version.

Funding: Publication costs of this work are supported by the Fondo de Investigación Sanitaria, Instituto de Salud Carlos III (Grants N°: PI17/00027, RD16/0012/0008).

Conflicts of Interest: The authors declare no conflict of interest.

Abbreviations

OA	Osteoarthritis
RA	Rheumatoid arthritis
ROS	Reactive oxygen species
SF	Synovial fibroblasts
IPFP	Infrapatellar fat pad
ECM	Extracellular matrix
MMPs	Matrix metalloproteinases
IL-1β	Interleukin-1β
TNF-α	Tumor necrosis factor-α
ACPA	Anti-citrullinated protein
RF	Rheumatoid factor
LMW	Low molecular weight
HMW	High molecular weight
LPS	Lipopolysaccharide
TLR	Toll-like receptor
DAS-28	28-joint disease activity score
OPN	Osteopontin
CIA	Collagen-induced arthritis
Tfh	T follicular helper cells
LEPR	Leptin receptor
NK	Natur killer
Th2	Type 2 T helper cells
Treg	T regulatory cells
SNP	Single nucleotide polymorphism
ADAMTS	A disintegrin and metalloproteinase with thrombospondin motifs
NOS2	Type 2 nitric oxide synthase
TGF-β	Transforming growth factor β
CCL3	Chemokine ligand 3
VCAM-1	Vascular cell adhesion molecule-1
COX-2	Catabolic cyclooxygenase-2
miRNA	MicroRNA
MCP-1	Monocyte chemoattractant protein-1
CPR	C-reactive protein
PBMC	Peripheral blood mononuclear cells
VEGF	Vascular endothelial growth factor

PBEF	Pre-B-cell colony-enhancing factor
Nampt	Nicotinamide phosphoribosyl-transferase
HIF-2α	Hypoxia-inducible factor 2alpha
IGF-1	Insulin-like growth factor-1
PGRN	Progranulin
TNFR	TNF-α receptors
PGRN-abs	Antibodies against Progranulin
CMKLR1	Chemokine-like receptor 1
LCN2	Lipocalin-2
PsA	Psoriatic arthritis
JIA	Juvenile idiopathic arthritis
WOMAC	Western Ontario and McMaster Universities Arthritis Index
PCC	Partial correlation coefficient

References

1. Yoshikawa, H.; Nara, K.; Suzuki, N. Recent Advances in Neuro-Endocrine-Immune Interactions in the Pathophysiology of Rheumatoid Arthritis. *Curr. Rheumatol. Rev.* **2006**, *2*, 191–205. [CrossRef]
2. Glyn-Jones, S.; Palmer, A.J.; Agricola, R.; Price, A.J.; Vincent, T.L.; Weinans, H.; Carr, A.J. Osteoarthritis. *Lancet* **2015**, *386*, 376–387. [CrossRef]
3. Mobasheri, A.; Batt, M. An update on the pathophysiology of osteoarthritis. *Ann. Phys. Rehabil. Med.* **2016**, *59*, 333–339. [CrossRef] [PubMed]
4. Felson, D.T.; Anderson, J.J.; Naimark, A.; Walker, A.M.; Meenan, R.F. Obesity and knee osteoarthritis. *Fram. Study Ann. Intern. Med.* **1988**, *109*, 18–24. [CrossRef] [PubMed]
5. Aspden, R.M.; Scheven, B.A.; Hutchison, J.D. Osteoarthritis as a systemic disorder including stromal cell differentiation and lipid metabolism. *Lancet* **2001**, *357*, 1118–1120. [CrossRef]
6. Rahmati, M.; Mobasheri, A.; Mozafari, M. Inflammatory mediators in osteoarthritis: A critical review of the state-of-the-art, current prospects, and future challenges. *Bone* **2016**, *85*, 81–90. [CrossRef] [PubMed]
7. Smolen, J.S.; Aletaha, D.; McInnes, I.B. Rheumatoid arthritis. *Lancet* **2016**, *388*, 2023–2038. [CrossRef]
8. Firestein, G.S.; McInnes, I.B. Immunopathogenesis of Rheumatoid Arthritis. *Immunity* **2017**, *46*, 183–196. [CrossRef]
9. Chen, Z.; Bozec, A.; Ramming, A.; Schett, G. Anti-inflammatory and immune-regulatory cytokines in rheumatoid arthritis. *Nat. Rev. Rheumatol.* **2019**, *15*, 9–17. [CrossRef]
10. Del Rey, A.; Besedovsky, H.O. Immune-Neuro-Endocrine Reflexes, Circuits, and Networks: Physiologic and Evolutionary Implications. *Front. Horm Res.* **2017**, *48*, 1–18.
11. Savino, W.; Mendes-da-Cruz, D.A.; Lepletier, A.; Dardenne, M. Hormonal control of T-cell development in health and disease. *Nat. Rev. Endocrinol.* **2016**, *12*, 77–89.
12. Silva, A.R.; Goncalves-de-Albuquerque, C.F.; Perez, A.R.; Carvalho, V.F. Immune-endocrine interactions related to a high risk of infections in chronic metabolic diseases: The role of PPAR gamma. *Eur. J. Pharm.* **2019**, *854*, 272–281. [CrossRef]
13. Pongratz, G.; Straub, R.H. The sympathetic nervous response in inflammation. *Arthritis Res.* **2014**, *16*, 504. [CrossRef]
14. Lowin, T.; Straub, R.H. Synovial fibroblasts integrate inflammatory and neuroendocrine stimuli to drive rheumatoid arthritis. *Expert Rev. Clin. Immunol.* **2015**, *11*, 1069–1071. [CrossRef]
15. Neumann, E.; Junker, S.; Schett, G.; Frommer, K.; Muller-Ladner, U. Adipokines in bone disease. *Nat. Rev. Rheumatol.* **2016**, *12*, 296–302. [CrossRef]
16. Azamar-Llamas, D.; Hernandez-Molina, G.; Ramos-Avalos, B.; Furuzawa-Carballeda, J. Adipokine Contribution to the Pathogenesis of Osteoarthritis. *Mediat. Inflamm.* **2017**, *2017*, 5468023. [CrossRef] [PubMed]
17. Schaffler, A.; Ehling, A.; Neumann, E.; Herfarth, H.; Tarner, I.; Scholmerich, J.; Muller-Ladner, U.; Gay, S. Adipocytokines in synovial fluid. *JAMA* **2003**, *290*, 1709–1710. [PubMed]
18. Sglunda, O.; Mann, H.; Hulejova, H.; Kuklova, M.; Pecha, O.; Plestilova, L.; Filkova, M.; Pavelka, K.; Vencovsky, J.; Senolt, L. Decreased circulating visfatin is associated with improved disease activity in early rheumatoid arthritis: Data from the PERAC cohort. *PLoS ONE* **2014**, *9*, e103495. [CrossRef] [PubMed]

19. Klein-Wieringa, I.R.; Kloppenburg, M.; Bastiaansen-Jenniskens, Y.M.; Yusuf, E.; Kwekkeboom, J.C.; El-Bannoudi, H.; Nelissen, R.G.; Zuurmond, A.; Stojanovic-Susulic, V.; Van Osch, G.J.; et al. The infrapatellar fat pad of patients with osteoarthritis has an inflammatory phenotype. *Ann. Rheum. Dis.* **2011**, *70*, 851–857. [CrossRef]
20. Brooks, P. Inflammation as an important feature of osteoarthritis. *Bull. World Health Organ.* **2003**, *81*, 689–690.
21. Goldring, M.B.; Goldring, S.R. Osteoarthritis. *J. Cell Physiol.* **2007**, *213*, 626–634. [CrossRef]
22. Abramson, S.B.; Attur, M. Developments in the scientific understanding of osteoarthritis. *Arthritis Res.* **2009**, *11*, 227. [CrossRef]
23. Hunter, D.J.; McDougall, J.J.; Keefe, F.J. The symptoms of osteoarthritis and the genesis of pain. *Rheum Dis Clin. North. Am.* **2008**, *34*, 623–643. [CrossRef] [PubMed]
24. Sharma, L. Osteoarthritis year in review 2015: Clinical. *Osteoarthr. Cart.* **2016**, *24*, 36–48. [CrossRef] [PubMed]
25. Goldring, M.B.; Marcu, K.B. Cartilage homeostasis in health and rheumatic diseases. *Arthritis Res.* **2009**, *11*, 224. [CrossRef]
26. Benito, M.J.; Veale, D.J.; FitzGerald, O.; van den Berg, W.B.; Bresnihan, B. Synovial tissue inflammation in early and late osteoarthritis. *Ann. Rheum. Dis.* **2005**, *64*, 1263–1267. [CrossRef]
27. Batlle-Gualda, E.; Benito-Ruiz, P.; Blanco, F.J.; Martín, E. *Manual SER de la Artrosis*; IM&C: Madrid, España, 2002.
28. Pérez-García, S.; Carrión, M.; Jimeno, R.; Ortiz, A.M.; González-Álvaro, I.; Fernández, J.; Gomariz, R.P.; Juarranz, Y. Urokinase plasminogen activator system in synovial fibroblasts from osteoarthritis patients: Modulation by inflammatory mediators and neuropeptides. *J. Mol. Neurosci.* **2014**, *52*, 18–27. [CrossRef] [PubMed]
29. Pérez-García, S.; Gutiérrez-Cañas, I.; Seoane, I.V.; Fernández, J.; Mellado, M.; Leceta, J.; Tío, L.; Villanueva-Romero, R.; Juarranz, Y.; Gomariz, R.P. Healthy and Osteoarthritic Synovial Fibroblasts Produce a Disintegrin and Metalloproteinase with Thrombospondin Motifs 4, 5, 7, and 12: Induction by IL-1beta and Fibronectin and Contribution to Cartilage Damage. *Am. J. Pathol.* **2016**, *186*, 2449–2461. [CrossRef] [PubMed]
30. Martel-Pelletier, J.; Pelletier, J.P. Is osteoarthritis a disease involving only cartilage or other articular tissues? *Eklem Hast. Cerrahisi* **2010**, *21*, 2–14.
31. Goldring, M.B.; Otero, M. Inflammation in osteoarthritis. *Curr. Opin. Rheumatol.* **2011**, *23*, 471–478. [CrossRef]
32. Loeser, R.F.; Goldring, S.R.; Scanzello, C.R.; Goldring, M.B. Osteoarthritis: A disease of the joint as an organ. *Arthritis Rheum.* **2012**, *64*, 1697–1707. [CrossRef] [PubMed]
33. Musumeci, G.; Castrogiovanni, P.; Leonardi, R.; Trovato, F.M.; Szychlinska, M.A.; Di Giunta, A.; Loreto, C.; Castorina, S. New perspectives for articular cartilage repair treatment through tissue engineering: A contemporary review. *World J. Orthop.* **2014**, *5*, 80–88. [CrossRef]
34. Pulai, J.I.; Chen, H.; Im, H.J.; Kumar, S.; Hanning, C.; Hegde, P.S.; Loeser, R.F. NF-kappa B mediates the stimulation of cytokine and chemokine expression by human articular chondrocytes in response to fibronectin fragments. *J. Immunol.* **2005**, *174*, 5781–5788. [CrossRef]
35. Millward-Sadler, S.J.; Salter, D.M. Integrin-dependent signal cascades in chondrocyte mechanotransduction. *Ann. Biomed. Eng.* **2004**, *32*, 435–446. [CrossRef] [PubMed]
36. Long, D.L.; Willey, J.S.; Loeser, R.F. Rac1 is required for matrix metalloproteinase-13 production by chondrocytes in response to fibronectin fragments. *Arthritis Rheum.* **2013**, *65*, 1561–1568. [CrossRef]
37. Bondeson, J.; Wainwright, S.; Hughes, C.; Caterson, B. The regulation of the ADAMTS4 and ADAMTS5 aggrecanases in osteoarthritis: A review. *Clin. Exp. Rheumatol.* **2008**, *26*, 139–145.
38. Huang, K.; Wu, L.D. Aggrecanase and aggrecan degradation in osteoarthritis: A review. *J. Int. Med. Res.* **2008**, *36*, 1149–1160. [CrossRef] [PubMed]
39. Piecha, D.; Weik, J.; Kheil, H.; Becher, G.; Timmermann, A.; Jaworski, A.; Burger, M.; Hofmann, M.W. Novel selective MMP-13 inhibitors reduce collagen degradation in bovine articular and human osteoarthritis cartilage explants. *Inflamm. Res.* **2010**, *59*, 379–389. [CrossRef]
40. Troeberg, L.; Nagase, H. Proteases involved in cartilage matrix degradation in osteoarthritis. *Biochim. Et Biophys. Acta* **2012**, *1824*, 133–145. [CrossRef]
41. Funck-Brentano, T.; Cohen-Solal, M. Crosstalk between cartilage and bone: When bone cytokines matter. *Cytokine Growth Factor Rev.* **2011**, *22*, 91–97. [CrossRef]
42. Sellam, J.; Berenbaum, F. The role of synovitis in pathophysiology and clinical symptoms of osteoarthritis. *Nat. Rev. Rheumatol.* **2010**, *6*, 625–635. [CrossRef] [PubMed]

43. Pelletier, J.P.; Martel-Pelletier, J.; Abramson, S.B. Osteoarthritis, an inflammatory disease: Potential implication for the selection of new therapeutic targets. *Arthritis Rheum.* **2001**, *44*, 1237–1247. [CrossRef]
44. Perez-Garcia, S.; Carrion, M.; Villanueva-Romero, R.; Hermida-Gomez, T.; Fernandez-Moreno, M.; Mellado, M.; Blanco, F.J.; Juarranz, Y.; Gomariz, R.P. Wnt and RUNX2 mediate cartilage breakdown by osteoarthritis synovial fibroblast-derived ADAMTS-7 and -12. *J. Cell Mol. Med.* **2019**, *23*, 3974–3983. [CrossRef] [PubMed]
45. Orr, C.; Vieira-Sousa, E.; Boyle, D.L.; Buch, M.H.; Buckley, C.D.; Canete, J.D.; Catrina, A.I.; Choy, E.H.S.; Emery, P.; Fearon, U.; et al. Synovial Tissue Research: A state-of-the-art review. *Nat. Rev. Rheumatol.* **2017**, *13*, 630. [CrossRef] [PubMed]
46. Dakin, S.G.; Coles, M.; Sherlock, J.P.; Powrie, F.; Carr, A.J.; Buckley, C.D. Pathogenic stromal cells as therapeutic targets in joint inflammation. *Nat. Rev. Rheumatol.* **2018**, *14*, 714–726. [CrossRef]
47. McGettrick, H.M.; Butler, L.M.; Buckley, C.D.; Rainger, G.E.; Nash, G.B. Tissue stroma as a regulator of leukocyte recruitment in inflammation. *J. Leukoc. Biol.* **2012**, *91*, 385–400. [CrossRef] [PubMed]
48. Ospelt, C.; Gay, S. The role of resident synovial cells in destructive arthritis. *Best Pr. Res. Clin. Rheumatol.* **2008**, *22*, 239–252. [CrossRef]
49. Neumann, E.; Lefevre, S.; Zimmermann, B.; Geyer, M.; Lehr, A.; Umscheid, T.; Schonburg, M.; Rehart, S.; Muller-Ladner, U. Migratory potential of rheumatoid arthritis synovial fibroblasts: Additional perspectives. *Cell Cycle* **2010**, *9*, 2286–2291. [CrossRef] [PubMed]
50. Mulherin, D.; Fitzgerald, O.; Bresnihan, B. Synovial tissue macrophage populations and articular damage in rheumatoid arthritis. *Arthritis Rheum.* **1996**, *39*, 115–124. [CrossRef] [PubMed]
51. Haringman, J.J.; Gerlag, D.M.; Zwinderman, A.H.; Smeets, T.J.; Kraan, M.C.; Baeten, D.; McInnes, I.B.; Bresnihan, B.; Tak, P.P. Synovial tissue macrophages: A sensitive biomarker for response to treatment in patients with rheumatoid arthritis. *Ann. Rheum. Dis.* **2005**, *64*, 834–838. [CrossRef]
52. Soler Palacios, B.; Estrada-Capetillo, L.; Izquierdo, E.; Criado, G.; Nieto, C.; Municio, C.; Gonzalez-Alvaro, I.; Sanchez-Mateos, P.; Pablos, J.L.; Corbi, A.L.; et al. Macrophages from the synovium of active rheumatoid arthritis exhibit an activin A-dependent pro-inflammatory profile. *J. Pathol.* **2015**, *235*, 515–526. [CrossRef] [PubMed]
53. Al-Soudi, A.; Kaaij, M.H.; Tas, S.W. Endothelial cells: From innocent bystanders to active participants in immune responses. *Autoimmun Rev.* **2017**, *16*, 951–962. [CrossRef] [PubMed]
54. Scherer, P.E.; Williams, S.; Fogliano, M.; Baldini, G.; Lodish, H.F. A novel serum protein similar to C1q, produced exclusively in adipocytes. *J. Biol. Chem.* **1995**, *270*, 26746–26749. [CrossRef] [PubMed]
55. Garaulet, M.; Hernandez-Morante, J.J.; de Heredia, F.P.; Tebar, F.J. Adiponectin, the controversial hormone. *Public Health Nutr.* **2007**, *10*, 1145–1150. [CrossRef] [PubMed]
56. Neumann, E.; Frommer, K.W.; Vasile, M.; Muller-Ladner, U. Adipocytokines as driving forces in rheumatoid arthritis and related inflammatory diseases? *Arthritis Rheum.* **2011**, *63*, 1159–1169. [CrossRef]
57. Tanaka, Y.; Kita, S.; Nishizawa, H.; Fukuda, S.; Fujishima, Y.; Obata, Y.; Nagao, H.; Masuda, S.; Nakamura, Y.; Shimizu, Y.; et al. Adiponectin promotes muscle regeneration through binding to T-cadherin. *Sci. Rep.* **2019**, *9*, 16. [CrossRef]
58. Fujishima, Y.; Maeda, N.; Matsuda, K.; Masuda, S.; Mori, T.; Fukuda, S.; Sekimoto, R.; Yamaoka, M.; Obata, Y.; Kita, S.; et al. Adiponectin association with T-cadherin protects against neointima proliferation and atherosclerosis. *Faseb J.* **2017**, *31*, 1571–1583. [CrossRef] [PubMed]
59. Obata, Y.; Kita, S.; Koyama, Y.; Fukuda, S.; Takeda, H.; Takahashi, M.; Fujishima, Y.; Nagao, H.; Masuda, S.; Tanaka, Y.; et al. Adiponectin/T-cadherin system enhances exosome biogenesis and decreases cellular ceramides by exosomal release. *Jci. Insight* **2018**, *3*, e99680. [CrossRef]
60. Parker-Duffen, J.L.; Nakamura, K.; Silver, M.; Kikuchi, R.; Tigges, U.; Yoshida, S.; Denzel, M.S.; Ranscht, B.; Walsh, K. T-cadherin is essential for adiponectin-mediated revascularization. *J. Biol. Chem.* **2013**, *288*, 24886–24897. [CrossRef]
61. Garitaonandia, I.; Smith, J.L.; Kupchak, B.R.; Lyons, T.J. Adiponectin identified as an agonist for PAQR3/RKTG using a yeast-based assay system. *J. Recept Signal. Transduct Res.* **2009**, *29*, 67–73. [CrossRef]
62. Fatel, E.C.S.; Rosa, F.T.; Simao, A.N.C.; Dichi, I. Adipokines in rheumatoid arthritis. *Adv. Rheumatol.* **2018**, *58*, 25. [CrossRef]

63. Neumeier, M.; Weigert, J.; Schaffler, A.; Wehrwein, G.; Muller-Ladner, U.; Scholmerich, J.; Wrede, C.; Buechler, C. Different effects of adiponectin isoforms in human monocytic cells. *J. Leukoc Biol.* **2006**, *79*, 803–808. [CrossRef]
64. Tang, Q.; Hu, Z.C.; Shen, L.Y.; Shang, P.; Xu, H.Z.; Liu, H.X. Association of osteoarthritis and circulating adiponectin levels: A systematic review and meta-analysis. *Lipids Health Dis.* **2018**, *17*, 189. [CrossRef]
65. Wu, J.; Xu, J.; Wang, K.; Zhu, Q.; Cai, J.; Ren, J.; Zheng, S.; Ding, C. Associations between circulating adipokines and bone mineral density in patients with knee osteoarthritis: A cross-sectional study. *BMC Musculoskelet Disord* **2018**, *19*, 16. [CrossRef]
66. Liu, B.; Gao, Y.H.; Dong, N.; Zhao, C.W.; Huang, Y.F.; Liu, J.G.; Qi, X. Differential expression of adipokines in the synovium and infrapatellar fat pad of osteoarthritis patients with and without metabolic syndrome. *Connect. Tissue Res.* **2019**, 1–8. [CrossRef]
67. Dong, N.; Gao, Y.H.; Liu, B.; Zhao, C.W.; Yang, C.; Li, S.Q.; Liu, J.G.; Qi, X. Differential expression of adipokines in knee osteoarthritis patients with and without metabolic syndrome. *Int. Orthop.* **2018**, *42*, 1283–1289. [CrossRef]
68. Calvet, J.; Orellana, C.; Albinana Gimenez, N.; Berenguer-Llergo, A.; Caixas, A.; Garcia-Manrique, M.; Galisteo Lencastre, C.; Navarro, N.; Larrosa, M.; Gratacos, J. Differential involvement of synovial adipokines in pain and physical function in female patients with knee osteoarthritis. A cross-sectional study. *Osteoarthr. Cartil.* **2018**, *26*, 276–284. [CrossRef]
69. Ruan, G.; Xu, J.; Wang, K.; Wu, J.; Zhu, Q.; Ren, J.; Bian, F.; Chang, B.; Bai, X.; Han, W.; et al. Associations between knee structural measures, circulating inflammatory factors and MMP13 in patients with knee osteoarthritis. *Osteoarthr. Cartil.* **2018**, *26*, 1063–1069. [CrossRef]
70. Harasymowicz, N.S.; Clement, N.D.; Azfer, A.; Burnett, R.; Salter, D.M.; Simpson, A. Regional Differences Between Perisynovial and Infrapatellar Adipose Tissue Depots and Their Response to Class II and Class III Obesity in Patients With Osteoarthritis. *Arthritis Rheumatol.* **2017**, *69*, 1396–1406. [CrossRef]
71. Alkady, E.A.; Ahmed, H.M.; Tag, L.; Abdou, M.A. Serum and synovial adiponectin, resistin, and visfatin levels in rheumatoid arthritis patients. Relation to disease activity. *Z Rheumatol.* **2011**, *70*, 602–608. [CrossRef]
72. Kontny, E.; Zielinska, A.; Ksiezopolska-Orlowska, K.; Gluszko, P. Secretory activity of subcutaneous abdominal adipose tissue in male patients with rheumatoid arthritis and osteoarthritis - association with clinical and laboratory data. *Reumatologia* **2016**, *54*, 227–235. [CrossRef] [PubMed]
73. Sikorska, D.; Rutkowski, R.; Luczak, J.; Samborski, W.; Witowski, J. Serum adiponectin as a predictor of laboratory response to anti-TNF-alpha therapy in rheumatoid arthritis. *Cent. Eur. J. Immunol.* **2018**, *43*, 289–294. [CrossRef] [PubMed]
74. Fioravanti, A.; Tenti, S.; Bacarelli, M.R.; Damiani, A.; Li Gobbi, F.; Bandinelli, F.; Cheleschi, S.; Galeazzi, M.; Benucci, M. Tocilizumab modulates serum levels of adiponectin and chemerin in patients with rheumatoid arthritis: Potential cardiovascular protective role of IL-6 inhibition. *Clin. Exp. Rheumatol.* **2019**, *37*, 293–300.
75. Liu, R.; Zhao, P.; Zhang, Q.; Che, N.; Xu, L.; Qian, J.; Tan, W.; Zhang, M. Adiponectin promotes fibroblast-like synoviocytes producing IL-6 to enhance T follicular helper cells response in rheumatoid arthritis. *Clin. Exp. Rheumatol.* **2019**, (in press).
76. Lee, Y.A.; Hahm, D.H.; Kim, J.Y.; Sur, B.; Lee, H.M.; Ryu, C.J.; Yang, H.I.; Kim, K.S. Potential therapeutic antibodies targeting specific adiponectin isoforms in rheumatoid arthritis. *Arthritis Res.* **2018**, *20*, 245. [CrossRef] [PubMed]
77. Qian, J.; Xu, L.; Sun, X.; Wang, Y.; Xuan, W.; Zhang, Q.; Zhao, P.; Wu, Q.; Liu, R.; Che, N.; et al. Adiponectin aggravates bone erosion by promoting osteopontin production in synovial tissue of rheumatoid arthritis. *Arthritis Res.* **2018**, *20*, 26. [CrossRef] [PubMed]
78. Zhang, Y.; Proenca, R.; Maffei, M.; Barone, M.; Leopold, L.; Friedman, J.M. Positional cloning of the mouse obese gene and its human homologue. *Nature* **1994**, *372*, 425–432. [CrossRef] [PubMed]
79. IJ, M.D.; Liu, S.C.; Huang, C.C.; Kuo, S.J.; Tsai, C.H.; Tang, C.H. Associations between Adipokines in Arthritic Disease and Implications for Obesity. *Int. J. Mol. Sci.* **2019**, *20*, 1505.
80. Abella, V.; Scotece, M.; Conde, J.; Pino, J.; Gonzalez-Gay, M.A.; Gomez-Reino, J.J.; Mera, A.; Lago, F.; Gomez, R.; Gualillo, O. Leptin in the interplay of inflammation, metabolism and immune system disorders. *Nat. Rev. Rheumatol.* **2017**, *13*, 100–109. [CrossRef]

81. Francisco, V.; Perez, T.; Pino, J.; Lopez, V.; Franco, E.; Alonso, A.; Gonzalez-Gay, M.A.; Mera, A.; Lago, F.; Gomez, R.; et al. Biomechanics, obesity, and osteoarthritis. The role of adipokines: When the levee breaks. *J. Orthop. Res.* **2018**, *36*, 594–604. [CrossRef]
82. Gualillo, O.; Eiras, S.; Lago, F.; Dieguez, C.; Casanueva, F.F. Elevated serum leptin concentrations induced by experimental acute inflammation. *Life Sci.* **2000**, *67*, 2433–2441. [CrossRef]
83. Tang, C.H.; Lu, D.Y.; Yang, R.S.; Tsai, H.Y.; Kao, M.C.; Fu, W.M.; Chen, Y.F. Leptin-induced IL-6 production is mediated by leptin receptor, insulin receptor substrate-1, phosphatidylinositol 3-kinase, Akt, NF-kappaB, and p300 pathway in microglia. *J. Immunol.* **2007**, *179*, 1292–1302. [CrossRef]
84. Lago, F.; Dieguez, C.; Gomez-Reino, J.; Gualillo, O. Adipokines as emerging mediators of immune response and inflammation. *Nat. Clin. Pr. Rheum.* **2007**, *3*, 716–724. [CrossRef]
85. Lago, F.; Gomez, R.; Gomez-Reino, J.J.; Dieguez, C.; Gualillo, O. Adipokines as novel modulators of lipid metabolism. *Trends Biochem. Sci.* **2009**, *34*, 500–510. [CrossRef]
86. Hasenkrug, K.J. The leptin connection: Regulatory T cells and autoimmunity. *Immunity* **2007**, *26*, 143–145. [CrossRef]
87. Conde, J.; Scotece, M.; Lopez, V.; Gomez, R.; Lago, F.; Pino, J.; Gomez-Reino, J.J.; Gualillo, O. Adiponectin and leptin induce VCAM-1 expression in human and murine chondrocytes. *PLoS ONE* **2012**, *7*, e52533. [CrossRef]
88. Procaccini, C.; Jirillo, E.; Matarese, G. Leptin as an immunomodulator. *Mol. Asp. Med.* **2012**, *33*, 35–45. [CrossRef]
89. Behnes, M.; Brueckmann, M.; Lang, S.; Putensen, C.; Saur, J.; Borggrefe, M.; Hoffmann, U. Alterations of leptin in the course of inflammation and severe sepsis. *BMC Infect. Dis.* **2012**, *12*, 217. [CrossRef]
90. Feijoo-Bandin, S.; Portoles, M.; Rosello-Lleti, E.; Rivera, M.; Gonzalez-Juanatey, J.R.; Lago, F. 20 years of leptin: Role of leptin in cardiomyocyte physiology and physiopathology. *Life Sci.* **2015**, *140*, 10–18. [CrossRef]
91. Chou, S.H.; Mantzoros, C. 20 years of leptin: Role of leptin in human reproductive disorders. *J. Endocrinol.* **2014**, *223*, T49–T62. [CrossRef]
92. Conde, J.; Scotece, M.; Abella, V.; Lopez, V.; Pino, J.; Gomez-Reino, J.J.; Gualillo, O. An update on leptin as immunomodulator. *Expert Rev. Clin. Immunol.* **2014**, *10*, 1165–1170. [CrossRef]
93. Scotece, M.; Conde, J.; Vuolteenaho, K.; Koskinen, A.; Lopez, V.; Gomez-Reino, J.; Lago, F.; Moilanen, E.; Gualillo, O. Adipokines as drug targets in joint and bone disease. *Drug Discov. Today* **2014**, *19*, 241–258. [CrossRef]
94. Gomez, R.; Conde, J.; Scotece, M.; Gomez-Reino, J.J.; Lago, F.; Gualillo, O. What's new in our understanding of the role of adipokines in rheumatic diseases? *Nat. Rev. Rheumatol.* **2011**, *7*, 528–536.
95. Scotece, M.; Conde, J.; Abella, V.; Lopez, V.; Lago, F.; Pino, J.; Gomez-Reino, J.J.; Gualillo, O. NUCB2/nesfatin-1: A new adipokine expressed in human and murine chondrocytes with pro-inflammatory properties, an in vitro study. *J. Orthop. Res.* **2014**, *32*, 653–660. [CrossRef]
96. Simopoulou, T.; Malizos, K.N.; Iliopoulos, D.; Stefanou, N.; Papatheodorou, L.; Ioannou, M.; Tsezou, A. Differential expression of leptin and leptin's receptor isoform (Ob-Rb) mRNA between advanced and minimally affected osteoarthritic cartilage; effect on cartilage metabolism. *Osteoarthr. Cartil.* **2007**, *15*, 872–883. [CrossRef]
97. Zheng, S.; Xu, J.; Xu, S.; Zhang, M.; Huang, S.; He, F.; Yang, X.; Xiao, H.; Zhang, H.; Ding, C. Association between circulating adipokines, radiographic changes, and knee cartilage volume in patients with knee osteoarthritis. *Scand. J. Rheumatol.* **2016**, *45*, 224–229. [CrossRef]
98. De Boer, T.N.; van Spil, W.E.; Huisman, A.M.; Polak, A.A.; Bijlsma, J.W.; Lafeber, F.P.; Mastbergen, S.C. Serum adipokines in osteoarthritis; comparison with controls and relationship with local parameters of synovial inflammation and cartilage damage. *Osteoarthr. Cartil.* **2012**, *20*, 846–853. [CrossRef]
99. Ku, J.H.; Lee, C.K.; Joo, B.S.; An, B.M.; Choi, S.H.; Wang, T.H.; Cho, H.L. Correlation of synovial fluid leptin concentrations with the severity of osteoarthritis. *Clin. Rheumatol.* **2009**, *28*, 1431–1435. [CrossRef]
100. Azim, S.; Nicholson, J.; Rebecchi, M.J.; Galbavy, W.; Feng, T.; Rizwan, S.; Reinsel, R.A.; Kaczocha, M.; Benveniste, H. Interleukin-6 and leptin levels are associated with preoperative pain severity in patients with osteoarthritis but not with acute pain after total knee arthroplasty. *Knee* **2018**, *25*, 25–33. [CrossRef]
101. Qin, J.; Shi, D.; Dai, J.; Zhu, L.; Tsezou, A.; Jiang, Q. Association of the leptin gene with knee osteoarthritis susceptibility in a Han Chinese population: A case-control study. *J. Hum. Genet.* **2010**, *55*, 704–706. [CrossRef]

102. Ma, X.J.; Guo, H.H.; Hao, S.W.; Sun, S.X.; Yang, X.C.; Yu, B.; Jin, Q.H. Association of single nucleotide polymorphisms (SNPs) in leptin receptor gene with knee osteoarthritis in the Ningxia Hui population. *Yi Chuan* **2013**, *35*, 359–364. [CrossRef]
103. Iliopoulos, D.; Malizos, K.N.; Tsezou, A. Epigenetic regulation of leptin affects MMP-13 expression in osteoarthritic chondrocytes: Possible molecular target for osteoarthritis therapeutic intervention. *Ann. Rheum. Dis.* **2007**, *66*, 1616–1621. [CrossRef]
104. Fan, Q.; Liu, Z.; Shen, C.; Li, H.; Ding, J.; Jin, F.; Sha, L.; Zhang, Z. Microarray study of gene expression profile to identify new candidate genes involved in the molecular mechanism of leptin-induced knee joint osteoarthritis in rat. *Hereditas* **2018**, *155*, 4. [CrossRef]
105. Bao, J.P.; Chen, W.P.; Feng, J.; Hu, P.F.; Shi, Z.L.; Wu, L.D. Leptin plays a catabolic role on articular cartilage. *Mol. Biol. Rep.* **2010**, *37*, 3265–3272. [CrossRef]
106. Otero, M.; Lago, R.; Lago, F.; Reino, J.J.; Gualillo, O. Signalling pathway involved in nitric oxide synthase type II activation in chondrocytes: Synergistic effect of leptin with interleukin-1. *Arthritis Res. Ther.* **2005**, *7*, R581–R591. [CrossRef]
107. Otero, M.; Gomez Reino, J.J.; Gualillo, O. Synergistic induction of nitric oxide synthase type II: In vitro effect of leptin and interferon-gamma in human chondrocytes and ATDC5 chondrogenic cells. *Arthritis Rheum.* **2003**, *48*, 404–409. [CrossRef]
108. Dumond, H.; Presle, N.; Terlain, B.; Mainard, D.; Loeuille, D.; Netter, P.; Pottie, P. Evidence for a key role of leptin in osteoarthritis. *Arthritis Rheum.* **2003**, *48*, 3118–3129. [CrossRef]
109. Zhao, X.; Dong, Y.; Zhang, J.; Li, D.; Hu, G.; Yao, J.; Li, Y.; Huang, P.; Zhang, M.; Zhang, J.; et al. Leptin changes differentiation fate and induces senescence in chondrogenic progenitor cells. *Cell Death Dis.* **2016**, *7*, e2188. [CrossRef]
110. Mutabaruka, M.S.; Aoulad Aissa, M.; Delalandre, A.; Lavigne, M.; Lajeunesse, D. Local leptin production in osteoarthritis subchondral osteoblasts may be responsible for their abnormal phenotypic expression. *Arthritis Res. Ther.* **2010**, *12*, R20. [CrossRef]
111. Scotece, M.; Perez, T.; Conde, J.; Abella, V.; Lopez, V.; Pino, J.; Gonzalez-Gay, M.A.; Gomez-Reino, J.J.; Mera, A.; Gomez, R.; et al. Adipokines induce pro-inflammatory factors in activated Cd4+ T cells from osteoarthritis patient. *J. Orthop. Res.* **2017**, *35*, 1299–1303. [CrossRef]
112. Griffin, T.M.; Huebner, J.L.; Kraus, V.B.; Guilak, F. Extreme obesity due to impaired leptin signaling in mice does not cause knee osteoarthritis. *Arthritis Rheum.* **2009**, *60*, 2935–2944. [CrossRef]
113. Yoshino, T.; Kusunoki, N.; Tanaka, N.; Kaneko, K.; Kusunoki, Y.; Endo, H.; Hasunuma, T.; Kawai, S. Elevated serum levels of resistin, leptin, and adiponectin are associated with C-reactive protein and also other clinical conditions in rheumatoid arthritis. *Intern. Med.* **2011**, *50*, 269–275. [CrossRef]
114. Lee, S.W.; Park, M.C.; Park, Y.B.; Lee, S.K. Measurement of the serum leptin level could assist disease activity monitoring in rheumatoid arthritis. *Rheumatol. Int.* **2007**, *27*, 537–540. [CrossRef]
115. Lee, Y.H.; Bae, S.C. Circulating leptin level in rheumatoid arthritis and its correlation with disease activity: A meta-analysis. *Z Rheumatol.* **2016**, *75*, 1021–1027. [CrossRef]
116. Cao, H.; Lin, J.; Chen, W.; Xu, G.; Sun, C. Baseline adiponectin and leptin levels in predicting an increased risk of disease activity in rheumatoid arthritis: A meta-analysis and systematic review. *Autoimmunity* **2016**, *49*, 547–553. [CrossRef]
117. Olama, S.M.; Senna, M.K.; Elarman, M. Synovial/serum leptin ratio in rheumatoid arthritis: The association with activity and erosion. *Rheumatol. Int.* **2012**, *32*, 683–690. [CrossRef]
118. Xibille-Friedmann, D.; Bustos-Bahena, C.; Hernandez-Gongora, S.; Burgos-Vargas, R.; Montiel-Hernandez, J.L. Two-year follow-up of plasma leptin and other cytokines in patients with rheumatoid arthritis. *Ann. Rheum. Dis.* **2010**, *69*, 930–931. [CrossRef]
119. Yang, W.H.; Liu, S.C.; Tsai, C.H.; Fong, Y.C.; Wang, S.J.; Chang, Y.S.; Tang, C.H. Leptin induces IL-6 expression through OBRl receptor signaling pathway in human synovial fibroblasts. *PLoS ONE* **2013**, *8*, e75551. [CrossRef]
120. Muraoka, S.; Kusunoki, N.; Takahashi, H.; Tsuchiya, K.; Kawai, S. Leptin stimulates interleukin-6 production via janus kinase 2/signal transducer and activator of transcription 3 in rheumatoid synovial fibroblasts. *Clin. Exp. Rheumatol.* **2013**, *31*, 589–595.

121. Busso, N.; So, A.; Chobaz-Peclat, V.; Morard, C.; Martinez-Soria, E.; Talabot-Ayer, D.; Gabay, C. Leptin signaling deficiency impairs humoral and cellular immune responses and attenuates experimental arthritis. *J. Immunol.* **2002**, *168*, 875–882. [CrossRef]
122. Deng, J.; Liu, Y.; Yang, M.; Wang, S.; Zhang, M.; Wang, X.; Ko, K.H.; Hua, Z.; Sun, L.; Cao, X.; et al. Leptin exacerbates collagen-induced arthritis via enhancement of Th17 cell response. *Arthritis Rheum.* **2012**, *64*, 3564–3573. [CrossRef] [PubMed]
123. Guimaraes, M.; de Andrade, M.V.M.; Machado, C.J.; Vieira, E.L.M.; Pinto, M.; Junior, A.L.T.; Kakehasi, A.M. Leptin as an obesity marker in rheumatoid arthritis. *Rheumatol. Int.* **2018**, *38*, 1671–1677. [CrossRef] [PubMed]
124. Batun-Garrido, J.A.J.; Salas-Magana, M.; Juarez-Rojop, I.E. Association between leptin and IL-6 concentrations with cardiovascular risk in patients with rheumatoid arthritis. *Clin. Rheumatol.* **2018**, *37*, 631–637. [CrossRef] [PubMed]
125. Zhao, C.W.; Gao, Y.H.; Song, W.X.; Liu, B.; Ding, L.; Dong, N.; Qi, X. An Update on the Emerging Role of Resistin on the Pathogenesis of Osteoarthritis. *Mediat. Inflamm.* **2019**, *2019*, 1532164. [CrossRef] [PubMed]
126. Steppan, C.M.; Bailey, S.T.; Bhat, S.; Brown, E.J.; Banerjee, R.R.; Wright, C.M.; Patel, H.R.; Ahima, R.S.; Lazar, M.A. The hormone resistin links obesity to diabetes. *Nature* **2001**, *409*, 307–312. [CrossRef] [PubMed]
127. Silswal, N.; Singh, A.K.; Aruna, B.; Mukhopadhyay, S.; Ghosh, S.; Ehtesham, N.Z. Human resistin stimulates the pro-inflammatory cytokines TNF-alpha and IL-12 in macrophages by NF-kappaB-dependent pathway. *Biochem. Biophys. Res. Commun.* **2005**, *334*, 1092–1101. [CrossRef] [PubMed]
128. Bokarewa, M.; Nagaev, I.; Dahlberg, L.; Smith, U.; Tarkowski, A. Resistin, an adipokine with potent proinflammatory properties. *J. Immunol.* **2005**, *174*, 5789–5795. [CrossRef]
129. Krysiak, R.; Handzlik-Orlik, G.; Okopien, B. The role of adipokines in connective tissue diseases. *Eur. J. Nutr.* **2012**, *51*, 513–528. [CrossRef]
130. Nakata, M.; Okada, T.; Ozawa, K.; Yada, T. Resistin induces insulin resistance in pancreatic islets to impair glucose-induced insulin release. *Biochem. Biophys. Res. Commun.* **2007**, *353*, 1046–1051. [CrossRef]
131. Li, F.P.; He, J.; Li, Z.Z.; Luo, Z.F.; Yan, L.; Li, Y. Effects of resistin expression on glucose metabolism and hepatic insulin resistance. *Endocrine* **2009**, *35*, 243–251. [CrossRef]
132. Emamalipour, M.; Seidi, K.; Jahanban-Esfahlan, A.; Jahanban-Esfahlan, R. Implications of resistin in type 2 diabetes mellitus and coronary artery disease: Impairing insulin function and inducing pro-inflammatory cytokines. *J. Cell Physiol.* **2019**. [CrossRef] [PubMed]
133. Jiang, Y.; Lu, L.; Hu, Y.; Li, Q.; An, C.; Yu, X.; Shu, L.; Chen, A.; Niu, C.; Zhou, L.; et al. Resistin Induces Hypertension and Insulin Resistance in Mice via a TLR4-Dependent Pathway. *Sci. Rep.* **2016**, *6*, 22193. [CrossRef]
134. He, Y.; Bai, X.J.; Li, F.X.; Fan, L.H.; Ren, J.; Liang, Q.; Li, H.B.; Bai, L.; Tian, H.Y.; Fan, F.L.; et al. Resistin may be an independent predictor of subclinical atherosclerosis formale smokers. *Biomarkers* **2017**, *22*, 291–295. [CrossRef]
135. Tu, C.; He, J.; Wu, B.; Wang, W.; Li, Z. An extensive review regarding the adipokines in the pathogenesis and progression of osteoarthritis. *Cytokine* **2019**, *113*, 1–12. [CrossRef] [PubMed]
136. Uyar, G.O.; Sanlier, N. Association of Adipokines and Insulin, Which Have a Role in Obesity, with Colorectal Cancer. *Eurasian J. Med.* **2019**, *51*, 191–195.
137. Li, X.C.; Tian, F.; Wang, F. Clinical significance of resistin expression in osteoarthritis: A meta-analysis. *Biomed. Res. Int.* **2014**, *2014*, 208016. [CrossRef] [PubMed]
138. Doherty, A.L.; Battaglino, R.A.; Donovan, J.; Gagnon, D.; Lazzari, A.A.; Garshick, E.; Zafonte, R.; Morse, L.R. Adiponectin is a candidate biomarker of lower extremity bone density in men with chronic spinal cord injury. *J. Bone Min. Res.* **2014**, *29*, 251–259. [CrossRef] [PubMed]
139. Berry, P.A.; Jones, S.W.; Cicuttini, F.M.; Wluka, A.E.; Maciewicz, R.A. Temporal relationship between serum adipokines, biomarkers of bone and cartilage turnover, and cartilage volume loss in a population with clinical knee osteoarthritis. *Arthritis Rheum.* **2011**, *63*, 700–707. [CrossRef]
140. Kontunen, P.; Vuolteenaho, K.; Nieminen, R.; Lehtimaki, L.; Kautiainen, H.; Kesaniemi, Y.; Ukkola, O.; Kauppi, M.; Hakala, M.; Moilanen, E. Resistin is linked to inflammation, and leptin to metabolic syndrome, in women with inflammatory arthritis. *Scand. J. Rheumatol.* **2011**, *40*, 256–262. [CrossRef] [PubMed]

141. Song, Y.Z.; Guan, J.; Wang, H.J.; Ma, W.; Li, F.; Xu, F.; Ding, L.B.; Xie, L.; Liu, B.; Liu, K.; et al. Possible Involvement of Serum and Synovial Fluid Resistin in Knee Osteoarthritis: Cartilage Damage, Clinical, and Radiological Links. *J. Clin. Lab. Anal.* **2016**, *30*, 437–443. [CrossRef]
142. Koskinen, A.; Vuolteenaho, K.; Moilanen, T.; Moilanen, E. Resistin as a factor in osteoarthritis: Synovial fluid resistin concentrations correlate positively with interleukin 6 and matrix metalloproteinases MMP-1 and MMP-3. *Scand. J. Rheumatol.* **2014**, *43*, 249–253. [CrossRef]
143. Calvet, J.; Orellana, C.; Gratacos, J.; Berenguer-Llergo, A.; Caixas, A.; Chillaron, J.J.; Pedro-Botet, J.; Garcia-Manrique, M.; Navarro, N.; Larrosa, M. Synovial fluid adipokines are associated with clinical severity in knee osteoarthritis: A cross-sectional study in female patients with joint effusion. *Arthritis Res.* **2016**, *18*, 207. [CrossRef]
144. Martel-Pelletier, J.; Raynauld, J.P.; Dorais, M.; Abram, F.; Pelletier, J.P. The levels of the adipokines adipsin and leptin are associated with knee osteoarthritis progression as assessed by MRI and incidence of total knee replacement in symptomatic osteoarthritis patients: A post hoc analysis. *Rheumatology (Oxf.)* **2016**, *55*, 680–688. [CrossRef]
145. Fang, W.Q.; Zhang, Q.; Peng, Y.B.; Chen, M.; Lin, X.P.; Wu, J.H.; Cai, C.H.; Mei, Y.F.; Jin, H. Resistin level is positively correlated with thrombotic complications in Southern Chinese metabolic syndrome patients. *J. Endocrinol. Invest.* **2011**, *34*, e36–42. [CrossRef]
146. Zhang, Z.; Xing, X.; Hensley, G.; Chang, L.W.; Liao, W.; Abu-Amer, Y.; Sandell, L.J. Resistin induces expression of proinflammatory cytokines and chemokines in human articular chondrocytes via transcription and messenger RNA stabilization. *Arthritis Rheum.* **2010**, *62*, 1993–2003.
147. Su, Y.P.; Chen, C.N.; Chang, H.I.; Huang, K.C.; Cheng, C.C.; Chiu, F.Y.; Lee, K.C.; Lo, C.M.; Chang, S.F. Low Shear Stress Attenuates COX-2 Expression Induced by Resistin in Human Osteoarthritic Chondrocytes. *J. Cell Physiol.* **2017**, *232*, 1448–1457. [CrossRef]
148. Lee, J.H.; Ort, T.; Ma, K.; Picha, K.; Carton, J.; Marsters, P.A.; Lohmander, L.S.; Baribaud, F.; Song, X.Y.; Blake, S. Resistin is elevated following traumatic joint injury and causes matrix degradation and release of inflammatory cytokines from articular cartilage in vitro. *Osteoarthr. Cartil.* **2009**, *17*, 613–620. [CrossRef]
149. Cheleschi, S.; Giordano, N.; Volpi, N.; Tenti, S.; Gallo, I.; Di Meglio, M.; Giannotti, S.; Fioravanti, A. A Complex Relationship between Visfatin and Resistin and microRNA: An In Vitro Study on Human Chondrocyte Cultures. *Int. J. Mol. Sci.* **2018**, *19*, 3909. [CrossRef]
150. Nishimuta, J.F.; Levenston, M.E. Meniscus is more susceptible than cartilage to catabolic and anti-anabolic effects of adipokines. *Osteoarthr. Cartil.* **2015**, *23*, 1551–1562. [CrossRef]
151. Chen, W.C.; Wang, S.W.; Lin, C.Y.; Tsai, C.H.; Fong, Y.C.; Lin, T.Y.; Weng, S.L.; Huang, H.D.; Liao, K.W.; Tang, C.H. Resistin Enhances Monocyte Chemoattractant Protein-1 Production in Human Synovial Fibroblasts and Facilitates Monocyte Migration. *Cell Physiol. Biochem.* **2019**, *52*, 408–420.
152. Wang, K.; Xu, J.; Cai, J.; Zheng, S.; Yang, X.; Ding, C. Serum levels of resistin and interleukin-17 are associated with increased cartilage defects and bone marrow lesions in patients with knee osteoarthritis. *Mod. Rheumatol.* **2017**, *27*, 339–344. [CrossRef] [PubMed]
153. Van Spil, W.E.; Welsing, P.M.; Kloppenburg, M.; Bierma-Zeinstra, S.M.; Bijlsma, J.W.; Mastbergen, S.C.; Lafeber, F.P. Cross-sectional and predictive associations between plasma adipokines and radiographic signs of early-stage knee osteoarthritis: Data from CHECK. *Osteoarthr. Cartil.* **2012**, *20*, 1278–1285. [CrossRef] [PubMed]
154. Gandhi, R.; Perruccio, A.V.; Rizek, R.; Dessouki, O.; Evans, H.M.; Mahomed, N.N. Obesity-related adipokines predict patient-reported shoulder pain. *Obes. Facts.* **2013**, *6*, 536–541. [CrossRef] [PubMed]
155. Senolt, L.; Housa, D.; Vernerova, Z.; Jirasek, T.; Svobodova, R.; Veigl, D.; Anderlova, K.; Muller-Ladner, U.; Pavelka, K.; Haluzik, M. Resistin in rheumatoid arthritis synovial tissue, synovial fluid and serum. *Ann. Rheum. Dis* **2007**, *66*, 458–463. [CrossRef] [PubMed]
156. Otero, M.; Lago, R.; Gomez, R.; Lago, F.; Dieguez, C.; Gomez-Reino, J.J.; Gualillo, O. Changes in plasma levels of fat-derived hormones adiponectin, leptin, resistin and visfatin in patients with rheumatoid arthritis. *Ann. Rheum. Dis* **2006**, *65*, 1198–1201. [CrossRef] [PubMed]
157. Fadda, S.M.; Gamal, S.M.; Elsaid, N.Y.; Mohy, A.M. Resistin in inflammatory and degenerative rheumatologic diseases. Relationship between resistin and rheumatoid arthritis disease progression. *Z. Rheumatol.* **2013**, *72*, 594–600. [CrossRef] [PubMed]

158. Forsblad d'Elia, H.; Pullerits, R.; Carlsten, H.; Bokarewa, M. Resistin in serum is associated with higher levels of IL-1Ra in post-menopausal women with rheumatoid arthritis. *Rheumatology (Oxf.)* **2008**, *47*, 1082–1087. [CrossRef] [PubMed]
159. Huang, Q.; Tao, S.S.; Zhang, Y.J.; Zhang, C.; Li, L.J.; Zhao, W.; Zhao, M.Q.; Li, P.; Pan, H.F.; Mao, C.; et al. Serum resistin levels in patients with rheumatoid arthritis and systemic lupus erythematosus: A meta-analysis. *Clin. Rheumatol.* **2015**, *34*, 1713–1720. [CrossRef]
160. Bustos Rivera-Bahena, C.; Xibille-Friedmann, D.X.; Gonzalez-Christen, J.; Carrillo-Vazquez, S.M.; Montiel-Hernandez, J.L. Peripheral blood leptin and resistin levels as clinical activity biomarkers in Mexican Rheumatoid Arthritis patients. *Reum. Clin.* **2016**, *12*, 323–326. [CrossRef]
161. Migita, K.; Maeda, Y.; Miyashita, T.; Kimura, H.; Nakamura, M.; Ishibashi, H.; Eguchi, K. The serum levels of resistin in rheumatoid arthritis patients. *Clin. Exp. Rheumatol.* **2006**, *24*, 698–701.
162. Sato, H.; Muraoka, S.; Kusunoki, N.; Masuoka, S.; Yamada, S.; Ogasawara, H.; Imai, T.; Akasaka, Y.; Tochigi, N.; Takahashi, H.; et al. Resistin upregulates chemokine production by fibroblast-like synoviocytes from patients with rheumatoid arthritis. *Arthritis Res.* **2017**, *19*, 263. [CrossRef] [PubMed]
163. Su, C.M.; Huang, C.Y.; Tang, C.H. Characteristics of resistin in rheumatoid arthritis angiogenesis. *Biomark Med.* **2016**, *10*, 651–660. [CrossRef] [PubMed]
164. Gonzalez-Gay, M.A.; Garcia-Unzueta, M.T.; Gonzalez-Juanatey, C.; Miranda-Filloy, J.A.; Vazquez-Rodriguez, T.R.; De Matias, J.M.; Martin, J.; Dessein, P.H.; Llorca, J. Anti-TNF-alpha therapy modulates resistin in patients with rheumatoid arthritis. *Clin. Exp. Rheumatol.* **2008**, *26*, 311–316. [PubMed]
165. Klaasen, R.; Herenius, M.M.; Wijbrandts, C.A.; de Jager, W.; van Tuyl, L.H.; Nurmohamed, M.T.; Prakken, B.J.; Gerlag, D.M.; Tak, P.P. Treatment-specific changes in circulating adipocytokines: A comparison between tumour necrosis factor blockade and glucocorticoid treatment for rheumatoid arthritis. *Ann. Rheum. Dis.* **2012**, *71*, 1510–1516. [CrossRef] [PubMed]
166. Nagaev, I.; Andersen, M.; Olesen, M.K.; Nagaeva, O.; Wikberg, J.; Mincheva-Nilsson, L.; Andersen, G.N. Resistin Gene Expression is Downregulated in CD4(+) T Helper Lymphocytes and CD14(+) Monocytes in Rheumatoid Arthritis Responding to TNF-alpha Inhibition. *Scand. J. Immunol.* **2016**, *84*, 229–236. [CrossRef]
167. Li, H.M.; Zhang, T.P.; Li, X.M.; Pan, H.F.; Ma, D.C. Association of single nucleotide polymorphisms in resistin gene with rheumatoid arthritis in a Chinese population. *J. Clin. Lab. Anal.* **2018**, *32*, e22595. [CrossRef] [PubMed]
168. Wang, L.; Tang, C.H.; Lu, T.; Sun, Y.; Xu, G.; Huang, C.C.; Yang, S.F.; Su, C.M. Resistin polymorphisms are associated with rheumatoid arthritis susceptibility in Chinese Han subjects. *Medicine (Baltimore)* **2018**, *97*, e0177. [CrossRef]
169. Yang, S.; Ryu, J.H.; Oh, H.; Jeon, J.; Kwak, J.S.; Kim, J.H.; Kim, H.A.; Chun, C.H.; Chun, J.S. NAMPT (visfatin), a direct target of hypoxia-inducible factor-2alpha, is an essential catabolic regulator of osteoarthritis. *Ann. Rheum. Dis.* **2015**, *74*, 595–602. [CrossRef]
170. Meier, F.M.; Frommer, K.W.; Peters, M.A.; Brentano, F.; Lefevre, S.; Schroder, D.; Kyburz, D.; Steinmeyer, J.; Rehart, S.; Gay, S.; et al. Visfatin/pre-B-cell colony-enhancing factor (PBEF), a proinflammatory and cell motility-changing factor in rheumatoid arthritis. *J. Biol. Chem.* **2012**, *287*, 28378–28385. [CrossRef]
171. Brown, J.E.; Onyango, D.J.; Ramanjaneya, M.; Conner, A.C.; Patel, S.T.; Dunmore, S.J.; Randeva, H.S. Visfatin regulates insulin secretion, insulin receptor signalling and mRNA expression of diabetes-related genes in mouse pancreatic beta-cells. *J. Mol. Endocrinol.* **2010**, *44*, 171–178. [CrossRef]
172. Revollo, J.R.; Korner, A.; Mills, K.F.; Satoh, A.; Wang, T.; Garten, A.; Dasgupta, B.; Sasaki, Y.; Wolberger, C.; Townsend, R.R.; et al. Nampt/PBEF/Visfatin regulates insulin secretion in beta cells as a systemic NAD biosynthetic enzyme. *Cell Metab* **2007**, *6*, 363–375. [CrossRef] [PubMed]
173. Busso, N.; Karababa, M.; Nobile, M.; Rolaz, A.; Van Gool, F.; Galli, M.; Leo, O.; So, A.; De Smedt, T. Pharmacological inhibition of nicotinamide phosphoribosyltransferase/visfatin enzymatic activity identifies a new inflammatory pathway linked to NAD. *PLoS ONE* **2008**, *3*, e2267. [CrossRef] [PubMed]
174. Yammani, R.R.; Loeser, R.F. Extracellular nicotinamide phosphoribosyltransferase (NAMPT/visfatin) inhibits insulin-like growth factor-1 signaling and proteoglycan synthesis in human articular chondrocytes. *Arthritis Res. Ther.* **2012**, *14*, R23. [CrossRef] [PubMed]
175. Liao, L.; Chen, Y.; Wang, W. The current progress in understanding the molecular functions and mechanisms of visfatin in osteoarthritis. *J. Bone Min. Metab.* **2016**, *34*, 485–490. [CrossRef] [PubMed]

176. Fioravanti, A.; Giannitti, C.; Cheleschi, S.; Simpatico, A.; Pascarelli, N.A.; Galeazzi, M. Circulating levels of adiponectin, resistin, and visfatin after mud-bath therapy in patients with bilateral knee osteoarthritis. *Int. J. Biometeorol.* **2015**, *59*, 1691–1700. [CrossRef] [PubMed]

177. Wu, M.H.; Tsai, C.H.; Huang, Y.L.; Fong, Y.C.; Tang, C.H. Visfatin Promotes IL-6 and TNF-alpha Production in Human Synovial Fibroblasts by Repressing miR-199a-5p through ERK, p38 and JNK Signaling Pathways. *Int. J. Mol. Sci.* **2018**, *19*, 190. [CrossRef] [PubMed]

178. Gosset, M.; Berenbaum, F.; Salvat, C.; Sautet, A.; Pigenet, A.; Tahiri, K.; Jacques, C. Crucial role of visfatin/pre-B cell colony-enhancing factor in matrix degradation and prostaglandin E2 synthesis in chondrocytes: Possible influence on osteoarthritis. *Arthritis Rheum.* **2008**, *58*, 1399–1409. [CrossRef]

179. Robinson, C.; Tsang, L.; Solomon, A.; Woodiwiss, A.J.; Gunter, S.; Mer, M.; Hsu, H.C.; Gomes, M.; Norton, G.R.; Millen, A.M.E.; et al. Nesfatin-1 and visfatin expression is associated with reduced atherosclerotic disease risk in patients with rheumatoid arthritis. *Peptides* **2018**, *102*, 31–37. [CrossRef]

180. Li, X.; Islam, S.; Xiong, M.; Nsumu, N.N.; Lee, M.W., Jr.; Zhang, L.Q.; Ueki, Y.; Heruth, D.P.; Lei, G.; Ye, S.Q. Epigenetic regulation of NfatC1 transcription and osteoclastogenesis by nicotinamide phosphoribosyl transferase in the pathogenesis of arthritis. *Cell Death Discov.* **2019**, *5*, 62. [CrossRef]

181. Wei, J.; Hettinghouse, A.; Liu, C. The role of progranulin in arthritis. *Ann. N. Y. Acad. Sci.* **2016**, *1383*, 5–20. [CrossRef]

182. Xu, K.; Zhang, Y.; Ilalov, K.; Carlson, C.S.; Feng, J.Q.; Di Cesare, P.E.; Liu, C.J. Cartilage oligomeric matrix protein associates with granulin-epithelin precursor (GEP) and potentiates GEP-stimulated chondrocyte proliferation. *J. Biol. Chem.* **2007**, *282*, 11347–11355. [CrossRef]

183. Zhao, Y.P.; Tian, Q.Y.; Frenkel, S.; Liu, C.J. The promotion of bone healing by progranulin, a downstream molecule of BMP-2, through interacting with TNF/TNFR signaling. *Biomaterials* **2013**, *34*, 6412–6421. [CrossRef] [PubMed]

184. Bai, X.H.; Wang, D.W.; Kong, L.; Zhang, Y.; Luan, Y.; Kobayashi, T.; Kronenberg, H.M.; Yu, X.P.; Liu, C.J. ADAMTS-7, a direct target of PTHrP, adversely regulates endochondral bone growth by associating with and inactivating GEP growth factor. *Mol. Cell Biol.* **2009**, *29*, 4201–4219. [CrossRef] [PubMed]

185. Tang, W.; Lu, Y.; Tian, Q.Y.; Zhang, Y.; Guo, F.J.; Liu, G.Y.; Syed, N.M.; Lai, Y.; Lin, E.A.; Kong, L.; et al. The growth factor progranulin binds to TNF receptors and is therapeutic against inflammatory arthritis in mice. *Science* **2011**, *332*, 478–484. [CrossRef]

186. Abella, V.; Scotece, M.; Conde, J.; Lopez, V.; Pirozzi, C.; Pino, J.; Gomez, R.; Lago, F.; Gonzalez-Gay, M.A.; Gualillo, O. The novel adipokine progranulin counteracts IL-1 and TLR4-driven inflammatory response in human and murine chondrocytes via TNFR1. *Sci. Rep.* **2016**, *6*, 20356. [CrossRef]

187. Cerezo, L.A.; Kuklova, M.; Hulejova, H.; Vernerova, Z.; Kasprikova, N.; Veigl, D.; Pavelka, K.; Vencovsky, J.; Senolt, L. Progranulin Is Associated with Disease Activity in Patients with Rheumatoid Arthritis. *Mediat. Inflamm.* **2015**, *2015*, 740357.

188. Yamamoto, Y.; Takemura, M.; Serrero, G.; Hayashi, J.; Yue, B.; Tsuboi, A.; Kubo, H.; Mitsuhashi, T.; Mannami, K.; Sato, M.; et al. Increased serum GP88 (Progranulin) concentrations in rheumatoid arthritis. *Inflammation* **2014**, *37*, 1806–1813. [CrossRef] [PubMed]

189. Chen, J.; Li, S.; Shi, J.; Zhang, L.; Li, J.; Chen, S.; Wu, C.; Shen, B. Serum progranulin irrelated with Breg cell levels, but elevated in RA patients, reflecting high disease activity. *Rheumatol. Int.* **2016**, *36*, 359–364. [CrossRef] [PubMed]

190. Johnson, J.; Yeter, K.; Rajbhandary, R.; Neal, R.; Tian, Q.; Jian, J.; Fadle, N.; Thurner, L.; Liu, C.; Stohl, W. Serum progranulin levels in Hispanic rheumatoid arthritis patients treated with TNF antagonists: A prospective, observational study. *Clin. Rheumatol.* **2017**, *36*, 507–516. [CrossRef] [PubMed]

191. Thurner, L.; Preuss, K.D.; Fadle, N.; Regitz, E.; Klemm, P.; Zaks, M.; Kemele, M.; Hasenfus, A.; Csernok, E.; Gross, W.L.; et al. Progranulin antibodies in autoimmune diseases. *J. Autoimmun.* **2013**, *42*, 29–38. [CrossRef] [PubMed]

192. Assmann, G.; Zinke, S.; Gerling, M.; Bittenbring, J.T.; Preuss, K.D.; Thurner, L. Progranulin-autoantibodies in sera of rheumatoid arthritis patients negative for rheumatoid factor and anti-citrullinated peptide antibodies. *Clin. Exp. Rheumatol.* **2019**, (in press).

193. Abella, V.; Pino, J.; Scotece, M.; Conde, J.; Lago, F.; Gonzalez-Gay, M.A.; Mera, A.; Gomez, R.; Mobasheri, A.; Gualillo, O. Progranulin as a biomarker and potential therapeutic agent. *Drug Discov. Today* **2017**, *22*, 1557–1564. [CrossRef] [PubMed]

194. He, Z.; Ong, C.H.; Halper, J.; Bateman, A. Progranulin is a mediator of the wound response. *Nat. Med.* **2003**, *9*, 225–229. [CrossRef]
195. Guo, F.; Lai, Y.; Tian, Q.; Lin, E.A.; Kong, L.; Liu, C. Granulin-epithelin precursor binds directly to ADAMTS-7 and ADAMTS-12 and inhibits their degradation of cartilage oligomeric matrix protein. *Arthritis Rheum.* **2010**, *62*, 2023–2036. [CrossRef]
196. Zhao, Y.; Liu, B.; Liu, C.J. Establishment of a surgically-induced model in mice to investigate the protective role of progranulin in osteoarthritis. *J. Vis. Exp.* **2014**, *84*, e50924. [CrossRef]
197. Xia, Q.; Zhu, S.; Wu, Y.; Wang, J.; Cai, Y.; Chen, P.; Li, J.; Heng, B.C.; Ouyang, H.W.; Lu, P. Intra-articular transplantation of atsttrin-transduced mesenchymal stem cells ameliorate osteoarthritis development. *Stem Cells Transl. Med.* **2015**, *4*, 523–531. [CrossRef]
198. Wang, M.; Tang, D.; Shu, B.; Wang, B.; Jin, H.; Hao, S.; Dresser, K.A.; Shen, J.; Im, H.J.; Sampson, E.R.; et al. Conditional activation of beta-catenin signaling in mice leads to severe defects in intervertebral disc tissue. *Arthritis Rheum.* **2012**, *64*, 2611–2623. [CrossRef]
199. Haynes, K.R.; Pettit, A.R.; Duan, R.; Tseng, H.W.; Glant, T.T.; Brown, M.A.; Thomas, G.P. Excessive bone formation in a mouse model of ankylosing spondylitis is associated with decreases in Wnt pathway inhibitors. *Arthritis Res. Ther.* **2012**, *14*, R253. [CrossRef] [PubMed]
200. Wang, N.; Zhang, J.; Yang, J.X. Growth factor progranulin blocks tumor necrosis factor-alpha-mediated inhibition of osteoblast differentiation. *Genet. Mol. Res.* **2016**, *15*, gmr.15038126.
201. Chen, L.; Li, Q.; Wang, J.; Jin, S.; Zheng, H.; Lin, J.; He, F.; Zhang, H.; Ma, S.; Mei, J.; et al. MiR-29b-3p promotes chondrocyte apoptosis and facilitates the occurrence and development of osteoarthritis by targeting PGRN. *J. Cell Mol. Med.* **2017**, *21*, 3347–3359. [CrossRef] [PubMed]
202. Wei, J.L.; Fu, W.; Ding, Y.J.; Hettinghouse, A.; Lendhey, M.; Schwarzkopf, R.; Kennedy, O.D.; Liu, C.J. Progranulin derivative Atsttrin protects against early osteoarthritis in mouse and rat models. *Arthritis Res. Ther.* **2017**, *19*, 280. [CrossRef] [PubMed]
203. Li, P.; Schwarz, E.M. The TNF-alpha transgenic mouse model of inflammatory arthritis. *Springer Semin. Immunopathol.* **2003**, *25*, 19–33. [CrossRef] [PubMed]
204. Thwin, M.M.; Douni, E.; Aidinis, V.; Kollias, G.; Kodama, K.; Sato, K.; Satish, R.L.; Mahendran, R.; Gopalakrishnakone, P. Effect of phospholipase A2 inhibitory peptide on inflammatory arthritis in a TNF transgenic mouse model: A time-course ultrastructural study. *Arthritis Res. Ther.* **2004**, *6*, R282–R294. [CrossRef] [PubMed]
205. Wei, F.; Zhang, Y.; Zhao, W.; Yu, X.; Liu, C.J. Progranulin facilitates conversion and function of regulatory T cells under inflammatory conditions. *PLoS ONE* **2014**, *9*, e112110. [CrossRef] [PubMed]
206. Wei, F.; Zhang, Y.; Jian, J.; Mundra, J.J.; Tian, Q.; Lin, J.; Lafaille, J.J.; Tang, W.; Zhao, W.; Yu, X.; et al. PGRN protects against colitis progression in mice in an IL-10 and TNFR2 dependent manner. *Sci. Rep.* **2014**, *4*, 7023. [CrossRef] [PubMed]
207. Roh, S.G.; Song, S.H.; Choi, K.C.; Katoh, K.; Wittamer, V.; Parmentier, M.; Sasaki, S. Chemerin—A new adipokine that modulates adipogenesis via its own receptor. *Biochem. Biophys. Res. Commun.* **2007**, *362*, 1013–1018. [CrossRef]
208. Zhao, L.; Yamaguchi, Y.; Ge, X.; Robinson, W.H.; Morser, J.; Leung, L.L.K. Chemerin 156F, generated by chymase cleavage of prochemerin, is elevated in joint fluids of arthritis patients. *Arthritis Res. Ther.* **2018**, *20*, 132. [CrossRef] [PubMed]
209. Yamaguchi, Y.; Du, X.Y.; Zhao, L.; Morser, J.; Leung, L.L. Proteolytic cleavage of chemerin protein is necessary for activation to the active form, Chem157S, which functions as a signaling molecule in glioblastoma. *J. Biol. Chem.* **2011**, *286*, 39510–39519. [CrossRef] [PubMed]
210. Cash, J.L.; Hart, R.; Russ, A.; Dixon, J.P.; Colledge, W.H.; Doran, J.; Hendrick, A.G.; Carlton, M.B.; Greaves, D.R. Synthetic chemerin-derived peptides suppress inflammation through ChemR23. *J. Exp. Med.* **2008**, *205*, 767–775. [CrossRef] [PubMed]
211. Luangsay, S.; Wittamer, V.; Bondue, B.; De Henau, O.; Rouger, L.; Brait, M.; Franssen, J.D.; de Nadai, P.; Huaux, F.; Parmentier, M. Mouse ChemR23 is expressed in dendritic cell subsets and macrophages, and mediates an anti-inflammatory activity of chemerin in a lung disease model. *J. Immunol.* **2009**, *183*, 6489–6499. [CrossRef]

212. Bozaoglu, K.; Segal, D.; Shields, K.A.; Cummings, N.; Curran, J.E.; Comuzzie, A.G.; Mahaney, M.C.; Rainwater, D.L.; VandeBerg, J.L.; MacCluer, J.W.; et al. Chemerin is associated with metabolic syndrome phenotypes in a Mexican-American population. *J. Clin. Endocrinol. Metab.* **2009**, *94*, 3085–3088. [CrossRef] [PubMed]
213. Wittamer, V.; Franssen, J.D.; Vulcano, M.; Mirjolet, J.F.; Le Poul, E.; Migeotte, I.; Brezillon, S.; Tyldesley, R.; Blanpain, C.; Detheux, M.; et al. Specific recruitment of antigen-presenting cells by chemerin, a novel processed ligand from human inflammatory fluids. *J. Exp. Med.* **2003**, *198*, 977–985. [CrossRef] [PubMed]
214. Meder, W.; Wendland, M.; Busmann, A.; Kutzleb, C.; Spodsberg, N.; John, H.; Richter, R.; Schleuder, D.; Meyer, M.; Forssmann, W.G. Characterization of human circulating TIG2 as a ligand for the orphan receptor ChemR23. *FEBS Lett.* **2003**, *555*, 495–499. [CrossRef]
215. Berg, V.; Sveinbjornsson, B.; Bendiksen, S.; Brox, J.; Meknas, K.; Figenschau, Y. Human articular chondrocytes express ChemR23 and chemerin; ChemR23 promotes inflammatory signalling upon binding the ligand chemerin(21-157). *Arthritis Res. Ther.* **2010**, *12*, R228. [CrossRef]
216. Kaneko, K.; Miyabe, Y.; Takayasu, A.; Fukuda, S.; Miyabe, C.; Ebisawa, M.; Yokoyama, W.; Watanabe, K.; Imai, T.; Muramoto, K.; et al. Chemerin activates fibroblast-like synoviocytes in patients with rheumatoid arthritis. *Arthritis Res. Ther.* **2011**, *13*, R158. [CrossRef]
217. Eisinger, K.; Bauer, S.; Schaffler, A.; Walter, R.; Neumann, E.; Buechler, C.; Muller-Ladner, U.; Frommer, K.W. Chemerin induces CCL2 and TLR4 in synovial fibroblasts of patients with rheumatoid arthritis and osteoarthritis. *Exp. Mol. Pathol.* **2012**, *92*, 90–96. [CrossRef]
218. Conde, J.; Gomez, R.; Bianco, G.; Scotece, M.; Lear, P.; Dieguez, C.; Gomez-Reino, J.; Lago, F.; Gualillo, O. Expanding the adipokine network in cartilage: Identification and regulation of novel factors in human and murine chondrocytes. *Ann. Rheum. Dis.* **2011**, *70*, 551–559. [CrossRef]
219. Ma, J.; Niu, D.S.; Wan, N.J.; Qin, Y.; Guo, C.J. Elevated chemerin levels in synovial fluid and synovial membrane from patients with knee osteoarthritis. *Int. J. Clin. Exp. Pathol.* **2015**, *8*, 13393–13398. [PubMed]
220. Huang, K.; Du, G.; Li, L.; Liang, H.; Zhang, B. Association of chemerin levels in synovial fluid with the severity of knee osteoarthritis. *Biomarkers* **2012**, *17*, 16–20. [CrossRef] [PubMed]
221. Simsek Kaya, G.; Yapici Yavuz, G.; Kiziltunc, A. Expression of chemerin in the synovial fluid of patients with temporomandibular joint disorders. *J. Oral. Rehabil.* **2018**, *45*, 289–294. [CrossRef] [PubMed]
222. Ma, J.; Ren, L.; Guo, C.J.; Wan, N.J.; Niu, D.S. Chemerin affects the metabolic and proliferative capabilities of chondrocytes by increasing the phosphorylation of AKT/ERK. *Eur. Rev. Med. Pharmacol. Sci.* **2018**, *22*, 3656–3662. [PubMed]
223. Tolusso, B.; Gigante, M.R.; Alivernini, S.; Petricca, L.; Fedele, A.L.; Di Mario, C.; Aquilanti, B.; Magurano, M.R.; Ferraccioli, G.; Gremese, E. Chemerin and PEDF Are Metaflammation-Related Biomarkers of Disease Activity and Obesity in Rheumatoid Arthritis. *Front Med (Lausanne)* **2018**, *5*, 207. [CrossRef]
224. Gupta, K.; Shukla, M.; Cowland, J.B.; Malemud, C.J.; Haqqi, T.M. Neutrophil gelatinase-associated lipocalin is expressed in osteoarthritis and forms a complex with matrix metalloproteinase 9. *Arthritis Rheum.* **2007**, *56*, 3326–3335. [CrossRef] [PubMed]
225. Katano, M.; Okamoto, K.; Arito, M.; Kawakami, Y.; Kurokawa, M.S.; Suematsu, N.; Shimada, S.; Nakamura, H.; Xiang, Y.; Masuko, K.; et al. Implication of granulocyte-macrophage colony-stimulating factor induced neutrophil gelatinase-associated lipocalin in pathogenesis of rheumatoid arthritis revealed by proteome analysis. *Arthritis Res. Ther.* **2009**, *11*, R3. [CrossRef] [PubMed]
226. Owen, H.C.; Roberts, S.J.; Ahmed, S.F.; Farquharson, C. Dexamethasone-induced expression of the glucocorticoid response gene lipocalin 2 in chondrocytes. *Am. J. Physiol. Endocrinol. Metab.* **2008**, *294*, E1023–E1034. [CrossRef] [PubMed]
227. Abella, V.; Scotece, M.; Conde, J.; Gomez, R.; Lois, A.; Pino, J.; Gomez-Reino, J.J.; Lago, F.; Mobasheri, A.; Gualillo, O. The potential of lipocalin-2/NGAL as biomarker for inflammatory and metabolic diseases. *Biomarkers* **2015**, *20*, 565–571. [CrossRef]
228. Villalvilla, A.; Garcia-Martin, A.; Largo, R.; Gualillo, O.; Herrero-Beaumont, G.; Gomez, R. The adipokine lipocalin-2 in the context of the osteoarthritic osteochondral junction. *Sci. Rep.* **2016**, *6*, 29243. [CrossRef] [PubMed]
229. Gomez, R.; Scotece, M.; Conde, J.; Lopez, V.; Pino, J.; Lago, F.; Gomez-Reino, J.J.; Gualillo, O. Nitric oxide boosts TLR-4 mediated lipocalin 2 expression in chondrocytes. *J. Orthop. Res.* **2013**, *31*, 1046–1052. [CrossRef]

230. Shen, F.; Ruddy, M.J.; Plamondon, P.; Gaffen, S.L. Cytokines link osteoblasts and inflammation: Microarray analysis of interleukin-17- and TNF-alpha-induced genes in bone cells. *J. Leukoc. Biol.* **2005**, *77*, 388–399. [CrossRef] [PubMed]
231. Rucci, N.; Capulli, M.; Piperni, S.G.; Cappariello, A.; Lau, P.; Frings-Meuthen, P.; Heer, M.; Teti, A. Lipocalin 2: A new mechanoresponding gene regulating bone homeostasis. *J. Bone Miner. Res.* **2015**, *30*, 357–368. [CrossRef] [PubMed]
232. Staikos, C.; Ververidis, A.; Drosos, G.; Manolopoulos, V.G.; Verettas, D.A.; Tavridou, A. The association of adipokine levels in plasma and synovial fluid with the severity of knee osteoarthritis. *Rheumatology (Oxford)* **2013**, *52*, 1077–1083. [CrossRef]
233. Choi, W.S.; Chun, J.S. Upregulation of lipocalin-2 (LCN2) in osteoarthritic cartilage is not necessary for cartilage destruction in mice. *Osteoarthr. Cartil.* **2017**, *25*, 401–405. [CrossRef] [PubMed]
234. Gulkesen, A.; Akgol, G.; Poyraz, A.K.; Aydin, S.; Denk, A.; Yildirim, T.; Kaya, A. Lipocalin 2 as a clinical significance in rheumatoid arthritis. *Cent. Eur. J. Immunol.* **2017**, *42*, 269–273. [CrossRef]
235. Conde, J.; Lazzaro, V.; Scotece, M.; Abella, V.; Villar, R.; Lopez, V.; Gonzalez-Gay, M.A.; Pino, J.; Gomez, R.; Mera, A.; et al. Corticoids synergize with IL-1 in the induction of LCN2. *Osteoarthr. Cartil.* **2017**, *25*, 1172–1178. [CrossRef]
236. Dimova, R.; Tankova, T. The role of vaspin in the development of metabolic and glucose tolerance disorders and atherosclerosis. *Biomed. Res. Int.* **2015**, *2015*, 823481. [CrossRef] [PubMed]
237. Choi, S.H.; Kwak, S.H.; Lee, Y.; Moon, M.K.; Lim, S.; Park, Y.J.; Jang, H.C.; Kim, M.S. Plasma vaspin concentrations are elevated in metabolic syndrome in men and are correlated with coronary atherosclerosis in women. *Clin. Endocrinol. (Oxf)* **2011**, *75*, 628–635. [CrossRef]
238. Nicholson, T.; Church, C.; Baker, D.J.; Jones, S.W. The role of adipokines in skeletal muscle inflammation and insulin sensitivity. *J. Inflamm. (Lond)* **2018**, *15*, 9. [CrossRef] [PubMed]
239. Bao, J.P.; Jiang, L.F.; Chen, W.P.; Hu, P.F.; Wu, L.D. Expression of vaspin in the joint and the levels in the serum and synovial fluid of patients with osteoarthritis. *Int. J. Clin. Exp. Med.* **2014**, *7*, 3447–3453.
240. Ozgen, M.; Koca, S.S.; Dagli, N.; Balin, M.; Ustundag, B.; Isik, A. Serum adiponectin and vaspin levels in rheumatoid arthritis. *Arch. Med. Res.* **2010**, *41*, 457–463. [CrossRef]
241. Maijer, K.I.; Neumann, E.; Muller-Ladner, U.; Drop, D.A.; Ramwadhdoebe, T.H.; Choi, I.Y.; Gerlag, D.M.; de Hair, M.J.; Tak, P.P. Serum Vaspin Levels Are Associated with the Development of Clinically Manifest Arthritis in Autoantibody-Positive Individuals. *PLoS ONE* **2015**, *10*, e0144932. [CrossRef] [PubMed]
242. Nakatsuka, A.; Wada, J.; Iseda, I.; Teshigawara, S.; Higashio, K.; Murakami, K.; Kanzaki, M.; Inoue, K.; Terami, T.; Katayama, A.; et al. Vaspin is an adipokine ameliorating ER stress in obesity as a ligand for cell-surface GRP78/MTJ-1 complex. *Diabetes* **2012**, *61*, 2823–2832. [CrossRef]
243. Hida, K.; Wada, J.; Eguchi, J.; Zhang, H.; Baba, M.; Seida, A.; Hashimoto, I.; Okada, T.; Yasuhara, A.; Nakatsuka, A.; et al. Visceral adipose tissue-derived serine protease inhibitor: A unique insulin-sensitizing adipocytokine in obesity. *Proc. Natl. Acad. Sci.* **2005**, *102*, 10610–10615. [CrossRef] [PubMed]
244. Sato, K.; Shirai, R.; Yamaguchi, M.; Yamashita, T.; Shibata, K.; Okano, T.; Mori, Y.; Matsuyama, T.A.; Ishibashi-Ueda, H.; Hirano, T.; et al. Anti-Atherogenic Effects of Vaspin on Human Aortic Smooth Muscle Cell/Macrophage Responses and Hyperlipidemic Mouse Plaque Phenotype. *Int. J. Mol. Sci.* **2018**, *19*, 1732. [CrossRef] [PubMed]
245. Colak, S.; Omma, A.; Sandikci, S.C.; Yucel, C.; Omma, T.; Turhan, T. Vaspin, neutrophil gelatinase-associated lipocalin and apolipoprotein levels in patients with psoriatic arthritis. *Bratisl. Lek. Listy* **2019**, *120*, 65–69. [CrossRef] [PubMed]
246. Senolt, L.; Polanska, M.; Filkova, M.; Cerezo, L.A.; Pavelka, K.; Gay, S.; Haluzik, M.; Vencovsky, J. Vaspin and omentin: New adipokines differentially regulated at the site of inflammation in rheumatoid arthritis. *Ann. Rheum. Dis.* **2010**, *69*, 1410–1411. [CrossRef] [PubMed]
247. Cantarini, L.; Simonini, G.; Fioravanti, A.; Generoso, M.; Bacarelli, M.R.; Dini, E.; Galeazzi, M.; Cimaz, R. Circulating levels of the adipokines vaspin and omentin in patients with juvenile idiopathic arthritis, and relation to disease activity. *Clin. Exp. Rheumatol.* **2011**, *29*, 1044–1048. [PubMed]
248. Xue, Y.; Jiang, L.; Cheng, Q.; Chen, H.; Yu, Y.; Lin, Y.; Yang, X.; Kong, N.; Zhu, X.; Xu, X.; et al. Adipokines in psoriatic arthritis patients: The correlations with osteoclast precursors and bone erosions. *PLoS ONE* **2012**, *7*, e46740. [CrossRef] [PubMed]

249. Wang, H.H.; Wang, Q.F. Low vaspin levels are related to endothelial dysfunction in patients with ankylosing spondylitis. *Braz. J. Med. Biol. Res.* **2016**, *49*, e5231. [CrossRef]
250. Zhu, X.; Jiang, Y.; Shan, P.F.; Shen, J.; Liang, Q.H.; Cui, R.R.; Liu, Y.; Liu, G.Y.; Wu, S.S.; Lu, Q.; et al. Vaspin attenuates the apoptosis of human osteoblasts through ERK signaling pathway. *Amino Acids* **2013**, *44*, 961–968. [CrossRef] [PubMed]
251. Liu, Y.; Xu, F.; Pei, H.X.; Zhu, X.; Lin, X.; Song, C.Y.; Liang, Q.H.; Liao, E.Y.; Yuan, L.Q. Vaspin regulates the osteogenic differentiation of MC3T3-E1 through the PI3K-Akt/miR-34c loop. *Sci. Rep.* **2016**, *6*, 25578. [CrossRef] [PubMed]
252. Kamio, N.; Kawato, T.; Tanabe, N.; Kitami, S.; Morita, T.; Ochiai, K.; Maeno, M. Vaspin attenuates RANKL-induced osteoclast formation in RAW264.7 cells. *Connect. Tissue Res.* **2013**, *54*, 147–152. [CrossRef] [PubMed]
253. Bao, J.P.; Jiang, L.F.; Li, J.; Chen, W.P.; Hu, P.F.; Wu, L.D. Visceral adipose tissue-derived serine protease inhibitor inhibits interleukin-1beta-induced catabolic and inflammatory responses in murine chondrocytes. *Mol. Med. Rep.* **2014**, *10*, 2191–2197. [CrossRef] [PubMed]
254. Bao, J.P.; Xu, L.H.; Ran, J.S.; Xiong, Y.; Wu, L.D. Vaspin prevents leptininduced inflammation and catabolism by inhibiting the activation of nuclear factorkappaB in rat chondrocytes. *Mol. Med. Rep.* **2017**, *16*, 2925–2930. [CrossRef]
255. Schaffler, A.; Neumeier, M.; Herfarth, H.; Furst, A.; Scholmerich, J.; Buchler, C. Genomic structure of human omentin, a new adipocytokine expressed in omental adipose tissue. *Biochim. et Biophys. Acta* **2005**, *1732*, 96–102. [CrossRef]
256. Zhou, J.Y.; Chan, L.; Zhou, S.W. Omentin: Linking metabolic syndrome and cardiovascular disease. *Curr. Vasc. Pharmacol.* **2014**, *12*, 136–143. [CrossRef]
257. Yin, J.; Hou, P.; Wu, Z.; Nie, Y. Decreased levels of serum omentin-1 in patients with inflammatory bowel disease. *Med. Sci. Monit.* **2015**, *21*, 118–122.
258. Jaikanth, C.; Gurumurthy, P.; Cherian, K.M.; Indhumathi, T. Emergence of omentin as a pleiotropic adipocytokine. *Exp. Clin. Endocrinol Diabetes* **2013**, *121*, 377–383. [CrossRef] [PubMed]
259. Li, Z.G.; Zhao, D.W.; Xia, C.J.; Wang, T.N.; Liu, Y.P.; Zhang, Y.; Wang, B.J. Decreased synovial fluid omentin-1 concentrations reflect symptomatic severity in patients with knee osteoarthritis. *Scand. J. Clin. Lab. Invest.* **2012**, *72*, 623–628. [CrossRef] [PubMed]
260. Xu, L.; Zhu, G.B.; Wang, L.; Wang, D.F.; Jiang, X.R. Synovial fluid omentin-1 levels are inversely correlated with radiographic severity of knee osteoarthritis. *J. Investig. Med.* **2012**, *60*, 583–586. [CrossRef]
261. Frommer, K.W.; Vasile, M.; Muller-Ladner, U.; Neumann, E. The Adipokine Omentin in Late-stage Rheumatoid Arthritis and Endstage Osteoarthritis. *J. Rheumatol.* **2017**, *44*, 539–541. [CrossRef]
262. Robinson, C.; Tsang, L.; Solomon, A.; Woodiwiss, A.J.; Gunter, S.; Millen, A.M.; Norton, G.R.; Fernandez-Lopez, M.J.; Hollan, I.; Dessein, P.H. Omentin concentrations are independently associated with those of matrix metalloproteinase-3 in patients with mild but not severe rheumatoid arthritis. *Rheumatol. Int.* **2017**, *37*, 3–11. [CrossRef] [PubMed]
263. Oh, I.S.; Shimizu, H.; Satoh, T.; Okada, S.; Adachi, S.; Inoue, K.; Eguchi, H.; Yamamoto, M.; Imaki, T.; Hashimoto, K.; et al. Identification of nesfatin-1 as a satiety molecule in the hypothalamus. *Nature* **2006**, *443*, 709–712. [CrossRef] [PubMed]
264. Ayada, C.; Toru, U.; Korkut, Y. Nesfatin-1 and its effects on different systems. *Hippokratia* **2015**, *19*, 4–10. [PubMed]
265. Zhang, Y.; Shui, X.; Lian, X.; Wang, G. Serum and synovial fluid nesfatin-1 concentration is associated with radiographic severity of knee osteoarthritis. *Med. Sci. Monit.* **2015**, *21*, 1078–1082. [PubMed]
266. Jiang, L.; Bao, J.; Zhou, X.; Xiong, Y.; Wu, L. Increased serum levels and chondrocyte expression of nesfatin-1 in patients with osteoarthritis and its relation with BMI, hsCRP, and IL-18. *Mediators Inflamm* **2013**, *2013*, 631251. [CrossRef] [PubMed]
267. Tang, C.H.; Fu, X.J.; Xu, X.L.; Wei, X.J.; Pan, H.S. The anti-inflammatory and anti-apoptotic effects of nesfatin-1 in the traumatic rat brain. *Peptides* **2012**, *36*, 39–45. [CrossRef]
268. Dai, H.; Li, X.; He, T.; Wang, Y.; Wang, Z.; Wang, S.; Xing, M.; Sun, W.; Ding, H. Decreased plasma nesfatin-1 levels in patients with acute myocardial infarction. *Peptides* **2013**, *46*, 167–171. [CrossRef] [PubMed]
269. Ding, S.; Qu, W.; Dang, S.; Xie, X.; Xu, J.; Wang, Y.; Jing, A.; Zhang, C.; Wang, J. Serum nesfatin-1 is reduced in type 2 diabetes mellitus patients with peripheral arterial disease. *Med. Sci. Monit.* **2015**, *21*, 987–991.

270. Akour, A.; Kasabri, V.; Boulatova, N.; Bustanji, Y.; Naffa, R.; Hyasat, D.; Khawaja, N.; Bustanji, H.; Zayed, A.; Momani, M. Levels of metabolic markers in drug-naive prediabetic and type 2 diabetic patients. *Acta. Diabetol.* **2017**, *54*, 163–170. [CrossRef]
271. Hulejova, H.; Andres Cerezo, L.; Kuklova, M.; Pecha, O.; Vondracek, T.; Pavelka, K.; Vencovsky, J.; Haluzik, M.; Senolt, L. Novel adipokine fibroblast growth factor 21 is increased in rheumatoid arthritis. *Physiol. Res.* **2012**, *61*, 489–494.
272. Yu, D.; Ye, X.; Che, R.; Wu, Q.; Qi, J.; Song, L.; Guo, X.; Zhang, S.; Wu, H.; Ren, G.; et al. FGF21 exerts comparable pharmacological efficacy with Adalimumab in ameliorating collagen-induced rheumatoid arthritis by regulating systematic inflammatory response. *Biomed. Pharm.* **2017**, *89*, 751–760. [CrossRef] [PubMed]
273. Yu, Y.; Li, S.; Liu, Y.; Tian, G.; Yuan, Q.; Bai, F.; Wang, W.; Zhang, Z.; Ren, G.; Zhang, Y.; et al. Fibroblast growth factor 21 (FGF21) ameliorates collagen-induced arthritis through modulating oxidative stress and suppressing nuclear factor-kappa B pathway. *Int. Immunopharmacol.* **2015**, *25*, 74–82. [CrossRef] [PubMed]
274. Yu, Y.; He, J.; Li, S.; Song, L.; Guo, X.; Yao, W.; Zou, D.; Gao, X.; Liu, Y.; Bai, F.; et al. Fibroblast growth factor 21 (FGF21) inhibits macrophage-mediated inflammation by activating Nrf2 and suppressing the NF-kappaB signaling pathway. *Int. Immunopharmacol.* **2016**, *38*, 144–152. [CrossRef] [PubMed]
275. Li, S.M.; Yu, Y.H.; Li, L.; Wang, W.F.; Li, D.S. Treatment of CIA Mice with FGF21 Down-regulates TH17-IL-17 Axis. *Inflammation* **2016**, *39*, 309–319. [CrossRef] [PubMed]
276. Li, Z.C.; Xiao, J.; Wang, G.; Li, M.Q.; Hu, K.Z.; Ma, T.; Wang, W.L.; Liu, Z.D.; Zhang, J.D. Fibroblast growth factor-21 concentration in serum and synovial fluid is associated with radiographic bone loss of knee osteoarthritis. *Scand. J. Clin. Lab. Invest.* **2015**, *75*, 121–125. [CrossRef] [PubMed]

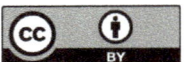

© 2019 by the authors. Licensee MDPI, Basel, Switzerland. This article is an open access article distributed under the terms and conditions of the Creative Commons Attribution (CC BY) license (http://creativecommons.org/licenses/by/4.0/).

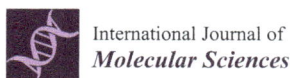

Article

Effects of Tocilizumab, an Anti-Interleukin-6 Receptor Antibody, on Serum Lipid and Adipokine Levels in Patients with Rheumatoid Arthritis

Elinoar Hoffman [1,2,3,†], Michal A. Rahat [2,3,†], Joy Feld [1], Muna Elias [1], Itzhak Rosner [3,4], Lisa Kaly [4], Idit Lavie [3,5], Tal Gazitt [1] and Devy Zisman [1,3,*]

1. Rheumatology Unit, Carmel Medical Center, Haifa 3436212, Israel; elinoard@gmail.com (E.H.); joyfeld@gmail.com (J.F.); MUNAEL@clalit.org.il (M.E.); tgazitt@gmail.com (T.G.)
2. The Immunotherapy Laboratory, Carmel Medical Center, Haifa 3436212, Israel; mrahat@netvision.net.il
3. The Ruth and Bruce Rappaport Faculty of Medicine, Technion, Haifa 3109601, Israel; itzhak.rosner@b-zion.org.il (I.R.); lavi_idit@clalit.org.il (I.L.)
4. Rheumatology Unit, Bnai Zion Medical Center, Haifa, 3339419, Israel; lisakaly@yahoo.fr
5. Department of Community Medicine and Epidemiology, Carmel Medical Center, Haifa 3436212, Israel
* Correspondence: devyzisman@gmail.com; Tel.: +972-4-8250486; Fax: +972-4-8260213
† These authors contributed equally to the manuscript.

Received: 17 August 2019; Accepted: 16 September 2019; Published: 18 September 2019

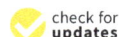

Abstract: Patients with rheumatoid arthritis (RA) are at increased risk of cardiovascular disease. Dyslipidemia is a known adverse effect of tocilizumab (TCZ), an anti-interleukin-6 receptor antibody used in RA treatment. We aimed to assess the effect of TCZ on lipid profile and adipokine levels in RA patients. Height, weight, disease activity scores, lipid profile and atherogenic indices (AI), leptin, adiponectin, resistin, interleukin-6, and high-sensitivity C-reactive protein (CRP) were measured before and four months after initiation of TCZ in 40 RA patients and 40 healthy controls. Following TCZ treatment, total cholesterol, high density lipoprotein (HDL), and triglycerides were significantly elevated, but no significant changes in weight, body mass index (BMI), low density lipoprotein (LDL), and AI were observed. Compared with controls, significantly higher adiponectin levels were measured in the RA group at baseline. Following TCZ treatment, resistin levels and the leptin-to-adiponectin ratio increased, adiponectin levels decreased, and leptin levels remained unchanged. No correlation was found between the change in adipokine serum levels and changes in the disease activity indices, nor the lipid profile. In conclusion, the changes observed suggest a protective role for TCZ on the metabolic and cardiovascular burden associated with RA, but does not provide a mechanistic explanation for this phenomenon.

Keywords: rheumatoid arthritis; tocilizumab; lipids; adipokines; adiponectin; resistin; leptin

1. Introduction

Rheumatoid arthritis (RA), a chronic inflammatory disease with typical bone erosion and damage, is also associated with an increased incidence of metabolic syndrome and cardiovascular disease (CVD). Although CVD risk factors such as obesity, smoking, hypertension, and diabetes are also increased in RA patients, systemic inflammation caused by RA itself seems to contribute to CVD risk in these patients. Chronic low-grade inflammation—often assessed by C-reactive protein (CRP), an acute phase reaction protein—is associated with accelerated atherosclerosis, increased CVD risk, and increased mortality [1]. Hence, it is suggested that successful treatment of RA patients so as to reduce the inflammatory burden may decrease CVD risk [2–4]. This has already been shown for the administration of tumor necrosis factor-alpha (TNF-α) inhibitors [5].

Adipokines, cytokines secreted mostly by white adipose tissue, are involved in inflammation, endothelial dysfunction, and atherosclerosis, placing them as possible molecular links between RA, the metabolic syndrome, and CVD risk [2,6–8]. However, their putative role as key inflammatory mediators contributing to CVD risk is still controversial, as their serum levels vary. For instance, the pro-inflammatory adipokine leptin has been shown to variably exhibit either elevated or similar serum levels in RA patients relative to healthy controls, while resistin, another pro-inflammatory adipokine, has been shown to have either elevated, similar, or reduced levels relative to healthy controls. Surprisingly, the serum and synovial fluid level of the anti-inflammatory adipokine adiponectin was found to be consistently elevated in RA patients [3,4,6,7,9–13]. Notably, the levels of these three major adipokines—leptin, resistin, and adiponectin—were shown to correlate with insulin resistance. The leptin-to-adiponectin ratio (LAR) is used to assess insulin resistance among type-2 diabetes mellitus patients and healthy individuals [14–18], while resistin levels were found to correlate with insulin resistance in septic patients [6].

Tocilizumab (TCZ), a human monoclonal antibody that targets the interleukin-6 (IL-6) receptor, is a novel biologic disease-modifying anti-rheumatic drug (bDMARD) effective in treating RA in humans [19]. TCZ has been shown to worsen dyslipidemia, a significant adverse metabolic effect that was attributed to the blockage of IL-6 and its ability to induce the expression of apolipoproteins in the liver [20]. However, despite that dyslipidemia is known to be associated with TCZ treatment, this biologic agent was not found to increase CVD risk in RA patients [21]. We hypothesized that TCZ might affect adipokine levels, thus exerting a cardioprotective role in RA patients.

Our aim in the present study was to evaluate the effects of TCZ treatment on serum lipid and adipokine levels in RA patients compared with healthy controls, and to evaluate whether any changes in adipokine profile mediated by TCZ are cardioprotective.

2. Results

2.1. Patient Characteristics

The average age of the 40 patients in the RA group was 57.5 years, and 82.5% were women, with a mean disease duration of 7.7 ± 5.6 years. All participants completed the four month follow-up. Their demographic and clinical characteristics are summarized by disease activity class (DAS28-CRP score) at baseline (Table 1).

Table 1. Patients demographic and clinical characteristics according to disease activity at baseline (disease activity score-28 joint count (DAS28)-C-reactive protein (CRP)).

Characteristic	Moderate Disease Activity (DAS ≤ 5.1) (n = 15)	High Disease Activity (DAS > 5.1) (n = 25)	Total (n = 40)	p Value
Age (years)	60 ± 14.96	56.04 ± 7.90	57.53 ± 11.07	NS
Gender (% female)	13 (86.7%)	20 (80%)	33 (82.5%)	NS
RF positive (%)	8 (53.3%)	13 (54.2%)	21 (53.8%)	NS
Anti-CCP positive (N) (%)	6 (10) (60.0%)	6 (13) (46.2%)	12/23 (52.2%)	NS
Disease duration (years)	6.46 ± 5.71	8.44 ± 5.52	7.7 ± 5.6	NS
Concomitant Diseases				
Ischemic heart disease (%)	1 (6.7%)	0 (0.0%)	1 (2.5%)	NS
Diabetes mellitus (%)	3 (20.0%)	5 (20.0%)	8 (20.0%)	NS
Hypertension (%)	5 (33.3%)	7 (28%)	12 (30%)	NS
Chronic obstructive lung disease (%)	1 (6.7%)	0 (0%)	1 (2.5%)	NS
Dyslipidemia (%)	6 (40.0%)	13 (52.0%)	19 (47.5%)	NS
Prior malignancy (%)	1 (6.7%)	0 (0.0%)	1 (2.5%)	NS

Table 1. Cont.

Characteristic	Moderate Disease Activity (DAS ≤ 5.1) (n = 15)	High Disease Activity (DAS > 5.1) (n = 25)	Total (n = 40)	p Value
Therapy at Baseline				
Methotrexate	8 (53.3%)	19 (76.0%)	27 (67.5%)	NS
Sulfasalazine	1 (6.7%)	4 (16.0%)	5 (12.5%)	NS
Hydroxycholoroquine	1 (6.7%)	3 (12.0%)	4 (10.0%)	NS
Leflunomide	0 (0.0%)	3 (12.0%)	3 (7.5%)	NS
Corticosteroid dose in milligrams (mean + SD)	3 ± 5.92	7.2 ± 10.52	5.63 ± 9.22	NS
Statin use	6 (40%)	15 (56%)	20 (50%)	NS
Anti-diabetic therapy	3 (20.0%)	5 (20.0%)	8 (20.0%)	NS

* anti-CCP = anti-cyclic citrullinated peptide, (N) = number, NS = not significant, RF = rheumatoid factor, SD = standard deviation.

There were no significant differences between the groups with respect to demographics, clinical parameters, comorbidities, and medical regimen.

The majority of the patients responded clinically to TCZ after four months of treatment (Table 2) with a reduction in disease activity as assessed by CDAI (25 patients, 62.5%) or DAS28-CRP (22 patients, 55%).

Table 2. Effect of tocilizumab (TCZ) on clinical and laboratory parameters.

Parameter	Before Treatment	After 4 Months of Treatment	p Value
Inflammation Scores and Markers			
DAS28-CRP score	5.45 ± 1.06	3.46 ± 1.37	<0.0001
CDAI score	36.59 ± 12.48	20.0 ± 12.56	<0.0001
28-tender joint count	12.48 ± 6.47	5.93 ± 5.21	<0.0001
28-swollen joint count	9.25 ± 5.39	4.06 ± 4.18	<0.0001
Patient global assessment of disease activity (0–100 mm)	76.45 ± 19.15	56.78 ± 23.18	<0.0001
Provider global assessment of disease activity (0–100 mm)	72.1 ± 15.5	44.1 ± 26.1	<0.0001
CRP (mg/dL)	1.33 ± 1.8	0.13 ± 0.42	<0.0001
hsCRP (mg/dL)	3.37 ± 2.0	0.74 ± 1.36	<0.001
IL-6 (pg/mL)	28.4 ± 94.42	69.28 ± 109.05	<0.001
Anthropometric Measurements			
Weight (kg)	74.5 ± 17.52	75.31 ± 16.91	NS*
BMI (kg/m^2)	27.77 ± 6.6	27.96 ± 6.45	NS
Lipid Profile and Atherogenic Indices			
Total cholesterol (mg/dl)	199.4 ± 52.71	220.83 ± 53.39	0.003
LDL (mg/dl)	123.67 ± 36.87	131.38 ± 36.95	NS
HDL (mg/dl)	54.53 ± 19.0	59.0 ± 23.27	0.039
TG (mg/dl)	139.56 ± 68.53	167.67 ± 106.93	0.04
AI (HDL/cholesterol)	3.79 ± 0.78	3.96 ± 1.13	NS
AI of plasma [log(TG/HDL)]	0.93 ± 0.09	0.95 ± 0.11	NS
RA Therapy			
Prednisone (Mean ± SD)	5.63 ± 9.21	5.13 ± 8.28	NS
Methotrexate (%)	27 (67.5%)	25 (62.5%)	NS
Sulfasalazine (%)	5 (12.5%)	1 (2.5%)	NS
Hydroxychloroquine (%)	4 (10%)	3 (7.5%)	NS
Leflunomide (%)	3 (7.5%)	1 (2.5%)	NS

AI = atherogenic index, BMI = body mass index, CDAI = clinical disease activity index, CRP = C-reactive protein, hsCRP = high sensitivity CRP, DAS28-CRP = disease activity score-28 joint count, HDL = high density lipoproteins, IL-6 = interleukin-6, LDL = low density lipoproteins, SD = standard deviation, TG = triglycerides. * not significant.

Following four months of treatment, 27.5% and 15% of the patients achieved low disease activity or remission by CDAI and DAS28-CRP criteria, respectively. There were no significant changes in concomitant medications including doses of corticosteroids, statins, or other disease modifying agents (DMARDs) during the four months of follow-up.

The effects of TCZ treatment on serum samples are summarized in Table 2. Following four months of treatment, CRP and hsCRP levels decreased significantly, while IL-6 levels increased significantly, demonstrating the predictable pharmacological effect of TCZ.

2.2. TCZ Effects on Metabolic Parameters

Upon recruitment, 25 RA patients were overweight (BMI > 25) and 11 were obese (BMI > 30). There were no significant changes in weight or BMI following four months of treatment. Total cholesterol, HDL, and TG levels increased significantly following treatment, with the increase in LDL not reaching statistical significance. Of note, three patients had incalculable LDL levels owing to hypertriglyceridemia. Atherogenic indices did not change significantly following treatment (Table 2).

2.3. TCZ Effects on Adipokine Levels

Before TCZ treatment, adiponectin levels adjusted to BMI and statin treatment were higher in RA patients compared with healthy controls ($p < 0.0001$), whereas LAR was decreased ($p = 0.03$) (Table 3). TCZ treatment normalized the adiponectin and resistin levels, which decreased to the levels observed in the healthy control group. Only leptin levels continued to increase after four months of treatment.

Table 3. Serum adipokine levels in healthy controls compared with RA patients before and after four months of tocilizumab (TCZ) treatment.

Cytokine	Control	Patients before Treatment	Patients after Treatment	p Value		
				Control vs. Patient before treatment*	Control vs. Patients after treatment*	Patients before treatment vs Patents following four months of treatment**
Adiponectin (ng/mL) Mean (± SD) Median	3.75 ± 1.63 3.56	5.59 ± 2.39 5.33	4.53 ± 2.12 4.44	<0.0001	0.17	0.0001
Leptin (pg/mL) Mean (± SD) Median	21.92 ± 21.63 15.05	25.15 ± 26.36 19.38	29.36 ± 30.25 15.95	0.84	0.92	0.125
Resistin (pg/mL) Mean (± SD) Median	21.53 ± 8.19 20.24	16.25 ± 7.17 14.73	20.42 ± 8.06 19.91	0.63	0.63	0.001
Leptin/ Adiponectin ratio Mean (± SD) Median	6.44 ± 6.44 4.36	5.52 ± 6.08 3.93	7.99 ± 7.84 4.90	0.03	0.59	0.002

SD = standard deviation; * p value adjusted to BMI and statin; ** p value adjusted to BMI, statin treatment, and disease duration.

Following four months of TCZ treatment, significant changes in the levels of adiponectin, resistin, and LAR were noted after adjustment to BMI, statin treatment, and disease duration. Adiponectin levels decreased ($p \leq 0.0001$), whereas resistin and LAR increased. The adipokine profile following four months of TCZ treatment trended to the levels measured in the control group, and no statistically significant differences were found between the patient group after treatment and controls in the three adipokine levels or the LAR measured in the study (Table 3).

The changes in the serum levels of the three adipokines prior to starting TCZ treatment and after four months of treatment did not correlate with the changes in the clinical and metabolic parameters that are associated with the risk of CVD (Table 4). The only significant correlation we found was a positive correlation between the changes in HDL values and levels of leptin.

Table 4. Correlation between the changes in adipokine levels and clinical and biochemical parameters of RA reflecting cardiovascular disease (CVD) risk and disease activity, before and after four months of TCZ treatment.

		ΔDAS28	ΔCDAI	ΔhsCRP	ΔHDL	ΔLDL	ΔTG	ΔCholesterol	ΔAI	ΔAI-Plasma
ΔAdiponectin	r	0.026	0.020	−0.045	0.160	0.162	−0.005	0.257	0.106	−0.085
	p	0.875	0.902	0.782	0.365	0.393	0.979	0.135	0.549	0.633
ΔLeptin	r	0.186	0.025	−0.009	0.390	0.208	−0.008	0.200	−0.196	−0.217
	p	0.250	0.879	0.957	0.023	0.270	0.964	0.248	0.267	0.218
ΔLAR	r	−0.026	−0.078	−0.041	0.177	0.157	0.013	0.000	−0.194	−0.121
	p	0.876	0.631	0.803	0.318	0.408	0.938	1.000	0.273	0.494
ΔResistin	r	0.068	0.096	−0.058	0.009	0.240	−0.086	0.165	0.097	−0.008
	p	0.679	0.555	0.722	0.961	0.201	0.619	0.345	0.586	0.963

AI = atherogenic index, CDAI = clinical disease activity index, hsCRP = high sensitive CRP, DAS28-CRP = disease activity score-28 joint count, HDL = high density lipoproteins, LDL = low density lipoproteins, SD = standard deviation, TG = triglycerides. r = Pearson's correlation coefficient, p = significance value.

There were no statistically significant differences in the adipokine levels when patients were stratified into responders and non-responders according to DAS28-CRP or CDAI score response after adjustment to BMI, statin treatment, and disease duration.

3. Discussion

In this study, we show that TCZ treatment improves disease activity and reduces the inflammatory burden in RA patients, as has been shown before. As expected, disease activity scores were significantly reduced with TCZ treatment, as were the values of hsCRP, a measure considered to reflect vascular inflammation and that serves as a predictor of cardiovascular events [1]. However, this improvement in disease activity was accompanied by increased dyslipidemia, as previously reported for TCZ. Therefore, we asked whether adipokines, which are the hypothesized link between inflammation and increased CVD risk, were responsible for this effect. Contrary to this hypothesis, we show that there is no correlation between changes in adipokine serum levels as a result of TCZ treatment and changes in the disease activity or lipid profile, indicating that the adipokines we examined do not directly regulate these parameters in our cohort.

Our RA study population was more overweight and obese (60% and 27.5%, respectively) than the general population in Israel (49% and 16%, respectively, in 2012) [22], and the four months of treatment with TCZ did not affect their BMI. The increased prevalence of obesity among our RA patients may be explained by the metabolic impact of the inflammatory state, which limits physical activity, as well as by prolonged corticosteroid treatment. However, the effects of TCZ on obesity are still controversial. Similar to our study, other studies found no significant change in weight or BMI in TCZ-treated non-diabetic RA patients over a period of three [23] or six months [24], or when patients were stratified to responders versus non-responders according to the DAS28-CRP criteria [25]. In contrast, Younis et al. demonstrated a significant rise in weight and BMI in TCZ-treated RA patients over a period of four months [26]. As TCZ blocks IL-6 signaling and leads to its elevated serum levels, as we demonstrated here, the metabolic effects of increased IL-6 should be taken into consideration. Elevated IL-6 levels in cancer patients are associated with cachexia, and IL-6 inhibitors have been suggested as possible treatment adjuncts in cancer patients in order to prevent this catabolic effect [27].

In line with the documented ability of TCZ to induce dyslipidemia, we observed significantly elevated levels of total cholesterol, HDL, and TG, as well as a rise in LDL that did not reach statistical significance in our RA patients following four months of TCZ treatment. While the elevated lipid profile raises concerns about its potential to increase CVD risk in RA patients, we did not detect changes in the two atherogenic indices we evaluated. Notably, atherogenic indices fluctuate less among RA patients and are considered more reliable in the assessment of CVD risk in these patients [28,29]. This finding is consistent with previous studies reporting elevation in the lipid profile with no change in atherogenic indices following TCZ treatment [23,28,30,31]. Moreover, the increase in HDL, which is considered to have a cardioprotective role in the general healthy population, could potentially mitigate this concern. The reported increase in RA patients of HDL particles, which might possess anti-inflammatory and athero-protective properties, indicates that the effects of TCZ on CVD risk are complex and still unclear [32].

Adipokines, and particularly leptin, are important mediators of the pathophysiology of RA and its comorbidities [10,12,33]. Xibillé-Friedmann et al. found that leptin, but not adiponectin, levels predict disease activity and response to conventional DMARD treatment in RA patients [34]. Indeed, many studies have shown elevated serum levels of adiponectin, leptin, and resistin in RA patients relative to healthy controls [3,4,6,7,9–13]. However, the literature is inconsistent regarding the effects of TCZ treatment on serum levels of adipokines in RA patients. We found that adiponectin levels decreased following therapy, while resistin levels and LAR increased following therapy. In contrast, Fioravanti et al. showed that after six months of TCZ treatment, resistin and leptin serum levels were not significantly changed, but the adiponectin level was increased [24]. Tournadre et al. showed no change in resistin and adiponectin levels, but a reduction in leptin serum levels [35]. Schultz et al. demonstrated that after three months of treatment, TCZ increased adiponectin levels, but did not change leptin levels, leading to a reduction in LAR [23]. In comparison, other treatments, such as infliximab (anti-TNFα), were found to decrease resistin levels [36], or did not have any effect on leptin and adiponectin levels in patients with RA [37,38]. Thus, the effects of TCZ are not straightforward, and may depend on additional, yet unknown factors.

Most of the above noted studies only compared the adipokine levels in RA patients before and after TCZ treatment. Therefore, it is noteworthy that we show here that in comparison with healthy controls, TCZ treatment normalized adipokine levels. The ability of TCZ to normalize adiponectin and resistin levels and to bring them closer to levels found in the healthy control group demonstrates a positive effect of TCZ on metabolism, in addition to its anti-inflammatory properties, and may hint at a putative cardioprotective role of this biologic agent. However, the increase in LAR and resistin levels, which have been shown to have pro-atherogenic and insulin resistant effects [5,14,17], cast doubt on this supposition.

Possible explanations for the differences between our study results and those of other studies include small sample sizes, demographic differences such as age and race, differences in disease duration, and treatment. BMI differences between study populations in the different studies may also be significant because BMI directly impacts leptin levels [6,10,23,34]. Of note, there were no significant changes in conventional DMARDs or prednisone dose in our RA patients throughout the study, suggesting that these medications were not confounding factors in our assessments.

Finally, we show that the change in the adipokine levels did not correlate with most of the known biochemical parameters that are associated with increased CVD risk or with RA disease activity. The only exception was the positive correlation found between the changes in HDL and leptin levels. HDL levels were previously found to negatively correlate with leptin and positively correlate with adiponectin in a healthy cohort, suggesting a link between leptin, insulin resistance, and the metabolic syndrome, as well as a cardioprotective role for adiponectin [39]. However, such a link would imply that other CVD risk factors, such as LDL, total cholesterol, or TG levels, should also correlate with leptin levels, which was not found in our study. Therefore, it is likely that the positive correlation between HDL and leptin levels that we observed is not representative, probably resulting from the small patient cohort. In contrast, the lack of correlation between adipokine levels with other parameters of CVD risk that we observed is similar to a previous study [24]. Taken together, our findings do not support a direct link between the adipokines leptin, resistin, and adiponectin and the reduction in CVD risk observed following initiation of TCZ treatment in RA patients, and may suggest that other adipokines or cytokines may play a greater role in mediating this effect, as was recently suggested [24], or that other mechanisms play a cardioprotective role in RA patients treated with this biologic agent.

Our results should be viewed with certain limitations, specifically the short follow-up period of four months and the relatively small sample size. Our study analyzed serum levels of only a few selected adipokines, and other adipokines could be included in a larger study. Because of the variation between serum and synovial fluid concentrations of various pro-inflammatory and anti-inflammatory mediators in RA patients [40], future studies should also include a comparison between serum and synovial fluid adipokine levels.

In conclusion, the impact of TCZ treatment on the metabolic profile of RA patients is complex. When taking all the changes recorded in our patients' lipid and adipokine profiles into consideration, the following findings should be highlighted: the rise in HDL, the lack of worsening in atherogenic indices, and the normalization of adiponectin and resistin levels in TCZ responders in comparison with healthy controls. These changes suggest a protective role for TCZ on the metabolic and cardiovascular burden associated with RA, but still do not provide a mechanistic explanation for this phenomenon.

4. Methods

4.1. Study Population

Forty RA patients with active disease who were suitable candidates for TCZ treatment were recruited from rheumatology clinics in two medical centers in Israel. All patients met the 2010 American College of Rheumatology/European League Against Rheumatism (ACR/EULAR) RA criteria [41]. Patients were treated with 8 mg/kg TCZ infusions every four weeks. All other medical decisions were at the treating physicians' discretion. Patients with diagnosis of another inflammatory arthritis or neoplastic disease were excluded. Parameters collected at baseline and after four months of TCZ treatment included demographic data, height, weight, calculated body mass index (BMI) (weight/height^2), patient comorbidities with emphasis on CVD risk factors, current medications, and physical examination data with a focus on swollen and tender joint counts.

Laboratory variables studied included complete blood count and chemistry panel, lipid panel, CRP, and rheumatoid factor (RF), all analyzed by standard methods in a central laboratory. Total cholesterol, high density lipoprotein (HDL), and triglyceride (TG) levels were used to calculate the atherogenic index (AI, total cholesterol/HDL) and the AI of plasma (the base 10 logarithm of TG/HDL). Blood samples were obtained for the analysis of adipokines (leptin, adiponectin, and resistin), as well as for measurement of IL-6 levels and high sensitivity CRP (hsCRP). Leptin and adiponectin levels were used to calculate the LAR.

The control group of 40 volunteers without inflammatory diseases, renal failure, CVD or malignancies was age-and gender-matched with the RA group. Blood samples from this group were drawn at recruitment and tested for leptin, adiponectin, resistin, LAR, IL-6, and hsCRP levels.

The study protocol was approved by the local institutional review boards of the participating medical centers, and informed consent was obtained from all participants at recruitment (approval number at Carmel Medical Center CMC-0018-11 on 23 March 2011; approval number at Bnei Zion Medical Center BNZ043-11 on 27 July 2011).

4.2. Assessment of Clinical Response

Clinical response was assessed using the disease activity score-28 joint count (DAS28-CRP) and clinical disease activity index (CDAI) scores. Patients were categorized as responders by DAS28-CRP if their score was reduced by more than 1.2 points (ΔDAS28-CRP $\geq$ 1.2), and their total DAS28-CRP score was <5.1 following four months of treatment; this represents moderate-to-large response to therapy according to the EULAR response criteria [42]. Patients were categorized as responders by CDAI if they demonstrated a reduction of at least one disease activity class after four months of treatment (i.e., from high disease activity (CDAI > 22) to moderate disease activity (CDAI 10–22) or from moderate disease activity to low disease activity or remission (CDAI < 10) [43,44].

4.3. Biochemical Analysis

Blood samples were drawn at baseline and after completing four months of TCZ therapy, immediately centrifuged at 1200 rpm, and stored at −80 °C until analysis. Serum concentrations of leptin, adiponectin, resistin, and IL-6 were determined using DuoSet enzyme-linked immunosorbent assay (ELISA) kits (R&D systems, Minneapolis, MN, USA), and hsCRP concentrations were determined using the hsCRP enzyme-linked immunosorbent assay (ELISA) kit (AssayPRO, St. Charles, MO, USA), according to manufacturer's instructions.

4.4. Statistical Analysis

Continuous data are presented as mean ± standard deviation (SD) and median; categorical variables as numbers and percentages. The changes in the DAS28-CRP and CDAI scores, total cholesterol, HDL, TG, weight, and BMI levels between baseline and follow-up visits in RA patients were analyzed by paired t-test.

ANCOVA models adjusted to baseline BMI and statin treatment were used to compare the log-transformed adipokine concentrations in the RA and control groups. Mann–Whitney test was used to compare serum concentrations of IL-6 and hsCRP between the two groups, as appropriate. Correlation between the changes in adipokine levels and clinical and biochemical parameters of RA reflecting CVD risk before and after four months of TCZ treatment was calculated using Pearson's correlation coefficient. The changes in adipokine serum concentrations in the RA group between baseline (before treatment) and follow-up time, four months after TCZ treatment, adjusted to BMI, statin treatment, and RA disease duration, were analyzed by linear mixed models with repeated measures. All tests were two-sided and p values of <0.05 were considered statistically significant. All statistical analyses were done using SPSS, version 24.0 (IBP Corp. Released 2016, IBM SPSS Statistics for Windows, version 24.0. Armonk, NY, USA: IBM Corp).

Author Contributions: Conceptualization, D.Z. and M.A.R.; Methodology, E.H., M.A.R., J.F., M.E., I.L., T.G. and D.Z.; Formal Analysis, E.H. and I.L.; Investigation, E.H., J.F., M.E., I.R. and L.K.; Writing—Original Draft Preparation, E.H. and M.A.R.; Writing—Review & Editing, D.Z., M.A.R., T.G., I.L., L.K. and I.R.; Visualization, D.Z. and M.A.R.; Supervision, M.A.R., I.R. and D.Z.; Project Administration, E.H. and L.K.

Funding: This research received no external funding.

Conflicts of Interest: The authors declare no conflict of interest.

References

1. Koenig, W. High-sensitivity C-reactive protein and atherosclerotic disease: From improved risk prediction to risk-guided therapy. *Int. J. Cardiol.* **2013**, *168*, 5126–5134. [CrossRef] [PubMed]
2. Sattar, N.; McCarey, D.W.; Capell, H.; McInnes, I.B. Explaining How "High-Grade" Systemic Inflammation Accelerates Vascular Risk in Rheumatoid Arthritis. *Circulation* **2003**, *108*, 2957–2963. [CrossRef] [PubMed]
3. Lago, F.; Gómez, R.; Conde, J.; Scotece, M.; Gómez-Reino, J.J.; Gualillo, O. Cardiometabolic comorbidities and rheumatic diseases: Focus on the role of fat mass and adipokines. *Arthritis Care Res.* **2011**, *63*, 1083–1090. [CrossRef] [PubMed]
4. Chung, C.P.; Oeser, A.; Solus, J.F.; Avalos, I.; Gebretsadik, T.; Shintani, A.; Raggi, P.; Sokka, T.; Pincus, T.; Stein, C.M. Prevalence of the metabolic syndrome is increased in rheumatoid arthritis and is associated with coronary atherosclerosis. *Atherosclerosis* **2008**, *196*, 756–763. [CrossRef] [PubMed]
5. Mahmoudi, M.; Aslani, S.; Fadaei, R.; Jamshidi, A.R. New insights to the mechanisms underlying atherosclerosis in rheumatoid arthritis. *Int. J. Rheum. Dis.* **2017**, *20*, 287–297. [CrossRef]
6. Otero, M.; Lago, R.; Gomez, R.; Lago, F.; Dieguez, C.; Gómez-Reino, J.J.; Gualillo, O. Changes in plasma levels of fat-derived hormones adiponectin, leptin, resistin and visfatin in patients with rheumatoid arthritis. *Ann. Rheum. Dis.* **2006**, *65*, 1198–1201. [CrossRef] [PubMed]
7. Abella, V.; Scotece, M.; Conde, J.; López, V.; Lazzaro, V.; Pino, J.; Gómez-Reino, J.J.; Gualillo, O. Adipokines, Metabolic Syndrome and Rheumatic Diseases. *J. Immunol. Res.* **2014**, *2014*, 343746. [CrossRef]

8. Francisco, V.; Ruiz-Fernández, C.; Pino, J.; Mera, A.; González-Gay, M.A.; Gómez, R.; Lago, F.; Mobasheri, A.; Gualillo, O. Adipokines: Linking metabolic syndrome, the immune system, and arthritic diseases. *Biochem. Pharmacol.* **2019**, *165*, 196–206. [CrossRef]
9. Del Prete, A.; Salvi, V.; Sozzani, S. Adipokines as Potential Biomarkers in Rheumatoid Arthritis. *Mediat. Inflamm.* **2014**, *2014*, 425068. [CrossRef]
10. Tian, G.; Liang, J.-N.; Pan, H.-F.; Zhou, D. Increased leptin levels in patients with rheumatoid arthritis: A meta-analysis. *Ir. J. Med. Sci.* **2014**, *183*, 659–666. [CrossRef]
11. Scotece, M.; Conde, J.; Gómez, R.; López, V.; Lago, F.; Gómez-Reino, J.J.; Gualillo, O. Beyond fat mass: Exploring the role of adipokines in rheumatic diseases. *ScientificWorldJournal* **2011**, *11*, 1932–1947. [CrossRef] [PubMed]
12. Tian, G.; Liang, J.-N.; Wang, Z.-Y.; Zhou, D. Emerging role of leptin in rheumatoid arthritis. *Clin. Exp. Immunol.* **2014**, *177*, 557–570. [CrossRef] [PubMed]
13. Toussirot, E.; Grandclément, E.; Gaugler, B.; Michel, F.; Wendling, D.; Saas, P.; Dumoulin, G. CBT-506 Serum adipokines and adipose tissue distribution in rheumatoid arthritis and ankylosing spondylitis. A comparative study. *Front. Immunol.* **2013**, *4*, 453. [CrossRef] [PubMed]
14. Zaletel, J.; Barlovic, D.P.; Prezelj, J. Adiponectin-leptin ratio: A useful estimate of insulin resistance in patients with Type 2 diabetes. *J. Endocrinol. Investig.* **2010**, *33*, 514–518. [CrossRef]
15. Finucane, F.M.; Luan, J.; Wareham, N.J.; Sharp, S.J.; O'Rahilly, S.; Balkau, B.; Flyvbjerg, A.; Walker, M.; Højlund, K.; Nolan, J.J.; et al. Correlation of the leptin:adiponectin ratio with measures of insulin resistance in non-diabetic individuals. *Diabetologia* **2009**, *52*, 2345–2349. [CrossRef] [PubMed]
16. Kang, Y.; Park, H.-J.; Kang, M.-I.; Lee, H.-S.; Lee, S.-W.; Lee, S.-K.; Park, Y.-B. Adipokines, inflammation, insulin resistance, and carotid atherosclerosis in patients with rheumatoid arthritis. *Arthritis Res. Ther.* **2013**, *15*, R194. [CrossRef]
17. Manrique-Arija, S.; Ureña, I.; Valdivielso, P.; Rioja, J.; Jiménez-Núñez, F.G.; Irigoyen, M.V.; Fernández-Nebro, A. Insulin resistance and levels of adipokines in patients with untreated early rheumatoid arthritis. *Clin. Rheumatol.* **2016**, *35*, 43–53. [CrossRef] [PubMed]
18. Shah, A.; St. Clair, E.W. Rheumatoid Arthritis. In *Harrison's Principles of Internal Medicine*; Jameson, J.L., Fauci, A.S., Kasper, D.L., Hauser, S.L., Longo, D.L., Loscalzo, J., Eds.; McGraw-Hill: New York, NY, USA, 2012.
19. Choy, E.H.S.; Isenberg, D.A.; Garrood, T.; Farrow, S.; Ioannou, Y.; Bird, H.; Cheung, N.; Williams, B.; Hazleman, B.; Price, R.; et al. Therapeutic benefit of blocking interleukin-6 activity with an anti-interleukin-6 receptor monoclonal antibody in rheumatoid arthritis: A randomized, double-blind, placebo-controlled, dose-escalation trial. *Arthritis Rheum.* **2002**, *46*, 3143–3150. [CrossRef]
20. Kawashiri, S.; Kawakami, A.; Yamasaki, S.; Imazato, T.; Iwamoto, N.; Fujikawa, K.; Aramaki, T.; Tamai, M.; Nakamura, H.; Ida, H.; et al. Effects of the anti-interleukin-6 receptor antibody, tocilizumab, on serum lipid levels in patients with rheumatoid arthritis. *Rheumatol. Int.* **2011**, *31*, 451–456. [CrossRef]
21. Rao, V.U.; Pavlov, A.; Klearman, M.; Musselman, D.; Giles, J.T.; Bathon, J.M.; Sattar, N.; Lee, J.S. An evaluation of risk factors for major adverse cardiovascular events during tocilizumab therapy. *Arthritis Rheumatol.* **2015**, *67*, 372–380. [CrossRef]
22. Central Bureau of Statistics. *Israel in Comparison with the OECD Countries & the EU*; CBS: Jerusalem, Israel, 2012.
23. Schultz, O.; Oberhauser, F.; Saech, J.; Rubbert-Roth, A.; Hahn, M.; Krone, W.; Laudes, M. Effects of inhibition of interleukin-6 signalling on insulin sensitivity and lipoprotein (a) levels in human subjects with rheumatoid diseases. *PLoS ONE* **2010**, *5*, e14328. [CrossRef] [PubMed]
24. Fioravanti, A.; Tenti, S.; Bacarelli, M.R.; Damiani, A.; Li Gobbi, F.; Bandinelli, F.; Cheleschi, S.; Galeazzi, M.; Benucci, M. Tocilizumab modulates serum levels of adiponectin and chemerin in patients with rheumatoid arthritis: Potential cardiovascular protective role of IL-6 inhibition. *Clin. Exp. Rheumatol.* **2019**, *37*, 293–300. [PubMed]
25. Gardette, A.; Ottaviani, S.; Sellam, J.; Berenbaum, F.; Lioté, F.; Meyer, A.; Sibilia, J.; Fautrel, B.; Palazzo, E.; Dieudé, P. Body mass index and response to tocilizumab in rheumatoid arthritis: A real life study. *Clin. Rheumatol.* **2016**, *35*, 857–861. [CrossRef]
26. Younis, S.; Rosner, I.; Rimar, D.; Boulman, N.; Rozenbaum, M.; Odeh, M.; Slobodin, G. Weight change during pharmacological blockade of interleukin-6 or tumor necrosis factor-α in patients with inflammatory rheumatic disorders: A 16-week comparative study. *Cytokine* **2013**, *61*, 353–355. [CrossRef] [PubMed]

27. Ando, K.; Takahashi, F.; Kato, M.; Kaneko, N.; Doi, T.; Ohe, Y.; Koizumi, F.; Nishio, K.; Takahashi, K. Tocilizumab, a proposed therapy for the cachexia of Interleukin6-expressing lung cancer. *PLoS ONE* **2014**, *9*, e102436. [CrossRef] [PubMed]
28. Popa, C.D.; Arts, E.; Fransen, J.; van Riel, P.L.C.M. Atherogenic index and high-density lipoprotein cholesterol as cardiovascular risk determinants in rheumatoid arthritis: The impact of therapy with biologicals. *Mediat. Inflamm.* **2012**, *2012*, 785946. [CrossRef] [PubMed]
29. Niroumand, S.; Khajedaluee, M.; Khadem-Rezaiyan, M.; Abrishami, M.; Juya, M.; Khodaee, G.; Dadgarmoghaddam, M. Atherogenic Index of Plasma (AIP): A marker of cardiovascular disease. *Med. J. Islam. Repub. Iran.* **2015**, *29*, 240.
30. Sweiss, N.; Shetty, A.; Hanson, R.; Korsten, P.; Arami, S.; Volkov, S.; Vila, O.; Swedler, W.; Shahrara, S.; Smadi, S.; et al. Tocilizumab in the treatment of rheumatoid arthritis and beyond. *Drug Des. Devel. Ther.* **2014**, *8*, 349–364. [CrossRef]
31. Ruscitti, P.; Di Benedetto, P.; Berardicurti, O.; Liakouli, V.; Cipriani, P.; Carubbi, F.; Giacomelli, R. Adipocytokines in Rheumatoid Arthritis: The Hidden Link between Inflammation and Cardiometabolic Comorbidities. *J. Immunol. Res.* **2018**, *2018*, 8410182. [CrossRef]
32. Choy, E.; Ganeshalingam, K.; Semb, A.G.; Szekanecz, Z.; Nurmohamed, M. Cardiovascular risk in rheumatoid arthritis: Recent advances in the understanding of the pivotal role of inflammation, risk predictors and the impact of treatment. *Rheumatology* **2014**, *53*, 2143–2154. [CrossRef]
33. Mac Donald, I.J.; Liu, S.C.; Huang, C.C.; Kuo, S.J.; Tsai, C.H.; Tang, C.H. Associations between adipokines in arthritic disease and implications for obesity. *Int. J. Mol. Sci.* **2019**, *20*, 1505. [CrossRef] [PubMed]
34. Xibillé-Friedmann, D.-X.; Ortiz-Panozo, E.; Bustos Rivera-Bahena, C.; Sandoval-Ríos, M.; Hernández-Góngora, S.-E.; Dominguez-Hernandez, L.; Montiel-Hernández, J.-L. Leptin and adiponectin as predictors of disease activity in rheumatoid arthritis. *Clin. Exp. Rheumatol.* **2015**, *33*, 471–477. [PubMed]
35. Tournadre, A.; Pereira, B.; Dutheil, F.; Giraud, C.; Courteix, D.; Sapin, V.; Frayssac, T.; Mathieu, S.; Malochet-Guinamand, S.; Soubrier, M. Changes in body composition and metabolic profile during interleukin 6 inhibition in rheumatoid arthritis. *J. Cachexia. Sarcopenia Muscle* **2017**, *8*, 639–646. [CrossRef] [PubMed]
36. Gonzalez-Gay, M.A.; Garcia-Unzueta, M.T.; Gonzalez-Juanatey, C.; Miranda-Filloy, J.A.; Vazquez-Rodriguez, T.R.; De Matias, J.M.; Martin, J.; Dessein, P.H.; Llorca, J. Anti-TNF-alpha therapy modulates resistin in patients with rheumatoid arthritis. *Clin. Exp. Rheumatol.* **2008**, *26*, 311–316. [PubMed]
37. Gonzalez-Gay, M.A.; Llorca, J.; Garcia-Unzueta, M.T.; Gonzalez-Juanatey, C.; De Matias, J.M.; Martin, J.; Redelinghuys, M.; Woodiwiss, A.J.; Norton, G.R.; Dessein, P.H. High-grade inflammation, circulating adiponectin concentrations and cardiovascular risk factors in severe rheumatoid arthritis. *Clin. Exp. Rheumatol.* **2008**, *26*, 596–603. [PubMed]
38. Gonzalez-Gay, M.A.; Garcia-Unzueta, M.T.; Berja, A.; Gonzalez-Juanatey, C.; Miranda-Filloy, J.A.; Vazquez-Rodriguez, T.R.; de Matias, J.M.; Martin, J.; Dessein, P.H.; Llorca, J. Anti-TNF-alpha therapy does not modulate leptin in patients with severe rheumatoid arthritis. *Clin. Exp. Rheumatol.* **2009**, *27*, 222–228.
39. Yadav, A.; Jyoti, P.; Jain, S.K.; Bhattacharjee, J. Correlation of adiponectin and leptin with insulin resistance: A pilot study in healthy North Indian population. *Indian J. Clin. Biochem.* **2011**, *26*, 193–196. [CrossRef]
40. Jones, J.; Laffafian, I.; Cooper, A.M.; Williams, B.D.; Morgan, B.P. Expression of complement regulatory molecules and other surface markers on neutrophils from synovial fluid and blood of patients with rheumatoid arthritis. *Br. J. Rheumatol.* **1994**, *33*, 707–712. [CrossRef]
41. Hobbs, K.F.; Cohen, M.D. Rheumatoid arthritis disease measurement: A new old idea. *Rheumatology* **2012**, *51* (Suppl. 6), vi21–vi27. [CrossRef]
42. Felson, D.T.; Anderson, J.J.; Boers, M.; Bombardier, C.; Furst, D.; Goldsmith, C.; Katz, L.M.; Lightfoot, R.; Paulus, H.; Strand, V. American College of Rheumatology. Preliminary definition of improvement in rheumatoid arthritis. *Arthritis Rheum.* **1995**, *38*, 727–735. [CrossRef]
43. Fransen, J.; van Riel, P.L.C.M. The Disease Activity Score and the EULAR Response Criteria. *Rheum. Dis. Clin. North. Am.* **2009**, *35*, 745–757. [CrossRef] [PubMed]
44. Van Riel, P.L.; Renskers, L. The Disease Activity Score (DAS) and the Disease Activity Score using 28 joint counts (DAS28) in the management of rheumatoid arthritis. *Clin. Exp. Rheumatol.* **2016**, *32*, S65–S74.

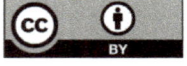

© 2019 by the authors. Licensee MDPI, Basel, Switzerland. This article is an open access article distributed under the terms and conditions of the Creative Commons Attribution (CC BY) license (http://creativecommons.org/licenses/by/4.0/).

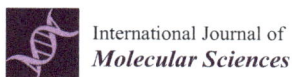

Review

The Role of Adipokines as Circulating Biomarkers in Critical Illness and Sepsis

Sven H. Loosen [1], Alexander Koch [1], Frank Tacke [2], Christoph Roderburg [2,*,†] and Tom Luedde [1,3,†]

1. Department of Medicine III, University Hospital RWTH Aachen, Pauwelsstrasse 30, 52074 Aachen, Germany; sloosen@ukaachen.de (S.H.L); akoch@ukaachen.de (A.K.); tluedde@ukaachen.de (T.L.)
2. Department of Hepatology and Gastroenterology, Charité University Medicine Berlin, Augustenburger Platz 1, 10117 Berlin, Germany; Frank.tacke@charite.de
3. Division of Gastroenterology, Hepatology and Hepatobiliary Oncology, University Hospital RWTH Aachen, Pauwelsstrasse 30, 52074 Aachen, Germany
* Correspondence: Christoph.roderburg@charite.de; Tel.: +49-3045-0653-022; Fax: +49-3045-0553-902
† These authors contributed equally to this work.

Received: 13 September 2019; Accepted: 26 September 2019; Published: 28 September 2019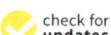

Abstract: Sepsis represents a major global health burden. Early diagnosis of sepsis as well as guiding early therapeutic decisions in septic patients still represent major clinical challenges. In this context, a whole plethora of different clinical and serum-based markers have been tested regarding their potential for early detection of sepsis and their ability to stratify patients according to their probability to survive critical illness and sepsis. Adipokines represent a fast-growing class of proteins that have gained an increasing interest with respect to their potential to modulate immune responses in inflammatory and infectious diseases. We review current knowledge on the role of different adipokines in diagnostic work-up and risk stratification of sepsis as well as critical illness. We discuss recent data from animal models as well as from clinical studies and finally highlight the limitations of these analyses that currently prevent the use of adipokines as biomarkers in daily practice.

Keywords: critical illness; sepsis; adipokines; biomarker; prognosis; ICU

---

1. Introduction

1.1. Critical Illness and Sepsis

Sepsis has recently been defined as "life-threatening organ dysfunction caused by a dysregulated host response to infection" [1–3]. In the United States, up to two percent of patients admitted to hospital suffer from sepsis. Half of these patients need treatment in an intensive care unit (ICU), representing 10% of all admissions [4]. Sepsis is still the leading cause of death among ICU patients. Between 28.3% and 41% of all sepsis patients will not survive their acute illness, with multi-organ failure being the most important cause of death [5]. In addition, survivors often show severe prolonged physical, neurological, and psychological limitations. Notably, the severity of sepsis correlates with the extent of post-sepsis disabilities in surviving patients [6], highlighting the need for early diagnosis and early treatment of this disease.

1.2. Biomarkers for Critical Illness and Sepsis

Adapting the diagnostic and therapeutic management to the personalized characteristics and needs of each individual patient represents one of the main challenges of precision medicine in the 21st century. In the last decade, many different treatment approaches were approved based on specific genetic characteristics such as anti-EGFR directed therapies in patients with *RAS wild-type* colorectal cancer [7]. Thus, providing individualized or personalized medicine requires the availability of specific "biomarkers" that allow stratification of patients into different subgroups [8]. The National Institutes of Health (NIH) define a biomarker as "any substance, structure, or process that can be measured in the body or its products and influence or predict the incidence or outcome of disease" or, more broadly, as "almost any measurement reflecting an interaction between a biological system and a potential hazard, which may be chemical, physical, or biological. The measured response may be functional and physiological, biochemical at the cellular level, or a molecular interaction" (reviewed in the work of [9]). Because, in recent years, manifold specific sepsis therapies have failed, current effective treatment strategies consist of detecting sepsis as early as possible, fluid resuscitation, and anti-infective treatments [1]. Especially easily accessible biomarkers, for example, from patients' serum, might provide an important tool in the diagnostic process of sepsis at an early stage, to detect subgroups of patients with a high-risk profile and to monitor disease progression [10]. At present, microbiological cultures are widely accepted as the gold standard for diagnosis of septic disease [11]. However, in most cases, the results from microbiological cultures are only available days after sample collection and are associated with high rates of false negative results, leading to an ongoing search for other markers that might serve as surrogate for the presence of sepsis [12]. The C-reactive protein (CRP) has been identified as an inexpensive, but sensitive surrogate for infection and inflammation [13]. Named for its ability to bind the C-polysaccharide of *Streptococcus pneumoniae*, it represents an acute-phase protein that is secreted by hepatocytes in response to infection, inflammation, and tissue damage [13]. However, to distinguish between sepsis and non-infectious disease etiology, CRP lacks specificity, and elevated CRP serum levels are also common in patients with inflammatory (but not infectious) diseases states such as cancer, thromboembolic- or cardiovascular diseases, and burns [13]. Moreover, owing to the hepatic provenience of CRP, in the case of severe liver failure, CRP levels may be falsely low and may rather reflect the degree of hepatic dysfunction than sepsis or inflammation [14], limiting its use in clinical routine. Besides CRP, procalcitonin (PCT) was more recently established in clinical routine to identify patients with septic disease. PCT represents a precursor-hormone of calcitonin. It is produced by various organs and, in healthy individuals, the liver is considered to be the most important source of PCT [15]. During infection, PCT is secreted by cytokine-activated macrophages as well as by the parenchyma of many organs, leading to a dramatic increase in circulating PCT levels [15]. Despite that different guidelines recommend the use of PCT to distinguish between sepsis and non-septic cause of disease in critically ill patients, recent meta-analyses have demonstrated that the use of PCT for guidance of therapy had no influence on further therapeutic procedures for ICU patients [11,16]. Moreover, the use of PCT is further hampered by the lack of a clear cut-off defining sepsis in patients with critical illness [17].

In addition to CRP and PCT, interleukin-6 (IL-6) has been suggested as a biomarker in the context of critical illness and sepsis. IL-6 represent the most potent inducer for the secretion of acute phase proteins in the liver. IL-6 serum concentrations were elevated in the blood of patients with septic disease and IL-6 concentrations were associated with the severity of sepsis. Moreover, patients with elevated IL-6 levels demonstrated an impaired prognosis compared with patients with lower levels [18]. However, similar to CRP and PCT, IL-6 concentrations were also elevated in non-septic disease states, limiting its specificity for the assessment of sepsis in patients with critical illness [19]. Therefore, owing to a lack in specificity and sensitivity of available markers for critical illness and sepsis, innovative biomarkers reflecting novel pathophysiological concepts are eagerly awaited to improve the outcome of patients treated on medical ICU. In this context, adipokines might represent biological plausible markers for diagnosis of sepsis and prognosis estimation in critically ill patients, because many processes that are regulated by or reflected by adipokines are involved in the pathophysiology of critical illness and sepsis. As an example, hyperglycemia, impaired glucose tolerance, and insulin resistance are commonly observed in critically ill patients with sepsis or septic shock and have been correlated with an impaired prognosis of these patients [20]. On the basis of these recent findings, many authors have measured serum concentrations of different adipokines in serum and plasma of critically ill patients with or without sepsis. Here, we review these previous data on the role of adipokines in diagnostic work-up and risk stratification of sepsis as well as critical illness.

2. Adipokines

Until recently, the adipose tissue was only considered an energy storage organ, but many novel studies have demonstrated that it is deeply integrated into different physiological and pathophysiological regulatory processes including the regulation of diseases associated with systemic inflammatory responses [21]. In this context, it became obvious that the adipose tissue is able to secrete different factors that are collectively referred to as adipokines [22]. In obese patients, the secretory profiles of adipose tissue are decisively altered dependent on the degree of overweight. Secretion of almost all known adipokines is upregulated in patients with obesity, promoting systemic inflammation and the development of metabolic diseases. In detail, next to leptin, TNF, and IL-6, elevated levels of a broad panel of other proinflammatory adipokines (resistin, retinol-binding protein 4 (RBP4), lipocalin 2, IL-18, angiopoietin-like protein 2 (ANGPTL2), monocyte chemoattractant protein 1 (MCP1), CXC-chemokine ligand 5 (CXCL5), nicotinamide phosphoribosyltransferase (NAmPT)) were found to be upregulated in obese patients (reviewed in the work of [21]). In contrast, adiponectin expression was shown to be lower in adipocytes of obese patients. In line, data from animal models revealed that adiponectin is protective against metabolic and cardiovascular diseases that might develop in the context of obesity. Thus, it seems likely that the inflammatory response and metabolic dysfunction occurring in patients with obesity represent the consequence of a disturbed balance in the secretion of pro- and anti-inflammatory adipokines.

The concept of adipokines as regulators of body homeostasis and responders to injurious threats might be of tremendous relevance for understanding the pathophysiology of critical illness and sepsis. Moreover, concentrations of adipokines can be easily determined in clinical routine, and different authors have suggested using adipokines as biomarkers in treated ICU patients. Within this review, we aim at summarizing available data on the most relevant adipokines in critical illness and sepsis and discuss limitations of the present analyses that have prevented the use of adipokine measurements in clinical routine until now.

3. Selected Adipokines with a Potential Role in Critical Illness and Sepsis

The following section will give an overview of the most relevant adipokines in the context of critical illness as sepsis. Table 1 summarizes the most significant findings with respect to adipokine regulation in critically ill patients.

3.1. Omentin

Omentin represents a relatively new member of the adipokine family and is mainly secreted by the visceral adipose tissue [23]. Experimental data support a decisive role of omentin in the inflammatory crosstalk. As such, it negatively influences a TNFa dependent activation of well-known inflammatory signaling pathways such as p38 or JNK. Clinical data further suggest aberrant omentin serum levels in patients with obesity, inflammatory bowel disease, diabetes mellitus, or coronary heart disease [24,25].

In patients with critical illness and/or sepsis, only little is known on a potential role of omentin as a biomarker for the assessment of disease severity or the patients' clinical outcome. Our group has assessed omentin serum levels in a cohort of $n = 117$ ICU patients with different disease etiologies. While serum omentin levels at admission to the ICU or 72 h after did not differ between ICU patients and healthy controls and were independent of disease etiology and the presence of sepsis, low omentin serum levels were an independent predictor for overall survival [26]. However, these data need further validation before omentin might be implemented into clinical risk prediction scores.

3.2. C1q/TNF-Related Protein 1 (CTRP1)

The CTRP1 represents a member of the CTRP family that consists of 15 proteins that are involved in numerous physiological and pathophysiological processes such as the immune defense, systemic inflammation, cell differentiation and apoptosis, and autoimmunity [27]. CTRP1 is known to regulate important processes within the systemic energy homeostasis and insulin sensitivity and is, for example, involved in PI3K-dependent signaling pathways to induce intracellular glucose transport by insulin [28,29]. Moreover, CTRP1 stimulates human vascular smooth muscle cells, which results in an upregulation of pro-inflammatory cytokines such as interleukin 6 (IL-6), monocyte chemoattractant protein 1 (MCP1), and intracellular adhesion molecule 1 (ICAM1) [30].

In critically ill patients, recent data suggest a significant upregulation of CTRP1 compared with healthy controls [31]. Moreover, CTRP1 levels were significantly higher in patients who fulfilled the criteria of sepsis compared with non-sepsis patients. Importantly, our group showed a strong correlation with markers of systemic inflammation (CRP, IL-6, and PCT), obesity/diabetes (BMI and HbA1c), liver function and cholestasis (bilirubin, GGT, GLDH, AP), and renal function (creatinine, urea). Although these data clearly link CTRP1 to inflammatory and metabolic disturbance in critically ill patients, especially in those patients with septic disease stage, circulating CTRP1 levels were not indicative for the patients' short- or long-term mortality [31]. In a different cohort of $n = 539$ patients undergoing coronary angiography for the evaluation of coronary artery disease, CTRP1 was likewise correlated to obesity and the presence of metabolic syndrome or type 2 diabetes, but circulating levels of CTRP were also a significant predictor of major adverse cardiovascular events such as cardiovascular death, non-fatal myocardial infarction, and non-fatal stroke over a follow-up period of eight years [32].

3.3. C1q/TNFa-Related Protein 3 (CTRP3)

Similar to CTRP1, CTRP3 is a recently recognized adipokine that is also involved in various physiological and pathophysiological processes such as food intake and metabolism, inflammation, vascular disorders, and tumor metastases [33]. CTRP3 is expressed by visceral and subcutaneous adipose tissue [34] and is generally referred to as a "beneficial" mediator as it lowers levels of glucose, inhibits gluconeogenesis, and exerts anti-inflammatory effects [35,36]. In line, serum levels of CTRP3 are reduced in patients with obesity or diabetes [29].

In terms of septic disease, animal models suggest an anti-inflammatory and protective role of CTRP3. As an example, intramyocardial overexpression of CTRP3 in mice resulted in a significantly attenuated myocardial dysfunction in an LPS-induced model of sepsis [37]. In human critical illness, circulating CTRP3 levels were found to be reduced. In a cohort of $n = 218$ patients, both critically ill patients with ($n = 145$) or without ($n = 73$) sepsis had significantly decreased plasma CTRP3 levels compared with healthy controls [38]. Moreover, low CTRP3 levels were directly associated with the presence of sepsis among ICU patients. Interestingly, we did not observe an association of CTRP3 levels with obesity or diabetes in ICU patients, arguing that critical illness might overrule the regulation mechanisms of CTRP3 in non-critically ill patients. In line, CTRP3 plasma concentrations were inversely correlated with inflammatory cytokines and standard markers of sepsis such as CRP and PCT. Importantly, the authors described a direct association between low CTRP3 levels (<620.6 ng/mL) and an increased overall mortality [38]. Although these data need to be confirmed in further trials, it suggests a clinically relevant role of CTRP3 as a potential new diagnostic and prognostic biomarker in patients with critical illness and sepsis.

3.4. Leptin and Leptin-Receptor

Leptin represents a 16 kDa hormone that was initially described in 1994 and has since been extensively studied for its regulatory role with respect to food intake, glucose homeostasis, and energy expenditure [39,40]. It mainly originates from adipocytes and was also found to be involved in cell-mediated immunity as well as inflammatory cytokine crosstalk [41]. There is a direct correlation of circulating leptin levels with body fat mass; starvation or malnutrition leads to low serum concentrations, while obesity increases leptin serum levels [42].

Several clinical studies have evaluated the role of circulating leptin as a biomarker in the context of critical illness, but the results are partly inconclusive. In a first study of $n = 137$ critically ill patients (95 with sepsis, 42 without sepsis), serum leptin concentrations at admission to ICU were similar compared with healthy controls and did not differ between septic and non-septic patients [43]. Similar results were obtained for the soluble leptin receptor, which is known to form complexes with circulating leptin. In line, a smaller series of patients with severe sepsis revealed no significant regulation of serum leptin levels in septic disease [44]. Contrarily, serum leptin levels were significantly elevated in septic patients compared with non-septic patients in a cohort of $n = 331$ patients with critical illness from a medical ICU [41]. In a longitudinal study including patients with sepsis, leptin levels were significantly higher compared with controls and showed a positive correlation with insulin levels and insulin resistance. Interestingly, a decline of leptin serum levels was found during prolonged sepsis, which was, however, not related to survival [45]. A potential explanation for these contradictory results might relate to different sampling time points, divergent BMI or feeding state prior and during sepsis, or from heterogeneous cohorts in terms of disease etiology.

In terms of a prognostic marker, low leptin serum levels (<10 ng/mL) were associated with an adverse outcome in a cohort of 230 adult patients with severe secondary peritonitis [46]. Moreover, elevated leptin-receptor receptor levels (>32 ng/mL) were associated with an impaired overall survival compared with patients with low serum levels (<32 ng/mL) [44].

3.5. Visfatin

Visfatin, which is also referred to as pre-B-cell colony-enhancing factor (PBEF) given its initial identification in lymphocytes, represents an adipokine with key functions in the process of systemic inflammation. It was shown that visfatin acts as a chemoattractant to recruit neutrophils and promotes their survival [47,48], and is further capable of stimulating cytokine release from monocytes [49]. Visfatin has also been associated with human critical illness and sepsis and was primarily suggested as a diagnostic marker. In septic infants, visfatin serum levels were significantly elevated compared with healthy controls and showed a positive correlation with CRP, PCT, and IL-6 [50]. At a cut-off value of 10 ng/mL, visfatin revealed a sensitivity and specificity of 92% and 94%, respectively, for the diagnosis of neonatal sepsis.

In a larger study including 229 critically ill medical ICU patients, circulating visfatin levels were also significantly higher in ICU patients when compared with healthy controls [51]. Visfatin serum levels were highest in patients who fulfilled the diagnostic criteria for sepsis, and visfatin concentrations strongly correlated with disease severity and organ failure. Although visfatin serum levels were comparable between patients with or without type 2 diabetes or obesity, the authors observed a significant correlation between visfatin levels and biomarkers of liver and kidney dysfunction and other adipokines such as resistin and leptin. Most importantly, high visfatin levels upon admission to ICU were associated with both an increased ICU as well as long-term mortality [51].

3.6. Resistin

Resistin was first described in 2001 as an adipokine. Data from rodent models revealed an association between resistin and the presence of metabolic diseases including obesity and type 2 diabetes. In these studies, elevated serum levels of glucose as well as hyperinsulinemia correlated with an increase in resistin [52]. When translating data from animal models to humans, it is important to consider that the protein sequences of murine and human resistin demonstrate important differences [53]. Moreover, in mice, adipocytes represent the main source of circulating resistin, while in humans, resistin seems to be mainly secreted by macrophages [54,55], suggesting that the role of resistin in humans and mice may vary. In this context, data from a 'humanized mouse' model in which only human resistin was produced by macrophages suggested that human resistin might display pro-inflammatory characteristics mediating insulin resistance [56]. Therefore, a role of resistin in the pathophysiology of critical illness and sepsis seemed likely. Just recently, it was demonstrated that serum levels of resistin are elevated in patients with critical illness compared with controls [20]. Moreover, patients with sepsis displayed further elevated resistin concentrations compared with non-septic patients, suggesting a link between inflammation and infection and the secretion of resistin in humans. In line, serum resistin concentrations were closely correlated to inflammatory parameters such as CRP, the leukocyte count, PCT, and cytokines such as IL6 and TNF [20]. Moreover, elevated resistin levels indicated an impaired prognosis [20]. Notably, these data were subsequently corroborated by similar findings of different groups, demonstrating that elevated resistin concentrations correlate with disease severity, inflammatory cytokine, lactate levels, and serum creatinine concentrations in patients with severe sepsis and septic shock [57,58]. These data might at least partly be explained by the fact that resistin represents a uremic toxin, inhibiting neutrophils and thereby modulating sepsis-related immune responses at concentrations that can be found in patients with end-stage kidney failure [59]. In line with these data from adult patients, recently, Gokmen et al. demonstrated that resistin levels are elevated in preterm infants with sepsis, concluding that resistin may represent a marker for sepsis in premature infants [60].

3.7. Adiponectin

Adiponectin represents an adipokine of 30 kDa that is exclusively secreted by adipocytes and has been extensively studied for its role in glucose and lipid metabolism and in the context of insulin resistance [61]. In obese and patients with diabetes mellitus, circulating levels of adiponectin are reduced compared with healthy individuals [62]. Moreover, circulating adiponectin levels negatively correlate with serum levels of low-density lipoprotein cholesterol and triglycerides, blood pressure, and insulin resistance [63], arguing for a protective function of adiponectin in human metabolic homoeostasis. This concept is supported by animal studies suggesting an anti-inflammatory and protective role of adiponectin in mouse models of sepsis [64,65].

Only limited data on a regulation of adiponectin in critical illness and sepsis are available. In a study evaluating circulating levels of adiponectin in 170 critically ill patients at admission to the ICU, the authors found comparable adiponectin levels in ICU patients with or without sepsis and healthy controls [66]. Similar to patients without critical illness, ICU patients with obesity or preexisting diabetes mellitus displayed significantly reduced levels of circulating adiponectin. Interestingly, although not regulated in ICU patients, the authors found that low adiponectin levels at ICU admission are an independent positive predictive marker for short-term and overall survival [66]. During the clinical course of critical illness, two studies have reported low to normal levels of circulating adiponectin. In a small series of patients, plasma adiponectin concentrations in an ICU cohort at day 3 and day 7 after admission were significantly lower compared with healthy control samples [67]. In line, a study including 318 patients with respiratory critical illness revealed low adiponectin levels, which were enhanced by insulin therapy and returned to normal when critical illness was sustained [68].

3.8. Retinol Binding Protein 4

Retinol binding protein 4 (RBP4) is involved in the transport of hepatic retinol to distant organs. Levels of circulating RBP4 have been linked to metabolic diseases such as insulin resistance, obesity, metabolic syndrome, diabetes, and fatty liver disease, representing chronic inflammatory diseases [68]. Recently, the group of Langouche et al. demonstrated in 318 critically ill patients that those patients with sepsis had significantly lower RBP4 levels than those with other disease etiologies [68]. In a different study, RBP4 levels were also lower in ICU patients, regardless of whether or not sepsis was present, compared with controls [69]. Interestingly, in these patients, liver cirrhosis was associated with further reduced RBP4 concentrations and RBP4 was correlated with markers of liver dysfunction. Interestingly, RBP4 concentrations were independent on the presence of obesity or preexisting diabetes and were not associated with overall survival in the analyzed cohort. In contrast, Chen et al. demonstrated that baseline RBP levels predicted short-term mortality in critically ill patients with underlying liver disease. Interestingly, in this analysis, those patients that survived ICU treatment displayed significantly increased RBP4 levels after ICU discharge [70], highlighting the potential of this biomarker in predicting survival in patients treated on a medical ICU.

Table 1. Overview of regulated adipokines in critically illness and sepsis.

	Adipokine	Circulating Adipokine Levels in Critical Illness and/or Sepsis	Prognostic Relevance?	Reference
1	Omentin	−	+	[26]
2	CTRP1	↑	−/(+)	[31,32]
3	CTRP3	↓	+	[38]
4	Leptin and Leptin Receptor	−/↑	+	[41,43–46]
5	Visfatin	↑	+	[50,51]
6	Resistin	↑	+	[20,57,58]
7	Adiponectin	−/↓	+	[66–68]
8	RBP4	↓	−/(+)	[68–70]

CTRP1: C1q/TNFa-related protein 1, CTRP3: C1q/TNFa-related protein 3, RBP4: retinol binding protein 4, −: no regulation/no prognostic relevance, +: prognostic relevance, ↑: elevated circulating levels, ↓: decreased circulating levels.

4. Discussion and Outlook

Adipokines represent a growing class of proteins that exert a wide range of metabolic effects. Moreover, adipokines have been shown to withhold regulatory effects in immune responses during inflammation and infectious disease. Because adipokines are secreted into the blood, recent studies have analyzed their potential as biomarkers in many different pathological conditions. While many papers found an association between serum levels of adipokines and the presence of sepsis and/or the prognosis of patients with critical illness, it is important to highlight some limitations that apply at least for most of the available studies. Many of the available studies featured a retrospective design and the missing longitudinal approach may have induced a bias. Moreover, some of the analyzed cohorts were extremely heterogeneous and relatively small in terms of patients' numbers; therefore, larger prospective studies are needed to finally infer about the role of circulating adipokines in patients with critical illness, a collective of patients with a still unacceptably poor prognosis. Within this review, we summarized available data on the potential role of these proteins in critically ill and septic patients. We highlight that, despite that their use as single marker might be limited owing to a lack of sensitivity and specificity, measurements of circulating adipokines might be integrated into available and future scoring systems for the diagnosis of sepsis and risk stratification of critically ill patients.

Author Contributions: C.R., S.H.L., T.L., F.T., and A.K. designed the review. S.H.L., C.R., and T.L. performed literature review and drafted the manuscript. F.T. and A.K. provided intellectual input. All authors approved the paper.

Funding: Work in the lab of T.L. was funded from the European Research Council (ERC) under the European Union's Horizon 2020 research and innovation program through the ERC Consolidator Grant PhaseControl (Grant Agreement n 771083). The lab of T.L. was further supported by the German Cancer Aid (Deutsche Krebshilfe 110043 and a Mildred-Scheel-Professorship), the German-Research-Foundation (SFB-TRR57/P06 and LU 1360/3-1), the Ernst-Jung-Foundation Hamburg, the IZKF (interdisciplinary centre of clinical research) Aachen, and a grant from the medical faculty of the RWTH Aachen.

Conflicts of Interest: The authors declare no conflict of interest.

References

1. Singer, M.; Deutschman, C.S.; Seymour, C.W.; Shankar-Hari, M.; Annane, D.; Bauer, M.; Bellomo, R.; Bernard, G.R.; Chiche, J.-D.; Coopersmith, C.M.; et al. The Third International Consensus Definitions for Sepsis and Septic Shock (Sepsis-3). *JAMA* **2016**, *315*, 801–810. [CrossRef] [PubMed]
2. Shankar-Hari, M.; Phillips, G.S.; Levy, M.L.; Seymour, C.W.; Liu, V.X.; Deutschman, C.S.; Angus, D.C.; Rubenfeld, G.D.; Singer, M. Developing a New Definition and Assessing New Clinical Criteria for Septic Shock. *JAMA* **2016**, *315*, 775. [CrossRef] [PubMed]
3. Seymour, C.W.; Liu, V.X.; Iwashyna, T.J.; Brunkhorst, F.M.; Rea, T.D.; Scherag, A.; Rubenfeld, G.; Kahn, J.M.; Shankar-Hari, M.; Singer, M.; et al. Assessment of Clinical Criteria for Sepsis: For the Third International Consensus Definitions for Sepsis and Septic Shock (Sepsis-3). *JAMA* **2016**, *315*, 762–774. [CrossRef] [PubMed]
4. Angus, D.C.; van der Poll, T. Severe sepsis and septic shock. *N. Engl. J. Med.* **2013**, *369*, 840–851. [CrossRef] [PubMed]
5. Levy, M.M.; Artigas, A.; Phillips, G.S.; Rhodes, A.; Beale, R.; Osborn, T.; Vincent, J.-L.; Townsend, S.; Lemeshow, S.; Dellinger, R.P. Outcomes of the Surviving Sepsis Campaign in intensive care units in the USA and Europe: A prospective cohort study. *Lancet. Infect. Dis.* **2012**, *12*, 919–924. [CrossRef]
6. Iwashyna, T.J.; Ely, E.W.; Smith, D.M.; Langa, K.M. Long-term Cognitive Impairment and Functional Disability Among Survivors of Severe Sepsis. *JAMA* **2010**, *304*, 1787. [CrossRef] [PubMed]
7. Van Cutsem, E.; Köhne, C.-H.; Hitre, E.; Zaluski, J.; Chang Chien, C.-R.; Makhson, A.; D'Haens, G.; Pintér, T.; Lim, R.; Bodoky, G.; et al. Cetuximab and Chemotherapy as Initial Treatment for Metastatic Colorectal Cancer. *N. Engl. J. Med.* **2009**, *360*, 1408–1417. [CrossRef]
8. Vanden Berghe, T.; Hoste, E. Paving the way for precision medicine v2.0 in intensive care by profiling necroinflammation in biofluids. *Cell Death Differ.* **2019**, *26*, 83–98. [CrossRef]
9. Strimbu, K.; Tavel, J.A. What are biomarkers? *Curr. Opin. HIV AIDS* **2010**, *5*, 463–466. [CrossRef]
10. Samraj, R.S.; Zingarelli, B.; Wong, H.R. Role of biomarkers in sepsis care. *Shock* **2013**, *40*, 358–365. [CrossRef]
11. Rhodes, A.; Evans, L.E.; Alhazzani, W.; Levy, M.M.; Antonelli, M.; Ferrer, R.; Kumar, A.; Sevransky, J.E.; Sprung, C.L.; Nunnally, M.E.; et al. Surviving Sepsis Campaign: International Guidelines for Management of Sepsis and Septic Shock: 2016. *Intensive Care Med.* **2017**, *43*, 304–377. [CrossRef] [PubMed]
12. Van Engelen, T.S.R.; Wiersinga, W.J.; Scicluna, B.P.; van der Poll, T. Biomarkers in Sepsis. *Crit. Care Clin.* **2018**, *34*, 139–152. [CrossRef] [PubMed]
13. Pepys, M.B.; Hirschfield, G.M. C-reactive protein: A critical update. *J. Clin. Investig.* **2003**, *111*, 1805–1812. [CrossRef]
14. Silvestre, J.P.; Coelho, L.M.; Póvoa, P.M. Impact of fulminant hepatic failure in C-reactive protein? *J. Crit. Care* **2010**, *25*, e7–e12. [CrossRef] [PubMed]
15. Wacker, C.; Prkno, A.; Brunkhorst, F.M.; Schlattmann, P. Procalcitonin as a diagnostic marker for sepsis: A systematic review and meta-analysis. *Lancet. Infect. Dis.* **2013**, *13*, 426–435. [CrossRef]
16. Bloos, F.; Trips, E.; Nierhaus, A.; Briegel, J.; Heyland, D.K.; Jaschinski, U.; Moerer, O.; Weyland, A.; Marx, G.; Gründling, M.; et al. Effect of Sodium Selenite Administration and Procalcitonin-Guided Therapy on Mortality in Patients With Severe Sepsis or Septic Shock: A Randomized Clinical Trial. *JAMA Intern. Med.* **2016**, *176*, 1266–1276. [CrossRef] [PubMed]
17. Cohn, B. Can procalcitonin differentiate sepsis from systemic inflammatory response syndrome without infection? *Ann. Emerg. Med.* **2014**, *63*, 631–632. [CrossRef] [PubMed]
18. Selberg, O.; Hecker, H.; Martin, M.; Klos, A.; Bautsch, W.; Köhl, J. Discrimination of sepsis and systemic inflammatory response syndrome by determination of circulating plasma concentrations of procalcitonin, protein complement 3a, and interleukin-6. *Crit. Care Med.* **2000**, *28*, 2793–2798. [CrossRef]
19. Jawa, R.S.; Anillo, S.; Huntoon, K.; Baumann, H.; Kulaylat, M. Analytic Review: Interleukin-6 in Surgery, Trauma, and Critical Care: Part I: Basic Science. *J. Intensive Care Med.* **2011**, *26*, 3–12. [CrossRef]
20. Koch, A.; Gressner, O.A.; Sanson, E.; Tacke, F.; Trautwein, C. Serum resistin levels in critically ill patients are associated with inflammation, organ dysfunction and metabolism and may predict survival of non-septic patients. *Crit. Care* **2009**, *13*, R95. [CrossRef]
21. Ouchi, N.; Parker, J.L.; Lugus, J.J.; Walsh, K. Adipokines in inflammation and metabolic disease. *Nat. Rev. Immunol.* **2011**, *11*, 85–97. [CrossRef] [PubMed]

22. Ouchi, N.; Kihara, S.; Funahashi, T.; Matsuzawa, Y.; Walsh, K. Obesity, adiponectin and vascular inflammatory disease. *Curr. Opin. Lipidol.* **2003**, *14*, 561–566. [CrossRef] [PubMed]
23. Tan, B.K.; Adya, R.; Randeva, H.S. Omentin: A Novel Link Between Inflammation, Diabesity, and Cardiovascular Disease. *Trends Cardiovasc. Med.* **2010**, *20*, 143–148. [CrossRef] [PubMed]
24. Ohashi, K.; Shibata, R.; Murohara, T.; Ouchi, N. Role of anti-inflammatory adipokines in obesity-related diseases. *Trends Endocrinol. Metab.* **2014**, *25*, 348–355. [CrossRef]
25. Herder, C.; Carstensen, M.; Ouwens, D.M. Anti-inflammatory cytokines and risk of type 2 diabetes. *Diabetes Obes. Metab.* **2013**, *15*, 39–50. [CrossRef]
26. Luedde, M.; Benz, F.; Niedeggen, J.; Vucur, M.; Hippe, H.-J.; Spehlmann, M.E.; Schueller, F.; Loosen, S.; Frey, N.; Trautwein, C.; et al. Elevated Omentin Serum Levels Predict Long-Term Survival in Critically Ill Patients. *Dis. Markers* **2016**, *2016*, 3149243. [CrossRef]
27. Chen, L.; Wu, F.; Yuan, S.; Feng, B. Identification and characteristic of three members of the C1q/TNF-related proteins (CTRPs) superfamily in Eudontomyzon morii. *Fish Shellfish Immunol.* **2016**, *59*, 233–240. [CrossRef]
28. Han, S.; Yang, Y. A novel blood pressure modulator C1q/TNF-α-related protein 1 (CTRP1). *BMB Rep.* **2018**, *51*, 611–612. [CrossRef]
29. Chen, H.; Gao, L.; Huang, Z.; Liu, Y.; Guo, S.; Xing, J.; Meng, Z.; Liang, C.; Li, Y.; Yao, R.; et al. C1qTNF-related protein 1 attenuates doxorubicin-induced cardiac injury via activation of AKT. *Life Sci.* **2018**, *207*, 492–498. [CrossRef]
30. Kim, D.; Park, S.-Y. C1q and TNF related protein 1 regulates expression of inflammatory genes in vascular smooth muscle cells. *Genes Genomics* **2019**, *41*, 397–406. [CrossRef]
31. Yagmur, E.; Buergerhausen, D.; Koek, G.H.; Weiskirchen, R.; Trautwein, C.; Koch, A.; Tacke, F. Elevated CTRP1 Plasma Concentration Is Associated with Sepsis and Pre-Existing Type 2 Diabetes Mellitus in Critically Ill Patients. *J. Clin. Med.* **2019**, *8*, 661. [CrossRef] [PubMed]
32. Muendlein, A.; Leiherer, A.; Saely, C.; Ebner, J.; Geiger, K.; Brandtner, E.M.; Vonbank, A.; Fraunberger, P.; Drexel, H. The novel adipokine CTRP1 is significantly associated with the incidence of major adverse cardiovascular events. *Atherosclerosis* **2019**, *286*, 1–6. [CrossRef] [PubMed]
33. Seldin, M.M.; Tan, S.Y.; Wong, G.W. Metabolic function of the CTRP family of hormones. *Rev. Endocr. Metab. Disord.* **2014**, *15*, 111–123. [CrossRef] [PubMed]
34. Li, Y.; Wright, G.L.; Peterson, J.M. C1q/TNF-Related Protein 3 (CTRP3) Function and Regulation. *Compr. Physiol.* **2017**, *7*, 863–878. [PubMed]
35. Yi, W.; Sun, Y.; Yuan, Y.; Lau, W.B.; Zheng, Q.; Wang, X.; Wang, Y.; Shang, X.; Gao, E.; Koch, W.J.; et al. C1q/Tumor Necrosis Factor-Related Protein-3, a Newly Identified Adipokine, Is a Novel Antiapoptotic, Proangiogenic, and Cardioprotective Molecule in the Ischemic Mouse Heart. *Circulation* **2012**, *125*, 3159–3169. [CrossRef] [PubMed]
36. Peterson, J.M.; Wei, Z.; Wong, G.W. C1q/TNF-related Protein-3 (CTRP3), a Novel Adipokine That Regulates Hepatic Glucose Output. *J. Biol. Chem.* **2010**, *285*, 39691–39701. [CrossRef] [PubMed]
37. Wei, W.-Y.; Ma, Z.-G.; Zhang, N.; Xu, S.-C.; Yuan, Y.-P.; Zeng, X.-F.; Tang, Q.-Z. Overexpression of CTRP3 protects against sepsis-induced myocardial dysfunction in mice. *Mol. Cell. Endocrinol.* **2018**, *476*, 27–36. [CrossRef]
38. Yagmur, E.; Otto, S.; Koek, G.H.; Weiskirchen, R.; Trautwein, C.; Koch, A.; Tacke, F. Decreased CTRP3 Plasma Concentrations Are Associated with Sepsis and Predict Mortality in Critically Ill Patients. *Diagnostics* **2019**, *9*, 63. [CrossRef]
39. Bates, S.H.; Myers, M.G. The role of leptin receptor signaling in feeding and neuroendocrine function. *Trends Endocrinol. Metab.* **2003**, *14*, 447–452. [CrossRef]
40. Friedman, J.M.; Halaas, J.L. Leptin and the regulation of body weight in mammals. *Nature* **1998**, *395*, 763–770. [CrossRef]
41. Chen, M.; Wang, B.; Xu, Y.; Deng, Z.; Xue, H.; Wang, L.; He, L. Diagnostic value of serum leptin and a promising novel diagnostic model for sepsis. *Exp. Ther. Med.* **2014**, *7*, 881–886. [CrossRef] [PubMed]
42. Friedman, J.M. The function of leptin in nutrition, weight, and physiology. *Nutr. Rev.* **2002**, *60*, S1–S14; discussion S68–S84, S85–S87. [CrossRef] [PubMed]
43. Koch, A.; Weiskirchen, R.; Zimmermann, H.W.; Sanson, E.; Trautwein, C.; Tacke, F. Relevance of Serum Leptin and Leptin-Receptor Concentrations in Critically Ill Patients. *Mediators Inflamm.* **2010**, *2010*, 1–9. [CrossRef] [PubMed]

44. Hillenbrand, A.; Knippschild, U.; Weiss, M.; Schrezenmeier, H.; Henne-Bruns, D.; Huber-Lang, M.; Wolf, A.M. Sepsis induced changes of adipokines and cytokines - septic patients compared to morbidly obese patients. *BMC Surg.* **2010**, *10*, 26. [CrossRef] [PubMed]
45. Tzanela, M.; Orfanos, S.E.; Tsirantonaki, M.; Kotanidou, A.; Sotiropoulou, C.; Christophoraki, M.; Vassiliadi, D.; Thalassinos, N.C.; Roussos, C. Leptin alterations in the course of sepsis in humans. *In Vivo* **2006**, *20*, 565–570. [PubMed]
46. Bracho-Riquelme, R.L.; Reyes-Romero, M.A.; Pescador, N.; Flores-García, A.I. A leptin serum concentration less than 10 ng/mL is a predictive marker of outcome in patients with moderate to severe secondary peritonitis. *Eur. Surg. Res.* **2008**, *41*, 238–244. [CrossRef]
47. Jia, S.H.; Li, Y.; Parodo, J.; Kapus, A.; Fan, L.; Rotstein, O.D.; Marshall, J.C. Pre–B cell colony–enhancing factor inhibits neutrophil apoptosis in experimental inflammation and clinical sepsis. *J. Clin. Investig.* **2004**, *113*, 1318–1327. [CrossRef]
48. Hong, S.-B.; Huang, Y.; Moreno-Vinasco, L.; Sammani, S.; Moitra, J.; Barnard, J.W.; Ma, S.-F.; Mirzapoiazova, T.; Evenoski, C.; Reeves, R.R.; et al. Essential Role of Pre–B-Cell Colony Enhancing Factor in Ventilator-induced Lung Injury. *Am. J. Respir. Crit. Care Med.* **2008**, *178*, 605–617. [CrossRef]
49. Moschen, A.R.; Kaser, A.; Enrich, B.; Mosheimer, B.; Theurl, M.; Niederegger, H.; Tilg, H. Visfatin, an Adipocytokine with Proinflammatory and Immunomodulating Properties. *J. Immunol.* **2007**, *178*, 1748–1758. [CrossRef]
50. Cekmez, F.; Canpolat, F.E.; Cetinkaya, M.; Aydinöz, S.; Aydemir, G.; Karademir, F.; Ipcioglu, O.M.; Sarici, S.Ü. Diagnostic value of resistin and visfatin, in comparison with C-reactive protein, procalcitonin and interleukin-6 in neonatal sepsis. *Eur. Cytokine Netw.* **2011**, *22*, 113–117. [CrossRef]
51. Koch, A.; Weiskirchen, R.; Krusch, A.; Bruensing, J.; Buendgens, L.; Herbers, U.; Yagmur, E.; Koek, G.H.; Trautwein, C.; Tacke, F. Visfatin Serum Levels Predict Mortality in Critically Ill Patients. *Dis. Markers* **2018**, *2018*, 1–8. [CrossRef] [PubMed]
52. Steppan, C.M.; Bailey, S.T.; Bhat, S.; Brown, E.J.; Banerjee, R.R.; Wright, C.M.; Patel, H.R.; Ahima, R.S.; Lazar, M.A. The hormone resistin links obesity to diabetes. *Nature* **2001**, *409*, 307–312. [CrossRef] [PubMed]
53. Youn, B.-S.; Yu, K.-Y.; Park, H.J.; Lee, N.S.; Min, S.S.; Youn, M.Y.; Cho, Y.M.; Park, Y.J.; Kim, S.Y.; Lee, H.K.; et al. Plasma resistin concentrations measured by enzyme-linked immunosorbent assay using a newly developed monoclonal antibody are elevated in individuals with type 2 diabetes mellitus. *J. Clin. Endocrinol. Metab.* **2004**, *89*, 150–156. [CrossRef] [PubMed]
54. Patel, L.; Buckels, A.C.; Kinghorn, I.J.; Murdock, P.R.; Holbrook, J.D.; Plumpton, C.; Macphee, C.H.; Smith, S.A. Resistin is expressed in human macrophages and directly regulated by PPAR gamma activators. *Biochem. Biophys. Res. Commun.* **2003**, *300*, 472–476. [CrossRef]
55. Savage, D.B.; Sewter, C.P.; Klenk, E.S.; Segal, D.G.; Vidal-Puig, A.; Considine, R.V.; O'Rahilly, S. Resistin/Fizz3 expression in relation to obesity and peroxisome proliferator-activated receptor-gamma action in humans. *Diabetes* **2001**, *50*, 2199–2202. [CrossRef] [PubMed]
56. Qatanani, M.; Szwergold, N.R.; Greaves, D.R.; Ahima, R.S.; Lazar, M.A. Macrophage-derived human resistin exacerbates adipose tissue inflammation and insulin resistance in mice. *J. Clin. Investig.* **2009**, *119*, 531–539. [CrossRef] [PubMed]
57. Vassiliadi, D.A.; Tzanela, M.; Kotanidou, A.; Orfanos, S.E.; Nikitas, N.; Armaganidis, A.; Koutsilieris, M.; Roussos, C.; Tsagarakis, S.; Dimopoulou, I. Serial changes in adiponectin and resistin in critically ill patients with sepsis: Associations with sepsis phase, severity, and circulating cytokine levels. *J. Crit. Care* **2012**, *27*, 400–409. [CrossRef]
58. Macdonald, S.P.J.; Stone, S.F.; Neil, C.L.; van Eeden, P.E.; Fatovich, D.M.; Arendts, G.; Brown, S.G.A. Sustained elevation of resistin, NGAL and IL-8 are associated with severe sepsis/septic shock in the emergency department. *PLoS ONE* **2014**, *9*, e110678. [CrossRef]
59. Cohen, G.; Ilic, D.; Raupachova, J.; Hörl, W.H. Resistin inhibits essential functions of polymorphonuclear leukocytes. *J. Immunol.* **2008**, *181*, 3761–3768. [CrossRef]
60. Gokmen, Z.; Ozkiraz, S.; Kulaksizoglu, S.; Kilicdag, H.; Ozel, D.; Ecevit, A.; Tarcan, A. Resistin—A novel feature in the diagnosis of sepsis in premature neonates. *Am. J. Perinatol.* **2013**, *30*, 513–517. [CrossRef]
61. Berg, A.H.; Combs, T.P.; Scherer, P.E. ACRP30/adiponectin: An adipokine regulating glucose and lipid metabolism. *Trends Endocrinol. Metab.* **2002**, *13*, 84–89. [CrossRef]

62. Kern, P.A.; Di Gregorio, G.B.; Lu, T.; Rassouli, N.; Ranganathan, G. Adiponectin Expression From Human Adipose Tissue: Relation to Obesity, Insulin Resistance, and Tumor Necrosis Factor- Expression. *Diabetes* **2003**, *52*, 1779–1785. [CrossRef] [PubMed]
63. Yamamoto, Y.; Hirose, H.; Saito, I.; Tomita, M.; Taniyama, M.; Matsubara, K.; Okazaki, Y.; Ishii, T.; Nishikai, K.; Saruta, T. Correlation of the adipocyte-derived protein adiponectin with insulin resistance index and serum high-density lipoprotein-cholesterol, independent of body mass index, in the Japanese population. *Clin. Sci.* **2002**, *103*, 137–142. [CrossRef] [PubMed]
64. Teoh, H.; Quan, A.; Bang, K.W.A.; Wang, G.; Lovren, F.; Vu, V.; Haitsma, J.J.; Szmitko, P.E.; Al-Omran, M.; Wang, C.-H.; et al. Adiponectin deficiency promotes endothelial activation and profoundly exacerbates sepsis-related mortality. *Am. J. Physiol. Metab.* **2008**, *295*, E658–E664. [CrossRef] [PubMed]
65. Uji, Y.; Yamamoto, H.; Tsuchihashi, H.; Maeda, K.; Funahashi, T.; Shimomura, I.; Shimizu, T.; Endo, Y.; Tani, T. Adiponectin deficiency is associated with severe polymicrobial sepsis, high inflammatory cytokine levels, and high mortality. *Surgery* **2009**, *145*, 550–557. [CrossRef]
66. Koch, A.; Sanson, E.; Voigt, S.; Helm, A.; Trautwein, C.; Tacke, F. Serum adiponectin upon admission to the intensive care unit may predict mortality in critically ill patients. *J. Crit. Care* **2011**, *26*, 166–174. [CrossRef] [PubMed]
67. Venkatesh, B.; Hickman, I.; Nisbet, J.; Cohen, J.; Prins, J. Changes in serum adiponectin concentrations in critical illness: A preliminary investigation. *Crit. Care* **2009**, *13*, R105. [CrossRef]
68. Langouche, L.; Vander Perre, S.; Frystyk, J.; Flyvbjerg, A.; Hansen, T.K.; Van den Berghe, G. Adiponectin, retinol-binding protein 4, and leptin in protracted critical illness of pulmonary origin. *Crit. Care* **2009**, *13*, R112. [CrossRef]
69. Koch, A.; Weiskirchen, R.; Sanson, E.; Zimmermann, H.W.; Voigt, S.; Dückers, H.; Trautwein, C.; Tacke, F. Circulating retinol binding protein 4 in critically ill patients before specific treatment: Prognostic impact and correlation with organ function, metabolism and inflammation. *Crit. Care* **2010**, *14*, R179. [CrossRef]
70. Chen, W.-T.; Lee, M.-S.; Chang, C.-L.; Chiu, C.-T.; Chang, M.-L. Retinol-binding protein-4 expression marks the short-term mortality of critically ill patients with underlying liver disease: Lipid, but not glucose, matters. *Sci. Rep.* **2017**, *7*, 2881. [CrossRef]

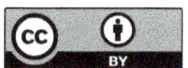

© 2019 by the authors. Licensee MDPI, Basel, Switzerland. This article is an open access article distributed under the terms and conditions of the Creative Commons Attribution (CC BY) license (http://creativecommons.org/licenses/by/4.0/).

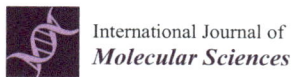

Article

Adiponectin Reverses the Hypothalamic Microglial Inflammation during Short-Term Exposure to Fat-Rich Diet

Hannah Lee [1,†], Thai Hien Tu [1,†], Byong Seo Park [1], Sunggu Yang [2] and Jae Geun Kim [1,3,*]

1. Division of Life Sciences, College of Life Sciences and Bioengineering, Incheon National University, Incheon 406-772, Korea; 8973215@hanmail.net (H.L.); thaihientu@gmail.com (T.H.T.); bbs0808@naver.com (B.S.P.)
2. Department of Nano-Bioengineering, Incheon National University, Incheon 406-772, Korea; abiyang9@gmail.com
3. Institute for New Drug Development, Division of Life Sciences, Incheon National University, Incheon 406-772, Korea
* Correspondence: jgkim@inu.ac.kr; Tel.: +82-32-835-8256
† These authors contributed equally to this work.

Received: 7 November 2019; Accepted: 12 November 2019; Published: 15 November 2019

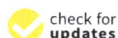

Abstract: Adiponectin, an adipokine derived from the adipose tissue, manifests anti-inflammatory effects in the metabolically active organs and is, therefore, beneficial in various metabolic diseases associated with inflammation. However, the role of adiponectin in alleviating the hypothalamic inflammation connected to the pathogenesis of obesity has not yet been clearly interrogated. Here, we identified that the systemic administration of adiponectin suppresses the activation of microglia and thereby reverses the hypothalamic inflammation during short-term exposure to a high-fat diet. Additionally, we show that adiponectin induces anti-inflammatory effects in the microglial cell line subjected to an exogenous treatment with a saturated free fatty acid. In conclusion, the current study suggests that adiponectin suppresses the saturated free fatty acid-triggered the hypothalamic inflammation by modulating the microglial activation and thus maintains energy homeostasis.

Keywords: energy metabolism; inflammation; hypothalamus; microglia; adiponectin

1. Introduction

Inflammation is one of the major pathological causes implicated in the development of obesity and its related metabolic disorders [1–3]. Chronic inflammation triggered by over-nutrition results in perturbation of the activity of hypothalamic neurons, which govern the whole-body energy balance [4–6]. Recent studies report that microglia, the resident macrophages of the central nervous system (CNS), respond to the elevation of saturated free fatty acid (FFA) following consumption of the fat-rich diet and thereby trigger the hypothalamic inflammation [6]. This results in abnormal functioning of the neuronal circuit that controls the energy homeostasis.

Adiponectin, an adipokine derived from adipose tissue, has been reported as beneficial in alleviating multiple physiological disturbances [7–9]. It helps in alleviating a variety of metabolic diseases by ameliorating the cellular stresses including inflammation, oxidative stress, and endoplasmic reticulum stress [7,8,10–12]. Although, a recent study identified an anti-inflammatory effect of adiponectin in the CNS [11], the role of adiponectin in rectifying the hypothalamic inflammation during early over-nutrition period remains elusive. Therefore, this study was aimed at identification of the contribution of adiponectin in regulating the hypothalamic inflammation and the microglial function. We evaluated the inflammatory responses and microglial activation utilizing mice model

2. Results

2.1. Adiponectin Reverses the Hypothalamic Inflammation Induced by Short-Term Exposure to High Fat Diet

In order to verify if adiponectin exerts anti-inflammatory effect in the hypothalamus during the early over-nutrition period, we evaluated the pattern of the hypothalamic inflammation after treatment with high fat diet (HFD) for 4 weeks combined with the systemic administration of globular adiponectin, which has a more potent effect on their identified functions [13]. In line with the previous finding that identified a reduction in circulating adiponectin level during short-term exposure to a fat-rich diet [13], we also confirmed a reduction in adiponectin mRNA level in epididymal white adipose tissue (eWAT) 4 weeks after high-fat diet treatment (Figure 1A). In accordance with the previous reports, we observed that HFD treatment resulted in a drastic increase in the expression levels of mRNA encoding inflammatory cytokines such as IL-1β (Figure 1B), IL-6 (Figure 1C), TNF-α (Figure 1D) as well as *Cox-2* gene (Figure 1E), the rate-limiting enzyme involved in the synthesis of the prostaglandin E2, which controls the cellular inflammatory process. This elevation of mRNA levels was effectively reversed by a systemic treatment with adiponectin for five days. Furthermore, we observed that an elevation in the levels of hypothalamic *Iba-1* and *CD11b mRNA*, the molecular markers of microglia, in HFD-treated group was almost completely rescued by the systemic treatment with adiponectin (Figure 1F,G). These findings suggest that adiponectin treatment exerts anti-inflammatory effects on the hypothalamus following short-term HFD exposure, at least in part, via targeting the microglial cells.

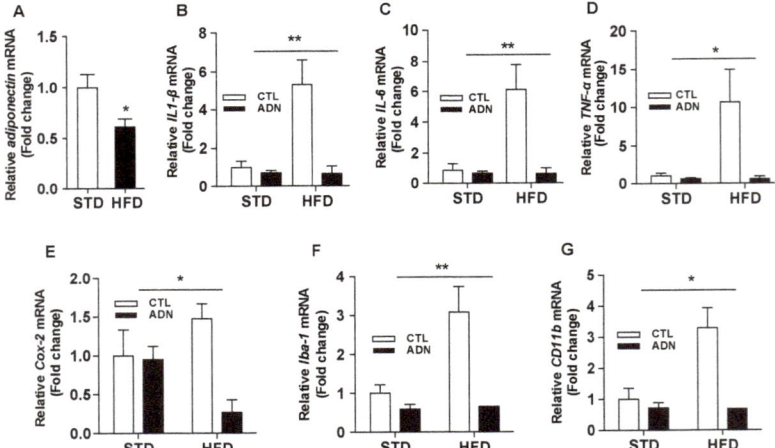

Figure 1. Systemic administration of adiponectin reverses the hypothalamic inflammation in response to short-term HFD treatment. C57BL/6 mice were fed either a Standard diet (STD) or a HFD for 4 weeks followed by i.p. injection of adiponectin or saline (as a control group) for 5 days. (**A**) The level of *adiponectin* mRNA in eWAT was significantly elevated 4 weeks after HFD treatment. The elevated mRNA levels of hypothalamic genes involved in inflammatory processes such as (**B**) *IL-1β*, (**C**) *IL-6*, and (**D**) *TNF-α* and (**E**) *Cox-2* observed in HFD-treated group were significantly reversed by i.p administration of adiponectin. Adiponectin treatment dampened the increase in the mRNA levels of hypothalamic (**F**) *Iba-1* and (**G**) *CD11b*, markers for microglia activation, in response to HFD treatment. Results are presented as mean ± SEM. n = at least 5 mice per group. * $p < 0.05$, ** $p < 0.01$ for effects of adiponectin on HFD-treated group versus effects of adiponectin on STD-treated group. CTL, control group; ADN, adiponectin-treated group.

2.2. Adiponectin Suppresses the Microglial Activation Induced by Short-Term Exposure to HFD

To determine whether adiponectin relieves the development of HFD-triggered hypothalamic inflammation by targeting the hypothalamic microglial cells, we identified the presence of adiponectin receptor 1 (*AdipoR1*) and adiponectin receptor 2 (*AdipoR2*) in the hypothalamic glial cells utilizing cultured primary microglia and astrocytes (Figure 2A). We also validated the purification of a single cell type determined by a strong expression of Iba-1, a molecular marker for microglia participating in membrane ruffling and phagocytosis in activated microglia (Figure 2B) [14], or GFAP, a molecular marker for astrocytes (Figure 2C). Based on the anti-inflammatory effects of adiponectin on hypothalamic inflammation triggered by short-term HFD treatment, we next performed immunohistochemistry (IHC) using an antibody against Iba-1 on brain slices from mice fed either a STD or a HFD combined with adiponectin to evaluate the impact of adiponectin treatment on microglia activation in the hypothalamus. We observed that the HFD treatment resulted in an increase in body weight (Figure 2D) and WAT weight (Figure 2E) as compared to the STD-treated group. On the contrary, the systemic administration of adiponectin for 7 days did not alter the increase in the body weight and WAT weight seen in the HFD-treated group (Figure 2D,E). Consistent with our cellular data, we observed that adiponectin treatment effectively reverses the microglial activation in the hypothalamus characterized by increased in a number of microglia (Figure 2F,G). In addition, we found that systemic treatment of adiponectin blocked the increase in microglia soma area in the HFD-treated hypothalamus (Figure 2H). However, adiponectin did not rescue the elevated of Iba-1 intensity seen in the HFD-treated hypothalamus (Figure 2I). These findings indicate that adiponectin reverses the effects of HFD on the hypothalamic inflammation by ameliorating the microglial activation during the early over-nutrition period.

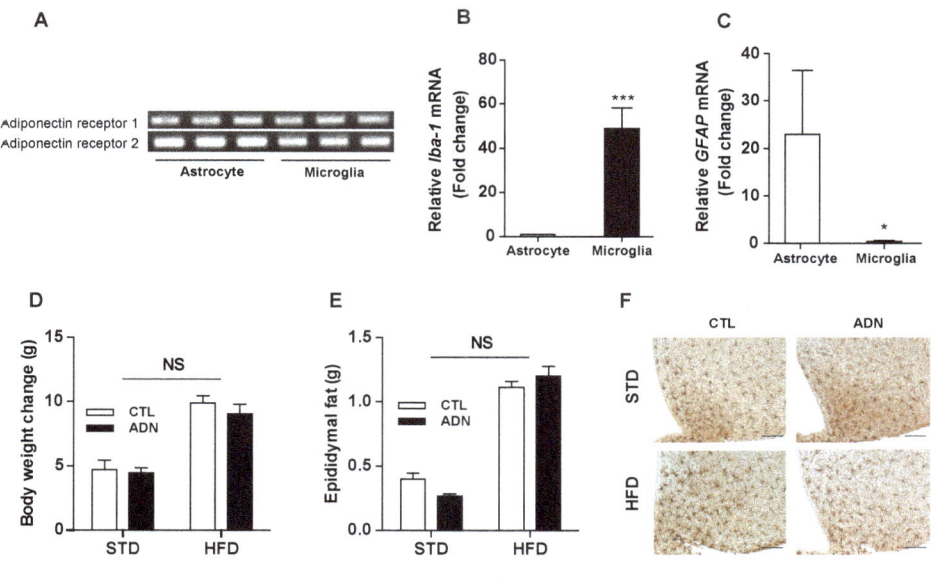

Figure 2. Cont.

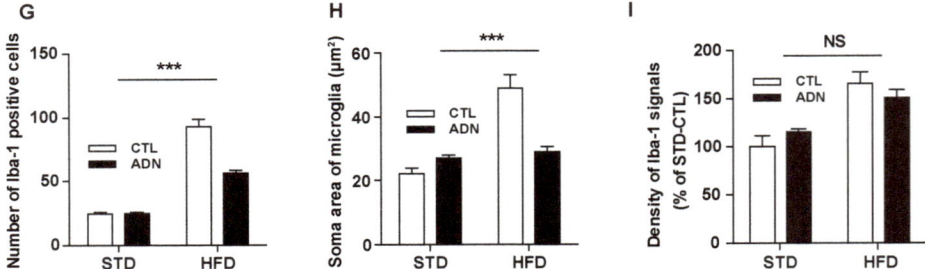

Figure 2. Adiponectin rescues the microglial activation caused by short-term exposure to high fat diet. (**A**) RT-PCR bands indicate the presence of AdipoR1 and AdipoR2 in both primary microglia and astrocytes. Confirmation of purification of microglia and astrocytes, as determined by levels of (**B**) *Iba-1* and (**C**) *GFAP* mRNAs. (**D**) Changes of body weight and (**E**) white adipose tissue weight seen in mice fed with either a STD or a HFD for 4 weeks followed by i.p. injection of adiponectin or saline (as a control group) for 5 days. (**F**) Representative images showing immunohistochemistry staining of Iba-1 in the sections of the hypothalamus from each group. Scale bar = 100 μm. The increased (**G**) number of microglial cells, and (**H**) soma area of microglia, observed in the hypothalamus of mice exposed to HFD were reversed by systemic adiponectin administration. (**I**) Adiponectin treatment did not alter the increased intensity of Iba-1 signals seen in the hypothalamus of mice fed a HFD. Results are presented as mean ± SEM. n = 5 mice per group. *** $p < 0.001$ for effects of adiponectin on HFD-treated group versus effects of adiponectin on STD-treated group or *Iba-1* mRNA level in astrocyte versus *Iba-1* mRNA level in microglia; * $p < 0.05$ for *GFAP* mRNA level in astrocyte versus *GFAP* mRNA level in microglia. NS, not significant; CTL, control group; ADN, adiponectin-treated group.

2.3. Adiponectin Improves Palmitic Acid-Induced Inflammatory Responses in the Microglial Cells

The consumption of fat-rich diet results in an elevation in the levels of circulating free fatty acids which cause the obesity pathogenesis linked to the hypothalamic inflammation [15,16]. Our previous study identified that the levels of saturated free fatty acid were elevated in both the hypothalamus and sera of mice fed a HFD for 4 weeks [17]. Therefore, to verify the anti-inflammatory role of adiponectin in alleviating the microglial inflammation induced by over-nutrition, we further evaluated the anti-inflammatory effect of adiponectin in the BV-2 microglial cell line by an administration of palmitic acid, a saturated free fatty acid followed by adiponectin treatment. We confirmed that single treatment of adiponectin did not alter cell viability (Figure 3A) or IL-1β release (Figure 3B) in cultured BV-2 microglial cells. However, adiponectin treatment led to a reduction in IL-6 secretion (Figure 3C). These findings indicated that adiponectin itself did not affect cellular inflammation and degeneration. In accordance with previous reports, palmitic acid treatment induced increase in the mRNA levels of inflammatory cytokines such as IL-1β (Figure 3D), IL-6 (Figure 3E) and TNF-α (Figure 3F), and *Cox-2* gene (Figure 3G) in cultured BV-2 microglial cells. This elevation of inflammatory responses triggered by palmitic acid was completely rescued by an exogenous adiponectin treatment. Moreover, the administration of adiponectin reversed the palmitic acid-induced release of IL-1β (Figure 3H) and IL-6 (Figure 3I) in the BV-2 microglial cells. These observations confirmed that adiponectin treatment reverses the development of hypothalamic inflammation and the associated microglial activation.

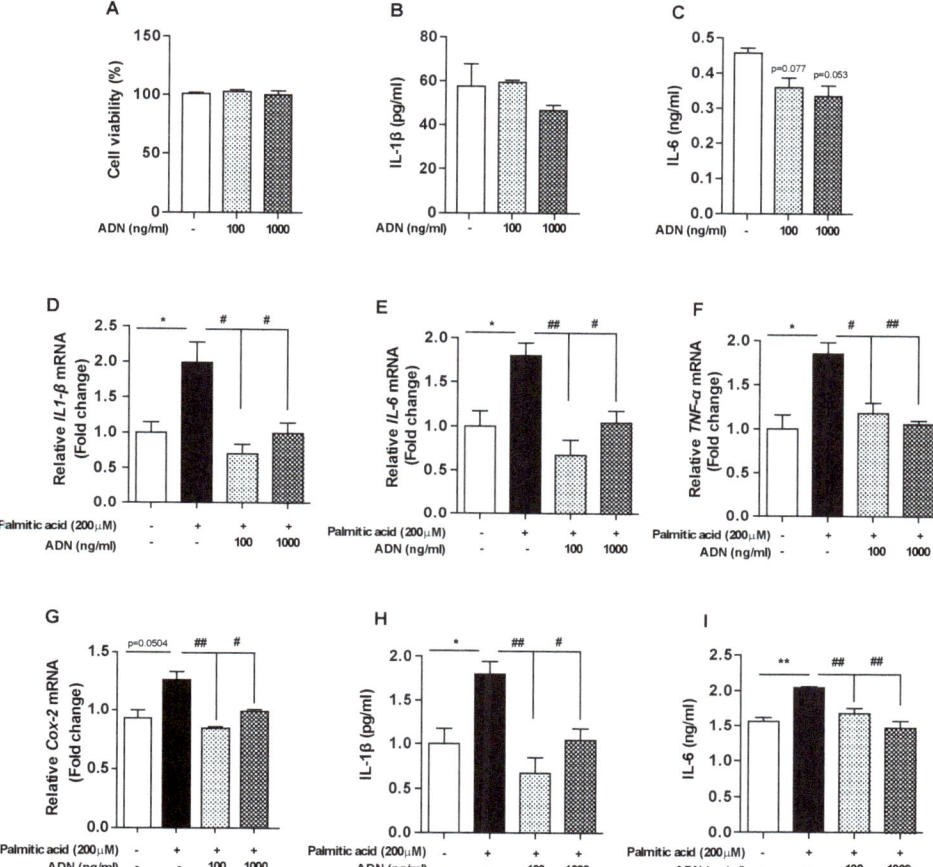

Figure 3. Adiponectin rescues the palmitic acid-induced inflammation in the microglial cell line. The BV-2 cells were seeded at a density of 5×10^5 cells/well and pretreated with adiponectin at indicated concentration for 1 h followed by palmitic acid (200 μM) treatment for 4 h. Exogenous treatment of adiponectin did not change cell viability (**A**) or IL-1β release (**B**), but reduced IL-6 secretion (**C**). The palmitic acid-induced elevations of *IL-1β* (**D**), *IL-6* (**E**) *TNF-α* (**F**) and *Cox-2* (**G**) mRNA levels were reversed by adiponectin treatment in the BV-2 cells as determined by qPCR analysis. The palmitic acid-induced increase of IL-1β (**H**) and IL-6 (**I**) cytokine release was reversed by adiponectin treatment in the BV-2 cells as determined by ELISA. Results are presented as mean ± SEM. * $p < 0.05$ and ** $p < 0.01$ for palmitic acid-treated group versus vehicle-treated group; # $p < 0.05$ and ## $p < 0.01$ for palmitic acid + adiponectin (ADN)-treated group versus palmitic acid-treated group.

2.4. Adiponectin Reverses the Palmitic Acid-Induced Alterations in the Intracellular Signaling Molecules Involved in Inflammation

In order to further verify anti-inflammatory functions of adiponectin, we evaluated the phosphorylation of ERK, a molecular component of intracellular signal transduction in the inflammatory signaling pathway [18,19], and the level of IkB-α protein, which inhibits the activity of NF-κB transcription factor regulating the expression of multiple inflammatory cytokines [20]. As shown in the Figure 4, adiponectin reversed the palmitic acid-induced phosphorylation of ERK (Figure 4A) and degradation of IkB-α (Figure 4B). These observations suggest that adiponectin treatment suppresses the microglial inflammation in response to saturated FFA, at least in part, via modulating the general signaling molecules linked to the development of cellular inflammation.

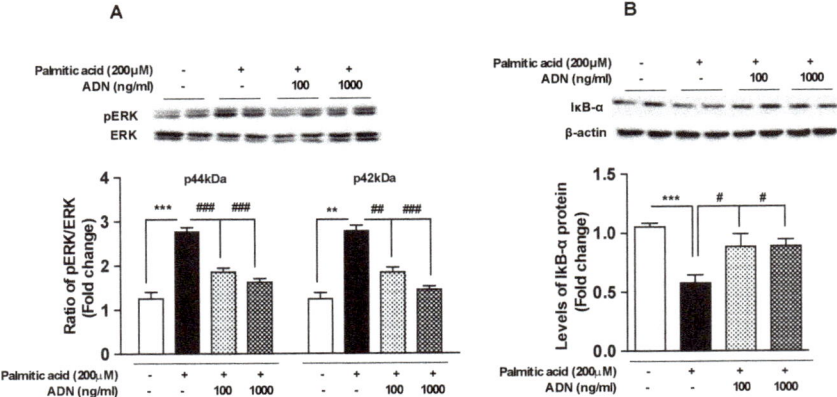

Figure 4. Adiponectin reverses palmitic acid-induced changes of the inflammatory mediators in the microglial cells. The BV-2 cells were seeded at a density of 1×10^6 cells/well and pretreated with adiponectin for 1 h followed by a palmitic acid (200 µM) treatment for 30 min or 4 h. Palmitic acid-induced phosphorylation of ERK (**A**) and reduction of IkB-α synthesis (**B**) were reversed by adiponectin treatment at indicated concentration. Results are presented as mean ± SEM. ** $p < 0.01$ and *** $p < 0.005$ for palmitic acid-treated group versus vehicle-treated group; # $p < 0.05$, ## $p < 0.01$ and ### $p < 0.005$ for palmitic acid + adiponectin (AND)-treated group versus palmitic acid-treated group.

3. Discussion

The present study highlights the beneficial effects of adiponectin in the alleviating the hypothalamic inflammation triggered by the over-nutrition that causes the disturbance in the functioning of hypothalamic neurons that regulate the whole-body energy metabolism.

Multiple lines of evidence have suggested that chronic inflammation in the hypothalamic neuronal circuit, which controls the appetite and energy expenditure, causes a variety of cellular stresses and thereby results in the energy imbalance [4–6]. The adipose tissue is a specialized connective tissue that functions as a major storage site for fats in the body [21–23]. However, it has been well established that the adipose tissue also acts as an endocrine organ besides regulating the energy balance [22,24,25]. The adipose tissue communicated with the hypothalamus by releasing multiple chemical messengers that systemically propagate the signals reflecting nutrient availability for the homeostatic control of energy homeostasis [21,22,26]. In addition, the adipose tissue also regulates the obesity pathogenesis by secreting a variety of inflammatory cytokines and adipokines that deteriorate the cellular stresses such as inflammation, endoplasmic reticulum stress, and oxidative stresses [21,22]. Although majority of the adipokines act as proinflammatory factors, adiponectin displays anti-inflammatory properties that potentially improve the dysfunction of metabolic controls in the body [8,27,28]. In the CNS, adiponectin inhibits neuronal degeneration by ameliorating the cellular stresses including inflammation [10,11,29].

A growing body of evidence suggested that the microglial cells essentially participates in the development of the neuronal inflammation [16,30,31] and the reactive gliosis is an important cellular event for both acute and chronic inflammation triggered by the over-nutrition [32,33]. Therefore, it is not surprising that the anti-inflammatory role of adiponectin in the microglial cells is coupled to the improvement of metabolic abnormalities. Since adiponectin binds via adiponectin receptors, AdipoR1 and AdipoR2 in the microglial cells, we confirmed the presence of these receptors in the microglial cells.

It has been quite well established that the short-term exposure of HFD results in an increased hypothalamic inflammation accompanied by the reactive gliosis of both microglia and astrocytes [5,6,34].

Intriguingly, mice having HFD for a couple of days displayed a significant increase in the inflammatory cytokines expression in the hypothalamus [5,6]. In line with this notion, we verified the role of adiponectin in ameliorating the hypothalamic inflammation during the consumption of the short-term fat-rich diet. Furthermore, we verified that adiponectin successfully reverses the inflammatory responses in the hypothalamic microglia during early over-nutrition period by observing the reduced microgliosis as determined by the accumulation of Iba-1 protein and the altered number and morphology of microglial cells.

A variety of substances are involved in the obesity-related pathogenesis. Among them, saturated FFAs are critical substances that trigger the inflammation in brain during early obesity period [16]. We observed that adiponectin effectively rescues the palmitic acid-induced microglial inflammation via regulation of the intracellular signaling molecules that mediate the inflammatory responses. Although there are substantial evidences highlighting the pathogenic factors associated with obesity and their impact on the development of metabolic dysfunction [35,36], the pathogenic substances involved in the initiation of hypothalamic inflammation during early over-nutrition period remain unexplored. Thus, it is also valuable to investigate the cellular and molecular responses following induction or prevention of the hypothalamic inflammation during early over-nutrition period. Indeed, previous studies indicated that adiponectin levels are slightly elevated during short-term exposure to HFD [37]. Therefore, we suggest that the anti-inflammatory effects of adiponectin might be due to the homeostatic response to suppress the hypothalamic inflammation induced by the multiple humoral factors such as saturated FFAs and adipokines. However, the beneficial effects of adiponectin treatment on the severe obesity associated with the chronic inflammation need to be determined. Therefore, further studies are required to identify the beneficial effects of adiponectin in alleviating the cellular stresses following long-term treatment of adiponectin to the obesity model accompanied by chronic hypothalamic inflammation and the cellular lipotoxicity. Collectively, the current study identifies a reversible effect exerted by adiponectin treatment on the initiation of the hypothalamic inflammation during early over-nutrition period and provides novel insight into the strategies to prevent early disruption of the energy homeostasis.

4. Materials and Methods

4.1. Animals

Seven-week-old C57B/L6 mice (Dae Han Bio Link, Eumseong, Korea) were maintained under specific pathogen-free conditions at 22 °C and given access to food and water ad libitum. To examine the effects of adiponectin on early obesity stage-induced hypothalamic inflammation, mice were adapted for a week, randomly divided into two groups and fed either a standard diet (STD, 10% calories from fat, Research Diet Inc., New Brunswick, NJ, USA) or a high-fat diet (HFD, 60% of calories from fat, Research Diets Inc.) for four weeks. The components of the HFD and STD are indicated in Table 1. For adiponectin treatment, mice were given intraperitoneal (i.p) injections of globular adiponectin (3 mg/kg, Lugen Sci, Bucheon, Korea) for five days. Brains and serum were collected 3 h after last injection. In addition, body weight and epididymal fat weight were measured when tissue was harvested. The experimental procedure is described in a flowchart (Figure 5). All the animal care and experimental procedures were performed in accordance with the protocols approved by the Institutional Animal Care and Use Committee (IACUC) at the Incheon National University (permission number: INU-2016-001).

Table 1. Components of the HFD and STD.

	High-Fat Diet (5.24 kcal/g)		Standard Diet (3.85 kcal/g)	
	g%	kcal%	g%	kcal%
Protein	26.2	20	19.2	20
Carbohydrate	26.3	20	67.3	70
Fat	34.9	60	4.3	10
	g	kcal	g	kcal
Casein80-mesh	200	800	200	800
L-Cystine	3	12	3	12
Cornstarch	0	0	315	1260
Maltodextrin 10	125	500	35	140
Sucrose	68.8	275.2	350	1400
Cellulose BW200	50	0	50	0
Soybean oil	25	225	25	225
Lard	245	2205	20	180
Mineral mix S10026	10	0	10	0
Dicalcium phosphate	13	0	13	0
Calcium carbonate	5.5	0	5.5	0
Potassium citrate	16.5	0	16.5	0
Vitamin mix V10001	10	40	10	40
Choline bitartrate	2	0	2	0
FD and C dye	0.05	0	0.05	0

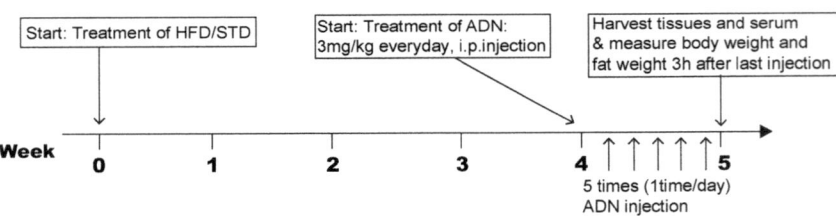

Figure 5. Flowchart showing the experimental procedure. Arrows indicate the start of treatment, sample preparation and analysis.

4.2. Immunohistochemistry

Mice were anesthetized and perfused transcardially with 0.9% saline (*w/v*), followed by fixation with 4% paraformaldehyde in phosphate buffer (PB, 0.1 M, pH 7.4). Brains were isolated and post-fixed overnight with 4% paraformaldehyde PB buffer before the coronal sections (50 μm thickness) were prepared using a vibratome (5100 mz Campden Instruments; Leicestershire, UK). After washing in PB several times, the sections were preincubated with 0.3% Triton X-100 (Sigma-Aldrich, St. Louis, MO, USA) for 30 min at room temperature (RT) and then incubated with Iba-1 antibody (1:1000 dilution, Wako, Osaka, Japan) for overnight at RT. For diaminobenzidine- (DAB-) based Iba-1 IHC, sections were extensively washed and incubated with biotinylated anti-rabbit secondary antibody, ABC reagent (Vector Laboratories, Burlingame, CA, USA), and DAB substrate (Vector Laboratories).

4.3. Cell Culture and Treatments

The murine microglial BV-2 cells were maintained in Dulbecco's modified Eagle medium (DMEM) with high glucose (Gibco BRL, Grand Island NY, USA), containing 5% (*v/v*) fetal bovine serum (Gibco BRL, Grand Island NY, USA) and incubated at 37 °C in humidified 5% CO_2. For gene expression assay, cells were seeded at a density of 5×10^5 cells/well in 12-well plate. After 24 h, the attached cells were pre-treated with adiponectin (100 ng/mL or 1000 ng/mL) for 1 h followed by the treatment with 200 μM palmitic acid (Sigma-Aldrich) for 4 h. The palmitic acid was dissolved in ethanol and conjugated into 10% bovine serum albumin (BSA).

4.4. Primary Astrocyte Culture

Following decapitation of five-day-old C57BL/6 mice, the diencephalon was removed under sterile conditions and triturated in Dulbecco's modified Eagle's medium (DMEM) F-12 containing 1% penicillin-streptomycin. The cell suspension was filtered through a 100-µm sterile cell strainer to remove debris and fibrous layers. The suspension was centrifuged, and the pellet resuspended in DMEM F-12, containing 10% fetal bovine serum (FBS) and 1% penicillin-streptomycin. The cells were then grown in this culture medium in 75-cm^3 culture flasks at 37 °C and 5% CO_2. When the cells reached confluence (at approximately nine days), microglia were separated from adhered astrocytes by shaking the culture at approximately 250 rpm for 2 h. The cells were then seeded onto 12-well tissue culture plates, previously coated with poly-D-lysine hydrobromide (50 µg/mL), after which they were distributed at 7.5×10^4 cells/well and incubated at 37 °C with 5% CO_2. For the astrocyte primary culture, the adhered cells were harvested using 0.05% trypsin-ethylenediamine tetraacetic acid, resuspended in DMEM F-12 containing 10% FBS and 1% penicillin-streptomycin, and centrifuged for 5 min at 1000 rpm. The cells were then seeded at a concentration of 5×10^5 cells/mL in culture plates previously treated with poly-L-lysine hydrobromide (50 µg/mL), and grown for 24 h.

4.5. Quantitative Real-Time PCR (qRT-PCR)

Total RNA was isolated from the hypothalamus, cultured BV-2 cells, primary microglia and primary astrocytes, and reverse-transcribed to make cDNA using maxime RT PreMix kit (Intron Biotechnology, Seoul, Korea). Real-time PCR amplification of the cDNA was analyzed with SYBR Green Real-time PCR Master Mix (Toyobo Co., Ltd., Osaka, Japan) in a Bio-Rad CFX 96 Real-Time Detection System (Bio-Rad Laboratories, Hercules, CA, USA). The results were analyzed by the CFX Manager software and normalized to the housekeeping gene β-actin. Primer sequences used are *IL-1β* F-AGGGCTGCTTCCAAACCTTTGAC, R-ATACTGCCTGCCTGAAGCTCTTGT; *IL-6* F-CCACTTCACAAGTCGGAGGCTTA, R-GCAAGTGCATCATCGTTGTTCATAC; *TNF-α* F-TGGGACAGTGACCTGGACTGT, R-TTCGGAAAGCCCATTTGAGT; *Cox-2* F-TGCTGTACAA GCAGTGGCAA, R-AGGGCTTTCAATTCTGCAGCC; *Iba-1* F-AGCTTTTGGACTGCTGAAGG, R-TTTGGACGGCAGATCCTCATC; *CD11b* F-CCACTCATTGTGGGCAGCTC, R-GGGCAGCTT CATTCATCATGTC; *Adiponectin* F-GTTGCAAGCTCTCCTGTTCC, R-TCTCCA GGAGTGCCATCTCT; *GFAP* F-TCAATGACCGCTTTG CTAGC, R-ACTCGTGCAGCCTTACACAG; *β-Actin* F-TGGAATCCT GTGGCATCCATGAAAC, R-TAAAACGCAGCTCAGTAACAGTAACAGTCCG.

4.6. Measurement of Cytokine Levels

Supernatant from cultured BV-2 cells were collected 1 h after adiponectin (100 ng/mL or 1000 ng/mL) treatment followed by administration of palmitic acid (200 µM) for 24 h. The concentration of released cytokines was measured using mouse IL-1β and IL-6 DuoSet (R&D Systems, Minneapolis, MN, USA) according to the manufacturer's instructions.

4.7. Immunoblot Analysis

BV-2 cells were seeded at a density of 1×10^6 cells/well in 6-well plate and pre-treated with adiponectin (100 ng/mL or 1000 ng/mL) for 1 h followed by palmitic acid treatment for 30 min or 4 h. The cells were rinsed with phosphate buffered saline (PBS), followed by scraping and resuspension of the cell pellet in RIPA lysis buffer containing protease inhibitors, and centrifuged to remove debris, unbroken cells and cellular nuclei. The samples containing 20 µg of total protein were subjected to immunoblot analysis using polyclonal antibodies including anti-phospho-ERK, anti-ERK (Cell Signaling, Danvers, MA, USA), anti-IκBα (Santa Cruz Biotechnology, Santa Cruz, CA, USA), and anti-β-actin (Sigma-Aldrich, St. Louis, MO, USA). Quantification of band intensity was conducted using Image J software. The band intensities were normalized by dividing their values by the value for the total ERK protein, or β-actin protein, for the same sample on the same blot.

4.8. Statistical Analysis

Statistical analyses were performed by Prism 6.0 software (GraphPad Software, San Diego, CA, USA). All the data are expressed as mean ± SEM. An unpaired t test was performed to analyze the significance between the two experimental groups. Two-way ANOVA analysis was performed to detect the interaction between two treatments. Significance was taken at $p < 0.05$.

Author Contributions: Data curation, B.S.P.; Funding acquisition, J.G.K.; Investigation, H.L., T.H.T. and J.G.K.; Validation, J.G.K.; Writing – original draft, T.H.T. and J.G.K.; Writing – review & editing, S.Y.

Funding: This work was supported by a grant of the Korea Health Technology R&D Project through the Korea Health Industry Development Institute (KHIDI), funded by the Ministry of Health & Welfare, Republic of Korea (grant number: HI17C1600) and supported by an Incheon National University (International Cooperative) Research Grant for Jae Geun Kim.

Conflicts of Interest: The authors declare no conflicts of interest.

References

1. Lumeng, C.N.; Saltiel, A.R. Inflammatory links between obesity and metabolic disease. *J. Clin. Investig.* **2011**, *121*, 2111–2117. [CrossRef] [PubMed]
2. Posey, K.A.; Clegg, D.J.; Printz, R.L.; Byun, J.; Morton, G.J.; Vivekanandan-Giri, A.; Pennathur, S.; Baskin, D.G.; Heinecke, J.W.; Woods, S.C.; et al. Hypothalamic proinflammatory lipid accumulation, inflammation, and insulin resistance in rats fed a high-fat diet. *Am. J. Physiol. Endocrinol. Metab.* **2009**, *296*, E1003–E1012. [CrossRef] [PubMed]
3. Esser, N.; Legrand-Poels, S.; Piette, J.; Scheen, A.J.; Paquot, N. Inflammation as a link between obesity, metabolic syndrome and type 2 diabetes. *Diabetes Res. Clin. Pract.* **2014**, *105*, 141–150. [CrossRef] [PubMed]
4. Thaler, J.P.; Guyenet, S.J.; Dorfman, M.D.; Wisse, B.E.; Schwartz, M.W. Hypothalamic inflammation: Marker or mechanism of obesity pathogenesis? *Diabetes* **2013**, *62*, 2629–2634. [CrossRef]
5. Thaler, J.P.; Yi, C.-X.; Schur, E.A.; Guyenet, S.J.; Hwang, B.H.; Dietrich, M.O.; Zhao, X.; Sarruf, D.A.; Izgur, V.; Maravilla, K.R.; et al. Obesity is associated with hypothalamic injury in rodents and humans. *J. Clin. Investig.* **2012**, *122*, 153–162. [CrossRef]
6. Valdearcos, M.; Douglass, J.D.; Robblee, M.M.; Dorfman, M.D.; Stifler, D.R.; Bennett, M.L.; Gerritse, I.; Fasnacht, R.; Barres, B.A.; Thaler, J.P.; et al. Microglial inflammatory signaling orchestrates the hypothalamic immune response to dietary excess and mediates obesity susceptibility. *Cell Metab.* **2017**, *26*, 185–197. [CrossRef]
7. Koch, C.E.; Lowe, C.; Legler, K.; Benzler, J.; Boucsein, A.; Böttiger, G.; Grattan, D.R.; Williams, L.M.; Tups, A. Central adiponectin acutely improves glucose tolerance in male mice. *Endocrinology* **2014**, *155*, 1806–1816. [CrossRef]
8. Liu, Y.; Turdi, S.; Park, T.; Morris, N.J.; Deshaies, Y.; Xu, A.; Sweeney, G. Adiponectin corrects high-fat diet-induced disturbances in muscle metabolomic profile and whole-body glucose homeostasis. *Diabetes* **2013**, *62*, 743–752. [CrossRef]
9. Song, J.; Lee, J.E. Adiponectin as a new paradigm for approaching Alzheimer's disease. *Anat. Cell Biol.* **2013**, *46*, 229–234. [CrossRef]
10. Chan, K.-H.; Lam, K.S.-L.; Cheng, O.-Y.; Kwan, J.S.-C.; Ho, P.W.-L.; Cheng, K.K.-Y.; Chung, S.K.; Ho, J.W.-M.; Guo, V.Y.; Xu, A. Adiponectin is protective against oxidative stress induced cytotoxicity in amyloid-beta neurotoxicity. *PLoS ONE* **2012**, *7*, e52354. [CrossRef]
11. Chen, B.; Liao, W.-Q.; Xu, N.; Xu, H.; Wen, J.-Y.; Yu, C.-A.; Liu, X.-Y.; Li, C.-L.; Zhao, S.-M.; Campbell, W. Adiponectin protects against cerebral ischemia-reperfusion injury through anti-inflammatory action. *Brain Res.* **2009**, *1273*, 129–137. [CrossRef] [PubMed]
12. Ding, W.; Zhang, X.; Huang, H.; Ding, N.; Zhang, S.; Hutchinson, S.Z.; Zhang, X. Adiponectin protects rat myocardium against chronic intermittent hypoxia-induced injury via inhibition of endoplasmic reticulum stress. *PLoS ONE* **2014**, *9*, e94545. [CrossRef] [PubMed]

13. Naitoh, R.; Miyawaki, K.; Harada, N.; Mizunoya, W.; Toyoda, K.; Fushiki, T.; Yamada, Y.; Seino, Y.; Inagaki, N. Inhibition of GIP signaling modulates adiponectin levels under high-fat diet in mice. *Biochem. Biophys. Res. Commun.* **2008**, *376*, 21–25. [CrossRef]
14. Ohsawa, K.; Imai, Y.; Kanazawa, H.; Sasaki, Y.; Kohsaka, S. Involvement of Iba1 in membrane ruffling and phagocytosis of macrophages/microglia. *J. Cell Sci.* **2000**, *113*, 1–12.
15. Tanaka, Y.; Aleksunes, L.M.; Yeager, R.L.; Gyamfi, M.A.; Esterly, N.; Guo, G.L.; Klaassen, C.D. NF-E2-related factor 2 inhibits lipid accumulation and oxidative stress in mice fed a high-fat diet. *J. Pharmacol. Exp. Ther.* **2008**, *325*, 655–664. [CrossRef] [PubMed]
16. Valdearcos, M.; Robblee, M.M.; Benjamin, D.I.; Nomura, D.K.; Xu, A.W.; Koliwad, S.K. Microglia dictate the impact of saturated fat consumption on hypothalamic inflammation and neuronal function. *Cell Rep.* **2014**, *9*, 2124–2138. [CrossRef]
17. Tu, T.H.; Kim, H.; Yang, S.; Kim, J.K.; Kim, J.G. Linoleic acid rescues microglia inflammation triggered by saturated fatty acid. *Biochem. Biophys. Res. Commun.* **2019**, *513*, 1–6. [CrossRef]
18. Jiang, B.; Xu, S.; Hou, X.; Pimentel, D.R.; Brecher, P.; Cohen, R.A. Temporal control of NF-kappaB activation by ERK differentially regulates interleukin-1beta-induced gene expression. *J. Biol. Chem.* **2004**, *279*, 1323–1329. [CrossRef]
19. Dumitru, C.D.; Ceci, J.D.; Tsatsanis, C.; Kontoyiannis, D.; Stamatakis, K.; Lin, J.H.; Patriotis, C.; Jenkins, N.A.; Copeland, N.G.; Kollias, G.; et al. TNF-alpha induction by LPS is regulated posttranscriptionally via a Tpl2/ERK-dependent pathway. *Cell* **2000**, *103*, 1071–1083. [CrossRef]
20. Yamamoto, Y.; Gaynor, R.B. IkappaB kinases: Key regulators of the NF-kappaB pathway. *Trends Biochem. Sci.* **2004**, *29*, 72–79. [CrossRef]
21. Greenberg, A.S.; Obin, M.S. Obesity and the role of adipose tissue in inflammation and metabolism. *Am. J. Clin. Nutr.* **2006**, *83*, 461S–465S. [CrossRef] [PubMed]
22. Kershaw, E.E.; Flier, J.S. Adipose tissue as an endocrine organ. *J. Clin. Endocrinol. Metab.* **2004**, *89*, 2548–2556. [CrossRef]
23. Shadid, S.; Koutsari, C.; Jensen, M.D. Direct free fatty acid uptake into human adipocytes in vivo: Relation to body fat distribution. *Diabetes* **2007**, *56*, 1369–1375. [CrossRef] [PubMed]
24. Mohamed-Ali, V.; Pinkney, J.H.; Coppack, S.W. Adipose tissue as an endocrine and paracrine organ. *Int. J. Obes. Relat. Metab. Disord.* **1998**, *22*, 1145–1158. [CrossRef]
25. Rosen, E.D.; Spiegelman, B.M. Adipocytes as regulators of energy balance and glucose homeostasis. *Nature* **2006**, *444*, 847–853. [CrossRef] [PubMed]
26. Woods, S.C.; Seeley, R.J.; Porte, D.; Schwartz, M.W. Signals that regulate food intake and energy homeostasis. *Science* **1998**, *280*, 1378–1383. [CrossRef] [PubMed]
27. Ouchi, N.; Walsh, K. Adiponectin as an anti-inflammatory factor. *Clin. Chim. Acta* **2007**, *380*, 24–30. [CrossRef]
28. Whitehead, J.P.; Richards, A.A.; Hickman, I.J.; Macdonald, G.A.; Prins, J.B. Adiponectin—A key adipokine in the metabolic syndrome. *Diabetes Obes. Metab.* **2006**, *8*, 264–280. [CrossRef]
29. Ng, R.; Chan, K.-H. Potential neuroprotective effects of adiponectin in Alzheimer's disease. *Int. J. Mol. Sci.* **2017**, *18*, 592. [CrossRef]
30. Graeber, M.B.; Li, W.; Rodriguez, M.L. Role of microglia in CNS inflammation. *FEBS Lett.* **2011**, *585*, 3798–3805. [CrossRef]
31. Wang, W.-Y.; Tan, M.-S.; Yu, J.-T.; Tan, L. Role of pro-inflammatory cytokines released from microglia in Alzheimer's disease. *Ann. Transl. Med.* **2015**, *3*, 136. [PubMed]
32. Pistell, P.J.; Morrison, C.D.; Gupta, S.; Knight, A.G.; Keller, J.N.; Ingram, D.K.; Bruce-Keller, A.J. Cognitive impairment following high fat diet consumption is associated with brain inflammation. *J. Neuroimmunol.* **2010**, *219*, 25–32. [CrossRef] [PubMed]
33. Williams, L.M. Hypothalamic dysfunction in obesity. *Proc. Nutr. Soc.* **2012**, *71*, 521–533. [CrossRef] [PubMed]
34. André, C.; Guzman-Quevedo, O.; Rey, C.; Rémus-Borel, J.; Clark, S.; Castellanos-Jankiewicz, A.; Ladeveze, E.; Leste-Lasserre, T.; Nadjar, A.; Abrous, D.N.; et al. Inhibiting microglia expansion prevents diet-induced hypothalamic and peripheral inflammation. *Diabetes* **2017**, *66*, 908–919. [CrossRef] [PubMed]
35. Milanski, M.; Degasperi, G.; Coope, A.; Morari, J.; Denis, R.; Cintra, D.E.; Tsukumo, D.M.L.; Anhe, G.; Amaral, M.E.; Takahashi, H.K.; et al. Saturated fatty acids produce an inflammatory response predominantly through the activation of TLR4 signaling in hypothalamus: Implications for the pathogenesis of obesity. *J. Neurosci.* **2009**, *29*, 359–370. [CrossRef] [PubMed]

36. Ouchi, N.; Parker, J.L.; Lugus, J.J.; Walsh, K. Adipokines in inflammation and metabolic disease. *Nat. Rev. Immunol.* **2011**, *11*, 85–97. [CrossRef]
37. Cahill, F.; Amini, P.; Wadden, D.; Khalili, S.; Randell, E.; Vasdev, S.; Gulliver, W.; Sun, G. Short-Term overfeeding increases circulating adiponectin independent of obesity status. *PLoS ONE* **2013**, *8*, e74215. [CrossRef]

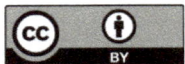

© 2019 by the authors. Licensee MDPI, Basel, Switzerland. This article is an open access article distributed under the terms and conditions of the Creative Commons Attribution (CC BY) license (http://creativecommons.org/licenses/by/4.0/).

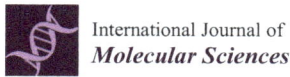 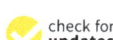

Review

The Novel Perspectives of Adipokines on Brain Health

Thomas Ho-yin Lee [1], Kenneth King-yip Cheng [2], Ruby Lai-chong Hoo [3], Parco Ming-fai Siu [4] and Suk-yu Yau [1,*]

1. Department of Rehabilitation Sciences, Faculty of Health and Social Sciences, The Hong Kong Polytechnic University, 11 Yuk Choi Road, Hung Hum, Hong Kong; thomas.hy.lee@connect.polyu.hk
2. Department of Health Technology and Informatics, Faculty of Health and Social Sciences, The Hong Kong Polytechnic University, 11 Yuk Choi Road, Hung Hom, Hong Kong; kenneth.ky.cheng@polyu.edu.hk
3. Department of Pharmacology and Pharmacy, Li Ka Shing Faculty of Medicine, The University of Hong Kong, 11 Sassoon Road, Pokfulam, Hong Kong; rubyhoo@hku.hk
4. Division of Kinesiology, School of Public Health, Li Ka Shing Faculty of Medicine, The University of Hong Kong, 5 Sassoon Road, Pokfulam, Hong Kong; pmsiu@hku.hk
* Correspondence: sonata.yau@polyu.edu.hk

Received: 16 October 2019; Accepted: 6 November 2019; Published: 11 November 2019

Abstract: First seen as a fat-storage tissue, the adipose tissue is considered as a critical player in the endocrine system. Precisely, adipose tissue can produce an array of bioactive factors, including cytokines, lipids, and extracellular vesicles, which target various systemic organ systems to regulate metabolism, homeostasis, and immune response. The global effects of adipokines on metabolic events are well defined, but their impacts on brain function and pathology remain poorly defined. Receptors of adipokines are widely expressed in the brain. Mounting evidence has shown that leptin and adiponectin can cross the blood–brain barrier, while evidence for newly identified adipokines is limited. Significantly, adipocyte secretion is liable to nutritional and metabolic states, where defective circuitry, impaired neuroplasticity, and elevated neuroinflammation are symptomatic. Essentially, neurotrophic and anti-inflammatory properties of adipokines underlie their neuroprotective roles in neurodegenerative diseases. Besides, adipocyte-secreted lipids in the bloodstream can act endocrine on the distant organs. In this article, we have reviewed five adipokines (leptin, adiponectin, chemerin, apelin, visfatin) and two lipokines (palmitoleic acid and lysophosphatidic acid) on their roles involving in eating behavior, neurotrophic and neuroprotective factors in the brain. Understanding and regulating these adipokines can lead to novel therapeutic strategies to counteract metabolic associated eating disorders and neurodegenerative diseases, thus promote brain health.

Keywords: adipokine; adipose-brain axis; brain health; neurodegeneration; depression

1. Introduction

Adipose tissues are recognized as highly dynamic endocrine tissues exhibiting extensive physiological functions [1]. Adipose tissue is composed of mature adipocytes as well as the stromal vascular fraction, where adipose-derived stem cells, blood cells, fibroblasts, and nerves reside [2]. White and brown adipose tissues are the two fat tissues in mammals. The adipocytes in white and brown adipose tissues are morphologically and functionally distinct. Brown adipose tissues are accountable for thermogenesis by their abundant mitochondria and extensive vascularization [3,4], whereas white adipose tissues are preferably responsible for energy storage in the form of triglycerides. During fasting conditions, insulin inhibits lipolysis in white adipose tissues, where triglycerides are hydrolyzed into fatty acids and glycerol to generate energy [5]. In response to the nutritional states, adipose tissue plays an endocrine role by synthesizing and secreting bioactive compounds termed adipokines. Adipokine secretion is essential to energy and metabolic homeostasis [6]. Adipsin and leptin are the first adipokines identified [7,8]. Since then, many pivotal adipokines, such as adiponectin, resistin, and tumor necrosis factor α (TNF-α), have been extensively studied in metabolism and metabolic syndromes [9]. Novel adipokines, including chemerin, omentin, apelin, and adipocyte fatty acid-binding protein, have been identified by their metabolic functions resembling former adipokines and their alterations afflicted by metabolic diseases in humans [10].

The adipose-brain axis was first established with the discovery of leptin as an endocrine hormone targeting the hypothalamus to regulate energy balance, satiety, metabolism, and body weight [11]. It was later demonstrated that leptin signaling is also involved in hippocampal neuroplasticity [12]. De la Monte et al. have suggested that energy metabolism, glucose utilization, and insulin sensitization are compromised in Alzheimer's disease (AD) patients, whereas these pathological symptoms may contribute to AD neuropathology [13–16]. Since AD neuropathology highly resembles the pathology of diabetes mellitus, AD is now recognized as the 'type 3 diabetes'. Adiponectin promotes insulin sensitivity [17], whereas adiponectin deficiency exacerbates insulin resistance [18] and AD neuropathology [19]. Concerns are raised regarding how metabolic syndromes are linked to neurodegenerative diseases and mood disorders [20,21]. Given that adipose tissue is a major organ to regulate metabolism through adipokines, understanding the central function of adipokines in the brain can illustrate how the adipose-brain crosstalk works to prevent metabolic diseases and to promote brain health.

Metabolic dysfunction could share common molecular mechanisms with neurodegenerative diseases [22]. Therefore, emerging studies aim at investigating how adipose tissue exerts neuroprotective effects and influences neuroplasticity through secreting adipokines. Notably, several adipokines can cross the blood–brain barrier and act on the brain directly [1], while a damaged barrier will hinder adipose-secreting compounds entering the brain [23]. At present, it is noticeable that adipokines can modulate neuroplasticity. Accumulated studies have shown that leptin and adiponectin pathways can regulate cell proliferation [24,25], survival [19,26,27], and synaptic plasticity [12,28] by modulating cellular metabolism [29,30] and suppressing inflammatory response [31–33] in the brain. Previous studies focus on the acute action of leptin on synaptic plasticity, whereas recent studies report insulin resistance afflicts circulating leptin levels and affects central neuroplasticity and cognitive functions. Besides, animal studies have demonstrated a possible link between metabolic disorders with aberrant circulating adipokine levels and cognitive behavioral deficits [34–38] or neuropathology [39–41].

This review summarizes the emerging evidence on the roles of five adipokines, including leptin, adiponectin, chemerin, apelin, and visfatin, on promoting neuroplasticity. Furthermore, this review will discuss how diet-, obesity-, and diabetes-related conditions alter the adipokine levels and impair neuroplasticity and cognitive function in terms of mood as well as learning and memory.

2. Effects of Conventional and Novel Adipokines on the Brain

The neuroendocrine roles of leptin and adiponectin have been widely studied. Leptin and adiponectin receptors are widely expressed across many brain regions, in particular, the hippocampus, a critical region for spatial learning and memory formation, and emotional regulation [42]. Both leptin and adiponectin are shown to affect synaptic plasticity in the hippocampus. However, the neuroprotective effects of other adipokines, including chemerin, apelin, and visfatin, are mostly unknown.

2.1. Leptin

Leptin is mostly secreted by white adipose tissue to regulate energy homeostasis by suppressing food intake and thereby reducing weight loss [43]. Circulating leptin levels are positively correlated with adiposity [44] and caloric intake [45–49]. In the obese population, increased adiposity is the primary cause of hyperleptinemia, a condition with high circulating leptin levels [44]. Obese subjects are refractory to the anorexigenic effect of leptin due to leptin resistance in the brain and peripheral tissues [50]. Similarly, patients with type 2 diabetes mellitus comorbid with obesity show both insulin-resistance and hyperleptinemia [51]. Multiple studies have demonstrated the effectiveness of exogenous leptin administration on improving insulin resistance in different obese and diabetic rodent models. Mouse models that feature obesity, hyperglycemia, hyperinsulinemia, particularly db/db (leptin-deficient) mice, and Zucker fa/fa (loss-of-function leptin receptor) rats resemble type 2 diabetic conditions in humans. Infusion of recombinant leptin for seven days is sufficient to ameliorate hyperglycemia and hyperinsulinemia in leptin-deficient ob/ob mice [52]. Leptin treatment can also improve insulin resistance, and glucose and lipid imbalances in some type 2 diabetic models [53–56]. However, mice receiving chronic (>20 weeks) high-fat diet are resistant to leptin even when leptin is directly infused into the cerebral ventricle of the brain [57–60]. Prominently, leptin also fails to improve diabetes and insulin resistance in type 2 diabetic patients comorbid with obesity [61,62]. These suggest that leptin replacement therapy is feasible when deficient. However, further elevation in the leptin-resistant state will not improve metabolic syndrome.

Adiposity hinges on excessive caloric intake and accumulation, whereas food consumption is a complex behavior integrating energy homeostasis, reward system, and stress. Leptin is an appetite hormone, where leptin receptors are expressed in multiple brain regions [63]. Leptin exerts dual actions to regulate anorexigenic-mediated energy homeostasis [64] as well as to suppress the food-cued reward circuit in the hypothalamus [65,66]. Hypothalamus is the main target of leptin in the brain by eliciting a homeostatic response to energy accumulation in accord with nutritional states. In response to energy accumulation, leptin inhibits orexigenic neurons expressing neuropeptide Y (NPY) and agouti-related peptide (AgRP) as well as activates the anorexigenic proopiomelanocortin (POMC) neurons in the hypothalamic arcuate nucleus (ARC). The inclusive anorexigenic effect prevails during energy accumulation after feeding together with an increased body fat oxidation, and hence suppresses leptin synthesis and secretion in a negative feedback loop [67]. On the other hand, plasma leptin levels are decreased by fasting before fat depletion [68], which in turn, disinhibits orexigenic action and stimulates the appetite.

Hedonic behavior in response to food is mediated by the mesolimbic circuit involving endocannabinoid [69], orexinergic [70], and dopaminergic signaling. The food-induced hedonic circuit can possibly override homeostatic feeding. The lateral hypothalamic (LH) together with the mesolimbic reward circuit, which involves the ventral tegmental area (VTA) and nucleus accumbens (NAc) predominate the hedonic circuit, where leptin elicits anorectic action by inhibiting multiple signaling along the circuit [71–73]. Orexin is a neuropeptide that mediates energy sensing, appetite, body weight, and reinforces reward behaviors [74–76]. Orexin-expressing neurons located in the LH innervate in the VTA, where leptin receptors are expressed [77]. Leptin can suppress activities of orexin-expressing neurons in the LH, as shown in electrophysiological recordings [77]. Besides, intra-LH leptin infusion abolishes high-fat diet-conditioned place preference mediated by orexin-expressing neurons [77]. Of note, endocannabinoid signaling is in part involved in the leptin inhibitory action on orexin-expressing neurons. Leptin deficiency and high-fat diet could enhance cannabinoid receptor-mediated presynaptic inhibitory control of orexin-expressing neurons in the hypothalamic ARC [69]. These findings taken together suggest the leptin suppresses hedonic behavior in the hypothalamus involving orexigenic and endocannabinoid signaling. In addition, dopamine release in the NAc is an adaptive response to palatable food consumption in association with reward learning and incentive salience [78–80]. A recent review has comprehensively addressed the crosstalk of leptin and dopamine signaling in inhibiting the food reward system through the LH-VTA-NAc neural circuit [81]. The LH GABA-ergic projection to the VTA expresses leptin receptors [82]. Leptin promotes GABA release from the LH to VTA is associated with reduced food consumption in leptin-deficient mice [82]. The inhibitory effect of leptin in the reward circuit is further supported by the lentiviral-mediated knockdown of the leptin receptor in the LH [83]. Finally, leptin receptors are also expressed in dopaminergic innervation from the VTA to the NAc. Intra-VTA infusion of leptin suppresses food intake [84]. Inhibition of dopaminergic neuron activity in the VTA neurons [85] and the reduced dopamine levels in the NAc [86] may downregulate the reward system. The underlying molecular signaling for leptin inhibition in the VTA dopaminergic neuron may activate the Janus kinase-signal transducer and activator of transcription proteins JAK/STAT/PI3K/mTOR pathway [84,87]. Significantly, long-term overexpression of leptin in the VTA causes leptin receptor desensitization [88]. Conversely, adenoviral-mediated knockdown of leptin receptor in the VTA promotes food intake and sucrose preference [89], and leptin antagonism or knockout in the VTA increases NAc dopamine levels [90]. The abovementioned studies concertedly suggest the overconsumption behavior and continuous body weight gain regardless of hyperleptinemia in obese subjects [91]. Enlarged adipocyte is the culprit of hyperleptinemia. And potentially, instead of exhibiting a stronger anorexigenic effect or a stronger inhibition of hedonic reward, prolonged hyperleptinemia may desensitize the leptin receptor-mediated signaling [60]. These result in a vicious cycle of hedonic eating and obesity.

Excessive caloric intake and energy accumulation are not the only causes of obesity. Chronic atypical antipsychotic medication is obesogenic in association with severe metabolic disorders, including hyperglycemia, insulin resistance, and hyperleptinemia [92–98]. In particular, weight gain, increased food consumption, and hyperleptinemia are frequently reported in psychotic patients receiving olanzapine medication [99,100]. Significant elevation of circulating leptin is detected in schizophrenic subjects receiving haloperidol medication (pre, typical antipsychotic treatment) versus risperidone and clozapine medication (post, atypical antipsychotic treatment) [101]. Elevated leptin levels and weight gain in schizophrenic patients treated with atypical antipsychotics may be involved in an adiposity-induced feedback mechanism [102]. Rodent studies further support the fact that the atypical antipsychotics, namely risperidone and olanzapine, are obesogenic as well as induce leptin expression and secretion [103–106]. Essentially, antipsychotics can act on multiple neuroendocrine pathways. Alongside with serotoninergic antagonism that may underline hedonic feeding behaviors and atypical weight gain [107–109], some atypical antipsychotics can contravene energy homeostasis by inhibiting peripheral adrenergic system [97]. β-3 antagonism by atypical antipsychotics can not only disrupt energy homeostasis [110,111] but also induce hyperleptinemia [112]. In sum, atypical antipsychotics are obesogenic by contravening brain anorexigenic and reward circuit as well as disrupting normal adipocyte functioning.

Besides, leptin receptors are found in the hippocampus and neocortex, suggesting their possible roles in the cognitive process [63]. Leptin resistance in obese and diabetic patients can be linked to impaired leptin receptor signaling [64] and leptin insensitivity at the blood–brain barrier [50,113]. Although both leptin mRNA and protein expressions are widely detected in the brain [114,115], circulating leptin can pass through the blood–brain barrier [116] and could function as a neurotrophic factor in modulating neuroplasticity and cognitive functions [117]. *db/db* mice, which show loss of function in leptin receptor signaling, display neuronal atrophy in the hippocampus, including reduced hippocampal progenitor cell proliferation [118], reduced dendritic branching and dendritic spine [119]. Besides, both *db/db* mice and Zucker *fa/fa* rats show spatial memory deficits in the Morris water maze task [118,120,121] and exhibit despair behaviors [122], suggesting that impaired leptin signaling could affect structural plasticity in the hippocampus. HFD-induced diabetic model [123] and *db/db* mice [124] display hyperleptinemia and leptin resistance. Enhancing leptin levels enhances neuroplasticity and cognitive function in rodents under physiological conditions. For example, intraperitoneal injection with 1 mg/kg recombinant leptin continuously for 14 days promotes hippocampal cell proliferation and survival of newborn neurons in healthy male mice [24]. An in vitro study has demonstrated that leptin promotes dendritic branching and spine maturation in cultured primary neurons [125]. Moreover, leptin elicits a rapid antidepressant effect by reducing depression-like behavior in the forced swim test and tail suspension test [126]. Intrahippocampal infusion with leptin immediately after training improves memory processing in T-maze footshock avoidance and step down passive avoidance tests [127], suggesting that leptin has a direct effect on influencing hippocampal function and enhances behavioral outcome. Notably, previous studies have shown that leptin treatment via systemic injection or intra-hippocampus injection to the dorsal part can improve spatial and context-cued learning and memory. Nonetheless, a study has reported that leptin infusion in the ventral hippocampus, but not in the dorsal hippocampus, impairs memory consolidation for the spatial location of food [128]. A recent review suggests that activating the leptin signaling pathway, specifically in the ventral hippocampus, could suppress spatial working memory [129]. Mechanisms of how leptin affects structural plasticity in the hippocampus are still unclear. Leptin receptors are coupled to JAK/STAT and PI3K/Akt signaling cascades in hippocampal neurons. Activation of the above cascades increases the production of manganese superoxide dismutase (Mn-SOD), an antioxidant enzyme, as well as the anti-apoptotic protein Bcl-xL. The synergistic antioxidant and anti-apoptotic effects may stabilize the mitochondrial membrane potential, and hence lessen mitochondrial oxidative stress to promote neuronal proliferation in the hippocampus [26]. Leptin treatment could increase hippocampal cell proliferation and survival by increasing mitochondrial functioning. In addition, leptin can also promote synaptogenesis via increasing expression of microRNA-132 (miR-132) [119]. Leptin induces long-term potentiation (LTP) by modulating post-synaptic signaling pathway and glutamatergic N-methyl-D-aspartate (NMDA) receptor. LTP is considered as a cellular mechanism of learning and memory formation. The NMDA receptor-dependent LTP in the CA1 region of the hippocampus underlies spatial memory formation [130]. Both db/db mice and Zucker fa/fa rats with defective leptin receptors impair hippocampal LTP formation [120], whereas infusion of 1 µM leptin into the hippocampal dentate gyrus enhances LTP [131]. Ex vivo studies also show that leptin can increase pharmacologically-isolated NMDA receptor-mediated excitatory postsynaptic currents (EPSCs) in the CA1 region in acute rat hippocampal slices [132] (Table 1).

Neuroprotective effects of leptin have also been shown in animal models. Eight weeks of systemic infusion with leptin reduces amyloid-β levels in the brain and serum of six-month old CRND8 transgenic mouse model of AD. Leptin treatment also improves object recognition and contextual fear learning [133]. Moreover, intracerebroventricular injection of leptin (1 µg) for ten days improves spatial memory in Y-maze and water maze tasks, as well as restores LTP in the CA1 region in an Aβ-induced AD rat model [134]. The neuroprotective effects of leptin could be linked to a leptin/JAK2/STAT3 signaling pathway [135] or leptin mediated PI3K/Akt/mTOR signaling pathway [136]. In sum, leptin can directly modulate structural and synaptic plasticity, however prolonged elevation in leptin levels could be detrimental to neuroplasticity under hyperleptinemia condition.

2.2. Adiponectin

Adiponectin is secreted by white adipose tissue and exerts anti-inflammatory effects on both endocrine and cardiovascular systems [137,138]. Adiponectin receptors (AdipoRs) express differentially in peripheral tissues. AdipoR1 is highly expressed in skeletal muscle, while AdipoR2 is abundant in the liver [139]. Hypoadiponectinemia, a condition of low circulating adiponectin, is commonly observed in obese and type 2 diabetic patients [140–142]. In line with clinical evidence, diabetic and obese mice also have reduced adiponectin expression in adipose tissues as well as the blood [143–146]. Circulating adiponectin levels are reduced in obesity [140–142], whereas the expressions of adiponectin receptors are increased, as evidenced by higher mRNA expressions of AdipoR1 in skeletal muscle in obese subjects [147] and AdipoR2 in insulin-resistant subjects [148]. Recombinant adiponectin treatment can reduce body weight and increase hepatic and muscular insulin sensitivity in an adiponectin-deficient mouse model [149]. Similarly, patients receiving rosiglitazone, an insulin sensitizer targeting the adipose tissue, experience increased plasma adiponectin by approximately two-fold [150]. These findings indicate that upregulating adiponectin expression can improve insulin sensitivity. Adiponectin receptors (AdipoR) are widely expressed in rodent brains, including the hypothalamus, brainstem, prefrontal cortex, and hippocampus, suggesting its role in the CNS in addition to its role in metabolism [27,139,151–159]. Overnight fasting by food deprivation for sixteen hours concomitantly downregulates mRNA expression of adiponectin and upregulates mRNA expression levels of AdipoR1 and APPL1 in the hypothalamic ARC [160], a brain area in the mediobasal hypothalamus regulating energy and glucose homeostasis [161].

Adiponectin could enter the blood–brain barrier since the low-molecular weight trimeric form of adiponectin is detectable in cerebrospinal fluid after intravenous injection in adiponectin-deficient mice [25,162]. Prominently, adiponectin is involved in energy homeostasis and appetite in concordance with leptin. A recent investigation shows that adiponectin promotes anorexigenic POMC activity in the hypothalamic ARC [163] possibly through PI3-K signaling [164]. Adiponectin elicits an excitatory effect on POMC neurons in a leptin-receptor dependent manner [163], whereas leptin synergistically potentiates adiponectin excitatory effect on POMC neuronal activity [163]. Simultaneously, adiponectin inhibits the neighboring orexigenic NPY/AgRP neurons, which then disinhibit POMC activity [163]. Further studies show that adiponectin action on the hypothalamic POMC activity may occur in a glucose-dependent reciprocal manner. Adiponectin infusion in the cerebral ventricle exerts an orexigenic effect at high glucose levels but is anorexigenic at low glucose levels [165]. Moreover, adiponectin increases the anorexigenic POMC activity at low glucose levels (2.5–5 mM), mimicking the fasting and physiological states, but decreases the POMC activity at high glucose levels (10 mM), mimicking a fed state [165] in electrophysiological recordings. The state-dependent adiponectin mechanism of action may act differentially on different molecular pathways: Adiponectin inhibits POMC neurons at high glucose via AMPK signaling, while it activates POMC neurons at low glucose via PI3-K signaling [165]. In contrast to the glucose-dependent effect in POMC, adiponectin enhances the activity of inhibitory GABA-ergic NPY neurons in a glucose-independent fashion [166]. Altogether, at low glucose conditions, adiponectin suppresses orexigenic NPY neurons and activates anorexigenic POMC neurons to attenuate appetite and food intake under conditions of fasting or low blood glucose. On the other hand, at high glucose levels, feeding behavior is nullified [165] as adiponectin inhibits both anorexigenic and orexigenic activities. Since leptin resistance and hypoadiponectinemia are symptomatic in obese and type 2 diabetic subjects, disrupted interplay of leptin and adiponectin may collectively impair anorectic actions and thus promote caloric intake and energy accumulation in obese and diabetic conditions. Hypoadiponectinemia is often documented in patients receiving atypical antipsychotics medication, including olanzapine and clozapine, in association with increased adiposity and hyperleptinemia [68,167,168]. Specifically, clozapine medication leads to body weight gain, high triglyceride profile, and hypoadiponectinemia [169,170]. GABA-facilitated orexigenic NPY activation and the subsequent suppression of anorexigenic POMC activity is suggested to be a potential mechanism of olanzapine-induced obesity [171]. The disrupted hypothalamic control of energy homeostasis may, therefore, lead to hyperleptinemia and hypoadiponectinemia. Still, some atypical antipsychotics, including risperidone and quetiapine, do not affect adiponectin levels [168,172–174].

AdipoR1 is expressed in dopaminergic neurons in the VTA [175]. The adiponectin receptor expression implicates the crosstalk of adiponectin and dopamine signaling pathways. Hedonic behaviors and affective behaviors are intertwined by dopamine signaling [176–179]. Recent research dissecting the role of adiponectin receptor in mediating anxiety reveals that intra-VTA infusion of adiponectin or the adiponectin receptor agonist AdipoRon suppresses dopaminergic neuron firing in an AdipoR1-dependent manner [175]. However, impaired adiponectin signaling due to adiponectin haploinsufficiency or AdipoR1 ablation increases dopaminergic activity and anxiety behavior. Adiponectin action shares similarities with the inhibitory action of leptin on the VTA dopaminergic neurons. Importantly, anxiety symptoms are often comorbid with metabolic disorders [180], where hypoadiponectinemia is indicative in obese and type 2 diabetic subjects [140,141,181]. It is speculated that the interplay of leptin and adiponectin may also exist in the VTA dopaminergic neurons to modulate reward and affective behaviors.

Patients with type 2 diabetes or dementia display decreased adiponectin levels [182–184]. High fat diet-induced and streptozotocin-induced diabetic conditions reduce AdipoR1 and AdipoR2 expressions in the hippocampus [27]. Adiponectin knockout reduces proliferating cells, differentiating cells, and cell survival in the hippocampus [185]. Adiponectin stimulates the proliferation of hippocampal progenitors through p38MAPK/GSK-3β/β-catenin cascade [157]. Moreover, adiponectin deficiency reduces the dendritic length, branching, and spine density of dentate granule neurons, particularly in early-born granule neurons in the hippocampal dentate gyrus [185]. Low levels of adiponectin are associated with cognitive dysfunction [184]. Chronic adiponectin deficiency impairs spatial memory and learning and induces anxiety-like behavior [19]. Moreover, AdipoR1 knockdown causes metabolic dysfunction and neurodegeneration in an association with the cognitive deficit in Morris water maze [186]. Overexpression of adiponectin in the brain [25] or infusion of recombinant adiponectin into the cerebral ventricle induces antidepressant effects [158,187,188]. The antidepressant effect could be linked to the activation of the AdipoR1/APPL1/AMPK pathway [25]. Rosiglitazone, a blood–brain barrier-impermeable PPARγ-selective agonist, enhances adiponectin levels and elicits antidepressant- and anxiolytic-like effects in wild-type mice, but not adiponectin-deficient mice or mice pretreated with PPARγ-selective antagonist [189].

The pro-cognitive effect of adiponectin in AD could be linked to its anti-inflammatory effect and enhanced effects on synaptic plasticity. Globular adiponectin predominantly binds to AdipoR1 and inhibits nuclear factor-κB (NF-κB) activation in macrophages, which in turn, suppresses its production of pro-inflammatory cytokines [190,191]. Therefore, adiponectin may reduce the extracellular deposition of amyloid-β via its suppressive effect on microglial activation. Moreover, adiponectin attenuates streptozotocin-induced Tau hyperphosphorylation and cognitive deficits through PI3K/Akt/GSK-3β pathway [192]. Activating AMPK can suppress GSK-3β action on Tau phosphorylation, whereas chronic adiponectin deficiency fails to phosphorylate AMPK, which in turn, enables GSK3β action on promoting Tau hyperphosphorylation, and subsequently results in AD-like neuropathology [19]. Nine-month-old adiponectin-deficient, 5×FAD mice show microglia activation together with elevated TNFα and IL-1β levels in the cortex and hippocampus [193]. In accordance with the previous study, an in vivo study illustrates that globular adiponectin exerts anti-inflammatory effects on microglia by reducing IL-1β, IL-6, and TNFα [33]. Pre-treatment with adiponectin can diminish TNFα and IL-1β release in vitro [193]. Adiponectin potentially exerts anti-inflammatory action on microglia via AdipoR1/NF-κB signaling [33,193]. Other studies have further demonstrated that adiponectin exhibits anti-inflammatory response dependent on PPARγ [194] or IL-4/STAT6 signaling pathway [191]. Recently, an ex vivo study has demonstrated that adiponectin exhibits a beneficial effect on hippocampal synaptic plasticity in 5×FAD mice. Acute perfusion for 10-min or 2-h incubation of 2.7 nM adiponectin can induce LTP in the hippocampal CA1 region in five to six months old 5×FAD mice. Acute incubation of adiponectin also increases expressions of AdipoR1 and AdipoR2, increases protein expressions of GluA1, GluN1, GluN2B, and PSD-95 as well as elicits anti-apoptotic and anti-inflammatory effects [195]. These findings suggest that adiponectin inhibits neuronal apoptosis and inflammatory mechanisms and promotes hippocampal long-term potentiation. Taken together, these data have suggested the neuroprotective and neurogenic effects of adiponectin in the hippocampus (Table 1).

2.3. Chemerin

Chemerin is a novel adipokine that acts autocrine, paracrine, and endocrine on different tissues [196] by binding to either chemokine-like receptor 1 [197], chemokine receptor-like receptor 2 [198] or G protein-coupled receptor 1 [199]. Chemerin is highly expressed in white adipose tissue [200] and acts as a pro-inflammatory cytokine [201] and anti-inflammatory cytokine. It promotes adipogenesis [200], angiogenesis [202], and inflammation [203]. Clinical study has shown that change of chemerin levels is linked to obesity because the circulating levels of chemerin is positively correlated with high body-mass index and elevated obesity-related biomarkers [204–206]. Similarly, high fat diet-induced obese mice display an increase in plasma chemerin levels, and this increase can be reduced by overnight fasting [207]. Another study has shown that chemerin administration exacerbates the glucose intolerance in obese and diabetic mice by reducing hepatic glucose uptake [208]. Chemerin deficiency results in insulin resistance in adipose tissue and liver, leading to elevated hepatic glucose production and increased blood glucose levels [209]. On the other hand, chemokine-like receptor 1 knockout mice have reduced glucose uptake in adipose tissue and skeletal muscle [210], whereas high-fat diet further exacerbates glucose intolerance, hyperinsulinemia and enhances insulin resistance in these mice [211].

Activation of the chemerin signaling pathway plays a vital role in the neuroendocrine axis by regulating appetite. Chemerin receptors are highly expressed in multiple rodent brain regions, including the prefrontal cortex, hippocampus, and hypothalamus [212]. Continuous intracerebral infusion of chemerin into photoperiodic-sensitive F344 rats can promote food intake [213], whereas chemokine-like receptor 1 deficiency reduces food intake and body weight [210]. Chemerin can also aggravate glucose intolerance [208]. Consistently, clinical data indicate that circulating chemerin levels are increased in patients with obesity, diabetes, and cardiovascular diseases [214].

A recent study has shown that intranasal administration of human recombinant chemerin (rh-chemerin) exerts neuroprotective effects in a rat model of neonatal hypoxia-ischemia brain injury [215]. Intranasal treatment with chemerin significantly reduces infarct volume and attenuates developmental delay 24 h after hypoxic-ischemic encephalopathy. Chemerin treatment significantly improves cognitive and sensorimotor performance in animals with hypoxic-ischemic encephalopathy. Moreover, recombinant chemerin treatment significantly reduces apoptosis and the expressions of pro-apoptotic markers [215], suggesting a neuroprotective role of chemerin. Chemerin signaling is proposed to mediate neuro-inflammatory action in the brain. It is reported that the expression of chemokine like receptor 1 (CMKLR1) is upregulated in AD patients, suggesting the role of central chemerin signaling in the progression of AD [216]. Systemic lipopolysaccharide administration is known to upregulate CMKLR1 expression and promote neuroinflammation [216]. This study has reported that CMKLR1 and Aβ42 are colocalized in hippocampal neurons of APP/PS1 AD mice, and CMKLR1 is involved in Aβ processing and clearance. CMKLR1 is detected in the hippocampus and prefrontal cortex, two critical brain regions involved in the pathology of depression [217]. Intracerebral administration of chemerin elicits antidepressant effects [218]. In the lipopolysaccharide-induced depression mouse model, intracerebral administrations of chemerin receptor agonist: Eicosapentaenoic acid-derived resolvins E1 (1 ng) or E2 (10 ng) produce antidepressant effects depending on ChemR23/mTORC1 pathway in the medial prefrontal cortex and hippocampal dentate gyrus [218] (Table 1), suggesting activating chemerin signaling could be a novel antidepressant target.

2.4. Apelin

Apelin, a peptide hormone secreted by adipocytes, is involved in insulin secretion [219], glucose and lipid metabolism [220], angiogenesis [221], blood pressure regulation [222], and food intake [223]. Apelin has similar properties as physical exercise does in metabolism, and so given entitled it as an exerkine [224]. Apelin can be proteolytically cleaved into several bioactive forms, including apelin-13, -17, and -36, as well as the pyroglutaminated apelin-13 isoform [225]. Apelin receptors are widely distributed in rodent brain and systemic tissues [226].

Apelin is necessary for balancing the fat composition and promoting insulin sensitivity. Apelin-knockout mice exhibit obese and diabetic symptoms, including increased abdominal fat mass, glucose intolerance, hyperinsulinemia, and hypo-adiponectinemia [227]. High-fat diet and high-sucrose consumption aggravate glucose and insulin intolerance in apelin-deficient mice [228]. Clinical study has reported a positive correlation between plasma insulin levels and apelin expression in adipocytes from obese subjects. Given this insulin-sensitizing property, apelin has become a promising therapeutic target for treating obesity and diabetes. Single intravenous injection of 200 pmol/kg Pyr(1)-apelin-13 can improve glucose intolerance in high-fat diet-induced obese and insulin-resistant mice [229]. Chronic apelin treatment (two to four weeks) improves insulin sensitivity, lowers blood glucose levels, and protect the animals from hyperinsulinemia and glucose intolerance in mice with obesity or insulin resistance [228,230]. Apelin treatment can also significantly reduce adiposity and plasma triglycerides [230]. Apelin is involved in lipid metabolism by inhibiting isoproterenol-induced lipolysis in cultured adipocytes [227]. Moreover, exogenous apelin reduces the number of differentiated adipocytes and increases the size of lipid droplets inside the cells, suggesting that apelin might suppress lipolysis [231]. In vitro studies reveal that apelin-13 and [Pyr1]-apelin-13 improve glycemia in an AMPK/eNOS-dependent [229] and PI3K/Akt-dependent [232] pathways respectively. These findings have collectively suggested that apelin treatment could be useful in reducing adiposity, improving insulin sensitivity, and improving diabetic conditions.

Similar to other adipokines, apelin exhibits anti-inflammatory properties [232] and possesses neuroprotective effects [233]. In an ischemia/reperfusion (I/R) stroke rat model, the post-stroke intracerebral injection of apelin-13 can significantly reduce the infarct volume [234]. Similarly, intracerebral infusion of apelin-13 significantly decreases blood–brain barrier permeability and increases vascular endothelial growth factor levels in post-stroke mice [235]. Furthermore, post-stroke treatment with intranasal apelin-13 for three days can reduce infarct volume, reduce neuronal apoptosis, suppress inflammation, and increase angiogenesis [236]. In mice with traumatic brain injury, intracerebral administration of apelin-13 reduces brain damage via suppressing autophagy [237]. Apelin-13 also elicits an anti-inflammatory effect by inhibiting microglia and astrocyte activation and upregulates hippocampal BDNF and TrkB expression in streptozotocin-induced sporadic AD rats. Furthermore, the apelin-13 treatment also promotes learning and memory performance, as evidenced by its effect on improving novel object recognition and spatial recognition through the BDNF/TrkB pathway [238]. In a rat model of depression, apelin-13 treatment elicits antidepressant effect and improves recognition memory via activating phosphatidylinositol 3-kinases (PI3K) and extracellular signal-regulated kinase 1/2 (ERK1/2) signaling pathways. The hippocampus is thought to be the critical brain region mediating the antidepressant-like response of apelin [239,240]. Similarly, intracerebral infusion of apelin-13 can ameliorate depression-like phenotypes in rats subjected to chronic restraint stress. Apelin-13 can also suppress hypothalamic-pituitary-adrenal axis hyperactivity, promote hippocampal BDNF expression, and restore hippocampal glucocorticoid receptor functions in rats with chronic stress [241] (Table 1).

2.5. Visfatin (Nicotinamide phosphoribosyltransferase, NAMPT)

Nicotinamide phosphoribosyltransferase (NAMPT) is an enzyme which catalyzes the biosynthesis of nicotinamide adenine dinucleotide (NAD^+) in mammals [242]. There are two isoforms of NAMPT: Intracellular NAMPT (iNAMPT) and extracellular NAMPT (eNAMPT or visfatin) [242]. Growing evidence shows that NAD^+/NADH metabolism in adipose tissue is linked to obesity and insulin resistance. In humans, visceral adipose NAMPT expression and serum NAMPT levels are positively correlated with obesity [243]. In mice, adipose NAMPT expression and NAD^+ contents are markedly reduced by high-fat diet feeding [244,245], but increased by caloric restriction [246,247]. Adipocyte-specific *Nampt* knockout mice show severe insulin resistance in multiple organs under a chow-fed condition, which is independent of body weight and adiposity [248]. Loss of *Nampt* causes adipose tissue inflammation, increases plasma free fatty acid concentrations, and decreases adiponectin. Notably, oral administration with nicotinamide mononucleotide, a key NAD^+ intermediate, can restore adipose tissue NAD^+ biosynthesis and significantly restore insulin resistance, plasma adiponectin and free fatty acid concentrations in adipocyte-specific *Nampt* knockout mice. On the other hand, visfatin is secreted from white adipose tissue through sirtuin1 (SIRT1)-mediated deacetylation of iNAMPT [249]. At present, it remains uncertain whether visfatin can cross the blood–brain barrier. However, adipose-secreted visfatin serves as a neuroendocrine factor. Adipose tissue-specific *Nampt* knockout mice display a significant reduction in circulating visfatin, as well as reduced hypothalamic NAD^+ content and SIRT1 activity [249]. On the other hand, adipose-specific *Nampt* knock-in mice show increases in hypothalamic NAD^+ content, SIRT1 activity, and neural activity in response to fasting. Therefore, adipose-secreted visfatin has a strong implication on modulating brain functions.

Visfatin protects neurons against ischemia-induced injury because NAMPT overexpression can reduce infarct volume and improve long-term neurologic outcomes [250]. In a transient global cerebral ischemia model with 20-min carotid arteries occlusion, intracerebral infusion of 100 ng visfatin in the hippocampal CA3 region during cerebral reperfusion can reduce the caspase-3 activation and Bax/Bcl-2 ratio [251]. Visfatin can significantly reduce apoptosis and necrotic cell death in the CA1 region of the hippocampus, with improved memory deficits in I/R rats. The suppressed pro-apoptotic and enhanced anti-apoptotic mechanisms could contribute to the neuroprotective effects of visfatin [250]. In another study, transgenic mice overexpressing NAMPT globally increase NAD^+ content and neuronal survival in the hippocampal dentate gyrus [252]. These mice also display better learning and memory performance in the water maze test upon middle cerebral artery occlusion. Post-ischemic intraperitoneal administration with nicotinamide mononucleotide for seven days can improve adult hippocampal neurogenesis [252]. Nicotinamide mononucleotide and NAD^+ promotes proliferation and differentiation of neural stem cells in a NAMPT/NAD^+/SIRT manner [252]. An in vitro study has concluded that cultured glia, but not neuron, can secrete visfatin under oxygen-glucose deprivation stress. Treatment of wild-type visfatin, but not H247A-mutant enzymatic-dead visfatin, can significantly attenuate oxygen-glucose deprivation-elicited cell death in both cultured mouse neuron and glia. Treatment of neutralizing antibody can, in turn, abolish the protective effect of extracellular visfatin on cell viability [253].

Although the neuroprotective benefits of visfatin towards neurodegenerative diseases require further investigation, growing evidence has indicated that NAD^+ administration can improve cellular energetics and extend life span in rodents [254]. The evidence leads to the idea that the administration of NAD^+ precursors, including nicotinamide mononucleotide and nicotinamide riboside, is a potential treatment to forestall disease progress in AD by improving brain energetics [255]. In the AD rat model with an intracerebral infusion with Aβ amyloid, intraperitoneal administration of 500 mg/kg nicotinamide mononucleotide improves learning and memory performance in water maze task [256]. Nicotinamide mononucleotide also attenuates Aβ oligomer-induced neuronal cell death, prevents long-term potentiation deficit, restores NAD^+ and ATP levels, and eliminates reactive oxygen species in organotypic hippocampal slices [256]. Moreover, nicotinamide riboside treatment exhibits pro-cognitive function by increasing cortical NAD^+ content and restoring long-term potentiation deficit in the hippocampal CA1 region of the Tg2576 AD mouse model. This study has suggested that treatment upregulating the NAMPT/NAD^+ axis could prevent Aβ accumulation in the brain [257] (Table 1).

Table 1. Effects of adipokines on neuroplasticity, neuroprotection, and cognitive behaviors.

Animal Model		Treatment	Delivery Route	Neurological Effects	References	Year
Leptin						
C57BL/6J (healthy)	mice	14 days 1 mg/kg recombinant rat leptin	i.p.	• Increased cell proliferation and survival in the hippocampal dentate gyrus	Garza et al. [24]	2008
C57BL/6J (healthy)	mice	30 min after injecting 1 mg/kg leptin	i.p.	• Reduced depressive behavior in forced swim and tail suspension tests	Liu et al. [127]	2010
4 and 12 m.o. SAM-P8	mice	0.25–0.5 μg mouse recombinant leptin post-training	Intra-hippo	• Improved memory retention in T-maze footshock avoidance and step-down inhibitory avoidance.	Farr et al. [118]	2006
Sprague-Dawleyl (healthy)	rats	1.0 μM leptin	Intra-DG	• Enhanced LTP	Wayner et al. [151]	2004
6 m.o. TgCRND8 AD	mice	8 weeks 20 μg leptin daily	Systemic infusion by osmotic pump	• Improved object recognition • Improved fear-associated learning	Greco et al. [133]	2010
Aβ1-42-assaulted	rat	10 days 1 μg leptin daily	i.c.v.	• Improved spatial memory in Y maze and water maze • Enhanced LTP	Tong et al. [134]	2015
Adiponectin						
HFD-induced stress and naive C57BL/6J	mice	0.1–0.3 μg globular adiponectin	i.c.v	• Reduced depressive behavior	Liu et al. [158]	2012
C57BL/6J (healthy) Sedentary or environmentally enriched C57BL/6J	mice	Overexpression of adiponectin by adenovirus	i.c.v	• Reduced depressive behavior in forced swim test	Yau et al. [25]	2014
	mice	1 mg/kg globular adiponectin	i.v.	• Reduced depressive behavior in forced swim test • Reduced microglial response	Nicolas et al. [187]	2015
Corticosterone-induced stress C57BL/6J	mice	0.3 μg globular adiponectin	i.c.v.	• Reduced pro-inflammatory cytokine secretion from microglia	Chabry et al. [188]	2015
Adipo⁺/⁺ & ⁺/⁻ C57BL/6J mice	mice	10 mg/kg rosiglitazone 1 or 3 h before test	i.p.	• Reduced depressive and anxiety-like behavior	Guo et al. [189]	2017
STZ infused Sprague-Dawley	rats	0.1 μg/g adiponectin	i.c.v.	• Improved learning and memory • Increased hippocampal dendritic spine complexities • Reduced tau hyperphosphorylation	Xu et al. [192]	2018

Table 1. Cont.

Animal Model		Treatment	Delivery Route	Neurological Effects	References	Year
Chemerin						
Hypoxic-ischemic encephalopathy in P10 Sprague–Dawley	rats	9 µg/kg rh-chemerin, 3 doses	i.n.	• Better learning and memory functions • Reduced apoptosis	Zhang et al. [215]	2019
LPS-induced depression BALB/c	mice	500 ng chemerin	i.c.v.	• Reduced depressive behavior in forced swim and tail suspension tests	Deyama et al. [218]	2018
LPS-induced depression BALB/c	mice	Resolvin E1	i.c.v. (1 ng) and bilateral intra-mPFC and intra-DG (50 pg/side)	• Reduced depressive behavior in forced swim and tail suspension tests	Deyama et al. [218]	2018
LPS-induced depression BALB/c	mice	10 ng resolvin E2	i.c.v.	• Reduced depressive behavior in forced swim and tail suspension tests	Deyama et al. [218]	2018
Apelin						
Cerebral I/R Wistar	rats	50 ng/kg apelin-13 post-ischemia	i.c.v.	• Reduced infarct volume	Xin et al. [234]	2015
Cerebral I/R AQP4+/+ & -/-	mice	50 ng/kg apelin-13 post-ischemia	i.c.v.	• Decreased BBB permeability	Chu et al. [235]	2017
Cerebral I/R C57BL/6J	mice	4 mg/kg, 3 doses for three days post-ischemia	i.n.	• Reduced infarct • Reduced neuronal apoptosis	Chen et al. [236]	2015
TBI CD-1	mice	50 µg apelin-13	i.c.v.	• Suppressed autophagy	Bao et al. [237]	2015
STZ-infused AD Sprague–Dawley	rats	2 µg, daily for 4 weeks	i.c.v.	• Improved object and spatial recognition • Suppressed neuroinflammation	Luo et al. [238]	2019
Forced-swimming stressed Wistar	rats	2 µg, three doses in 24 h before FST	i.c.v.	• Reduced hedonic deficit in learned helplessness • Improve object recognition	Li et al. [238]	2016
Chronic water-immersion restraint stress Wistar	rats	2 µg, daily for 7 days	i.c.v.	• Reduced depressive behavior in sucrose preference and tail suspension tests	Dai et al. [241]	2018

Table 1. Cont.

Animal Model		Treatment	Delivery Route	Neurological Effects	References	Year
			Visfatin			
Cerebral I/R	mice	pThy1:NAMPT	transgenic	• Reduced infarct volume • Reduced neurological deficits • Increased striatal and corpus callosum myelination	Jing et al. [250]	2014
Cerebral I/R Wistar	rats	100 ng visfatin during reperfusion	Intra-CA	• Suppressed apoptosis • Enhanced anti-apoptotic mechanism	Erfani et al. [251]	2015
Cerebral I/R C57BL/6J	mice	pIRES2::NAMPT	transgenic	• Improved learning and memory	Zhao et al. [252]	2015
Cerebral I/R C57BL/6J	mice	500 mg/kg NMN daily for 7 days	i.p.	• Promoted hippocampal neurogenesis	Zhao et al. [252]	2015
Aβ-infused AD Sprague-Dawley	rats	500 mg/kg NMN daily for 10 days	i.p.	• Improved learning and memory	Wang et al. [256]	2016
Tg2576 AD	mice	250 mg/kg nicotinamide riboside daily for 3 months	i.p.	• Improved object recognition • Increased cortical NAD$^+$ • Abolished long-term potentiation deficits	Gong et al. [257]	2013

3. Novel Adipocyte-Derived Messengers on Brain Health

Lipokine refers to fatty acids that act like hormones and modulate lipid metabolism [258]. Notably, adipose tissue, which is one of the systemic sites with active lipid metabolism, secretes various lipids into the bloodstream to communicate with distant organs. Coincidentally, alterations in lipid metabolism may implicate the onset of brain diseases. For example, apolipoprotein E (ApoE) mediates systemic cholesterol metabolism and acts as a cholesterol carrier to neurons in the central nervous system. Human carriers of mutated apolipoprotein E allele ε4 are associated with an increased risk of AD [259]. Moreover, post-mortem studies have shown that AD patients display abnormal levels of ceramides, n-3 polyunsaturated fatty acids (PUFA), and PUFA-derived signaling lipids [260–264].

Lipokines, including monounsaturated palmitoleic acid and lysophosphatidic acid (LPA can exert endocrine effects on systemic tissues and have potential crosstalk with the central nervous system. Palmitoleic acid is a highly abundant fatty acid in the serum. Its circulating levels fluctuate dependent on metabolic states. Obese children and adults exhibit a higher plasma palmitoleic acid content compared to healthy control [265,266]. Besides, the change of palmitoleate could be associated with an increased risk of obesity, dyslipidemia, and insulin resistance [265–268]. On the other hand, lysophospholipid is a prominent class of lipid signaling molecules, whereas LPA is a crucial member. Circulating LPAs are synthesized by autotaxin, a phosphodiesterase produced by adipocytes [269]. Circulating autotaxin levels increase in obesity and insulin resistance [270–276], which is positively correlated with an increase in circulating lysophosphatidic acid [277,278]. A high-fat diet can perturb lipid composition in the brain. The altered lipid composition is evidenced by a surge of palmitoleic acid composition in the mouse brain after 14 days of high carbohydrate and high fatty acid diets [279]. Congruently, high-fat diet causes a significant elevation of LPA in mouse cortex after eight weeks of high-fat diet [280]. Importantly, over-nutritious food has detrimental effects on brain plasticity because brain diseases could be linked to dysregulated lipid metabolism [281–286]. The effects of palmitoleic acid and lysophosphatidic acid on brain health warrant further investigation.

3.1. Palmitoleic Acid (16:1n7)

Palmitic acid (16:0) is the most common saturated fatty acid in the human body. It can be consumed through diet or synthesized from other fatty acids, carbohydrates, and amino acids endogenously [287]. Under normal physiological conditions, palmitic acid accumulation is prevented by desaturation to palmitoleic acid (16:1n7) or by elongation to stearic acid (18:0), then further desaturation to oleic acid (18:1) [288,289]. Abnormal levels of palmitic acid have been documented in neurodegenerative diseases [290–292] that are related to dysregulated palmitic acid biosynthesis. Palmitoleic acid, a monounsaturated fatty acid, primarily originates from stearoyl-CoA desaturase 1-mediated de novo lipogenesis from palmitic acid in humans [287]. Palmitoleic acid is highly abundant in serum and adipose tissues [293]. cis-palmitoleate has been associated with increased insulin sensitivity and decreased lipid accumulation in the liver [258]. Various animal models have illustrated that cis-palmitoleate reduces the expressions of pro-inflammatory cytokines and adipokines in association with metabolic syndromes [258,294,295]. In vitro study also shows that palmitoleic acid increases lipolysis and lipase content in white adipose tissue in a PPARα-dependent manner [296]. Other than adipose tissues, palmitoleic acid can enhance whole-body glucose disposal [297] and improve circulating lipid profiles in both rodents and humans [298]. Therefore, palmitoleic acid is considered a lipokine.

Fatty acid-binding proteins (FABP) are lipid chaperones that regulate lipid trafficking and responses in cells [299,300]. In humans, circulating adipose-derived fatty acid-binding protein (A-FABP) levels are substantially higher than other adipokines, including leptin, resistin, TNF-α, and IL-6 [301–303]. Circulating A-FABP is markedly increased in both obese men and women [304], suggesting that A-FABP may involve in modulating insulin sensitivity and lipid metabolism in distant organs. Of note, A-FABP is also considered as an adipokine, which is secreted from adipocyte-derived exosomes by exocytosis [305]. Critically, deficiencies in A-FABP and epidermal fatty acid-binding protein (E-FABP) can activate SCD1 activity, leading to a subsequent elevation in palmitoleate concentration in adipose tissue [306,307]. A-FABP deficient mice exhibit improvement in systemic glucose, lipid metabolism and insulin resistance in association with diet-induced and genetically-disposed obesity [308]. The A-FABP and E-FABP double mutant mice are resistant to diet-induced obesity, insulinemia, type 2 diabetes, dyslipidemia, and fatty liver disease [309,310]. The dysregulated SCD1-mediated de novo synthesis of palmitoleic acid enhances whole-body glucose and fatty acid metabolism [311].

Although it requires more solid evidence to demonstrate the effect of adipocyte-secreted palmitoleic acid and A-FABP on brain health, it is reported that stearoyl-CoA desaturase activity and levels of palmitoleic acid in the brain are associated with AD [312]. Liquid chromatography-mass spectrometry analysis has revealed elevated levels of several monounsaturated fatty acids, including palmitoleic acid, in the mid-frontal cortex, temporal cortex, and hippocampus of AD patients as compared to their age-matched counterparts [312]. This increase is strongly associated with cognitive dysfunction and the increased expression of stearoyl-CoA desaturase in the brain [266,313–317]. Further studies have shown that AD patients have increased expressions of various stearoyl-CoA desaturase isoforms, including SCD-1 [312]. Coherently, stearoyl-CoA desaturase activity is negatively correlated to cognitive measures [312]. Levels of free palmitoleic acid and the desaturation index are decreased in frontal cortices in aged dogs treated with antioxidant, and vice versa [318]. The study implicates that altering stearoyl-CoA desaturase activity and reducing palmitoleic acid levels in the brain may improve cognitive performance [318].

3.2. Lysophosphatidic Acid

Neuroinflammation is commonly associated with type 2 diabetes [319], and obesity [320]. High-fat diet feeding results in profound central and peripheral inflammation [321,322]. Autotaxin is a lysophospholipase that synthesizes lysophosphatidic acid (LPA). Autotaxin is also regarded as an adipokine due to its role in promoting adipocyte differentiation [269]. Evidence suggests that the autotaxin-mediated LPA biosynthesis contributes to the majority of extracellular LPA, in which adipocyte-specific autotaxin contributes to most of the circulating LPA [269,272]. Further investigations suggest that circulating LPA and autotaxin levels are linked to adipocyte differentiation and obesity [269,271]. Autotaxin expression is upregulated in obese patients and obese *db/db* mice due to the accumulation of triglycerides in the adipocytes [271]. A recent study has reported that adipose-derived autotaxin serves as an inflammatory cytokine of diet-induced obesity [323].

LPA signaling mediates inflammation [324], angiogenesis [325], brain development [326], and neurogenesis [327] in the brain. Specifically, LPA exerts a pleiotropic effect on various brain cell types, including neurons, astrocytes, microglia, and oligodendrocytes that show LPA receptors expression [328]. LPA promotes neuronal differentiation in cortical neural progenitor cells through LPA1 receptor/$G_{i/o}$ pathway [329], whereas axonal branching is induced in hippocampal cell cultures through LPA3 receptor/G_q/Rho family GTPase 2 (Rnd2) pathway [330]. Mainly, LPA1 is essential in mediating synaptic plasticity and learning. In vitro studies have shown that overexpression of LPA1 increases dendritic spine density and size [331], potentially through protein kinase C (PKC)/Rho and PKC/Rac cascades [332,333]. It is speculated that LPA1 deficiency can cause schizophrenia-like behaviors, including impaired spatial memory retention and increased anxiety-like behavior [334–336]. Furthermore, the role of LPA and its receptors in anxiety-like behavior and learning has been confirmed by later studies using LPA1-null mice. These mice show normal survival but display aberrant hippocampal neurogenesis and decreased BDNF levels [327], as well as increased anxiety-like behavior and memory deficits [337]. LPA mediates astrocyte proliferation through the LPA1 receptor [338]. Interestingly, LPA promotes astrocyte-neuronal crosstalk through laminin-mediated EGFR/MAPK signaling to facilitate neuronal differentiation [339]. LPA triggers microglial migration through a Ca^{2+}-dependent K^+ channel [340,341], and reduces oxidative stress [342,343]. Moreover, LPA can promote the retraction of oligodendrocyte processes in mature oligodendrocytes [344] as well as promotes the formation of oligodendrocyte processes in differentiating oligodendrocytes [345].

In addition to a metabolic disorder, an altered systemic lipid metabolism may have a neurological impact [346] through autotaxin-LPA signaling. Clinical study has reported that mild cognitive impairment and AD patients have significantly higher levels of autotaxin in cerebrospinal fluid [347]. Furthermore, the autotaxin levels are positively correlated to neuroinflammatory markers, β-amyloid, and tau in the cerebrospinal fluid [347]. In vitro study has shown that LPA could increase Aβ production by upregulating the expression of β-secretase expressions in the N2a neuroblastoma cell line expressing wild-type presenilin 1 and Swedish mutant APP [348]. Potentially, LPA-induced BACE1 promoter activation is mediated by PKCδ/MEK/MAPK/p90RSk/CREB signaling cascades [348–353]. Moreover, LPA may be involved in tau hyperphosphorylation and paired helical filaments formation, which are the pathological patterns in AD brains through $G\alpha_{12/13}$/RhoA/Rock/GSK-3β pathway [354,355], suggesting potential connection among LPA, microfilament dynamics, and AD pathogenesis.

4. Conclusions

It is an emerging research field to understand the functions of different adipokines in regulating eating behavior, hippocampal plasticity, and neuronal protection. This review has denoted five adipokines (leptin, adiponectin, chemerin, apelin, and visfatin) and two lipokines (palmitoleic acid and lysophosphatidic acid) (Figure 1). The review has summarized the currently available evidence for their novel function in the brain. First, it is evident that the aberrant adipokine production not only renders the susceptibility to metabolic syndromes in genetically deficient rodent models of various adipokines but also the vulnerability to neurodegeneration, especially in models of impaired leptin-signaling. Accumulated evidence has indicated that diet-induced obese or diabetic rodent models show abnormal levels of leptin, adiponectin, chemerin, apelin, and visfatin. Notably, circulating adiponectin and visfatin levels are reduced in diet-induced obesity, with associated impairments in hippocampal plasticity and cognitive behaviors [356]. Due to the multifaceted effect of adipokines on systemic and brain health, dysregulated adipokine secretion could be one of the causes that underlie the comorbidity of metabolic syndromes with neurodegenerative disorders [357,358]. Thus, all these investigations have highlighted the prominent roles of adipokines on brain health. Second, evidence also shows that leptin and adiponectin can elicit their action directly in the brain by crossing the blood–brain barrier. Leptin is not only a satiety regulator through anorexigenic and dopaminergic controls, but ample evidence also supports its role in promoting neuroplasticity in the hippocampus [12]. On the other hand, adiponectin is a chief metabolic regulator in glucose and fatty acid metabolism with insulin-sensitizing ability in both peripheral and central systems. Current findings have suggested the direct effect of adiponectin on synaptic plasticity [195,359] and microglial activation [193]. Both exogenous leptin and adiponectin can exert pro-cognitive effects in mouse models. Besides, leptin and adiponectin signaling pathways are defective in AD brains [360]. Hence, increasing leptin and adiponectin signaling can be a potential therapeutic target for AD [361,362]. Third, emerging literature has also revealed the central function of three novel adipokines: Chemerin, apelin, and visfatin. Inflammatory response and apoptosis are typical in neurodegenerative diseases [363,364] and ischaemic stroke [365,366]. These novel adipokines are potential therapeutic targets, which modulate anti-inflammatory and anti-apoptotic effects in the hippocampus. Finally, this review has highlighted lipokines are a lipid signaling molecule secreted by adipocytes with potential endocrine effect acting on the brain [367]. Still, the potential of lipokines is mostly unknown, future studies will be required to illustrate its properties and function in neuroplasticity and cognitive functions.

Overall, adipokines emerge as viable therapeutic targets towards neurodegenerative diseases. Adipokine-based therapeutic approaches could be future pharmaceuticals to obliterate neurodegenerative disorders. More in-depth investigations on the above-mentioned adipokines and its crosstalk with the brain can open up new therapeutic targets to treat neurodegenerative diseases.

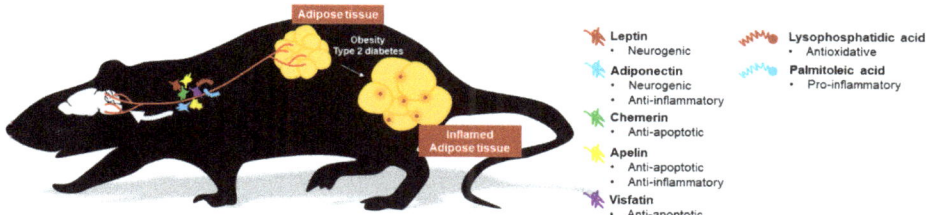

Figure 1. Potential mechanism of adipokine actions on brain health. Adiponectin and leptin can cross the blood–brain barrier to promote neuroplasticity. Other adipokines and lipokines show profound effects on mediating neurogenic and neuroinflammatory mechanisms.

Author Contributions: T.H.-y.L. wrote the manuscript. S.-y.Y., K.K.y.C., R.L.-c.H., and P.M.-f.S. revised and edited the manuscript.

Funding: This work is supported by the Hong Kong Research Council Early Career Scheme (project No. 25100217) and National Natural Science Foundation of China (Project No. 81801346) awarded to S.-y.Y.

Conflicts of Interest: The authors declare no conflict of interest.

References

1. Kershaw, E.E.; Flier, J.S. Adipose tissue as an endocrine organ. *J. Clin. Endocrinol. Metab.* **2004**, *89*, 2548–2556. [CrossRef] [PubMed]
2. Han, S.; Sun, H.M.; Hwang, K.C.; Kim, S.W. Adipose-derived stromal vascular fraction cells: Update on clinical utility and efficacy. *Crit. Rev. Eukaryot. Gene Expr.* **2015**, *25*, 145–152. [CrossRef] [PubMed]
3. Warner, A.; Mittag, J. Brown fat and vascular heat dissipation: The new cautionary tail. *Adipocyte* **2014**, *3*, 221–223. [CrossRef] [PubMed]
4. Cedikova, M.; Kripnerova, M.; Dvorakova, J.; Pitule, P.; Grundmanova, M.; Babuska, V.; Mullerova, D.; Kuncova, J. Mitochondria in white, brown, and beige adipocytes. *Stem Cells Int.* **2016**, *2016*, 6067349. [CrossRef] [PubMed]
5. Duncan, R.E.; Ahmadian, M.; Jaworski, K.; Sarkadi-Nagy, E.; Sul, H.S. Regulation of lipolysis in adipocytes. *Annu. Rev. Nutr.* **2007**, *27*, 79–101. [CrossRef] [PubMed]
6. Choe, S.S.; Huh, J.Y.; Hwang, I.J.; Kim, J.I.; Kim, J.B. Adipose tissue remodeling: Its role in energy metabolism and metabolic disorders. *Front. Endocrinol.* **2016**, *7*, 30. [CrossRef] [PubMed]
7. Cook, K.S.; Min, H.Y.; Johnson, D.; Chaplinsky, R.J.; Flier, J.S.; Hunt, C.R.; Spiegelman, B.M. Adipsin: A circulating serine protease homolog secreted by adipose tissue and sciatic nerve. *Science* **1987**, *237*, 402–405. [CrossRef] [PubMed]
8. Zhang, Y.; Proenca, R.; Maffei, M.; Barone, M.; Leopold, L.; Friedman, J.M. Positional cloning of the mouse obese gene and its human homologue. *Nature* **1994**, *372*, 425–432. [CrossRef] [PubMed]
9. Rosen, E.D.; Spiegelman, B.M. What we talk about when we talk about fat. *Cell* **2014**, *156*, 20–44. [CrossRef] [PubMed]
10. Bergmann, K.; Sypniewska, G. Diabetes as a complication of adipose tissue dysfunction. Is there a role for potential new biomarkers? *Clin. Chem. Lab. Med.* **2013**, *51*, 177–185. [CrossRef] [PubMed]
11. Flier, J.S.; Maratos-Flier, E. Lasker lauds leptin. *Cell* **2010**, *143*, 9–12. [CrossRef] [PubMed]
12. Harvey, J.; Solovyova, N.; Irving, A. Leptin and its role in hippocampal synaptic plasticity. *Prog. Lipid Res.* **2006**, *45*, 369–378. [CrossRef] [PubMed]
13. De la Monte, S.M.; Wands, J.R. Review of insulin and insulin-like growth factor expression, signaling, and malfunction in the central nervous system: Relevance to Alzheimer's disease. *J. Alzheimers Dis.* **2005**, *7*, 45–61. [CrossRef] [PubMed]
14. Steen, E.; Terry, B.M.; Rivera, E.J.; Cannon, J.L.; Neely, T.R.; Tavares, R.; Xu, X.J.; Wands, J.R.; de la Monte, S.M. Impaired insulin and insulin-like growth factor expression and signaling mechanisms in Alzheimer's disease—Is this type 3 diabetes? *J. Alzheimers Dis.* **2005**, *7*, 63–80. [CrossRef] [PubMed]

15. Schioth, H.B.; Craft, S.; Brooks, S.J.; Frey, W.H., 2nd; Benedict, C. Brain insulin signaling and Alzheimer's disease: Current evidence and future directions. *Mol. Neurobiol.* **2012**, *46*, 4–10. [CrossRef] [PubMed]
16. Craft, S. Alzheimer disease: Insulin resistance and AD—Extending the translational path. *Nat. Rev. Neurol.* **2012**, *8*, 360–362. [CrossRef] [PubMed]
17. Ye, R.; Scherer, P.E. Adiponectin, driver or passenger on the road to insulin sensitivity? *Mol. Metab.* **2013**, *2*, 133–141. [CrossRef] [PubMed]
18. Maeda, N.; Shimomura, I.; Kishida, K.; Nishizawa, H.; Matsuda, M.; Nagaretani, H.; Furuyama, N.; Kondo, H.; Takahashi, M.; Arita, Y.; et al. Diet-induced insulin resistance in mice lacking adiponectin/ACRP30. *Nat. Med.* **2002**, *8*, 731–737. [CrossRef] [PubMed]
19. Ng, R.C.; Cheng, O.Y.; Jian, M.; Kwan, J.S.; Ho, P.W.; Cheng, K.K.; Yeung, P.K.; Zhou, L.L.; Hoo, R.L.; Chung, S.K.; et al. Chronic adiponectin deficiency leads to Alzheimer's disease-like cognitive impairments and pathologies through AMPK inactivation and cerebral insulin resistance in aged mice. *Mol. Neurodegener.* **2016**, *11*, 71. [CrossRef] [PubMed]
20. Yaffe, K. Metabolic syndrome and cognitive decline. *Curr. Alzheimer Res.* **2007**, *4*, 123–126. [CrossRef] [PubMed]
21. Biessels, G.J.; Despa, F. Cognitive decline and dementia in diabetes mellitus: Mechanisms and clinical implications. *Nat. Rev. Endocrinol.* **2018**, *14*, 591–604. [CrossRef] [PubMed]
22. Stoeckel, L.E.; Arvanitakis, Z.; Gandy, S.; Small, D.; Kahn, C.R.; Pascual-Leone, A.; Sherwin, R.; Smith, P. Complex mechanisms linking neurocognitive dysfunction to insulin resistance and other metabolic dysfunction. *F1000Research* **2016**, *5*, 353. [CrossRef] [PubMed]
23. Gustafson, D. Adiposity indices and dementia. *Lancet Neurol.* **2006**, *5*, 713–720. [CrossRef]
24. Garza, J.C.; Guo, M.; Zhang, W.; Lu, X.Y. Leptin increases adult hippocampal neurogenesis in vivo and in vitro. *J. Biol. Chem.* **2008**, *283*, 18238–18247. [CrossRef] [PubMed]
25. Yau, S.Y.; Li, A.; Hoo, R.L.; Ching, Y.P.; Christie, B.R.; Lee, T.M.; Xu, A.; So, K.F. Physical exercise-induced hippocampal neurogenesis and antidepressant effects are mediated by the adipocyte hormone adiponectin. *Proc. Natl. Acad. Sci. USA* **2014**, *111*, 15810–15815. [CrossRef] [PubMed]
26. Guo, Z.; Jiang, H.; Xu, X.; Duan, W.; Mattson, M.P. Leptin-mediated cell survival signaling in hippocampal neurons mediated by JAK STAT3 and mitochondrial stabilization. *J. Biol. Chem.* **2008**, *283*, 1754–1763. [CrossRef] [PubMed]
27. Song, J.; Kang, S.M.; Kim, E.; Kim, C.H.; Song, H.T.; Lee, J.E. Adiponectin receptor-mediated signaling ameliorates cerebral cell damage and regulates the neurogenesis of neural stem cells at high glucose concentrations: An in vivo and in vitro study. *Cell Death Dis.* **2015**, *6*, e1844. [CrossRef] [PubMed]
28. Formolo, D.A.; Lee, T.H.; Yau, S.Y. Increasing adiponergic system activity as a potential treatment for depressive disorders. *Mol. Neurobiol.* **2019**. [CrossRef] [PubMed]
29. Huang, S.; Wang, Y.; Gan, X.; Fang, D.; Zhong, C.; Wu, L.; Hu, G.; Sosunov, A.A.; McKhann, G.M.; Yu, H.; et al. Drp1-mediated mitochondrial abnormalities link to synaptic injury in diabetes model. *Diabetes* **2015**, *64*, 1728–1742. [CrossRef] [PubMed]
30. Wang, B.; Guo, H.; Li, X.; Yue, L.; Liu, H.; Zhao, L.; Bai, H.; Liu, X.; Wu, X.; Qu, Y. Adiponectin attenuates oxygen-glucose deprivation-induced mitochondrial oxidative injury and apoptosis in hippocampal HT22 cells via the JAK2/STAT3 pathway. *Cell Transpl.* **2018**, *27*, 1731–1743. [CrossRef] [PubMed]
31. Qiu, G.; Wan, R.; Hu, J.; Mattson, M.P.; Spangler, E.; Liu, S.; Yau, S.Y.; Lee, T.M.; Gleichmann, M.; Ingram, D.K.; et al. Adiponectin protects rat hippocampal neurons against excitotoxicity. *Age* **2011**, *33*, 155–165. [CrossRef] [PubMed]
32. Song, J.; Choi, S.M.; Whitcomb, D.J.; Kim, B.C. Adiponectin controls the apoptosis and the expression of tight junction proteins in brain endothelial cells through AdipoR1 under beta amyloid toxicity. *Cell Death Dis.* **2017**, *8*, e3102. [CrossRef] [PubMed]
33. Nicolas, S.; Cazareth, J.; Zarif, H.; Guyon, A.; Heurteaux, C.; Chabry, J.; Petit-Paitel, A. Globular adiponectin limits microglia pro-inflammatory phenotype through an AdipoR1/NF-kappaB signaling pathway. *Front. Cell Neurosci.* **2017**, *11*, 352. [CrossRef] [PubMed]
34. Zuloaga, K.L.; Johnson, L.A.; Roese, N.E.; Marzulla, T.; Zhang, W.; Nie, X.; Alkayed, F.N.; Hong, C.; Grafe, M.R.; Pike, M.M.; et al. High fat diet-induced diabetes in mice exacerbates cognitive deficit due to chronic hypoperfusion. *J. Cereb. Blood Flow Metab.* **2016**, *36*, 1257–1270. [CrossRef] [PubMed]

35. Li, Z.; Hao, S.; Yin, H.; Gao, J.; Yang, Z. Autophagy ameliorates cognitive impairment through activation of PVT1 and apoptosis in diabetes mice. *Behav. Brain Res.* **2016**, *305*, 265–277. [CrossRef] [PubMed]
36. Yan, S.; Du, F.; Wu, L.; Zhang, Z.; Zhong, C.; Yu, Q.; Wang, Y.; Lue, L.F.; Walker, D.G.; Douglas, J.T.; et al. F1F0 ATP synthase-cyclophilin D interaction contributes to diabetes-induced synaptic dysfunction and cognitive decline. *Diabetes* **2016**, *65*, 3482–3494. [CrossRef] [PubMed]
37. Kong, F.J.; Wu, J.H.; Sun, S.Y.; Ma, L.L.; Zhou, J.Q. Liraglutide ameliorates cognitive decline by promoting autophagy via the AMP-activated protein kinase/mammalian target of rapamycin pathway in a streptozotocin-induced mouse model of diabetes. *Neuropharmacology* **2018**, *131*, 316–325. [CrossRef] [PubMed]
38. Wang, K.; Song, F.; Xu, K.; Liu, Z.; Han, S.; Li, F.; Sun, Y. Irisin attenuates neuroinflammation and prevents the memory and cognitive deterioration in streptozotocin-induced diabetic mice. *Mediators Inflamm.* **2019**, *2019*, 1567179. [CrossRef] [PubMed]
39. Saravia, F.E.; Beauquis, J.; Revsin, Y.; Homo-Delarche, F.; de Kloet, E.R.; De Nicola, A.F. Hippocampal neuropathology of diabetes mellitus is relieved by estrogen treatment. *Cell Mol. Neurobiol.* **2006**, *26*, 943–957. [CrossRef] [PubMed]
40. Li, J.; Deng, J.; Sheng, W.; Zuo, Z. Metformin attenuates Alzheimer's disease-like neuropathology in obese, leptin-resistant mice. *Pharmacol. Biochem. Behav.* **2012**, *101*, 564–574. [CrossRef] [PubMed]
41. Hayashi-Park, E.; Ozment, B.N.; Griffith, C.M.; Zhang, H.; Patrylo, P.R.; Rose, G.M. Experimentally induced diabetes worsens neuropathology, but not learning and memory, in middle aged 3xTg mice. *Behav. Brain Res.* **2017**, *322*, 280–287. [CrossRef] [PubMed]
42. Leuner, B.; Gould, E. Structural plasticity and hippocampal function. *Annu. Rev. Psychol.* **2010**, *61*, 111–140. [CrossRef] [PubMed]
43. Brunner, L.; Nick, H.P.; Cumin, F.; Chiesi, M.; Baum, H.P.; Whitebread, S.; Stricker-Krongrad, A.; Levens, N. Leptin is a physiologically important regulator of food intake. *Int. J. Obes. Relat. Metab. Disord.* **1997**, *21*, 1152–1160. [CrossRef] [PubMed]
44. Considine, R.V.; Sinha, M.K.; Heiman, M.L.; Kriauciunas, A.; Stephens, T.W.; Nyce, M.R.; Ohannesian, J.P.; Marco, C.C.; McKee, L.J.; Bauer, T.L.; et al. Serum immunoreactive-leptin concentrations in normal-weight and obese humans. *N. Engl. J. Med.* **1996**, *334*, 292–295. [CrossRef] [PubMed]
45. Licinio, J.; Mantzoros, C.; Negrao, A.B.; Cizza, G.; Wong, M.L.; Bongiorno, P.B.; Chrousos, G.P.; Karp, B.; Allen, C.; Flier, J.S.; et al. Human leptin levels are pulsatile and inversely related to pituitary-adrenal function. *Nat. Med.* **1997**, *3*, 575–579. [CrossRef] [PubMed]
46. Sinha, M.K.; Ohannesian, J.P.; Heiman, M.L.; Kriauciunas, A.; Stephens, T.W.; Magosin, S.; Marco, C.; Caro, J.F. Nocturnal rise of leptin in lean, obese, and non-insulin-dependent diabetes mellitus subjects. *J. Clin. Investig.* **1996**, *97*, 1344–1347. [CrossRef] [PubMed]
47. Boden, G.; Chen, X.; Mozzoli, M.; Ryan, I. Effect of fasting on serum leptin in normal human subjects. *J. Clin. Endocrinol. Metab.* **1996**, *81*, 3419–3423. [PubMed]
48. Chan, J.L.; Heist, K.; DePaoli, A.M.; Veldhuis, J.D.; Mantzoros, C.S. The role of falling leptin levels in the neuroendocrine and metabolic adaptation to short-term starvation in healthy men. *J. Clin. Investig.* **2003**, *111*, 1409–1421. [CrossRef] [PubMed]
49. Chan, J.L.; Mantzoros, C.S. Role of leptin in energy-deprivation states: Normal human physiology and clinical implications for hypothalamic amenorrhoea and anorexia nervosa. *Lancet* **2005**, *366*, 74–85. [CrossRef]
50. Myers, M.G.; Cowley, M.A.; Munzberg, H. Mechanisms of leptin action and leptin resistance. *Annu. Rev. Physiol.* **2008**, *70*, 537–556. [CrossRef] [PubMed]
51. Fischer, S.; Hanefeld, M.; Haffner, S.M.; Fusch, C.; Schwanebeck, U.; Kohler, C.; Fucker, K.; Julius, U. Insulin-resistant patients with type 2 diabetes mellitus have higher serum leptin levels independently of body fat mass. *Acta Diabetol.* **2002**, *39*, 105–110. [CrossRef] [PubMed]
52. Harris, R.B.; Zhou, J.; Redmann, S.M., Jr.; Smagin, G.N.; Smith, S.R.; Rodgers, E.; Zachwieja, J.J. A leptin dose-response study in obese (ob/ob) and lean (+/?) mice. *Endocrinology* **1998**, *139*, 8–19. [CrossRef] [PubMed]
53. Berglund, E.D.; Vianna, C.R.; Donato, J., Jr.; Kim, M.H.; Chuang, J.C.; Lee, C.E.; Lauzon, D.A.; Lin, P.; Brule, L.J.; Scott, M.M.; et al. Direct leptin action on POMC neurons regulates glucose homeostasis and hepatic insulin sensitivity in mice. *J. Clin. Investig.* **2012**, *122*, 1000–1009. [CrossRef] [PubMed]

54. Cummings, B.P.; Bettaieb, A.; Graham, J.L.; Stanhope, K.L.; Dill, R.; Morton, G.J.; Haj, F.G.; Havel, P.J. Subcutaneous administration of leptin normalizes fasting plasma glucose in obese type 2 diabetic UCD-T2DM rats. *Proc. Natl. Acad. Sci. USA* **2011**, *108*, 14670–14675. [CrossRef] [PubMed]
55. Morton, G.J.; Gelling, R.W.; Niswender, K.D.; Morrison, C.D.; Rhodes, C.J.; Schwartz, M.W. Leptin regulates insulin sensitivity via phosphatidylinositol-3-OH kinase signaling in mediobasal hypothalamic neurons. *Cell Metab.* **2005**, *2*, 411–420. [CrossRef] [PubMed]
56. Coppari, R.; Ichinose, M.; Lee, C.E.; Pullen, A.E.; Kenny, C.D.; McGovern, R.A.; Tang, V.; Liu, S.M.; Ludwig, T.; Chua, S.C., Jr.; et al. The hypothalamic arcuate nucleus: A key site for mediating leptin's effects on glucose homeostasis and locomotor activity. *Cell Metab.* **2005**, *1*, 63–72. [CrossRef] [PubMed]
57. Enriori, P.J.; Evans, A.E.; Sinnayah, P.; Jobst, E.E.; Tonelli-Lemos, L.; Billes, S.K.; Glavas, M.M.; Grayson, B.E.; Perello, M.; Nillni, E.A.; et al. Diet-induced obesity causes severe but reversible leptin resistance in arcuate melanocortin neurons. *Cell Metab.* **2007**, *5*, 181–194. [CrossRef] [PubMed]
58. El-Haschimi, K.; Pierroz, D.D.; Hileman, S.M.; Bjorbaek, C.; Flier, J.S. Two defects contribute to hypothalamic leptin resistance in mice with diet-induced obesity. *J. Clin. Investig.* **2000**, *105*, 1827–1832. [CrossRef] [PubMed]
59. Munzberg, H.; Flier, J.S.; Bjorbaek, C. Region-specific leptin resistance within the hypothalamus of diet-induced obese mice. *Endocrinology* **2004**, *145*, 4880–4889. [CrossRef] [PubMed]
60. Lin, S.; Thomas, T.C.; Storlien, L.H.; Huang, X.F. Development of high fat diet-induced obesity and leptin resistance in C57Bl/6J mice. *Int. J. Obes. Relat. Metab. Disord.* **2000**, *24*, 639–646. [CrossRef] [PubMed]
61. Mittendorfer, B.; Horowitz, J.F.; DePaoli, A.M.; McCamish, M.A.; Patterson, B.W.; Klein, S. Recombinant human leptin treatment does not improve insulin action in obese subjects with type 2 diabetes. *Diabetes* **2011**, *60*, 1474–1477. [CrossRef] [PubMed]
62. Moon, H.S.; Matarese, G.; Brennan, A.M.; Chamberland, J.P.; Liu, X.; Fiorenza, C.G.; Mylvaganam, G.H.; Abanni, L.; Carbone, F.; Williams, C.J.; et al. Efficacy of metreleptin in obese patients with type 2 diabetes: Cellular and molecular pathways underlying leptin tolerance. *Diabetes* **2011**, *60*, 1647–1656. [CrossRef] [PubMed]
63. Funahashi, H.; Yada, T.; Suzuki, R.; Shioda, S. Distribution, function, and properties of leptin receptors in the brain. *Int. Rev. Cytol.* **2003**, *224*, 1–27. [PubMed]
64. Zhou, Y.; Rui, L. Leptin signaling and leptin resistance. *Front. Med.* **2013**, *7*, 207–222. [CrossRef] [PubMed]
65. Morrison, C.D. Leptin signaling in brain: A link between nutrition and cognition? *Biochim. Biophys. Acta* **2009**, *1792*, 401–408. [CrossRef] [PubMed]
66. Farr, O.M.; Tsoukas, M.A.; Mantzoros, C.S. Leptin and the brain: Influences on brain development, cognitive functioning and psychiatric disorders. *Metabolism* **2015**, *64*, 114–130. [CrossRef] [PubMed]
67. Coll, A.P.; Farooqi, I.S.; O'Rahilly, S. The hormonal control of food intake. *Cell* **2007**, *129*, 251–262. [CrossRef] [PubMed]
68. Ahima, R.S.; Prabakaran, D.; Mantzoros, C.; Qu, D.; Lowell, B.; Maratos-Flier, E.; Flier, J.S. Role of leptin in the neuroendocrine response to fasting. *Nature* **1996**, *382*, 250–252. [CrossRef] [PubMed]
69. Cristino, L.; Busetto, G.; Imperatore, R.; Ferrandino, I.; Palomba, L.; Silvestri, C.; Petrosino, S.; Orlando, P.; Bentivoglio, M.; Mackie, K.; et al. Obesity-driven synaptic remodeling affects endocannabinoid control of orexinergic neurons. *Proc. Natl. Acad. Sci. USA* **2013**, *110*, E2229–E2238. [CrossRef] [PubMed]
70. Cason, A.M.; Smith, R.J.; Tahsili-Fahadan, P.; Moorman, D.E.; Sartor, G.C.; Aston-Jones, G. Role of orexin/hypocretin in reward-seeking and addiction: Implications for obesity. *Physiol. Behav.* **2010**, *100*, 419–428. [CrossRef] [PubMed]
71. Hay-Schmidt, A.; Helboe, L.; Larsen, P.J. Leptin receptor immunoreactivity is present in ascending serotonergic and catecholaminergic neurons of the rat. *Neuroendocrinology* **2001**, *73*, 215–226. [CrossRef] [PubMed]
72. Figlewicz, D.P.; Evans, S.B.; Murphy, J.; Hoen, M.; Baskin, D.G. Expression of receptors for insulin and leptin in the ventral tegmental area/substantia nigra (VTA/SN) of the rat. *Brain Res.* **2003**, *964*, 107–115. [CrossRef]
73. Balland, E.; Cowley, M.A. New insights in leptin resistance mechanisms in mice. *Front. Neuroendocrinol.* **2015**, *39*, 59–65. [CrossRef] [PubMed]
74. Hara, J.; Beuckmann, C.T.; Nambu, T.; Willie, J.T.; Chemelli, R.M.; Sinton, C.M.; Sugiyama, F.; Yagami, K.; Goto, K.; Yanagisawa, M.; et al. Genetic ablation of orexin neurons in mice results in narcolepsy, hypophagia, and obesity. *Neuron* **2001**, *30*, 345–354. [CrossRef]

75. Harris, G.C.; Wimmer, M.; Aston-Jones, G. A role for lateral hypothalamic orexin neurons in reward seeking. *Nature* **2005**, *437*, 556–559. [CrossRef] [PubMed]
76. Narita, M.; Nagumo, Y.; Hashimoto, S.; Narita, M.; Khotib, J.; Miyatake, M.; Sakurai, T.; Yanagisawa, M.; Nakamachi, T.; Shioda, S.; et al. Direct involvement of orexinergic systems in the activation of the mesolimbic dopamine pathway and related behaviors induced by morphine. *J. Neurosci.* **2006**, *26*, 398–405. [CrossRef] [PubMed]
77. Liu, J.J.; Bello, N.T.; Pang, Z.P. Presynaptic regulation of leptin in a defined lateral hypothalamus-ventral tegmental area neurocircuitry depends on energy state. *J. Neurosci.* **2017**, *37*, 11854–11866. [CrossRef] [PubMed]
78. Salamone, J.D.; Correa, M.; Mingote, S.M.; Weber, S.M. Beyond the reward hypothesis: Alternative functions of nucleus accumbens dopamine. *Curr. Opin. Pharmacol.* **2005**, *5*, 34–41. [CrossRef] [PubMed]
79. Kelley, A.E.; Baldo, B.A.; Pratt, W.E.; Will, M.J. Corticostriatal-hypothalamic circuitry and food motivation: Integration of energy, action and reward. *Physiol. Behav.* **2005**, *86*, 773–795. [CrossRef] [PubMed]
80. Schultz, W. Behavioral dopamine signals. *Trends Neurosci.* **2007**, *30*, 203–210. [CrossRef] [PubMed]
81. Coccurello, R.; Maccarrone, M. Hedonic eating and the "Delicious circle": From lipid-derived mediators to brain dopamine and back. *Front. Neurosci.* **2018**, *12*, 271. [CrossRef] [PubMed]
82. Leinninger, G.M.; Jo, Y.H.; Leshan, R.L.; Louis, G.W.; Yang, H.; Barrera, J.G.; Wilson, H.; Opland, D.M.; Faouzi, M.A.; Gong, Y.; et al. Leptin acts via leptin receptor-expressing lateral hypothalamic neurons to modulate the mesolimbic dopamine system and suppress feeding. *Cell Metab.* **2009**, *10*, 89–98. [CrossRef] [PubMed]
83. Davis, J.F.; Choi, D.L.; Schurdak, J.D.; Fitzgerald, M.F.; Clegg, D.J.; Lipton, J.W.; Figlewicz, D.P.; Benoit, S.C. Leptin regulates energy balance and motivation through action at distinct neural circuits. *Biol. Psychiatry* **2011**, *69*, 668–674. [CrossRef] [PubMed]
84. Fulton, S.; Pissios, P.; Manchon, R.P.; Stiles, L.; Frank, L.; Pothos, E.N.; Maratos-Flier, E.; Flier, J.S. Leptin regulation of the mesoaccumbens dopamine pathway. *Neuron* **2006**, *51*, 811–822. [CrossRef] [PubMed]
85. Korotkova, T.M.; Brown, R.E.; Sergeeva, O.A.; Ponomarenko, A.A.; Haas, H.L. Effects of arousal- and feeding-related neuropeptides on dopaminergic and GABAergic neurons in the ventral tegmental area of the rat. *Eur. J. Neurosci.* **2006**, *23*, 2677–2685. [CrossRef] [PubMed]
86. Krugel, U.; Schraft, T.; Kittner, H.; Kiess, W.; Illes, P. Basal and feeding-evoked dopamine release in the rat nucleus accumbens is depressed by leptin. *Eur. J. Pharmacol.* **2003**, *482*, 185–187. [CrossRef] [PubMed]
87. Morton, G.J.; Blevins, J.E.; Kim, F.; Matsen, M.; Figlewicz, D.P. The action of leptin in the ventral tegmental area to decrease food intake is dependent on Jak-2 signaling. *Am. J. Physiol. Endocrinol. Metab.* **2009**, *297*, E202–E210. [CrossRef] [PubMed]
88. Scarpace, P.J.; Matheny, M.; Kirichenko, N.; Gao, Y.X.; Tumer, N.; Zhang, Y. Leptin overexpression in VTA trans-activates the hypothalamus whereas prolonged leptin action in either region cross-desensitizes. *Neuropharmacology* **2013**, *65*, 90–100. [CrossRef] [PubMed]
89. Hommel, J.D.; Trinko, R.; Sears, R.M.; Georgescu, D.; Liu, Z.W.; Gao, X.B.; Thurmon, J.J.; Marinelli, M.; DiLeone, R.J. Leptin receptor signaling in midbrain dopamine neurons regulates feeding. *Neuron* **2006**, *51*, 801–810. [CrossRef] [PubMed]
90. Shen, M.; Jiang, C.; Liu, P.; Wang, F.; Ma, L. Mesolimbic leptin signaling negatively regulates cocaine-conditioned reward. *Transl. Psychiatry* **2016**, *6*, e972. [CrossRef] [PubMed]
91. Haass-Koffler, C.L.; Aoun, E.G.; Swift, R.M.; de la Monte, S.M.; Kenna, G.A.; Leggio, L. Leptin levels are reduced by intravenous ghrelin administration and correlated with cue-induced alcohol craving. *Transl. Psychiatry* **2015**, *5*, e646. [CrossRef] [PubMed]
92. Maes, M.; Bocchio Chiavetto, L.; Bignotti, S.; Battisa Tura, G.; Pioli, R.; Boin, F.; Kenis, G.; Bosmans, E.; de Jongh, R.; Lin, A.; et al. Effects of atypical antipsychotics on the inflammatory response system in schizophrenic patients resistant to treatment with typical neuroleptics. *Eur. Neuropsychopharmacol.* **2000**, *10*, 119–124. [CrossRef]
93. Coccurello, R.; Moles, A. Potential mechanisms of atypical antipsychotic-induced metabolic derangement: Clues for understanding obesity and novel drug design. *Pharmacol. Ther.* **2010**, *127*, 210–251. [CrossRef] [PubMed]

94. Sapra, M.; Lawson, D.; Iranmanesh, A.; Varma, A. Adiposity-independent hypoadiponectinemia as a potential marker of insulin resistance and inflammation in schizophrenia patients treated with second generation antipsychotics. *Schizophr. Res.* **2016**, *174*, 132–136. [CrossRef] [PubMed]
95. Flowers, S.A.; Evans, S.J.; Ward, K.M.; McInnis, M.G.; Ellingrod, V.L. Interaction between atypical antipsychotics and the gut microbiome in a bipolar disease cohort. *Pharmacotherapy* **2017**, *37*, 261–267. [CrossRef] [PubMed]
96. Chen, J.; Huang, X.F.; Shao, R.; Chen, C.; Deng, C. Molecular mechanisms of antipsychotic drug-induced diabetes. *Front. Neurosci.* **2017**, *11*, 643. [CrossRef] [PubMed]
97. Singh, R.; Bansal, Y.; Medhi, B.; Kuhad, A. Antipsychotics-induced metabolic alterations: Recounting the mechanistic insights, therapeutic targets and pharmacological alternatives. *Eur. J. Pharmacol.* **2019**, *844*, 231–240. [CrossRef] [PubMed]
98. Xu, H.; Zhuang, X. Atypical antipsychotics-induced metabolic syndrome and nonalcoholic fatty liver disease: A critical review. *Neuropsychiatr. Dis. Treat.* **2019**, *15*, 2087–2099. [CrossRef] [PubMed]
99. Kraus, T.; Haack, M.; Schuld, A.; Hinze-Selch, D.; Kühn, M.; Uhr, M.; Pollmächer, T. Body weight and leptin plasma levels during treatment with antipsychotic drugs. *Am. J. Psychiatry* **1999**, *156*, 312–314. [PubMed]
100. McIntyre, R.S.; Mancini, D.A.; Basile, V.S.; Srinivasan, J.; Kennedy, S.H. Antipsychotic-induced weight gain: Bipolar disorder and leptin. *J. Clin. Psychopharmacol.* **2003**, *23*, 323–327. [CrossRef] [PubMed]
101. Popovic, V.; Doknic, M.; Maric, N.; Pekic, S.; Damjanovic, A.; Miljic, D.; Popovic, S.; Miljic, N.; Djurovic, M.; Jasovic-Gasic, M.; et al. Changes in neuroendocrine and metabolic hormones induced by atypical antipsychotics in normal-weight patients with schizophrenia. *Neuroendocrinology* **2007**, *85*, 249–256. [CrossRef] [PubMed]
102. Potvin, S.; Zhornitsky, S.; Stip, E. Antipsychotic-induced changes in blood levels of leptin in schizophrenia: A meta-analysis. *Can. J. Psychiatry* **2015**, *60* (Suppl. 2), S26–S34.
103. Ota, M.; Mori, K.; Nakashima, A.; Kaneko, Y.S.; Fujiwara, K.; Itoh, M.; Nagasaka, A.; Ota, A. Peripheral injection of risperidone, an atypical antipsychotic, alters the bodyweight gain of rats. *Clin. Exp. Pharmacol. Physiol.* **2002**, *29*, 980–989. [CrossRef] [PubMed]
104. Albaugh, V.L.; Henry, C.R.; Bello, N.T.; Hajnal, A.; Lynch, S.L.; Halle, B.; Lynch, C.J. Hormonal and metabolic effects of olanzapine and clozapine related to body weight in rodents. *Obesity* **2006**, *14*, 36–51. [CrossRef] [PubMed]
105. Minet-Ringuet, J.; Even, P.C.; Goubern, M.; Tome, D.; de Beaurepaire, R. Long term treatment with olanzapine mixed with the food in male rats induces body fat deposition with no increase in body weight and no thermogenic alteration. *Appetite* **2006**, *46*, 254–262. [CrossRef] [PubMed]
106. Minet-Ringuet, J.; Even, P.C.; Lacroix, M.; Tome, D.; de Beaurepaire, R. A model for antipsychotic-induced obesity in the male rat. *Psychopharmacology* **2006**, *187*, 447–454. [CrossRef] [PubMed]
107. Lord, C.C.; Wyler, S.C.; Wan, R.; Castorena, C.M.; Ahmed, N.; Mathew, D.; Lee, S.; Liu, C.; Elmquist, J.K. The atypical antipsychotic olanzapine causes weight gain by targeting serotonin receptor, 2C. *J. Clin. Investig.* **2017**, *127*, 3402–3406. [CrossRef] [PubMed]
108. Kusumi, I.; Boku, S.; Takahashi, Y. Psychopharmacology of atypical antipsychotic drugs: From the receptor binding profile to neuroprotection and neurogenesis. *Psychiatry Clin. Neurosci.* **2015**, *69*, 243–258. [CrossRef] [PubMed]
109. Meltzer, H.Y. What's atypical about atypical antipsychotic drugs? *Curr. Opin. Pharmacol.* **2004**, *4*, 53–57. [CrossRef] [PubMed]
110. Basile, V.S.; Masellis, M.; McIntyre, R.S.; Meltzer, H.Y.; Lieberman, J.A.; Kennedy, J.L. Genetic dissection of atypical antipsychotic-induced weight gain: Novel preliminary data on the pharmacogenetic puzzle. *J. Clin. Psychiatry* **2001**, *62* (Suppl. 23), 45–66. [PubMed]
111. Starrenburg, F.C.; Bogers, J.P. How can antipsychotics cause Diabetes Mellitus? Insights based on receptor-binding profiles, humoral factors and transporter proteins. *Eur. Psychiatry* **2009**, *24*, 164–170. [CrossRef] [PubMed]
112. Gettys, T.W.; Harkness, P.J.; Watson, P.M. The beta 3-adrenergic receptor inhibits insulin-stimulated leptin secretion from isolated rat adipocytes. *Endocrinology* **1996**, *137*, 4054–4057. [CrossRef] [PubMed]
113. Munzberg, H. Differential leptin access into the brain—A hierarchical organization of hypothalamic leptin target sites? *Physiol. Behav.* **2008**, *94*, 664–669. [CrossRef] [PubMed]

114. Morash, B.; Li, A.; Murphy, P.R.; Wilkinson, M.; Ur, E. Leptin gene expression in the brain and pituitary gland. *Endocrinology* **1999**, *140*, 5995–5998. [CrossRef] [PubMed]
115. Ur, E.; Wilkinson, D.A.; Morash, B.A.; Wilkinson, M. Leptin immunoreactivity is localized to neurons in rat brain. *Neuroendocrinology* **2002**, *75*, 264–272. [CrossRef] [PubMed]
116. Banks, W.A.; Clever, C.M.; Farrell, C.L. Partial saturation and regional variation in the blood-to-brain transport of leptin in normal weight mice. *Am. J. Physiol. Endocrinol. Metab.* **2000**, *278*, E1158–E1165. [CrossRef] [PubMed]
117. Van Doorn, C.; Macht, V.A.; Grillo, C.A.; Reagan, L.P. Leptin resistance and hippocampal behavioral deficits. *Physiol. Behav.* **2017**, *176*, 207–213. [CrossRef] [PubMed]
118. Stranahan, A.M.; Arumugam, T.V.; Cutler, R.G.; Lee, K.; Egan, J.M.; Mattson, M.P. Diabetes impairs hippocampal function through glucocorticoid-mediated effects on new and mature neurons. *Nat. Neurosci.* **2008**, *11*, 309–317. [CrossRef] [PubMed]
119. Dhar, M.; Zhu, M.; Impey, S.; Lambert, T.J.; Bland, T.; Karatsoreos, I.N.; Nakazawa, T.; Appleyard, S.M.; Wayman, G.A. Leptin induces hippocampal synaptogenesis via CREB-regulated microRNA-132 suppression of, p.2.5.0.G.A.P. *Mol. Endocrinol.* **2014**, *28*, 1073–1087. [CrossRef] [PubMed]
120. Li, X.L.; Aou, S.; Oomura, Y.; Hori, N.; Fukunaga, K.; Hori, T. Impairment of long-term potentiation and spatial memory in leptin receptor-deficient rodents. *Neuroscience* **2002**, *113*, 607–615. [CrossRef]
121. Gerges, N.Z.; Aleisa, A.M.; Alkadhi, K.A. Impaired long-term potentiation in obese zucker rats: Possible involvement of presynaptic mechanism. *Neuroscience* **2003**, *120*, 535–539. [CrossRef]
122. Guo, M.; Lu, Y.; Garza, J.C.; Li, Y.; Chua, S.C.; Zhang, W.; Lu, B.; Lu, X.Y. Forebrain glutamatergic neurons mediate leptin action on depression-like behaviors and synaptic depression. *Transl. Psychiatry* **2012**, *2*, e83. [CrossRef] [PubMed]
123. Koch, C.E.; Lowe, C.; Pretz, D.; Steger, J.; Williams, L.M.; Tups, A. High-fat diet induces leptin resistance in leptin-deficient mice. *J. Neuroendocrinol.* **2014**, *26*, 58–67. [CrossRef] [PubMed]
124. Wang, B.; Chandrasekera, P.C.; Pippin, J.J. Leptin- and leptin receptor-deficient rodent models: Relevance for human type 2 diabetes. *Curr. Diabetes Rev.* **2014**, *10*, 131–145. [CrossRef] [PubMed]
125. O'Malley, D.; MacDonald, N.; Mizielinska, S.; Connolly, C.N.; Irving, A.J.; Harvey, J. Leptin promotes rapid dynamic changes in hippocampal dendritic morphology. *Mol. Cell. Neurosci.* **2007**, *35*, 559–572. [CrossRef] [PubMed]
126. Liu, J.; Garza, J.C.; Bronner, J.; Kim, C.S.; Zhang, W.; Lu, X.Y. Acute administration of leptin produces anxiolytic-like effects: A comparison with fluoxetine. *Psychopharmacology* **2010**, *207*, 535–545. [CrossRef] [PubMed]
127. Farr, S.A.; Banks, W.A.; Morley, J.E. Effects of leptin on memory processing. *Peptides* **2006**, *27*, 1420–1425. [CrossRef] [PubMed]
128. Kanoski, S.E.; Hayes, M.R.; Greenwald, H.S.; Fortin, S.M.; Gianessi, C.A.; Gilbert, J.R.; Grill, H.J. Hippocampal leptin signaling reduces food intake and modulates food-related memory processing. *Neuropsychopharmacology* **2011**, *36*, 1859–1870. [CrossRef] [PubMed]
129. Suarez, A.N.; Noble, E.E.; Kanoski, S.E. Regulation of memory function by feeding-relevant biological systems: following the breadcrumbs to the hippocampus. *Front. Mol. Neurosci.* **2019**, *12*, 101. [CrossRef] [PubMed]
130. Bliss, T.V.; Collingridge, G.L. A synaptic model of memory: Long-term potentiation in the hippocampus. *Nature* **1993**, *361*, 31–39. [CrossRef] [PubMed]
131. Wayner, M.J.; Armstrong, D.L.; Phelix, C.F.; Oomura, Y. Orexin-A (Hypocretin-1) and leptin enhance LTP in the dentate gyrus of rats in vivo. *Peptides* **2004**, *25*, 991–996. [CrossRef] [PubMed]
132. Malenka, R.C. Postsynaptic factors control the duration of synaptic enhancement in area CA1 of the hippocampus. *Neuron* **1991**, *6*, 53–60. [CrossRef]
133. Greco, S.J.; Bryan, K.J.; Sarkar, S.; Zhu, X.; Smith, M.A.; Ashford, J.W.; Johnston, J.M.; Tezapsidis, N.; Casadesus, G. Leptin reduces pathology and improves memory in a transgenic mouse model of Alzheimer's disease. *J. Alzheimers Dis.* **2010**, *19*, 1155–1167. [CrossRef] [PubMed]
134. Tong, J.Q.; Zhang, J.; Hao, M.; Yang, J.; Han, Y.F.; Liu, X.J.; Shi, H.; Wu, M.N.; Liu, Q.S.; Qi, J.S. Leptin attenuates the detrimental effects of beta-amyloid on spatial memory and hippocampal later-phase long term potentiation in rats. *Horm. Behav.* **2015**, *73*, 125–130. [CrossRef] [PubMed]

135. Liu, Z.; Zhang, Y.; Liu, J.; Yin, F. Geniposide attenuates the level of Aβ1-42 via enhancing leptin signaling in cellular and APP/PS1 transgenic mice. *Arch. Pharmacal Res.* **2017**, *40*, 571–578. [CrossRef] [PubMed]
136. Yamamoto, N.; Tanida, M.; Kasahara, R.; Sobue, K.; Suzuki, K. Leptin inhibits amyloid beta-protein fibrillogenesis by decreasing GM1 gangliosides on the neuronal cell surface through PI3K/Akt/mTOR pathway. *J. Neurochem.* **2014**, *131*, 323–332. [CrossRef] [PubMed]
137. Chandran, M.; Phillips, S.A.; Ciaraldi, T.; Henry, R.R. Adiponectin: More than just another fat cell hormone? *Diabetes Care* **2003**, *26*, 2442–2450. [CrossRef] [PubMed]
138. Kawano, J.; Arora, R. The role of adiponectin in obesity, diabetes, and cardiovascular disease. *J. Cardiometab. Syndr.* **2009**, *4*, 44–49. [CrossRef] [PubMed]
139. Yamauchi, T.; Kamon, J.; Ito, Y.; Tsuchida, A.; Yokomizo, T.; Kita, S.; Sugiyama, T.; Miyagishi, M.; Hara, K.; Tsunoda, M.; et al. Cloning of adiponectin receptors that mediate antidiabetic metabolic effects. *Nature* **2003**, *423*, 762–769. [CrossRef] [PubMed]
140. Arita, Y.; Kihara, S.; Ouchi, N.; Takahashi, M.; Maeda, K.; Miyagawa, J.; Hotta, K.; Shimomura, I.; Nakamura, T.; Miyaoka, K.; et al. Paradoxical decrease of an adipose-specific protein, adiponectin, in obesity. *Biochem. Biophys. Res. Commun.* **1999**, *257*, 79–83. [CrossRef] [PubMed]
141. Hotta, K.; Funahashi, T.; Arita, Y.; Takahashi, M.; Matsuda, M.; Okamoto, Y.; Iwahashi, H.; Kuriyama, H.; Ouchi, N.; Maeda, K.; et al. Plasma concentrations of a novel, adipose-specific protein, adiponectin, in type 2 diabetic patients. *Arterioscler. Thromb. Vasc. Biol.* **2000**, *20*, 1595–1599. [CrossRef] [PubMed]
142. Guenther, M.; James, R.; Marks, J.; Zhao, S.; Szabo, A.; Kidambi, S. Adiposity distribution influences circulating adiponectin levels. *Transl. Res.* **2014**, *164*, 270–277. [CrossRef] [PubMed]
143. Kim, J.Y.; van de Wall, E.; Laplante, M.; Azzara, A.; Trujillo, M.E.; Hofmann, S.M.; Schraw, T.; Durand, J.L.; Li, H.; Li, G.; et al. Obesity-associated improvements in metabolic profile through expansion of adipose tissue. *J. Clin. Investig.* **2007**, *117*, 2621–2637. [CrossRef] [PubMed]
144. Guo, C.; Ricchiuti, V.; Lian, B.Q.; Yao, T.M.; Coutinho, P.; Romero, J.R.; Li, J.; Williams, G.H.; Adler, G.K. Mineralocorticoid receptor blockade reverses obesity-related changes in expression of adiponectin, peroxisome proliferator-activated receptor-gamma, and proinflammatory adipokines. *Circulation* **2008**, *117*, 2253–2261. [CrossRef] [PubMed]
145. Saleh, S.; El-Maraghy, N.; Reda, E.; Barakat, W. Modulation of diabetes and dyslipidemia in diabetic insulin-resistant rats by mangiferin: Role of adiponectin and TNF-alpha. *An. Acad. Bras. Cienc.* **2014**, *86*, 1935–1948. [CrossRef] [PubMed]
146. Croze, M.L.; Geloen, A.; Soulage, C.O. Abnormalities in myo-inositol metabolism associated with type 2 diabetes in mice fed a high-fat diet: Benefits of a dietary myo-inositol supplementation. *Br. J. Nutr.* **2015**, *113*, 1862–1875. [CrossRef] [PubMed]
147. Holmes, R.M.; Yi, Z.; De Filippis, E.; Berria, R.; Shahani, S.; Sathyanarayana, P.; Sherman, V.; Fujiwara, K.; Meyer, C.; Christ-Roberts, C.; et al. Increased abundance of the adaptor protein containing pleckstrin homology domain, phosphotyrosine binding domain and leucine zipper motif (APPL1) in patients with obesity and type 2 diabetes: Evidence for altered adiponectin signalling. *Diabetologia* **2011**, *54*, 2122–2131. [CrossRef] [PubMed]
148. Felder, T.K.; Hahne, P.; Soyal, S.M.; Miller, K.; Hoffinger, H.; Oberkofler, H.; Krempler, F.; Patsch, W. Hepatic adiponectin receptors (ADIPOR) 1 and 2 mRNA and their relation to insulin resistance in obese humans. *Int. J. Obes.* **2010**, *34*, 846–851. [CrossRef] [PubMed]
149. Okamoto, Y.; Folco, E.J.; Minami, M.; Wara, A.K.; Feinberg, M.W.; Sukhova, G.K.; Colvin, R.A.; Kihara, S.; Funahashi, T.; Luster, A.D.; et al. Adiponectin inhibits the production of CXC receptor 3 chemokine ligands in macrophages and reduces T-lymphocyte recruitment in atherogenesis. *Circ. Res.* **2008**, *102*, 218–225. [CrossRef] [PubMed]
150. Yang, W.S.; Jeng, C.Y.; Wu, T.J.; Tanaka, S.; Funahashi, T.; Matsuzawa, Y.; Wang, J.P.; Chen, C.L.; Tai, T.Y.; Chuang, L.M. Synthetic peroxisome proliferator-activated receptor-gamma agonist, rosiglitazone, increases plasma levels of adiponectin in type 2 diabetic patients. *Diabetes Care* **2002**, *25*, 376–380. [CrossRef] [PubMed]
151. Fry, M.; Smith, P.M.; Hoyda, T.D.; Duncan, M.; Ahima, R.S.; Sharkey, K.A.; Ferguson, A.V. Area postrema neurons are modulated by the adipocyte hormone adiponectin. *J. Neurosci.* **2006**, *26*, 9695–9702. [CrossRef] [PubMed]
152. Hoyda, T.D.; Fry, M.; Ahima, R.S.; Ferguson, A.V. Adiponectin selectively inhibits oxytocin neurons of the paraventricular nucleus of the hypothalamus. *J. Physiol.* **2007**, *585*, 805–816. [CrossRef] [PubMed]

153. Neumeier, M.; Weigert, J.; Buettner, R.; Wanninger, J.; Schaffler, A.; Muller, A.M.; Killian, S.; Sauerbruch, S.; Schlachetzki, F.; Steinbrecher, A.; et al. Detection of adiponectin in cerebrospinal fluid in humans. *Am. J. Physiol. Endocrinol. Metab.* **2007**, *293*, E965–E969. [CrossRef] [PubMed]
154. Rodriguez-Pacheco, F.; Martinez-Fuentes, A.J.; Tovar, S.; Pinilla, L.; Tena-Sempere, M.; Dieguez, C.; Castano, J.P.; Malagon, M.M. Regulation of pituitary cell function by adiponectin. *Endocrinology* **2007**, *148*, 401–410. [CrossRef] [PubMed]
155. Thundyil, J.; Tang, S.C.; Okun, E.; Shah, K.; Karamyan, V.T.; Li, Y.I.; Woodruff, T.M.; Taylor, S.M.; Jo, D.G.; Mattson, M.P.; et al. Evidence that adiponectin receptor 1 activation exacerbates ischemic neuronal death. *Exp. Transl. Stroke Med.* **2010**, *2*, 15. [CrossRef] [PubMed]
156. Repunte-Canonigo, V.; Berton, F.; Cottone, P.; Reifel-Miller, A.; Roberts, A.J.; Morales, M.; Francesconi, W.; Sanna, P.P. A potential role for adiponectin receptor 2 (AdipoR2) in the regulation of alcohol intake. *Brain Res.* **2010**, *1339*, 11–17. [CrossRef] [PubMed]
157. Zhang, D.; Guo, M.; Zhang, W.; Lu, X.Y. Adiponectin stimulates proliferation of adult hippocampal neural stem/progenitor cells through activation of p38 mitogen-activated protein kinase (p38MAPK)/glycogen synthase kinase 3beta (GSK-3beta)/beta-catenin signaling cascade. *J. Biol. Chem.* **2011**, *286*, 44913–44920. [CrossRef] [PubMed]
158. Liu, J.; Guo, M.; Zhang, D.; Cheng, S.Y.; Liu, M.; Ding, J.; Scherer, P.E.; Liu, F.; Lu, X.Y. Adiponectin is critical in determining susceptibility to depressive behaviors and has antidepressant-like activity. *Proc. Natl. Acad. Sci. USA* **2012**, *109*, 12248–12253. [CrossRef] [PubMed]
159. Varhelyi, Z.P.; Kalman, J.; Olah, Z.; Ivitz, E.V.; Fodor, E.K.; Santha, M.; Datki, Z.L.; Pakaski, M. Adiponectin receptors are less sensitive to stress in a transgenic mouse model of Alzheimer's disease. *Front. Neurosci.* **2017**, *11*, 199. [CrossRef] [PubMed]
160. Koch, C.E.; Lowe, C.; Legler, K.; Benzler, J.; Boucsein, A.; Bottiger, G.; Grattan, D.R.; Williams, L.M.; Tups, A. Central adiponectin acutely improves glucose tolerance in male mice. *Endocrinology* **2014**, *155*, 1806–1816. [CrossRef] [PubMed]
161. Wang, B.; Cheng, K.K. Hypothalamic AMPK as a mediator of hormonal regulation of energy balance. *Int. J. Mol. Sci.* **2018**, *19*, 3552. [CrossRef] [PubMed]
162. Kubota, N.; Yano, W.; Kubota, T.; Yamauchi, T.; Itoh, S.; Kumagai, H.; Kozono, H.; Takamoto, I.; Okamoto, S.; Shiuchi, T.; et al. Adiponectin stimulates AMP-activated protein kinase in the hypothalamus and increases food intake. *Cell Metab.* **2007**, *6*, 55–68. [CrossRef] [PubMed]
163. Sun, J.; Gao, Y.; Yao, T.; Huang, Y.; He, Z.; Kong, X.; Yu, K.J.; Wang, R.T.; Guo, H.; Yan, J.; et al. Adiponectin potentiates the acute effects of leptin in arcuate Pomc neurons. *Mol. Metab.* **2016**, *5*, 882–891. [CrossRef] [PubMed]
164. Qi, Y.; Takahashi, N.; Hileman, S.M.; Patel, H.R.; Berg, A.H.; Pajvani, U.B.; Scherer, P.E.; Ahima, R.S. Adiponectin acts in the brain to decrease body weight. *Nat. Med.* **2004**, *10*, 524–529. [CrossRef] [PubMed]
165. Suyama, S.; Maekawa, F.; Maejima, Y.; Kubota, N.; Kadowaki, T.; Yada, T. Glucose level determines excitatory or inhibitory effects of adiponectin on arcuate POMC neuron activity and feeding. *Sci. Rep.* **2016**, *6*, 30796. [CrossRef] [PubMed]
166. Suyama, S.; Lei, W.; Kubota, N.; Kadowaki, T.; Yada, T. Adiponectin at physiological level glucose-independently enhances inhibitory postsynaptic current onto NPY neurons in the hypothalamic arcuate nucleus. *Neuropeptides* **2017**, *65*, 1–9. [CrossRef] [PubMed]
167. Hanssens, L.; van Winkel, R.; Wampers, M.; Van Eyck, D.; Scheen, A.; Reginster, J.Y.; Collette, J.; Peuskens, J.; De Hert, M. A cross-sectional evaluation of adiponectin plasma levels in patients with schizophrenia and schizoaffective disorder. *Schizophr. Res.* **2008**, *106*, 308–314. [CrossRef] [PubMed]
168. Bartoli, F.; Crocamo, C.; Clerici, M.; Carra, G. Second-generation antipsychotics and adiponectin levels in schizophrenia: A comparative meta-analysis. *Eur. Neuropsychopharmacol.* **2015**, *25*, 1767–1774. [CrossRef] [PubMed]
169. De Hert, M.; Schreurs, V.; Sweers, K.; Van Eyck, D.; Hanssens, L.; Sinko, S.; Wampers, M.; Scheen, A.; Peuskens, J.; van Winkel, R. Typical and atypical antipsychotics differentially affect long-term incidence rates of the metabolic syndrome in first-episode patients with schizophrenia: a retrospective chart review. *Schizophr. Res.* **2008**, *101*, 295–303. [CrossRef] [PubMed]

170. Bai, Y.M.; Chen, T.T.; Yang, W.S.; Chi, Y.C.; Lin, C.C.; Liou, Y.J.; Wang, Y.C.; Su, T.P.; Chou, P.; Chen, J.Y. Association of adiponectin and metabolic syndrome among patients taking atypical antipsychotics for schizophrenia: A cohort study. *Schizophr. Res.* **2009**, *111*, 1–8. [CrossRef] [PubMed]
171. Weston-Green, K.; Huang, X.F.; Deng, C. Alterations to melanocortinergic, GABAergic and cannabinoid neurotransmission associated with olanzapine-induced weight gain. *PLoS ONE* **2012**, *7*, e33548. [CrossRef] [PubMed]
172. Murashita, M.; Inoue, T.; Kusumi, I.; Nakagawa, S.; Itoh, K.; Tanaka, T.; Izumi, T.; Hosoda, H.; Kangawa, K.; Koyama, T. Glucose and lipid metabolism of long-term risperidone monotherapy in patients with schizophrenia. *Psychiatry Clin. Neurosci.* **2007**, *61*, 54–58. [CrossRef] [PubMed]
173. Wampers, M.; Hanssens, L.; van Winkel, R.; Heald, A.; Collette, J.; Peuskens, J.; Reginster, J.Y.; Scheen, A.; De Hert, M. Differential effects of olanzapine and risperidone on plasma adiponectin levels over time: Results from a 3-month prospective open-label study. *Eur. Neuropsychopharmacol.* **2012**, *22*, 17–26. [CrossRef] [PubMed]
174. Bartoli, F.; Lax, A.; Crocamo, C.; Clerici, M.; Carra, G. Plasma adiponectin levels in schizophrenia and role of second-generation antipsychotics: A meta-analysis. *Psychoneuroendocrinology* **2015**, *56*, 179–189. [CrossRef] [PubMed]
175. Sun, F.; Lei, Y.; You, J.; Li, C.; Sun, L.; Garza, J.; Zhang, D.; Guo, M.; Scherer, P.E.; Lodge, D.; et al. Adiponectin modulates ventral tegmental area dopamine neuron activity and anxiety-related behavior through AdipoR1. *Mol. Psychiatry* **2019**, *24*, 126–144. [CrossRef] [PubMed]
176. Nestler, E.J.; Carlezon, W.A., Jr. The mesolimbic dopamine reward circuit in depression. *Biol. Psychiatry* **2006**, *59*, 1151–1159. [CrossRef] [PubMed]
177. Coque, L.; Mukherjee, S.; Cao, J.L.; Spencer, S.; Marvin, M.; Falcon, E.; Sidor, M.M.; Birnbaum, S.G.; Graham, A.; Neve, R.L.; et al. Specific role of VTA dopamine neuronal firing rates and morphology in the reversal of anxiety-related, but not depression-related behavior in the ClockDelta19 mouse model of mania. *Neuropsychopharmacology* **2011**, *36*, 1478–1488. [CrossRef] [PubMed]
178. Tye, K.M.; Mirzabekov, J.J.; Warden, M.R.; Ferenczi, E.A.; Tsai, H.C.; Finkelstein, J.; Kim, S.Y.; Adhikari, A.; Thompson, K.R.; Andalman, A.S.; et al. Dopamine neurons modulate neural encoding and expression of depression-related behaviour. *Nature* **2013**, *493*, 537–541. [CrossRef] [PubMed]
179. Chaudhury, D.; Walsh, J.J.; Friedman, A.K.; Juarez, B.; Ku, S.M.; Koo, J.W.; Ferguson, D.; Tsai, H.C.; Pomeranz, L.; Christoffel, D.J.; et al. Rapid regulation of depression-related behaviours by control of midbrain dopamine neurons. *Nature* **2013**, *493*, 532–536. [CrossRef] [PubMed]
180. Kahl, K.G.; Schweiger, U.; Correll, C.; Muller, C.; Busch, M.L.; Bauer, M.; Schwarz, P. Depression, anxiety disorders, and metabolic syndrome in a population at risk for type 2 diabetes mellitus. *Brain Behav.* **2015**, *5*, e00306. [CrossRef] [PubMed]
181. Turer, A.T.; Khera, A.; Ayers, C.R.; Turer, C.B.; Grundy, S.M.; Vega, G.L.; Scherer, P.E. Adipose tissue mass and location affect circulating adiponectin levels. *Diabetologia* **2011**, *54*, 2515–2524. [CrossRef] [PubMed]
182. Okamoto, Y.; Kihara, S.; Funahashi, T.; Matsuzawa, Y.; Libby, P. Adiponectin: A key adipocytokine in metabolic syndrome. *Clin. Sci. (Lond.)* **2006**, *110*, 267–278. [CrossRef] [PubMed]
183. Garcia-Casares, N.; Garcia-Arnes, J.A.; Rioja, J.; Ariza, M.J.; Gutierrez, A.; Alfaro, F.; Nabrozidis, A.; Gonzalez-Alegre, P.; Gonzalez-Santos, P. Alzheimer's like brain changes correlate with low adiponectin plasma levels in type 2 diabetic patients. *J. Diabetes Complicat.* **2016**, *30*, 281–286. [CrossRef] [PubMed]
184. Teixeira, A.L.; Diniz, B.S.; Campos, A.C.; Miranda, A.S.; Rocha, N.P.; Talib, L.L.; Gattaz, W.F.; Forlenza, O.V. Decreased levels of circulating adiponectin in mild cognitive impairment and Alzheimer's disease. *Neuromolecular. Med.* **2013**, *15*, 115–121. [CrossRef] [PubMed]
185. Zhang, D.; Wang, X.; Lu, X.Y. Adiponectin Exerts Neurotrophic Effects on Dendritic Arborization, Spinogenesis, and Neurogenesis of the Dentate Gyrus of Male Mice. *Endocrinology* **2016**, *157*, 2853–2869. [CrossRef] [PubMed]
186. Kim, M.W.; Abid, N.B.; Jo, M.H.; Jo, M.G.; Yoon, G.H.; Kim, M.O. Suppression of adiponectin receptor 1 promotes memory dysfunction and Alzheimer's disease-like pathologies. *Sci. Rep.* **2017**, *7*, 12435. [CrossRef] [PubMed]
187. Nicolas, S.; Veyssiere, J.; Gandin, C.; Zsurger, N.; Pietri, M.; Heurteaux, C.; Glaichenhaus, N.; Petit-Paitel, A.; Chabry, J. Neurogenesis-independent antidepressant-like effects of enriched environment is dependent on adiponectin. *Psychoneuroendocrinology* **2015**, *57*, 72–83. [CrossRef] [PubMed]

188. Chabry, J.; Nicolas, S.; Cazareth, J.; Murris, E.; Guyon, A.; Glaichenhaus, N.; Heurteaux, C.; Petit-Paitel, A. Enriched environment decreases microglia and brain macrophages inflammatory phenotypes through adiponectin-dependent mechanisms: Relevance to depressive-like behavior. *Brain Behav. Immun.* **2015**, *50*, 275–287. [CrossRef] [PubMed]
189. Guo, M.; Li, C.; Lei, Y.; Xu, S.; Zhao, D.; Lu, X.Y. Role of the adipose PPARgamma-adiponectin axis in susceptibility to stress and depression/anxiety-related behaviors. *Mol. Psychiatry* **2017**, *22*, 1056–1068. [CrossRef] [PubMed]
190. Yamaguchi, N.; Argueta, J.G.; Masuhiro, Y.; Kagishita, M.; Nonaka, K.; Saito, T.; Hanazawa, S.; Yamashita, Y. Adiponectin inhibits Toll-like receptor family-induced signaling. *FEBS Lett.* **2005**, *579*, 6821–6826. [CrossRef] [PubMed]
191. Mandal, P.; Pratt, B.T.; Barnes, M.; McMullen, M.R.; Nagy, L.E. Molecular mechanism for adiponectin-dependent M2 macrophage polarization: Link between the metabolic and innate immune activity of full-length adiponectin. *J. Biol. Chem.* **2011**, *286*, 13460–13469. [CrossRef] [PubMed]
192. Xu, Z.P.; Gan, G.S.; Liu, Y.M.; Xiao, J.S.; Liu, H.X.; Mei, B.; Zhang, J.J. Adiponectin Attenuates Streptozotocin-Induced Tau Hyperphosphorylation and Cognitive Deficits by Rescuing PI3K/Akt/GSK-3beta Pathway. *Neurochem. Res.* **2018**, *43*, 316–323. [CrossRef] [PubMed]
193. Jian, M.; Kwan, J.S.; Bunting, M.; Ng, R.C.; Chan, K.H. Adiponectin suppresses amyloid-beta oligomer (AbetaO)-induced inflammatory response of microglia via AdipoR1-AMPK-NF-kappaB signaling pathway. *J. Neuroinflamm.* **2019**, *16*, 110. [CrossRef] [PubMed]
194. Song, J.; Choi, S.M.; Kim, B.C. Adiponectin Regulates the Polarization and Function of Microglia via PPAR-gamma Signaling Under Amyloid beta Toxicity. *Front. Cell Neurosci.* **2017**, *11*, 64. [CrossRef] [PubMed]
195. Wang, M.; Jo, J.; Song, J. Adiponectin improves long-term potentiation in the 5XFAD mouse brain. *Sci. Rep.* **2019**, *9*, 8918. [CrossRef] [PubMed]
196. Rourke, J.L.; Dranse, H.J.; Sinal, C.J. Towards an integrative approach to understanding the role of chemerin in human health and disease. *Obesity Rev.* **2013**, *14*, 245–262. [CrossRef] [PubMed]
197. Zabel, B.A.; Silverio, A.M.; Butcher, E.C. Chemokine-like receptor 1 expression and chemerin-directed chemotaxis distinguish plasmacytoid from myeloid dendritic cells in human blood. *J. Immunol.* **2005**, *174*, 244–251. [CrossRef] [PubMed]
198. Zabel, B.A.; Nakae, S.; Zuniga, L.; Kim, J.Y.; Ohyama, T.; Alt, C.; Pan, J.; Suto, H.; Soler, D.; Allen, S.J.; et al. Mast cell-expressed orphan receptor CCRL2 binds chemerin and is required for optimal induction of IgE-mediated passive cutaneous anaphylaxis. *J. Exp. Med.* **2008**, *205*, 2207–2220. [CrossRef] [PubMed]
199. Barnea, G.; Strapps, W.; Herrada, G.; Berman, Y.; Ong, J.; Kloss, B.; Axel, R.; Lee, K.J. The genetic design of signaling cascades to record receptor activation. *Proc. Natl. Acad. Sci. USA* **2008**, *105*, 64–69. [CrossRef] [PubMed]
200. Goralski, K.B.; McCarthy, T.C.; Hanniman, E.A.; Zabel, B.A.; Butcher, E.C.; Parlee, S.D.; Muruganandan, S.; Sinal, C.J. Chemerin, a novel adipokine that regulates adipogenesis and adipocyte metabolism. *J. Biol. Chem.* **2007**, *282*, 28175–28188. [CrossRef] [PubMed]
201. Nagpal, S.; Patel, S.; Jacobe, H.; DiSepio, D.; Ghosn, C.; Malhotra, M.; Teng, M.; Duvic, M.; Chandraratna, R.A. Tazarotene-induced gene 2 (TIG2), a novel retinoid-responsive gene in skin. *J. Investig. Dermatol.* **1997**, *109*, 91–95. [CrossRef] [PubMed]
202. Bozaoglu, K.; Curran, J.E.; Stocker, C.J.; Zaibi, M.S.; Segal, D.; Konstantopoulos, N.; Morrison, S.; Carless, M.; Dyer, T.D.; Cole, S.A.; et al. Chemerin, a novel adipokine in the regulation of angiogenesis. *J. Clin. Endocrinol. Metab.* **2010**, *95*, 2476–2485. [CrossRef] [PubMed]
203. Zabel, B.A.; Allen, S.J.; Kulig, P.; Allen, J.A.; Cichy, J.; Handel, T.M.; Butcher, E.C. Chemerin activation by serine proteases of the coagulation, fibrinolytic, and inflammatory cascades. *J. Biol. Chem.* **2005**, *280*, 34661–34666. [CrossRef] [PubMed]
204. Bozaoglu, K.; Bolton, K.; McMillan, J.; Zimmet, P.; Jowett, J.; Collier, G.; Walder, K.; Segal, D. Chemerin is a novel adipokine associated with obesity and metabolic syndrome. *Endocrinology* **2007**, *148*, 4687–4694. [CrossRef] [PubMed]
205. Sell, H.; Laurencikiene, J.; Taube, A.; Eckardt, K.; Cramer, A.; Horrighs, A.; Arner, P.; Eckel, J. Chemerin is a novel adipocyte-derived factor inducing insulin resistance in primary human skeletal muscle cells. *Diabetes* **2009**, *58*, 2731–2740. [CrossRef] [PubMed]

206. Chakaroun, R.; Raschpichler, M.; Kloting, N.; Oberbach, A.; Flehmig, G.; Kern, M.; Schon, M.R.; Shang, E.; Lohmann, T.; Dressler, M.; et al. Effects of weight loss and exercise on chemerin serum concentrations and adipose tissue expression in human obesity. *Metabolism* **2012**, *61*, 706–714. [CrossRef] [PubMed]
207. Wargent, E.T.; Zaibi, M.S.; O'Dowd, J.F.; Cawthorne, M.A.; Wang, S.J.; Arch, J.R.; Stocker, C.J. Evidence from studies in rodents and in isolated adipocytes that agonists of the chemerin receptor CMKLR1 may be beneficial in the treatment of type 2 diabetes. *PeerJ* **2015**, *3*, e753. [CrossRef] [PubMed]
208. Ernst, M.C.; Issa, M.; Goralski, K.B.; Sinal, C.J. Chemerin exacerbates glucose intolerance in mouse models of obesity and diabetes. *Endocrinology* **2010**, *151*, 1998–2007. [CrossRef] [PubMed]
209. Takahashi, M.; Okimura, Y.; Iguchi, G.; Nishizawa, H.; Yamamoto, M.; Suda, K.; Kitazawa, R.; Fujimoto, W.; Takahashi, K.; Zolotaryov, F.N.; et al. Chemerin regulates beta-cell function in mice. *Sci. Rep.* **2011**, *1*, 123. [CrossRef] [PubMed]
210. Ernst, M.C.; Haidl, I.D.; Zuniga, L.A.; Dranse, H.J.; Rourke, J.L.; Zabel, B.A.; Butcher, E.C.; Sinal, C.J. Disruption of the chemokine-like receptor-1 (CMKLR1) gene is associated with reduced adiposity and glucose intolerance. *Endocrinology* **2012**, *153*, 672–682. [CrossRef] [PubMed]
211. Huang, C.; Wang, M.; Ren, L.; Xiang, L.; Chen, J.; Li, M.; Xiao, T.; Ren, P.; Xiong, L.; Zhang, J.V. CMKLR1 deficiency influences glucose tolerance and thermogenesis in mice on high fat diet. *Biochem. Biophys. Res. Commun.* **2016**, *473*, 435–441. [CrossRef] [PubMed]
212. Rourke, J.L.; Muruganandan, S.; Dranse, H.J.; McMullen, N.M.; Sinal, C.J. Gpr1 is an active chemerin receptor influencing glucose homeostasis in obese mice. *J. Endocrinol.* **2014**, *222*, 201–215. [CrossRef] [PubMed]
213. Helfer, G.; Ross, A.W.; Thomson, L.M.; Mayer, C.D.; Stoney, P.N.; McCaffery, P.J.; Morgan, P.J. A neuroendocrine role for chemerin in hypothalamic remodelling and photoperiodic control of energy balance. *Sci. Rep.* **2016**, *6*, 26830. [CrossRef] [PubMed]
214. Perumalsamy, S.; Aqilah Mohd Zin, N.A.; Widodo, R.T.; Wan Ahmad, W.A.; Vethakkan, S.; Huri, H.Z. Chemokine Like Receptor-1 (CMKLR-1) Receptor: A Potential Therapeutic Target in Management of Chemerin Induced Type 2 Diabetes Mellitus and Cancer. *Curr. Pharm. Des.* **2017**, *23*, 3689–3698. [CrossRef] [PubMed]
215. Zhang, Y.; Xu, N.; Ding, Y.; Doycheva, D.M.; Zhang, Y.; Li, Q.; Flores, J.; Haghighiabyaneh, M.; Tang, J.; Zhang, J.H. Chemerin reverses neurological impairments and ameliorates neuronal apoptosis through ChemR23/CAMKK2/AMPK pathway in neonatal hypoxic-ischemic encephalopathy. *Cell Death Dis.* **2019**, *10*, 97. [CrossRef] [PubMed]
216. Peng, L.; Yu, Y.; Liu, J.; Li, S.; He, H.; Cheng, N.; Ye, R.D. The chemerin receptor CMKLR1 is a functional receptor for amyloid-beta peptide. *J. Alzheimers Dis.* **2015**, *43*, 227–242. [CrossRef] [PubMed]
217. Guo, X.; Fu, Y.; Xu, Y.; Weng, S.; Liu, D.; Cui, D.; Yu, S.; Liu, X.; Jiang, K.; Dong, Y. Chronic mild restraint stress rats decreased CMKLR1 expression in distinct brain region. *Neurosci. Lett.* **2012**, *524*, 25–29. [CrossRef] [PubMed]
218. Deyama, S.; Shimoda, K.; Suzuki, H.; Ishikawa, Y.; Ishimura, K.; Fukuda, H.; Hitora-Imamura, N.; Ide, S.; Satoh, M.; Kaneda, K.; et al. Resolvin E1/E2 ameliorate lipopolysaccharide-induced depression-like behaviors via ChemR23. *Psychopharmacology* **2018**, *235*, 329–336. [CrossRef] [PubMed]
219. Guo, L.; Li, Q.; Wang, W.; Yu, P.; Pan, H.; Li, P.; Sun, Y.; Zhang, J. Apelin inhibits insulin secretion in pancreatic beta-cells by activation of PI3-kinase-phosphodiesterase 3B. *Endocr Res.* **2009**, *34*, 142–154. [CrossRef] [PubMed]
220. Bertrand, C.; Valet, P.; Castan-Laurell, I. Apelin and energy metabolism. *Front. Physiol.* **2015**, *6*, 115. [CrossRef] [PubMed]
221. Wu, L.; Chen, L.; Li, L. Apelin/APJ system: A novel promising therapy target for pathological angiogenesis. *Clin. Chim. Acta* **2017**, *466*, 78–84. [CrossRef] [PubMed]
222. Yamaleyeva, L.M.; Shaltout, H.A.; Varagic, J. Apelin-13 in blood pressure regulation and cardiovascular disease. *Curr. Opin. Nephrol. Hypertens.* **2016**, *25*, 396–403. [CrossRef] [PubMed]
223. Valle, A.; Hoggard, N.; Adams, A.C.; Roca, P.; Speakman, J.R. Chronic central administration of apelin-13 over 10 days increases food intake, body weight, locomotor activity and body temperature in C57BL/6 mice. *J. Neuroendocrinol.* **2008**, *20*, 79–84. [CrossRef] [PubMed]
224. Vinel, C.; Lukjanenko, L.; Batut, A.; Deleruyelle, S.; Pradere, J.P.; Le Gonidec, S.; Dortignac, A.; Geoffre, N.; Pereira, O.; Karaz, S.; et al. The exerkine apelin reverses age-associated sarcopenia. *Nat. Med.* **2018**, *24*, 1360–1371. [CrossRef] [PubMed]

225. Castan-Laurell, I.; Dray, C.; Knauf, C.; Kunduzova, O.; Valet, P. Apelin, a promising target for type 2 diabetes treatment? *Trends Endocrinol. Metab.* **2012**, *23*, 234–241. [CrossRef] [PubMed]
226. Pope, G.R.; Roberts, E.M.; Lolait, S.J.; O'Carroll, A.M. Central and peripheral apelin receptor distribution in the mouse: Species differences with rat. *Peptides* **2012**, *33*, 139–148. [CrossRef] [PubMed]
227. Yue, P.; Jin, H.; Xu, S.; Aillaud, M.; Deng, A.C.; Azuma, J.; Kundu, R.K.; Reaven, G.M.; Quertermous, T.; Tsao, P.S. Apelin decreases lipolysis via G(q), G(i), and AMPK-Dependent Mechanisms. *Endocrinology* **2011**, *152*, 59–68. [CrossRef] [PubMed]
228. Yue, P.; Jin, H.; Aillaud, M.; Deng, A.C.; Azuma, J.; Asagami, T.; Kundu, R.K.; Reaven, G.M.; Quertermous, T.; Tsao, P.S. Apelin is necessary for the maintenance of insulin sensitivity. *Am. J. Physiol. Endocrinol. Metab.* **2010**, *298*, E59–E67. [CrossRef] [PubMed]
229. Dray, C.; Knauf, C.; Daviaud, D.; Waget, A.; Boucher, J.; Buleon, M.; Cani, P.D.; Attane, C.; Guigne, C.; Carpene, C.; et al. Apelin stimulates glucose utilization in normal and obese insulin-resistant mice. *Cell Metab.* **2008**, *8*, 437–445. [CrossRef] [PubMed]
230. Attane, C.; Foussal, C.; Le Gonidec, S.; Benani, A.; Daviaud, D.; Wanecq, E.; Guzman-Ruiz, R.; Dray, C.; Bezaire, V.; Rancoule, C.; et al. Apelin treatment increases complete Fatty Acid oxidation, mitochondrial oxidative capacity, and biogenesis in muscle of insulin-resistant mice. *Diabetes* **2012**, *61*, 310–320. [CrossRef] [PubMed]
231. Than, A.; Cheng, Y.; Foh, L.C.; Leow, M.K.; Lim, S.C.; Chuah, Y.J.; Kang, Y.; Chen, P. Apelin inhibits adipogenesis and lipolysis through distinct molecular pathways. *Mol. Cell Endocrinol.* **2012**, *362*, 227–241. [CrossRef] [PubMed]
232. Zhu, S.; Sun, F.; Li, W.; Cao, Y.; Wang, C.; Wang, Y.; Liang, D.; Zhang, R.; Zhang, S.; Wang, H.; et al. Apelin stimulates glucose uptake through the PI3K/Akt pathway and improves insulin resistance in 3T3-L1 adipocytes. *Mol. Cell Biochem.* **2011**, *353*, 305–313. [CrossRef] [PubMed]
233. Cheng, B.; Chen, J.; Bai, B.; Xin, Q. Neuroprotection of apelin and its signaling pathway. *Peptides* **2012**, *37*, 171–173. [CrossRef] [PubMed]
234. Xin, Q.; Cheng, B.; Pan, Y.; Liu, H.; Yang, C.; Chen, J.; Bai, B. Neuroprotective effects of apelin-13 on experimental ischemic stroke through suppression of inflammation. *Peptides* **2015**, *63*, 55–62. [CrossRef] [PubMed]
235. Chu, H.; Yang, X.; Huang, C.; Gao, Z.; Tang, Y.; Dong, Q. Apelin-13 Protects against Ischemic Blood-Brain Barrier Damage through the Effects of Aquaporin-4. *Cerebrovasc. Dis.* **2017**, *44*, 10–25. [CrossRef] [PubMed]
236. Chen, D.; Lee, J.; Gu, X.; Wei, L.; Yu, S.P. Intranasal Delivery of Apelin-13 Is Neuroprotective and Promotes Angiogenesis After Ischemic Stroke in Mice. *ASN Neuro* **2015**, *7*. [CrossRef] [PubMed]
237. Bao, H.J.; Zhang, L.; Han, W.C.; Dai, D.K. Apelin-13 attenuates traumatic brain injury-induced damage by suppressing autophagy. *Neurochem. Res.* **2015**, *40*, 89–97. [CrossRef] [PubMed]
238. Luo, H.; Xiang, Y.; Qu, X.; Liu, H.; Liu, C.; Li, G.; Han, L.; Qin, X. Apelin-13 Suppresses Neuroinflammation Against Cognitive Deficit in a Streptozotocin-Induced Rat Model of Alzheimer's Disease Through Activation of BDNF-TrkB Signaling Pathway. *Front. Pharmacol.* **2019**, *10*, 395. [CrossRef] [PubMed]
239. Li, E.; Deng, H.; Wang, B.; Fu, W.; You, Y.; Tian, S. Apelin-13 exerts antidepressant-like and recognition memory improving activities in stressed rats. *Eur. Neuropsychopharmacol.* **2016**, *26*, 420–430. [CrossRef] [PubMed]
240. Xiao, Z.Y.; Wang, B.; Fu, W.; Jin, X.; You, Y.; Tian, S.W.; Kuang, X. The Hippocampus is a Critical Site Mediating Antidepressant-like Activity of Apelin-13 in Rats. *Neuroscience* **2018**, *375*, 1–9. [CrossRef] [PubMed]
241. Dai, T.T.; Wang, B.; Xiao, Z.Y.; You, Y.; Tian, S.W. Apelin-13 Upregulates BDNF Against Chronic Stress-induced Depression-like Phenotypes by Ameliorating HPA Axis and Hippocampal Glucocorticoid Receptor Dysfunctions. *Neuroscience* **2018**, *390*, 151–159. [CrossRef] [PubMed]
242. Revollo, J.R.; Grimm, A.A.; Imai, S. The NAD biosynthesis pathway mediated by nicotinamide phosphoribosyltransferase regulates Sir2 activity in mammalian cells. *J. Biol. Chem.* **2004**, *279*, 50754–50763. [CrossRef] [PubMed]
243. Garten, A.; Schuster, S.; Penke, M.; Gorski, T.; de Giorgis, T.; Kiess, W. Physiological and pathophysiological roles of NAMPT and NAD metabolism. *Nat. Rev. Endocrinol.* **2015**, *11*, 535–546. [CrossRef] [PubMed]
244. Yoshino, J.; Mills, K.F.; Yoon, M.J.; Imai, S. Nicotinamide mononucleotide, a key NAD(+) intermediate, treats the pathophysiology of diet- and age-induced diabetes in mice. *Cell Metab.* **2011**, *14*, 528–536. [CrossRef] [PubMed]

245. Chalkiadaki, A.; Guarente, L. High-fat diet triggers inflammation-induced cleavage of SIRT1 in adipose tissue to promote metabolic dysfunction. *Cell Metab.* **2012**, *16*, 180–188. [CrossRef] [PubMed]
246. Chen, D.; Bruno, J.; Easlon, E.; Lin, S.J.; Cheng, H.L.; Alt, F.W.; Guarente, L. Tissue-specific regulation of SIRT1 by calorie restriction. *Genes Dev.* **2008**, *22*, 1753–1757. [CrossRef] [PubMed]
247. Song, J.; Ke, S.F.; Zhou, C.C.; Zhang, S.L.; Guan, Y.F.; Xu, T.Y.; Sheng, C.Q.; Wang, P.; Miao, C.Y. Nicotinamide phosphoribosyltransferase is required for the calorie restriction-mediated improvements in oxidative stress, mitochondrial biogenesis, and metabolic adaptation. *J. Gerontol. A Biol. Sci. Med. Sci.* **2014**, *69*, 44–57. [CrossRef] [PubMed]
248. Stromsdorfer, K.L.; Yamaguchi, S.; Yoon, M.J.; Moseley, A.C.; Franczyk, M.P.; Kelly, S.C.; Qi, N.; Imai, S.; Yoshino, J. NAMPT-Mediated NAD(+) Biosynthesis in Adipocytes Regulates Adipose Tissue Function and Multi-organ Insulin Sensitivity in Mice. *Cell Rep.* **2016**, *16*, 1851–1860. [CrossRef] [PubMed]
249. Yoon, M.J.; Yoshida, M.; Johnson, S.; Takikawa, A.; Usui, I.; Tobe, K.; Nakagawa, T.; Yoshino, J.; Imai, S. SIRT1-Mediated eNAMPT Secretion from Adipose Tissue Regulates Hypothalamic NAD+ and Function in Mice. *Cell Metab.* **2015**, *21*, 706–717. [CrossRef] [PubMed]
250. Jing, Z.; Xing, J.; Chen, X.; Stetler, R.A.; Weng, Z.; Gan, Y.; Zhang, F.; Gao, Y.; Chen, J.; Leak, R.K.; et al. Neuronal NAMPT is released after cerebral ischemia and protects against white matter injury. *J. Cereb Blood Flow Metab.* **2014**, *34*, 1613–1621. [CrossRef] [PubMed]
251. Erfani, S.; Khaksari, M.; Oryan, S.; Shamsaei, N.; Aboutaleb, N.; Nikbakht, F. Nampt/PBEF/visfatin exerts neuroprotective effects against ischemia/reperfusion injury via modulation of Bax/Bcl-2 ratio and prevention of caspase-3 activation. *J. Mol. Neurosci.* **2015**, *56*, 237–243. [CrossRef] [PubMed]
252. Zhao, Y.; Guan, Y.F.; Zhou, X.M.; Li, G.Q.; Li, Z.Y.; Zhou, C.C.; Wang, P.; Miao, C.Y. Regenerative Neurogenesis After Ischemic Stroke Promoted by Nicotinamide Phosphoribosyltransferase-Nicotinamide Adenine Dinucleotide Cascade. *Stroke* **2015**, *46*, 1966–1974. [CrossRef] [PubMed]
253. Zhao, Y.; Liu, X.Z.; Tian, W.W.; Guan, Y.F.; Wang, P.; Miao, C.Y. Extracellular visfatin has nicotinamide phosphoribosyltransferase enzymatic activity and is neuroprotective against ischemic injury. *CNS Neurosci. Ther.* **2014**, *20*, 539–547. [CrossRef] [PubMed]
254. Zhang, H.; Ryu, D.; Wu, Y.; Gariani, K.; Wang, X.; Luan, P.; D'Amico, D.; Ropelle, E.R.; Lutolf, M.P.; Aebersold, R.; et al. NAD(+) repletion improves mitochondrial and stem cell function and enhances life span in mice. *Science* **2016**, *352*, 1436–1443. [CrossRef] [PubMed]
255. Fricker, R.A.; Green, E.L.; Jenkins, S.I.; Griffin, S.M. The Influence of Nicotinamide on Health and Disease in the Central Nervous System. *Int. J. Tryptophan Res.* **2018**, *11*, 1178646918776658. [CrossRef] [PubMed]
256. Wang, X.; Hu, X.; Yang, Y.; Takata, T.; Sakurai, T. Nicotinamide mononucleotide protects against beta-amyloid oligomer-induced cognitive impairment and neuronal death. *Brain Res.* **2016**, *1643*, 1–9. [CrossRef] [PubMed]
257. Gong, B.; Pan, Y.; Vempati, P.; Zhao, W.; Knable, L.; Ho, L.; Wang, J.; Sastre, M.; Ono, K.; Sauve, A.A.; et al. Nicotinamide riboside restores cognition through an upregulation of proliferator-activated receptor-gamma coactivator 1alpha regulated beta-secretase 1 degradation and mitochondrial gene expression in Alzheimer's mouse models. *Neurobiol. Aging* **2013**, *34*, 1581–1588. [CrossRef] [PubMed]
258. Cao, H.; Gerhold, K.; Mayers, J.R.; Wiest, M.M.; Watkins, S.M.; Hotamisligil, G.S. Identification of a lipokine, a lipid hormone linking adipose tissue to systemic metabolism. *Cell* **2008**, *134*, 933–944. [CrossRef] [PubMed]
259. Saunders, A.M.; Strittmatter, W.J.; Schmechel, D.; George-Hyslop, P.H.; Pericak-Vance, M.A.; Joo, S.H.; Rosi, B.L.; Gusella, J.F.; Crapper-MacLachlan, D.R.; Alberts, M.J.; et al. Association of apolipoprotein E allele epsilon 4 with late-onset familial and sporadic Alzheimer's disease. *Neurology* **1993**, *43*, 1467–1472. [CrossRef] [PubMed]
260. Cutler, R.G.; Kelly, J.; Storie, K.; Pedersen, W.A.; Tammara, A.; Hatanpaa, K.; Troncoso, J.C.; Mattson, M.P. Involvement of oxidative stress-induced abnormalities in ceramide and cholesterol metabolism in brain aging and Alzheimer's disease. *Proc. Natl. Acad. Sci. USA* **2004**, *101*, 2070–2075. [CrossRef] [PubMed]
261. Lukiw, W.J.; Pappolla, M.; Pelaez, R.P.; Bazan, N.G. Alzheimer's disease–a dysfunction in cholesterol and lipid metabolism. *Cell Mol. Neurobiol.* **2005**, *25*, 475–483. [CrossRef] [PubMed]
262. Zhao, Y.; Calon, F.; Julien, C.; Winkler, J.W.; Petasis, N.A.; Lukiw, W.J.; Bazan, N.G. Docosahexaenoic acid-derived neuroprotectin D1 induces neuronal survival via secretase- and PPARgamma-mediated mechanisms in Alzheimer's disease models. *PLoS ONE* **2011**, *6*, e15816. [CrossRef]

263. Sanchez-Mejia, R.O.; Newman, J.W.; Toh, S.; Yu, G.Q.; Zhou, Y.; Halabisky, B.; Cisse, M.; Scearce-Levie, K.; Cheng, I.H.; Gan, L.; et al. Phospholipase A2 reduction ameliorates cognitive deficits in a mouse model of Alzheimer's disease. *Nat. Neurosci.* **2008**, *11*, 1311–1318. [CrossRef] [PubMed]
264. Grimm, M.O.; Grimm, H.S.; Patzold, A.J.; Zinser, E.G.; Halonen, R.; Duering, M.; Tschape, J.A.; De Strooper, B.; Muller, U.; Shen, J.; et al. Regulation of cholesterol and sphingomyelin metabolism by amyloid-beta and presenilin. *Nat. Cell Biol.* **2005**, *7*, 1118–1123. [CrossRef] [PubMed]
265. Okada, T.; Furuhashi, N.; Kuromori, Y.; Miyashita, M.; Iwata, F.; Harada, K. Plasma palmitoleic acid content and obesity in children. *Am. J. Clin. Nutr.* **2005**, *82*, 747–750. [CrossRef] [PubMed]
266. Paillard, F.; Catheline, D.; Duff, F.L.; Bouriel, M.; Deugnier, Y.; Pouchard, M.; Daubert, J.C.; Legrand, P. Plasma palmitoleic acid, a product of stearoyl-coA desaturase activity, is an independent marker of triglyceridemia and abdominal adiposity. *Nutr. Metab. Cardiovasc. Dis.* **2008**, *18*, 436–440. [CrossRef] [PubMed]
267. Warensjo, E.; Ohrvall, M.; Vessby, B. Fatty acid composition and estimated desaturase activities are associated with obesity and lifestyle variables in men and women. *Nutr. Metab. Cardiovasc. Dis.* **2006**, *16*, 128–136. [CrossRef] [PubMed]
268. Mozaffarian, D.; Cao, H.; King, I.B.; Lemaitre, R.N.; Song, X.; Siscovick, D.S.; Hotamisligil, G.S. Circulating palmitoleic acid and risk of metabolic abnormalities and new-onset diabetes. *Am. J. Clin. Nutr.* **2010**, *92*, 1350–1358. [CrossRef] [PubMed]
269. Ferry, G.; Tellier, E.; Try, A.; Gres, S.; Naime, I.; Simon, M.F.; Rodriguez, M.; Boucher, J.; Tack, I.; Gesta, S.; et al. Autotaxin is released from adipocytes, catalyzes lysophosphatidic acid synthesis, and activates preadipocyte proliferation. Up-regulated expression with adipocyte differentiation and obesity. *J. Biol. Chem.* **2003**, *278*, 18162–18169. [CrossRef] [PubMed]
270. Gesta, S.; Simon, M.F.; Rey, A.; Sibrac, D.; Girard, A.; Lafontan, M.; Valet, P.; Saulnier-Blache, J.S. Secretion of a lysophospholipase D activity by adipocytes: Involvement in lysophosphatidic acid synthesis. *J. Lipid Res.* **2002**, *43*, 904–910. [PubMed]
271. Boucher, J.; Quilliot, D.; Praderes, J.P.; Simon, M.F.; Gres, S.; Guigne, C.; Prevot, D.; Ferry, G.; Boutin, J.A.; Carpene, C.; et al. Potential involvement of adipocyte insulin resistance in obesity-associated up-regulation of adipocyte lysophospholipase D/autotaxin expression. *Diabetologia* **2005**, *48*, 569–577. [CrossRef] [PubMed]
272. Dusaulcy, R.; Rancoule, C.; Gres, S.; Wanecq, E.; Colom, A.; Guigne, C.; van Meeteren, L.A.; Moolenaar, W.H.; Valet, P.; Saulnier-Blache, J.S. Adipose-specific disruption of autotaxin enhances nutritional fattening and reduces plasma lysophosphatidic acid. *J. Lipid Res.* **2011**, *52*, 1247–1255. [CrossRef] [PubMed]
273. Rancoule, C.; Dusaulcy, R.; Treguer, K.; Gres, S.; Guigne, C.; Quilliot, D.; Valet, P.; Saulnier-Blache, J.S. Depot-specific regulation of autotaxin with obesity in human adipose tissue. *J. Physiol. Biochem.* **2012**, *68*, 635–644. [CrossRef] [PubMed]
274. Rachakonda, V.P.; Reeves, V.L.; Aljammal, J.; Wills, R.C.; Trybula, J.S.; DeLany, J.P.; Kienesberger, P.C.; Kershaw, E.E. Serum autotaxin is independently associated with hepatic steatosis in women with severe obesity. *Obesity (Silver Spring)* **2015**, *23*, 965–972. [CrossRef] [PubMed]
275. Reeves, V.L.; Trybula, J.S.; Wills, R.C.; Goodpaster, B.H.; Dube, J.J.; Kienesberger, P.C.; Kershaw, E.E. Serum Autotaxin/ENPP2 correlates with insulin resistance in older humans with obesity. *Obesity (Silver Spring)* **2015**, *23*, 2371–2376. [CrossRef] [PubMed]
276. D'Souza, K.; Kane, D.A.; Touaibia, M.; Kershaw, E.E.; Pulinilkunnil, T.; Kienesberger, P.C. Autotaxin Is Regulated by Glucose and Insulin in Adipocytes. *Endocrinology* **2017**, *158*, 791–803. [CrossRef] [PubMed]
277. Rancoule, C.; Attane, C.; Gres, S.; Fournel, A.; Dusaulcy, R.; Bertrand, C.; Vinel, C.; Treguer, K.; Prentki, M.; Valet, P.; et al. Lysophosphatidic acid impairs glucose homeostasis and inhibits insulin secretion in high-fat diet obese mice. *Diabetologia* **2013**, *56*, 1394–1402. [CrossRef] [PubMed]
278. Yung, Y.C.; Stoddard, N.C.; Chun, J. LPA receptor signaling: Pharmacology, physiology, and pathophysiology. *J. Lipid Res.* **2014**, *55*, 1192–1214. [CrossRef] [PubMed]
279. Gimenez da Silva-Santi, L.; Masetto Antunes, M.; Mori, M.A.; Biesdorf de Almeida-Souza, C.; Vergilio Visentainer, J.; Carbonera, F.; Rabello Crisma, A.; Nunes Masi, L.; Massao Hirabara, S.; Curi, R.; et al. Brain Fatty Acid Composition and Inflammation in Mice Fed with High-Carbohydrate Diet or High-Fat Diet. *Nutrients* **2018**, *10*. [CrossRef] [PubMed]
280. Lee, J.C.; Park, S.M.; Kim, I.Y.; Sung, H.; Seong, J.K.; Moon, M.H. High-fat diet-induced lipidome perturbations in the cortex, hippocampus, hypothalamus, and olfactory bulb of mice. *Biochim. Biophys. Acta Mol. Cell Biol. Lipids* **2018**, *1863*, 980–990. [CrossRef] [PubMed]

281. Agrawal, R.; Gomez-Pinilla, F. 'Metabolic syndrome' in the brain: Deficiency in omega-3 fatty acid exacerbates dysfunctions in insulin receptor signalling and cognition. *J. Physiol.* **2012**, *590*, 2485–2499. [CrossRef] [PubMed]
282. Sharma, S.; Zhuang, Y.; Gomez-Pinilla, F. High-fat diet transition reduces brain DHA levels associated with altered brain plasticity and behaviour. *Sci. Rep.* **2012**, *2*, 431. [CrossRef] [PubMed]
283. Sato, N.; Morishita, R. The roles of lipid and glucose metabolism in modulation of beta-amyloid, tau, and neurodegeneration in the pathogenesis of Alzheimer disease. *Front. Aging Neurosci.* **2015**, *7*, 199. [CrossRef] [PubMed]
284. Janssen, C.I.; Jansen, D.; Mutsaers, M.P.; Dederen, P.J.; Geenen, B.; Mulder, M.T.; Kiliaan, A.J. The Effect of a High-Fat Diet on Brain Plasticity, Inflammation and Cognition in Female ApoE4-Knockin and ApoE-Knockout Mice. *PLoS ONE* **2016**, *11*, e0155307. [CrossRef] [PubMed]
285. Zhu, T.B.; Zhang, Z.; Luo, P.; Wang, S.S.; Peng, Y.; Chu, S.F.; Chen, N.H. Lipid metabolism in Alzheimer's disease. *Brain Res. Bull.* **2019**, *144*, 68–74. [CrossRef] [PubMed]
286. Del Olmo, N.; Ruiz-Gayo, M. Influence of High-Fat Diets Consumed During the Juvenile Period on Hippocampal Morphology and Function. *Front. Cell Neurosci.* **2018**, *12*, 439. [CrossRef] [PubMed]
287. Carta, G.; Murru, E.; Banni, S.; Manca, C. Palmitic Acid: Physiological Role, Metabolism and Nutritional Implications. *Front. Physiol.* **2017**, *8*, 902. [CrossRef] [PubMed]
288. Strable, M.S.; Ntambi, J.M. Genetic control of de novo lipogenesis: Role in diet-induced obesity. *Crit. Rev. Biochem. Mol. Biol.* **2010**, *45*, 199–214. [CrossRef] [PubMed]
289. Silbernagel, G.; Kovarova, M.; Cegan, A.; Machann, J.; Schick, F.; Lehmann, R.; Haring, H.U.; Stefan, N.; Schleicher, E.; Fritsche, A.; et al. High hepatic SCD1 activity is associated with low liver fat content in healthy subjects under a lipogenic diet. *J. Clin. Endocrinol. Metab.* **2012**, *97*, E2288–E2292. [CrossRef] [PubMed]
290. Patil, S.; Balu, D.; Melrose, J.; Chan, C. Brain region-specificity of palmitic acid-induced abnormalities associated with Alzheimer's disease. *BMC Res. Notes* **2008**, *1*, 20. [CrossRef] [PubMed]
291. Hsiao, Y.H.; Lin, C.I.; Liao, H.; Chen, Y.H.; Lin, S.H. Palmitic acid-induced neuron cell cycle G2/M arrest and endoplasmic reticular stress through protein palmitoylation in SH-SY5Y human neuroblastoma cells. *Int. J. Mol. Sci.* **2014**, *15*, 20876–20899. [CrossRef] [PubMed]
292. Patil, S.; Melrose, J.; Chan, C. Involvement of astroglial ceramide in palmitic acid-induced Alzheimer-like changes in primary neurons. *Eur. J. Neurosci.* **2007**, *26*, 2131–2141. [CrossRef] [PubMed]
293. Frigolet, M.E.; Gutierrez-Aguilar, R. The Role of the Novel Lipokine Palmitoleic Acid in Health and Disease. *Adv. Nutr.* **2017**, *8*, 173S–181S. [CrossRef] [PubMed]
294. Guo, X.; Li, H.; Xu, H.; Halim, V.; Zhang, W.; Wang, H.; Ong, K.T.; Woo, S.L.; Walzem, R.L.; Mashek, D.G.; et al. Palmitoleate induces hepatic steatosis but suppresses liver inflammatory response in mice. *PLoS ONE* **2012**, *7*, e39286. [CrossRef] [PubMed]
295. Ouchi, N.; Parker, J.L.; Lugus, J.J.; Walsh, K. Adipokines in inflammation and metabolic disease. *Nat. Rev. Immunol.* **2011**, *11*, 85–97. [CrossRef] [PubMed]
296. Bolsoni-Lopes, A.; Festuccia, W.T.; Farias, T.S.; Chimin, P.; Torres-Leal, F.L.; Derogis, P.B.; de Andrade, P.B.; Miyamoto, S.; Lima, F.B.; Curi, R.; et al. Palmitoleic acid (n-7) increases white adipocyte lipolysis and lipase content in a PPARalpha-dependent manner. *Am. J. Physiol. Endocrinol. Metab.* **2013**, *305*, E1093–E1102. [CrossRef] [PubMed]
297. Dimopoulos, N.; Watson, M.; Sakamoto, K.; Hundal, H.S. Differential effects of palmitate and palmitoleate on insulin action and glucose utilization in rat L6 skeletal muscle cells. *Biochem. J.* **2006**, *399*, 473–481. [CrossRef] [PubMed]
298. Kuda, O.; Stankova, B.; Tvrzicka, E.; Hensler, M.; Jelenik, T.; Rossmeisl, M.; Flachs, P.; Kopecky, J. Prominent role of liver in elevated plasma palmitoleate levels in response to rosiglitazone in mice fed high-fat diet. *J. Physiol. Pharmacol.* **2009**, *60*, 135–140. [PubMed]
299. Furuhashi, M.; Hotamisligil, G.S. Fatty acid-binding proteins: Role in metabolic diseases and potential as drug targets. *Nat. Rev. Drug Discov.* **2008**, *7*, 489–503. [CrossRef] [PubMed]
300. Furuhashi, M.; Ishimura, S.; Ota, H.; Miura, T. Lipid chaperones and metabolic inflammation. *Int. J. Inflam.* **2011**, *2011*, 642612. [CrossRef] [PubMed]
301. Tan, K.C.; Wat, N.M.; Tam, S.C.; Janus, E.D.; Lam, T.H.; Lam, K.S. C-reactive protein predicts the deterioration of glycemia in chinese subjects with impaired glucose tolerance. *Diabetes Care* **2003**, *26*, 2323–2328. [CrossRef] [PubMed]

302. Liu, M.Y.; Xydakis, A.M.; Hoogeveen, R.C.; Jones, P.H.; Smith, E.O.; Nelson, K.W.; Ballantyne, C.M. Multiplexed analysis of biomarkers related to obesity and the metabolic syndrome in human plasma, using the Luminex-100 system. *Clin. Chem.* **2005**, *51*, 1102–1109. [CrossRef] [PubMed]
303. Degawa-Yamauchi, M.; Bovenkerk, J.E.; Juliar, B.E.; Watson, W.; Kerr, K.; Jones, R.; Zhu, Q.; Considine, R.V. Serum resistin (FIZZ3) protein is increased in obese humans. *J. Clin. Endocrinol. Metab.* **2003**, *88*, 5452–5455. [CrossRef] [PubMed]
304. Xu, A.; Wang, Y.; Xu, J.Y.; Stejskal, D.; Tam, S.; Zhang, J.; Wat, N.M.; Wong, W.K.; Lam, K.S. Adipocyte fatty acid-binding protein is a plasma biomarker closely associated with obesity and metabolic syndrome. *Clin. Chem.* **2006**, *52*, 405–413. [CrossRef] [PubMed]
305. Kralisch, S.; Ebert, T.; Lossner, U.; Jessnitzer, B.; Stumvoll, M.; Fasshauer, M. Adipocyte fatty acid-binding protein is released from adipocytes by a non-conventional mechanism. *Int J. Obes. (Lond.)* **2014**, *38*, 1251–1254. [CrossRef] [PubMed]
306. Erbay, E.; Babaev, V.R.; Mayers, J.R.; Makowski, L.; Charles, K.N.; Snitow, M.E.; Fazio, S.; Wiest, M.M.; Watkins, S.M.; Linton, M.F.; et al. Reducing endoplasmic reticulum stress through a macrophage lipid chaperone alleviates atherosclerosis. *Nat. Med.* **2009**, *15*, 1383–1391. [CrossRef] [PubMed]
307. Coleman, S.L.; Park, Y.K.; Lee, J.Y. Unsaturated fatty acids repress the expression of adipocyte fatty acid binding protein via the modulation of histone deacetylation in RAW 264.7 macrophages. *Eur. J. Nutr.* **2011**, *50*, 323–330. [CrossRef] [PubMed]
308. Uysal, K.T.; Scheja, L.; Wiesbrock, S.M.; Bonner-Weir, S.; Hotamisligil, G.S. Improved glucose and lipid metabolism in genetically obese mice lacking aP2. *Endocrinology* **2000**, *141*, 3388–3396. [CrossRef] [PubMed]
309. Maeda, K.; Cao, H.; Kono, K.; Gorgun, C.Z.; Furuhashi, M.; Uysal, K.T.; Cao, Q.; Atsumi, G.; Malone, H.; Krishnan, B.; et al. Adipocyte/macrophage fatty acid binding proteins control integrated metabolic responses in obesity and diabetes. *Cell Metab.* **2005**, *1*, 107–119. [CrossRef] [PubMed]
310. Cao, H.; Maeda, K.; Gorgun, C.Z.; Kim, H.J.; Park, S.Y.; Shulman, G.I.; Kim, J.K.; Hotamisligil, G.S. Regulation of metabolic responses by adipocyte/macrophage Fatty Acid-binding proteins in leptin-deficient mice. *Diabetes* **2006**, *55*, 1915–1922. [CrossRef] [PubMed]
311. Dobrzyn, P.; Jazurek, M.; Dobrzyn, A. Stearoyl-CoA desaturase and insulin signaling–what is the molecular switch? *Biochim. Biophys. Acta* **2010**, *1797*, 1189–1194. [CrossRef] [PubMed]
312. Astarita, G.; Jung, K.M.; Vasilevko, V.; Dipatrizio, N.V.; Martin, S.K.; Cribbs, D.H.; Head, E.; Cotman, C.W.; Piomelli, D. Elevated stearoyl-CoA desaturase in brains of patients with Alzheimer's disease. *PLoS ONE* **2011**, *6*, e24777. [CrossRef] [PubMed]
313. Cohen, P.; Miyazaki, M.; Socci, N.D.; Hagge-Greenberg, A.; Liedtke, W.; Soukas, A.A.; Sharma, R.; Hudgins, L.C.; Ntambi, J.M.; Friedman, J.M. Role for stearoyl-CoA desaturase-1 in leptin-mediated weight loss. *Science* **2002**, *297*, 240–243. [CrossRef] [PubMed]
314. Corpeleijn, E.; Feskens, E.J.; Jansen, E.H.; Mensink, M.; Saris, W.H.; de Bruin, T.W.; Blaak, E.E. Improvements in glucose tolerance and insulin sensitivity after lifestyle intervention are related to changes in serum fatty acid profile and desaturase activities: The SLIM study. *Diabetologia* **2006**, *49*, 2392–2401. [CrossRef] [PubMed]
315. Warensjo, E.; Ingelsson, E.; Lundmark, P.; Lannfelt, L.; Syvanen, A.C.; Vessby, B.; Riserus, U. Polymorphisms in the SCD1 gene: Associations with body fat distribution and insulin sensitivity. *Obesity (Silver Spring)* **2007**, *15*, 1732–1740. [CrossRef] [PubMed]
316. Warensjo, E.; Riserus, U.; Vessby, B. Fatty acid composition of serum lipids predicts the development of the metabolic syndrome in men. *Diabetologia* **2005**, *48*, 1999–2005. [CrossRef] [PubMed]
317. Mar-Heyming, R.; Miyazaki, M.; Weissglas-Volkov, D.; Kolaitis, N.A.; Sadaat, N.; Plaisier, C.; Pajukanta, P.; Cantor, R.M.; de Bruin, T.W.; Ntambi, J.M.; et al. Association of stearoyl-CoA desaturase 1 activity with familial combined hyperlipidemia. *Arterioscler. Thromb. Vasc. Biol.* **2008**, *28*, 1193–1199. [CrossRef] [PubMed]
318. Snigdha, S.; Astarita, G.; Piomelli, D.; Cotman, C.W. Effects of diet and behavioral enrichment on free fatty acids in the aged canine brain. *Neuroscience* **2012**, *202*, 326–333. [CrossRef] [PubMed]
319. Srodulski, S.; Sharma, S.; Bachstetter, A.B.; Brelsfoard, J.M.; Pascual, C.; Xie, X.S.; Saatman, K.E.; Van Eldik, L.J.; Despa, F. Neuroinflammation and neurologic deficits in diabetes linked to brain accumulation of amylin. *Mol. Neurodegener.* **2014**, *9*, 30. [CrossRef] [PubMed]
320. Miller, A.A.; Spencer, S.J. Obesity and neuroinflammation: A pathway to cognitive impairment. *Brain Behav. Immun.* **2014**, *42*, 10–21. [CrossRef] [PubMed]

321. Posey, K.A.; Clegg, D.J.; Printz, R.L.; Byun, J.; Morton, G.J.; Vivekanandan-Giri, A.; Pennathur, S.; Baskin, D.G.; Heinecke, J.W.; Woods, S.C.; et al. Hypothalamic proinflammatory lipid accumulation, inflammation, and insulin resistance in rats fed a high-fat diet. *Am. J. Physiol. Endocrinol. Metab.* **2009**, *296*, E1003–E1012. [CrossRef] [PubMed]
322. Pistell, P.J.; Morrison, C.D.; Gupta, S.; Knight, A.G.; Keller, J.N.; Ingram, D.K.; Bruce-Keller, A.J. Cognitive impairment following high fat diet consumption is associated with brain inflammation. *J. Neuroimmunol.* **2010**, *219*, 25–32. [CrossRef] [PubMed]
323. Brandon, J.A.; Kraemer, M.; Vandra, J.; Halder, S.; Ubele, M.; Morris, A.J.; Smyth, S.S. Adipose-derived autotaxin regulates inflammation and steatosis associated with diet-induced obesity. *PLoS ONE* **2019**, *14*, e0208099. [CrossRef] [PubMed]
324. Zhao, Y.; Natarajan, V. Lysophosphatidic acid (LPA) and its receptors: Role in airway inflammation and remodeling. *Biochim. Biophys. Acta* **2013**, *1831*, 86–92. [CrossRef] [PubMed]
325. Chen, Y.; Ramakrishnan, D.P.; Ren, B. Regulation of angiogenesis by phospholipid lysophosphatidic acid. *Front. Biosci. (Landmark Ed.)* **2013**, *18*, 852–861. [PubMed]
326. Estivill-Torrus, G.; Llebrez-Zayas, P.; Matas-Rico, E.; Santin, L.; Pedraza, C.; De Diego, I.; Del Arco, I.; Fernandez-Llebrez, P.; Chun, J.; De Fonseca, F.R. Absence of LPA1 signaling results in defective cortical development. *Cereb. Cortex* **2008**, *18*, 938–950. [CrossRef] [PubMed]
327. Matas-Rico, E.; Garcia-Diaz, B.; Llebrez-Zayas, P.; Lopez-Barroso, D.; Santin, L.; Pedraza, C.; Smith-Fernandez, A.; Fernandez-Llebrez, P.; Tellez, T.; Redondo, M.; et al. Deletion of lysophosphatidic acid receptor LPA1 reduces neurogenesis in the mouse dentate gyrus. *Mol. Cell Neurosci.* **2008**, *39*, 342–355. [CrossRef] [PubMed]
328. Dubin, A.E.; Herr, D.R.; Chun, J. Diversity of lysophosphatidic acid receptor-mediated intracellular calcium signaling in early cortical neurogenesis. *J. Neurosci.* **2010**, *30*, 7300–7309. [CrossRef] [PubMed]
329. Fukushima, N.; Shano, S.; Moriyama, R.; Chun, J. Lysophosphatidic acid stimulates neuronal differentiation of cortical neuroblasts through the LPA1-G(i/o) pathway. *Neurochem. Int.* **2007**, *50*, 302–307. [CrossRef] [PubMed]
330. Furuta, D.; Yamane, M.; Tsujiuchi, T.; Moriyama, R.; Fukushima, N. Lysophosphatidic acid induces neurite branch formation through LPA3. *Mol. Cell Neurosci.* **2012**, *50*, 21–34. [CrossRef] [PubMed]
331. Pilpel, Y.; Segal, M. The role of LPA1 in formation of synapses among cultured hippocampal neurons. *J. Neurochem.* **2006**, *97*, 1379–1392. [CrossRef] [PubMed]
332. Goldin, M.; Segal, M. Protein kinase C and ERK involvement in dendritic spine plasticity in cultured rodent hippocampal neurons. *Eur. J. Neurosci.* **2003**, *17*, 2529–2539. [CrossRef] [PubMed]
333. Pilpel, Y.; Segal, M. Activation of PKC induces rapid morphological plasticity in dendrites of hippocampal neurons via Rac and Rho-dependent mechanisms. *Eur. J. Neurosci.* **2004**, *19*, 3151–3164. [CrossRef] [PubMed]
334. Harrison, S.M.; Reavill, C.; Brown, G.; Brown, J.T.; Cluderay, J.E.; Crook, B.; Davies, C.H.; Dawson, L.A.; Grau, E.; Heidbreder, C.; et al. LPA1 receptor-deficient mice have phenotypic changes observed in psychiatric disease. *Mol. Cell Neurosci.* **2003**, *24*, 1170–1179. [CrossRef] [PubMed]
335. Roberts, C.; Winter, P.; Shilliam, C.S.; Hughes, Z.A.; Langmead, C.; Maycox, P.R.; Dawson, L.A. Neurochemical changes in LPA1 receptor deficient mice–a putative model of schizophrenia. *Neurochem. Res.* **2005**, *30*, 371–377. [CrossRef] [PubMed]
336. Castilla-Ortega, E.; Sanchez-Lopez, J.; Hoyo-Becerra, C.; Matas-Rico, E.; Zambrana-Infantes, E.; Chun, J.; De Fonseca, F.R.; Pedraza, C.; Estivill-Torrus, G.; Santin, L.J. Exploratory, anxiety and spatial memory impairments are dissociated in mice lacking the LPA1 receptor. *Neurobiol. Learn. Mem.* **2010**, *94*, 73–82. [CrossRef] [PubMed]
337. Santin, L.J.; Bilbao, A.; Pedraza, C.; Matas-Rico, E.; Lopez-Barroso, D.; Castilla-Ortega, E.; Sanchez-Lopez, J.; Riquelme, R.; Varela-Nieto, I.; de la Villa, P.; et al. Behavioral phenotype of maLPA1-null mice: Increased anxiety-like behavior and spatial memory deficits. *Genes Brain Behav.* **2009**, *8*, 772–784. [CrossRef] [PubMed]
338. Shano, S.; Moriyama, R.; Chun, J.; Fukushima, N. Lysophosphatidic acid stimulates astrocyte proliferation through LPA1. *Neurochem. Int.* **2008**, *52*, 216–220. [CrossRef] [PubMed]
339. TC, E.S.; Dezonne, R.S.; Rehen, S.K.; Gomes, F.C. Astrocytes treated by lysophosphatidic acid induce axonal outgrowth of cortical progenitors through extracellular matrix protein and epidermal growth factor signaling pathway. *J. Neurochem.* **2011**, *119*, 113–123. [CrossRef]

340. Schilling, T.; Repp, H.; Richter, H.; Koschinski, A.; Heinemann, U.; Dreyer, F.; Eder, C. Lysophospholipids induce membrane hyperpolarization in microglia by activation of IKCa1 Ca(2+)-dependent K(+) channels. *Neuroscience* **2002**, *109*, 827–835. [CrossRef]
341. Schilling, T.; Stock, C.; Schwab, A.; Eder, C. Functional importance of Ca2+-activated K+ channels for lysophosphatidic acid-induced microglial migration. *Eur. J. Neurosci.* **2004**, *19*, 1469–1474. [CrossRef] [PubMed]
342. Awada, R.; Rondeau, P.; Gres, S.; Saulnier-Blache, J.S.; Lefebvre d'Hellencourt, C.; Bourdon, E. Autotaxin protects microglial cells against oxidative stress. *Free Radic. Biol. Med.* **2012**, *52*, 516–526. [CrossRef] [PubMed]
343. Awada, R.; Saulnier-Blache, J.S.; Gres, S.; Bourdon, E.; Rondeau, P.; Parimisetty, A.; Orihuela, R.; Harry, G.J.; d'Hellencourt, C.L. Autotaxin downregulates LPS-induced microglia activation and pro-inflammatory cytokines production. *J. Cell Biochem.* **2014**, *115*, 2123–2132. [CrossRef] [PubMed]
344. Moller, T.; Musante, D.B.; Ransom, B.R. Lysophosphatidic acid-induced calcium signals in cultured rat oligodendrocytes. *Neuroreport* **1999**, *10*, 2929–2932. [CrossRef] [PubMed]
345. Nogaroli, L.; Yuelling, L.M.; Dennis, J.; Gorse, K.; Payne, S.G.; Fuss, B. Lysophosphatidic acid can support the formation of membranous structures and an increase in MBP mRNA levels in differentiating oligodendrocytes. *Neurochem. Res.* **2009**, *34*, 182–193. [CrossRef] [PubMed]
346. Castanon, N.; Luheshi, G.; Laye, S. Role of neuroinflammation in the emotional and cognitive alterations displayed by animal models of obesity. *Front. Neurosci.* **2015**, *9*, 229. [CrossRef] [PubMed]
347. McLimans, K.E.; Willette, A.A.; Alzheimer's Disease Neuroimaging, I. Autotaxin is Related to Metabolic Dysfunction and Predicts Alzheimer's Disease Outcomes. *J. Alzheimers Dis.* **2017**, *56*, 403–413. [CrossRef] [PubMed]
348. Shi, J.; Dong, Y.; Cui, M.Z.; Xu, X. Lysophosphatidic acid induces increased BACE1 expression and Abeta formation. *Biochim. Biophys. Acta* **2013**, *1832*, 29–38. [CrossRef] [PubMed]
349. Kinouchi, T.; Sorimachi, H.; Maruyama, K.; Mizuno, K.; Ohno, S.; Ishiura, S.; Suzuki, K. Conventional protein kinase C (PKC)-alpha and novel PKC epsilon, but not -delta, increase the secretion of an N-terminal fragment of Alzheimer's disease amyloid precursor protein from PKC cDNA transfected 3Y1 fibroblasts. *FEBS Lett.* **1995**, *364*, 203–206. [PubMed]
350. Jolly-Tornetta, C.; Wolf, B.A. Regulation of amyloid precursor protein (APP) secretion by protein kinase calpha in human ntera 2 neurons (NT2N). *Biochemistry* **2000**, *39*, 7428–7435. [CrossRef] [PubMed]
351. Rossner, S.; Mendla, K.; Schliebs, R.; Bigl, V. Protein kinase Calpha and beta1 isoforms are regulators of alpha-secretory proteolytic processing of amyloid precursor protein in vivo. *Eur J. Neurosci.* **2001**, *13*, 1644–1648. [CrossRef] [PubMed]
352. Zhu, G.; Wang, D.; Lin, Y.H.; McMahon, T.; Koo, E.H.; Messing, R.O. Protein kinase C epsilon suppresses Abeta production and promotes activation of alpha-secretase. *Biochem. Biophys. Res. Commun.* **2001**, *285*, 997–1006. [CrossRef] [PubMed]
353. Blois, J.T.; Mataraza, J.M.; Mecklenbrauker, I.; Tarakhovsky, A.; Chiles, T.C. B cell receptor-induced cAMP-response element-binding protein activation in B lymphocytes requires novel protein kinase Cdelta. *J. Biol. Chem.* **2004**, *279*, 30123–30132. [CrossRef] [PubMed]
354. Sayas, C.L.; Moreno-Flores, M.T.; Avila, J.; Wandosell, F. The neurite retraction induced by lysophosphatidic acid increases Alzheimer's disease-like Tau phosphorylation. *J. Biol. Chem.* **1999**, *274*, 37046–37052. [CrossRef] [PubMed]
355. Sayas, C.L.; Avila, J.; Wandosell, F. Regulation of neuronal cytoskeleton by lysophosphatidic acid: Role of GSK-3. *Biochim. Biophys. Acta* **2002**, *1582*, 144–153. [CrossRef]
356. Stranahan, A.M. Models and mechanisms for hippocampal dysfunction in obesity and diabetes. *Neuroscience* **2015**, *309*, 125–139. [CrossRef] [PubMed]
357. Li, X.; Li, X.; Lin, H.; Fu, X.; Lin, W.; Li, M.; Zeng, X.; Gao, Q. Metabolic syndrome and stroke: A meta-analysis of prospective cohort studies. *J. Clin. Neurosci.* **2017**, *40*, 34–38. [CrossRef] [PubMed]
358. Butterfield, D.A.; Halliwell, B. Oxidative stress, dysfunctional glucose metabolism and Alzheimer disease. *Nat. Rev. Neurosci.* **2019**, *20*, 148–160. [CrossRef] [PubMed]
359. Pousti, F.; Ahmadi, R.; Mirahmadi, F.; Hosseinmardi, N.; Rohampour, K. Adiponectin modulates synaptic plasticity in hippocampal dentate gyrus. *Neurosci. Lett.* **2018**, *662*, 227–232. [CrossRef] [PubMed]

360. Forny-Germano, L.; De Felice, F.G.; Vieira, M. The Role of Leptin and Adiponectin in Obesity-Associated Cognitive Decline and Alzheimer's Disease. *Front. Neurosci.* **2018**, *12*, 1027. [CrossRef] [PubMed]
361. Irving, A.J.; Harvey, J. Leptin regulation of hippocampal synaptic function in health and disease. *Philos. Trans. R. Soc. Lond. B Biol. Sci.* **2014**, *369*, 20130155. [CrossRef] [PubMed]
362. Sun, L.N.; Liu, X.L. Functions of adiponectin signaling in regulating neural plasticity and its application as the therapeutic target to neurological and psychiatric diseases. *Rev. Neurosci.* **2019**, *30*, 485–495. [CrossRef] [PubMed]
363. Ghavami, S.; Shojaei, S.; Yeganeh, B.; Ande, S.R.; Jangamreddy, J.R.; Mehrpour, M.; Christoffersson, J.; Chaabane, W.; Moghadam, A.R.; Kashani, H.H.; et al. Autophagy and apoptosis dysfunction in neurodegenerative disorders. *Prog. Neurobiol.* **2014**, *112*, 24–49. [CrossRef] [PubMed]
364. Stephenson, J.; Nutma, E.; van der Valk, P.; Amor, S. Inflammation in CNS neurodegenerative diseases. *Immunology* **2018**, *154*, 204–219. [CrossRef] [PubMed]
365. Radak, D.; Katsiki, N.; Resanovic, I.; Jovanovic, A.; Sudar-Milovanovic, E.; Zafirovic, S.; Mousad, S.A.; Isenovic, E.R. Apoptosis and Acute Brain Ischemia in Ischemic Stroke. *Curr. Vasc. Pharmacol.* **2017**, *15*, 115–122. [CrossRef] [PubMed]
366. Jayaraj, R.L.; Azimullah, S.; Beiram, R.; Jalal, F.Y.; Rosenberg, G.A. Neuroinflammation: Friend and foe for ischemic stroke. *J. Neuroinflamm.* **2019**, *16*, 142. [CrossRef] [PubMed]
367. Parimisetty, A.; Dorsemans, A.C.; Awada, R.; Ravanan, P.; Diotel, N.; Lefebvre d'Hellencourt, C. Secret talk between adipose tissue and central nervous system via secreted factors-an emerging frontier in the neurodegenerative research. *J. Neuroinflamm.* **2016**, *13*, 67. [CrossRef] [PubMed]

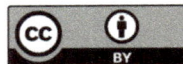

© 2019 by the authors. Licensee MDPI, Basel, Switzerland. This article is an open access article distributed under the terms and conditions of the Creative Commons Attribution (CC BY) license (http://creativecommons.org/licenses/by/4.0/).

MDPI
St. Alban-Anlage 66
4052 Basel
Switzerland
Tel. +41 61 683 77 34
Fax +41 61 302 89 18
www.mdpi.com

International Journal of Molecular Sciences Editorial Office
E-mail: ijms@mdpi.com
www.mdpi.com/journal/ijms

www.ingramcontent.com/pod-product-compliance
Lightning Source LLC
LaVergne TN
LVHW071935080526
838202LV00064B/6613